Augmentative &
Alternative Communication

Augmentative & Alternative Communication

Supporting Children and Adults
with Complex Communication Needs
Fourth Edition

by

David R. Beukelman, Ph.D.
University of Nebraska
Lincoln

and

Pat Mirenda, Ph.D.
University of British Columbia
Vancouver

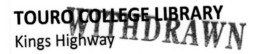
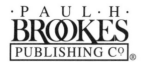
·P A U L·H·
BROOKES
PUBLISHING CO.®

Baltimore • London • Sydney

MW

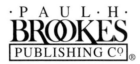

Paul H. Brookes Publishing Co.
Post Office Box 10624
Baltimore, Maryland 21285-0624

www.brookespublishing.com

Typeset by Network Publishing Partners, Inc., Glenview, Illinois.
Manufactured in the United States of America by
Sheridan Books, Inc., Chelsea, Michigan.

Photos are used by permission of the individuals pictured and/or their parents/guardians.

The individuals described in this book are composites or real people whose situations are masked and are based on the authors' experiences or real people whose names and identifying details are used by permission. Except where used by permission, names and identifying details have been changed to protect confidentiality.

Library of Congress Cataloging-in-Publication Data

Beukelman, David R., 1943–
   Augmentative and alternative communication: supporting children and adults with complex communication needs / by David R. Beukelman and Pat Mirenda.—4th ed.
      p.   cm.
   Rev. ed. of: Augmentative & alternative communication / by David R. Beukelman, Pat Mirenda. 3rd ed. c2005.
   Includes bibliographical references and index.
   ISBN 978-1-59857-196-7 (hardcover)—ISBN 1-59857-196-6 (hardcover)
   I. Mirenda, Pat. II. Beukelman, David R., 1943- Augmentative & alternative communication. III. Title.
   [DNLM: 1. Communication Disorders—rehabilitation.   2. Communication Aids for Disabled.
   3. Needs Assessment.   4. Nonverbal Communication.   WL 340.2]

616.85′503—dc23   2012015676

British Library Cataloguing in Publication data are available from the British Library.

2016   2015   2014   2013   2012

10   9   8   7   6   5   4   3   2   1

1/18/13

Contents

About the Authors

David R. Beukelman, Ph.D., Professor, Department of Special Education and Communication Disorders, University of Nebraska–Lincoln, 118 Barkley Memorial Center, Lincoln, NE 68583

Dr. Beukelman is the Barkley Professor of Communication Disorders at the University of Nebraska–Lincoln and a senior researcher in the Institute for Rehabilitation Science and Engineering at Madonna Rehabilitation Hospital. He is a research partner in the AAC-RERC (Rehabilitation Engineering Research Center on Communication Enhancement). He is coeditor of the Augmentative and Alternative Communication Series published by Paul H. Brookes Publishing Co. Previously, Dr. Beukelman was Director of Research and Education at the Munroe-Meyer Institute for Genetics and Rehabilitation at the University of Nebraska Medical Center. He was Director of the Communication Disorders and Augmentative Communication programs at the University of Washington Medical Center and Associate Professor in the Department of Rehabilitation Medicine at the University of Washington–Seattle. Dr. Beukelman specializes in the areas of augmentative communication and motor speech disorders of children and adults.

Pat Mirenda, Ph.D., Professor, Faculty of Education, University of British Columbia, 2125 Main Mall, Vancouver, British Columbia V6T 1Z4, Canada

Dr. Mirenda is a doctoral-level Board Certified Behavior Analyst (BCBA-D) who specializes in augmentative communication and positive behavior supports for individuals with developmental disabilities. She is a professor in the Department of Educational and Counseling Psychology and Special Education and director of the Centre for Interdisciplinary Research and Collaboration in Autism at the University of British Columbia. Previously, she was a faculty member in the Department of Special Education and Communication Disorders at the University of Nebraska–Lincoln. From 1998 to 2002, she was editor of the journal *Augmentative and Alternative Communication.* In 2004, she was named a Fellow of the American Speech-Language-Hearing Association and was awarded the Killam Teaching Prize at the University of British Columbia. In 2008, she was named a Fellow of the International Society for Augmentative and Alternative Communication. Dr. Mirenda is the author of numerous book chapters and research publications; she lectures widely and teaches courses on augmentative and alternative communication, inclusive education, developmental disabilities, autism, and positive behavior support. Her coedited book, *Autism Spectrum Disorders and AAC,* was published in December 2009.

About the Contributors

Laura J. Ball, Ph.D., Associate Professor, Department of Communication Sciences and Disorders, East Carolina University, 3310AE Allied Health Sciences, Mail Stop 668, Greenville, NC 27834

Dr. Ball completed her Ph.D. at the University of Nebraska–Lincoln and has focused research interests in augmentative and alternative communication (AAC) and motor speech disorders. Dr. Ball has more than 25 years' experience as a speech-language pathologist, working with people with complex communication needs who rely on AAC. She has strong research interest in amyotrophic lateral sclerosis and has authored publications in the areas of AAC, dysarthria, and apraxia.

Susan Fager, Ph.D., CCC-SLP, Assistant Director, Communication Center, Institute for Rehabilitation Science and Engineering, Madonna Rehabilitation Hospital, 5401 South Street, Lincoln, NE 68506

Dr. Fager is a researcher and augmentative and alternative communication specialist at the Institute for Rehabilitation Science and Engineering at Madonna Rehabilitation Hospital. She specializes in speech disorders of people with neurologic conditions such as traumatic brain injury, brainstem stroke, amyotrophic lateral sclerosis, and Parkinson's disease.

Kathryn L. Garrett, Ph.D., CCC-SLP, Alternative Communication Therapies, LLC, 1401 Forbes Avenue, Suite 201, Pittsburgh, PA 15219

Dr. Garrett currently treats individuals with complex communication disorders associated with aphasia and brain injury at her private practice in Pittsburgh, Pennsylvania. She collaborates on research projects in the area of severe aphasia, interaction, and supportive communication strategies with colleagues from Buffalo University and Florida State University.

Elizabeth K. Hanson, Ph.D., CCC-SLP, Associate Professor, Department of Communication Sciences and Disorders, University of South Dakota, 414 East Clark Street, Vermillion, SD 57069

Dr. Hanson earned her M.S. at the University of Wisconsin–Madison and her Ph.D. at the University of Nebraska–Lincoln. Her research interests are in augmentative and alternative communication (AAC) and motor speech disorders. Her clinical practice and supervision focuses on providing AAC services for people with complex communication needs across the life span.

Joanne P. Lasker, Ph.D., CCC-SLP, Associate Professor, School of Communication Science and Disorders, Florida State University, 127 Honors Way, Mail Code 32306-1200, Tallahassee, FL 32306

Dr. Lasker has published numerous papers and chapters related to assessment and treatment of adults living with acquired neurogenic communication disorders who may benefit from augmentative and alternative communication (AAC) techniques, in particular people living with aphasia. Her research has explored issues pertaining to AAC assessment protocols, context-based intervention practices, partner training, and the acceptance of AAC approaches by adults with severe communication disorders and their communication partners. She has presented nationally and internationally on these topics.

Janice C. Light, Ph.D., Department of Communication Sciences and Disorders, The Pennsylvania State University, 308G Ford Building, University Park, PA 16802

Dr. Light holds the Hintz Family Endowed Chair in Children's Communicative Competence in the Department of Communication Sciences and Disorders at the Pennsylvania State University. She is actively involved in research, personnel preparation, and service delivery in the area of augmentative and alternative communication (AAC). She is currently one of the project directors of the AAC-RERC (Rehabilitation Engineering Research Center on Communication Enhancement), a virtual research consortium funded by the National Institute on Disability and Rehabilitation Research. Dr. Light is the author of many peer-reviewed papers, book chapters, and books. She has received numerous awards in recognition of her research and teaching contributions to the field.

David B. McNaughton, Ph.D., Professor of Education, Department of Educational and School Psychology and Special Education, The Pennsylvania State University, 227 CEDAR Building, University Park, PA 16802

Dr. McNaughton teaches coursework in augmentative communication and assistive technology and collaboration skills for working with parents and educational team members. Dr. McNaughton's research interests include literacy instruction for individuals who rely on augmentative and alternative communication, and employment supports for individuals with severe disabilities.

Preface

As was the case for previous editions, the fourth edition of *Augmentative and Alternative Communication: Supporting Children and Adults with Complex Communication Needs* is an introductory text written for practicing professionals, preprofessional students, and others who are interested in learning more about communication options for people who are unable to meet their daily communication needs through natural modes such as speech, gestures, or handwriting. Because severe communication disorders can result from a variety of conditions, diseases, and syndromes that affect people of all ages, many individuals may be interested in these approaches. Several characteristics of the augmentative and alternative communication (AAC) field have shaped the format, content, and organization of this book. First, AAC is a multidisciplinary field in which individuals with complex communication needs (CCN) and their families, along with computer programmers, educators, engineers, linguists, occupational therapists, physical therapists, psychologists, speech-language pathologists, and many other professionals have contributed to the knowledge and practice base. We have attempted to be sensitive to these people's multiple perspectives and contributions by directly citing pertinent information from a wide variety of sources and by guiding the reader to appropriate additional resources when necessary.

Second, the AAC field has developed in many countries over the past six decades. For example, in 2011, individuals from more than 62 countries were members of the International Society for Augmentative and Alternative Communication. Although we are both from North America, we have made an effort to offer an international perspective in this book by including information about the contributions of researchers, clinicians, and people who rely on AAC from around the world. Unfortunately, within the constraints of an introductory textbook, only a limited number of these contributions can be cited specifically. Thus, we acknowledge that our primary sources of material have come from North America and hope that our AAC colleagues in other countries will tolerate our inability to represent multinational efforts more comprehensively.

Third, AAC interventions involve both electronic (i.e., digital) and nonelectronic systems. AAC technology changes very rapidly—products are being upgraded continually, and new products are always being introduced. Such product information presented in book form would be outdated very quickly. Therefore, we refer our readers to the AAC web site hosted by the Barkley AAC Center at the University of Nebraska–Lincoln (http://aac.unl.edu), which provides links to the web sites of manufacturers and publishers in the AAC field. Information on this web site is updated regularly. In addition, readers may refer to the Resources and Web Links section in this book for more information about the companies and organizations providing the AAC products and services that are mentioned in this book.

A fourth characteristic of the AAC field is that it incorporates three general areas of information. The first area relates to the processes of AAC: messages, symbols, alternative access, assessment, and intervention planning. The second area describes procedures that have been developed to serve individuals with developmental disabilities who require AAC services. The third area focuses on people with disabilities that are acquired later in life. In an effort to cover these areas, we have divided the book into three sections.

Specifically, the seven chapters in Part I are organized to introduce readers to AAC processes. Chapter 1 introduces the reader to AAC in general and to people with CCN in particular. Often using these individuals' own words, we attempt to convey what it means to communicate using AAC systems. Chapter 2 reviews the message types that are frequently communicated by people who rely on AAC and are thus stored in their systems. Chapter 3 is a detailed presentation of the most common aided and unaided symbol systems used to represent messages, as well as an introduction to the most common message encoding and rate-enhancement strategies. Chapter 4 discusses a range of alternative access options that are designed to accommodate a variety of motor, language, and cognitive impairments. Chapter 5 focuses on the various personnel involved in AAC interventions and their respective roles, as well as AAC assessment models and phases. This chapter also introduces the Participation Model for assessment and intervention planning that is used throughout the remainder of the book. Chapter 6 provides information about specific strategies for assessing the communication, language, motor, literacy, and sensory capabilities of people with CCN. Finally, Chapter 7 considers the principles of AAC intervention decision making to address both opportunity and access barriers, with emphasis on the importance of evidence-based practice and measurement of functional outcomes.

Part II contains six chapters that review AAC interventions for individuals with developmental disabilities. Specifically, Chapter 8 introduces AAC concerns unique to people with cerebral palsy, intellectual disabilities, autism spectrum disorders, deaf-blindness, and suspected childhood apraxia of speech. Chapter 9 introduces a number of strategies that can be used to resolve opportunity barriers and enhance the communicative participation of nonsymbolic communicators and those who are just beginning to use symbols to communicate. Chapter 10 summarizes what we know about the language development of people with CCN and how to support language learning and development in general. Chapter 11 builds on this discussion in order to discuss specific strategies that can be used to teach skills required for communicative competence, especially in the linguistic and social domains. Chapter 12, written by Janice C. Light and David B. McNaughton, focuses on the factors that affect literacy learning in people with CCN, strategies for fostering emergent literacy, and the key components of interventions for teaching conventional and advanced literacy skills. Finally, Chapter 13 provides guidelines for thinking about and planning for inclusive education for students with CCN, along with general strategies for how this might be accomplished.

Part III, composed of the last five chapters of the book, focuses on individuals with acquired communication disorders. Chapter 14, written with Laura J. Ball, reviews AAC interventions for adults with acquired physical disabilities, including amyotrophic lateral sclerosis, multiple sclerosis, Parkinson's disease, and brainstem stroke. Chapter 15, written by Kathryn L. Garrett and Joanne P. Lasker, describes a functional classification scheme for people with severe aphasia and contains related intervention strategies and techniques. Chapter 16, written with Elizabeth K. Hanson, introduces AAC strategies for people with degenerative language and cognitive disorders, including primary progressive aphasia and dementia. Chapter 17, written with Susan Fager, addresses AAC assessment and intervention techniques that are organized according to the cognitive levels of people with traumatic brain injury. Finally, Chapter 18 reviews a wide range of AAC interventions for people in intensive and acute care medical settings. Particular attention is focused on individuals who are unable to communicate because of respiratory impairments.

As we revised this book, we remained keenly aware of our dependence on those who have documented their experiences in the AAC field. In order to tell the "AAC story," we expected to cite traditional documents—professional research papers, scholarly books, and manuals. What we found is that we also made extensive use of the perspectives of people who rely on AAC, as documented in a variety of magazines, video recordings, web sites, and other popular sources. We also wish to thank those publishers, editors, associations, manufacturers, and institutions who supported the newsletters, bulletins, books, videos, magazines, web sites, and journals that now contain the historical record of the AAC field. Without these resources, we simply would have been unable to compile this book. We also want to acknowledge the role of the Barkley Trust in supporting AAC efforts at the University of Nebraska–Lincoln through the years. While we were revising this book, David R. Beukelman also served as Senior Researcher in the Research Institute for Rehabilitation Science and Engineering at Madonna Rehabilitation Hospital. In addition, we have appreciated the support, encouragement, and assistance we received from Astrid Zuckerman and Susan Hills at Paul H. Brookes Publishing Co., and Linda Wolf.

We note that this edition of this book and the previous three editions were collaborative efforts, with both of us completing those tasks that fit our areas of expertise and skills. Because we shared these tasks so completely, it was difficult to order the authorship for the first edition, and we had hoped to reverse the order for subsequent editions. We have not done so, however, in order not to confuse the status of this book as a fourth edition.

Acknowledgments

Special appreciation is due to a number of individuals with whom we have been fortunate to work before and during the production of this book. These include the students, families, staff, and administrators of the public school system in Lincoln, Nebraska; the Research Institute for Rehabilitation Science and Engineering at Madonna Rehabilitation Hospital; Quality Living, Inc.; Services for Students with Disabilities at the University of Nebraska–Lincoln; Special Education Technology–British Columbia; Communication Assistance for Youth and Adults; and the Sunny Hill Health Centre for Children. These individuals have collaborated with us extensively over the years and have thus greatly contributed to our augmentative and alternative communication (AAC) experiences and knowledge. Cay Holbrook, Janet Jamieson, and Brenda Fossett in the Department of Educational and Counselling Psychology and Special Education at the University of British Columbia also provided substantive input to one or more chapters in Part II of this book. Heidi Menard managed the reference list and proofed, checked, and rechecked the manuscript. Finally, we thank the many people who rely on AAC with whom we have worked, and their families—they have taught us about the AAC field and have allowed us to use their stories. May their voices grow ever stronger.

To the Barkley Board of Trustees, who determined nearly 30 years ago to allocate funds from the Barkley Trust to support a research, educational, and intervention emphasis on augmentative and alternative communication at the University of Nebraska–Lincoln. Through the years, this support has funded faculty and staff salaries as well as doctoral student scholarships.

I wish to thank my wife, Helen, who has been generous with her patience, understanding, and support over the years.

—David Beukelman

I am grateful beyond words to Jackie for her support and cheerleading through all four editions of this book. It never would have happened without you!

—Pat Mirenda

PART I

Introduction to Augmentative and Alternative Communication

CHAPTER 1

Augmentative and Alternative Communication Processes

The silence of speechlessness is never golden. We all need to communicate and connect with each other—not just in one way, but also in as many ways possible. It is a basic human need, a basic human right. And much more than this, it is a basic human power. (Bob Williams, 2000, p. 248)

Michael Williams has relied on augmentative and alternative communication (AAC) strategies throughout his life. To learn more about him and his communication strategies, access his webcast, *How Far We've Come, How Far We've Got to Go: Tales from the Trenches* (Williams, 2006).

For most of you who read this book, daily communication is so effortless and efficient that you hardly think about it when you interact with others face to face, over the phone, through e-mail, by texting, or through social media. You probably do not remember the effort that you initially expended as an infant and toddler to learn to speak because now these processes are largely automatic. Usually, you just "talk," formulating your messages and executing speech movements as you express yourself. However, effortless communication is not an option for all people (Beukelman & Ray, 2010) because some are unable to meet their daily communication needs through natural speech. Yet, effective communication is essential for learning and development, personal care, social engagement, education, and employment. It is also essential for medical care as noted in a statement from the Joint Commission titled *Advancing Effective Communication, Cultural Competence, and Patient- and Family-Centered Care: A Roadmap for Hospitals*:

No longer considered to be simply a patient's right, effective communication is now accepted as an essential component of quality care and patient safety [5,6]....Effective communication [is] the successful joint establishment of meaning wherein patients and health care providers exchange information, enabling patients to participate actively in their care from admission through discharge, and ensuring that the responsibilities of both patients and providers are understood. (2010, p. 1)

The purpose of this book is to introduce you to people who rely on AAC, to the AAC supports that they use to meet their communication needs, and to those who assist them. Approximately 1.3% of all people, or about 4 million Americans, cannot rely on their natural speech to meet their daily communication needs. Without access to speech, these people face severe restrictions in their communication and participation in all aspects of life—education, medical care, employment, family, and community involvement—unless they are provided with other communication supports. The development of AAC strategies offers great potential to enhance the communicative effectiveness of people with complex communication needs. However, for many, this potential has not been fully realized. There is an urgent need for people to assist those who rely on AAC strategies. In addition to helping those who rely on AAC and their families and caregivers, there is a continuing need to develop a range of competent AAC stakeholders, such as those who design new technologies; educators; speech-language pathologists; physical therapists; occupational therapists; rehabilitation engineers, and technicians who provide AAC intervention services; people who shape public policy and funding; and researchers who document AAC use and acceptance patterns as well as investigate communication processes when AAC strategies are used.

WHAT IS AUGMENTATIVE AND ALTERNATIVE COMMUNICATION?

The American Speech-Language-Hearing Association (ASHA) Special Interest Division 12: Augmentative and Alternative Communication (AAC) defined AAC as follows:

> Augmentative and alternative communication (AAC) refers to an area of research, clinical, and educational practice. AAC involves attempts to study and when necessary compensate for temporary or permanent impairments, activity limitations, and participation restrictions of individuals with severe disorders of speech-language production and/or comprehension, including spoken and written modes of communication. (2005, p. 1)

AAC intervention services and AAC technology are part of the habilitation and rehabilitation services and technology designation within the U.S. health care reform of 2010. *Rehabilitation* refers to intervention strategies and technologies that help someone who has an acquired disability regain a capability, whereas *habilitation* refers to intervention strategies and technologies that assist a person, such as someone with a developmental disability, to develop a capability for the first time.

WHO RELIES ON AUGMENTATIVE AND ALTERNATIVE COMMUNICATION?

There is no typical person who relies on AAC. They come from all age groups, socioeconomic groups, and ethnic and racial backgrounds. Their only unifying characteristic is the fact that they require adaptive assistance for speaking and/or writing because their gestural, spoken, and/or written communication is temporarily or permanently inadequate to meet all of their communication needs. Some of these individuals may be able to produce a limited amount of speech that is inadequate to meet their varied communication needs.

A variety of congenital or acquired conditions can cause the inability to speak or write without adaptive assistance. The most common congenital causes of such severe communication disorders include severe intellectual disability, cerebral palsy, autism, and developmental apraxia of speech. The acquired medical conditions that most often result in the need for AAC assistance include amyotrophic lateral sclerosis, multiple sclerosis, traumatic brain injury, and stroke. (See Parts II and III of this book for prevalence figures and demographic information related to each of these groups of people.)

Published prevalence reports of the number of people with severe speech and/or writing limitations vary to some extent depending on the country, age group, and type(s) of disability surveyed. In Canada, data from the 2001 Participation and Activity Limitation Survey suggested that approximately 318,000 Canadians older than age 4 years have difficulty speaking and being understood (Cossette & Duclos, 2003); this represents approximately 1.5% of the total population older than age 4 years. Paralleling the Canadian data, a study by Enderby and Philipp (1986) suggested that 800,000 individuals (1.4% of the total population) in the United Kingdom have a severe communication disorder that makes it difficult for them to be understood by anyone outside their immediate family. An Australian survey of the province of Victoria, which has more than 4 million residents, identified approximately 5,000 individuals who were unable to speak adequately for communication; this represents 1.2% of the population (Bloomberg & Johnson, 1990).

The prevalence of severe communication disorders appears to vary considerably with age. Based on the results of several studies, Blackstone (1990) suggested that 0.2%–0.6% of the total school-age population worldwide has a severe speech impairment. A Canadian study suggested that the prevalence increases to 0.8% of individuals from age 45 to 54 years and reaches a high of 4.2% for people age 85 years and older (Hirdes, Ellis-Hale, & Pearson Hirdes, 1993).

WHAT IS IT LIKE TO RELY ON AUGMENTATIVE AND ALTERNATIVE COMMUNICATION STRATEGIES?

Perhaps more relevant (certainly, more interesting) than demographic figures are the stories and experiences of people who rely on AAC. In Table 1.1, we provide resources that contain first-person accounts in the writings and presentations of people who rely on AAC. From these and other accounts, we can sense what it is like to be unable to communicate through traditional speech or writing and to rely on AAC. Rick Creech, a young man with cerebral palsy, provided a stark description of being unable to speak:

Table 1.1.   Selected first-person accounts by individuals who rely on augmentative and alternative communication

Brown, C. (1954). *My left foot.* London: Secker & Warburg.

Fried-Oken, M., & Bersani, H.A., Jr. (Eds.). (2000). *Speaking up and spelling it out: Personal essays on augmentative and alternative communication.* Baltimore: Paul H. Brookes Publishing Co.

Fried-Oken, M., Howard, J., & Stewart, S. (1991). Feedback on AAC intervention from adults who are temporarily unable to speak. *Augmentative and Alternative Communication, 7,* 43–50.

Mirenda, P., & Bopp, K. (2003). "Playing the game": Strategic competence in AAC. In J.C. Light, D.R. Beukelman, & J. Reichle (Eds.), *Communicative competence for individuals who use AAC: From research to effective practice* (pp. 401–437). Baltimore: Paul H. Brookes Publishing Co.

Nolan, C. (1987). *Under the eye of the clock.* New York: St. Martin's Press.

Williams, M., & Krezman, C. (Eds.). (2000). *Beneath the surface: Creative expression of augmented communicators.* Toronto: International Society for Augmentative and Alternative Communication.

> If you want to know what it is like to be unable to speak, there is a way. Go to a
> party and don't talk. Play mute. Use your hands if you wish but don't use paper and
> pencil. Paper and pencil are not always handy for a mute person. Here is what you
> will find: people talking; talking behind, beside, around, over, under, through, and
> even for you. But never with you. You are ignored until finally you feel like a piece
> of furniture. (Musselwhite & St. Louis, 1988, p. 104)

Jim Prentice, who has relied on AAC for years, wrote:

> Augmentative and alternative communication can provide a person with the ability
> to have and develop strong and rewarding relationships with others. Deny a person
> the ability to articulate intelligibly and that person is sentenced to live in social,
> intellectual and emotional isolation. (Prentice, 2000, p. 213)

In an early account of AAC, Christy Brown, who first communicated by writing with
chalk held in his left foot, recounted the day when he printed his first letter:

> I drew it—the letter "A." There it was on the floor before me….I looked up. I saw
> my mother's face for a moment, tears on her cheeks….I had done it! It had started—
> the thing that was to give my mind its chance of expressing itself….That one letter,
> scrawled on the floor with a broken bit of yellow chalk gripped between my toes,
> was my road to a new world, my key to mental freedom. (Brown, 1954, p. 17)

Janice Staehely commented eloquently on the limitations of one-way communication
as she writes:

> One day I was listening to…the radio, [and] the song ["Life's a Dance"] played. The
> words sounded so profound to me. Just as a dance couldn't possibly be a dance un-
> less people moved to it, so language doesn't become communication until people
> grow to express it back. It has to be a two-way exchange. (2000, p. 3)

Beyond having an interactive form, communication allows people to participate in
activities that are important to them. Gus Estrella and Janice Staehely provided insight into how their ability to rely on AAC affected their family relationships:

> So how important is augmentative communication technology to a person who has
> a severe speech disability? And when does the importance of augmentative com-
> munication technology become more evident to the person and to their family and
> friends? This may vary from person to person, and it could occur during different
> stages in a person's life. In my personal life, the importance became more evident
> at different points in my life. One was definitely when my father and I started talk-
> ing and sharing things that we couldn't before. We would talk about baseball, the
> Los Angeles Dodgers in particular. And who can forget basketball and the Arizona
> Wildcats? We were finally having father and son conversations, just like the other
> fathers and sons were having since the beginning of time. (Estrella, 2000, p. 40)

> With my new voice, my world began to open up. Cautiously at first, I went to work
> learning the [AAC device]….Soon even my family's skepticism toward [my AAC
> device] vanished as they saw my communication with people increase. I will never

forget the time when my sister was so pleased that she could keep a conversation with me going while tending her garden. (Staehely, 2000, p. 3)

AAC technology also allows people to develop social networks beyond their immediate families and those who are in face-to-face relationships with them. Three individuals described how they used AAC to expand their social networks and social roles:

> When I got my new computer, I also got hooked up to the Internet and to e-mail. My world changed overnight! At the time, I was very much involved with the local Disability Services Advisory Council. With my speech problem, they had a very hard time understanding me. When I got e-mail, I had no problems. When there were questions that the council wanted my input on, all they had to do was send an e-mail, and they would get an answer right back from me. (Price, 2000, p. 114)

> Currently, I use my [AAC device] to communicate at work, in meetings, and on the phone. At home, I usually communicate by facial expressions, letter signing, and typing notes on my computer. Usually when people get to know me and my communication methods, they have no trouble understanding me. Of course, some people learn faster than others. Also, e-mail plays a heavy role in my communication methods. There are many people to whom I only e-mail instead of picking up the phone and calling them. I feel e-mail is the most effective way for me to communicate. (Cardona, 2000, p. 244)

> Wendy recalled the difference it made for Leon when they had visitors. "It is very hard for some people to go visit a person who can't talk to them…but Leon communicated until the very end by using his device. His friends came regularly because he could communicate with them." (McKelvey, Evans, Kawai, & Beukelman, 2012)

Dattilo and colleagues (Dattilo et al., 2008; Dattilo, Benedek-Wood, & McLeod, 2010) documented the leisure and recreational activities of adults who rely on AAC. These people reported that leisure activities improved their physical and mental health, enhanced their social networks and personal independence, and provided them with ways to educate others about AAC and disabilities. However, the authors also documented the barriers encountered in the pursuit of leisure activities.

Although employment has been an elusive goal for many with complex communication needs, AAC strategies support efforts to enter or to maintain involvement in the employment arena. David Chapple, an individual with a developmental disability, and Stephen Hawking, the Nobel Prize–winning scientist who has an acquired disability, both provided some insight:

> With the help of augmentative and alternative communication (AAC), I have achieved my goal of starting my career as a software engineer. Although I have the strong computer skills to get a job and to work competitively, AAC has helped me with all the other facets of my job: my interview, my programming work, and my relationships with peers. At my interview, I was able to respond to the questions quickly and intelligently. With my voice output communication aid, I can store programming commands under icon sequences so I can type a programming line within seconds. Finally, AAC has helped me to express my sense of humor and technical ideas to my co-workers. (Chapple, 2000, p. 155)

> Without my computer, I cannot communicate....[It] has provided me with the means
> to continue working and researching....[It] also allows me to keep in touch with my
> family and friends; I can e-mail and make phone calls at any time using the mobile
> technology....It is vital for my security and safety that I can make calls for myself
> should the need arise. (Hawking, 2003)

AAC was initially considered essential to support social interactions among
people; however, DeRuyter, McNaughton, Caves, Bryen, and Williams (2007, p. 268)
described the future as they wrote:

> Full access to email, cell phones, digital music stores, e-commerce, digital photo albums,
> and e-books are all activities that require digital independence. These are fundamental
> communication activities in the twenty-first century and are necessary for full participa-
> tion in schools, the workplace, and the community-at-large. We must ensure that AAC
> technology...support[s] greater participation in today's Information Society.

Olinda Olson, a woman with ALS who uses mechanical ventilation for respiratory support, illustrated the multiple uses of eye-tracking AAC technology. She uses
it to communicate face-to-face with her family and residence staff, access the Internet,
and send and receive e-mail, which she uses to manage her personal and medical care
and to communicate with her children who live at a distance. In a webcast, she said:

> This is an eye gaze computer [AAC technology]. I use it to communicate with family
> and friends....I also use it to read books and my bible. [She then demonstrated using
> the AAC system to turn on her nurse call light.]...I love the eye gaze. It allows me to
> keep in contact with my children. (Fager & Beukelman, 2009, slide 42)

While this chapter was being written, she sent her AAC team an e-mail explain-
ing that her daughter-in-law was pregnant. Since her son and daughter-in-law live
a thousand miles from her, she had recently made the first use of Skype, a video-
calling application integrated into her AAC technology, so that she would be ready
to "meet" her first grandchild within a few hours of the child's birth (Susan Fager,
personal communication, October 2010).

PURPOSES OF COMMUNICATION INTERACTIONS

The ultimate goal of AAC is not to find a technological solution to communication
problems but to enable individuals to efficiently and effectively engage in a variety
of interactions and participate in activities of their choice. Light (1988), in an extensive review of AAC interaction research, identified four agendas or purposes that
communicative interactions fulfill: 1) communication of needs/wants, 2) information transfer, 3) social closeness, and 4) social etiquette (see Table 1.2). To Light's list,
we would add a fifth purpose—to communicate with oneself or conduct an internal
dialogue.

As shown in Table 1.2, the goal of expressing one's needs and wants is to regulate
the behavior of the listener toward an action-oriented response. Examples include
asking for help or ordering food in a restaurant. Here, the content of the message
is important, the vocabulary is relatively predictable, and the accuracy and rate of
message production are critical. The high degree of predictability and concreteness

Table 1.2. Characteristics of interactions intended to meet various social purposes

Characteristics	Social purpose of the interaction			
	Expression of needs/wants	Information transfer	Social closeness	Social etiquette
Goal of the interaction	To regulate the behavior of another as a means to fulfill needs/wants	To share information	To establish, maintain, and/ or develop personal relationships	To conform to social conventions of politeness
Focus of interaction	Desired object or action	Information	Interpersonal relationship	Social convention
Duration of the interaction	Limited. Emphasis is on initiating interaction.	May be lengthy. Emphasis is on developing interaction.	May be lengthy. Emphasis is on maintaining interaction.	Limited. Emphasis is on fulfilling designated turns.
Content of communication	Important	Important	Not important	Not important
Predictability of communication	Highly predictable	Not predictable	May be somewhat predictable	Highly predictable
Scope of communication	Limited scope	Wide scope	Wide scope	Very limited scope
Rate of communication	Important	Important	May not be important	Important
Tolerance for communication breakdown	Little tolerance	Little tolerance	Some tolerance	Little tolerance
Number of participants	Usually dyadic	Dyadic, small or large group	Usually dyadic or small group	Dyadic, small or large group
Independence of the communicator	Important	Important	Not important	Important
Partner	Familiar or unfamiliar	Familiar or unfamiliar	Usually familiar	Familiar or unfamiliar

From Light, J. (1988). Interaction involving individuals using augmentative and alternative communication systems: State of the art and future directions. *Augmentative and Alternative Communication, 4*, 76; reprinted by permission of Informa Healthcare.

inherent in these messages likely explains why needs/wants vocabulary often predominates in many communication systems. In fact, it is not unusual to see communication books or boards that consist almost entirely of such vocabulary, regardless of how motivating or relevant the person using the AAC system finds the messages.

The second area of interaction, information transfer, involves messages that are more complex and difficult to convey because the goal is to share information rather than to regulate behavior. Examples of people engaging in this kind of interaction include a child telling teachers what she did over the weekend, an adolescent talking with friends about the upcoming senior prom, an adult answering questions during a job interview, and a person with a medical condition communicating directly or over the Internet with a health care provider. As is the case with needs and wants, the content of the message is important. Information transfer messages, however, are likely to be composed of novel (rather than predictable) words and sentences that communicate a wide variety of topics. Accuracy and the rate of message production again remain paramount.

Communication related to social closeness greatly differs from the expression of needs and wants or the transfer of information. The goal of this type of interaction is establishing, maintaining, or developing social engagement. Thus, the content of the message is often less important than the interaction itself. Examples of people interacting in this way include a child greeting classmates, a group of teenagers cheering for their team at a basketball game, and an adult expressing feelings of sympathy to a friend whose mother recently died. In such interactions, the rate, accuracy, and content of the message, as well as the independence of the person communicating, are secondary to the feelings of connectedness and intimacy achieved through the interaction.

The goal of the fourth type of interaction listed in Table 1.2, social etiquette, is to conform to social conventions of politeness through interactions that are often brief and contain predictable vocabulary. Examples of people practicing social etiquette include a child saying "please" and "thank you" to his or her grandmother and an adult expressing appreciation to a caregiver. These messages resemble those that express needs and wants because rate, accuracy, and communicative independence all are important factors for success.

The fifth type of interaction is to communicate with oneself or to conduct an internal dialogue. To remain organized on a day-to-day basis, individuals often make lists, enter information into calendars, and prepare daily activity schedules. Diaries, journals of personal insights, lists of future plans, and records of personal reflections also fit into this category.

From the perspective of the person who uses AAC, communicative competence involves the ability to efficiently and effectively transmit messages in all of the interaction categories based on individual interests, circumstances, and abilities. Communication partners report that people who rely on AAC and are judged to be competent communicators also possess an additional set of skills. The research of Light (1988) and Light and Binger (1998) suggested that competent communicators are able to do the following:

- Portray a positive self-image to their communication partners
- Show interest in others and draw others into interactions
- Actively participate and take turns in a symmetrical fashion
- Be responsive to their communication partners by, for example, making relevant comments, asking partner-focused questions, and negotiating shared topics
- Put their partners at ease with the AAC system through the use of, for example, an introductory strategy (e.g., messages that say HI, MY NAME IS GORDON; I USE THIS MACHINE TO COMMUNICATE. I WILL TOUCH THE PICTURES OF WHAT I WANT TO SAY); humor and predictable, readable nonverbal signals might also serve this purpose.

AAC teams should be aware of the fact that different types of partners might perceive the importance of various strategies related to communicative competence differently. For example, Light, Binger, Bailey, and Millar (1997) found evidence that for both adults without prior AAC experience and professionals with prior AAC experience, nonverbal feedback from those who rely on AAC during conversational interactions was positively related to their perceptions of communicative competence. However, adolescents without experience did not find this factor to be critical. Clearly, part of every AAC intervention should involve 1) identification of critical skills for communicative competence from the perspective of relevant listeners and

2) strategic instruction to support the highest level of communicative competence possible. Such strategies are described in detail in Chapter 11.

ASSISTIVE TECHNOLOGY IS ONLY PART OF THE ANSWER

The personal accounts of the lived experiences of people who rely on AAC are encouraging. Certainly, assistive communication technology can change people's lives. However, AAC technology is not magic. A piano alone doesn't make a pianist, nor does a basketball make an athlete. Likewise, AAC technology alone doesn't make one a competent, proficient communicator (Beukelman, 1991). Those who rely on AAC strategies begin as AAC novices and evolve in competence to become AAC experts with appropriate support, instruction, practice, and encouragement. Therefore, AAC options must be provided to them in a timely manner so that they can become competent and proficient with AAC strategies.

Light and colleagues (Light, 1989b; Light, Arnold, & Clark, 2003; Light, Roberts, Dimarco, & Greiner, 1998) described in detail the components of communicative competence for those who rely on AAC. They identified four components: linguistic, operational, social, and strategic competence.

Linguistic Competence

Linguistic competence refers to the receptive and expressive language skills of one's native language(s). It also involves knowledge of the linguistic code unique to one's AAC system, such as line drawings, words, signs, and so forth. Equally important, the people who rely on AAC must learn the language spoken by communication partners in order to receive messages. In bilingual contexts, this may mean learning the family's native language as well as that of the community at large (Light, 1989b). For individuals with acquired disabilities, much of this learning may already be in place at the time of intervention, leaving only AAC-specific tasks to be mastered. For people with congenital disabilities, however, all of these skills must be learned within the accompanying physical, sensory, or cognitive constraints.

Parents, communication specialists, friends, and other facilitators can play a major role in assisting those who rely on AAC to master this formidable set of tasks. First, facilitators can offer ongoing opportunities for practicing expressive language (both native and augmentative) in natural contexts (Romski & Sevcik, 1996). In some cases, this may simply mean helping the person to learn the AAC symbol or code system. In other cases, especially if the individual has a history of poor generalization, facilitators may themselves have to learn the symbol system in order to provide sufficient opportunities for practice (e.g., manual signing; Loeding, Zangari, & Lloyd, 1990; Spragale & Micucci, 1990). It is also important for facilitators to provide augmented input models in the language of the community and family as well as in the symbols or codes used in the AAC display. Receptive language input strategies may include aided language stimulation vests or boards (Goossens', 1989), symbol song strips used with music (Musselwhite & St. Louis, 1988), joint use of the AAC display by the facilitator (Romski & Sevcik, 1996), or keyword input provided through manual signing (see Blackstone, Cassatt-James, & Bruskin, 1988, for additional strategies). Specific strategies for encouraging linguistic competence in relation to the AAC system are discussed in greater detail in Chapter 11. Blockberger and Sutton (2003) published a summary of research related to the development of linguistic competence by those who rely on AAC.

Operational Competence

Operational competence refers to the technical skills needed to operate the AAC system accurately and efficiently. The most immediate need for people who rely on AAC and those who support them is to acquire operational competence as quickly as possible when an AAC system is introduced. This requires instruction in all operational and maintenance aspects of the system (see Lee & Thomas, 1990, for details). Often, the person who relies on AAC is not the primary recipient of much of this instruction, and facilitators may take on much of the responsibility for operational competence. These facilitators may be parents, spouses, or other family members; educational, residential, or vocational staff; friends; and other people who are involved in and committed to the communicative well-being of the individual who relies on AAC. In school settings, new facilitators may have to be trained in AAC operation each school year to keep pace with staff turnover and teacher and staff rotations. For example, one fourth-grade student who has worked with the same speech-language pathologist and paraprofessional since kindergarten has nonetheless had 16 people trained in operational aspects of her system over a 5-year period (Beukelman, 1991). Specifically, the needs are to 1) keep the vocabulary in the technology up to date; 2) construct overlays or other displays as needed; 3) protect the technology against breakage, damage, or other problems; 4) secure necessary repairs; 5) modify the system for future needs; and 6) generally ensure day-to-day availability and operation of the technology. Generally, unaided or low-technology systems require less operational competence, which is one reason why they may be preferable when capable facilitators are not available.

Social Competence

Social competence refers to skills of social interaction such as initiating, maintaining, developing, and terminating communication interactions. Of the four areas of communicative competence identified by Light (1989b), social competence has been the focus of most of the research in the AAC field (e.g., Kraat, 1985; Light, 1988). Social competence requires the person who relies on AAC to have knowledge, judgment, and skills in both the sociolinguistic and sociorelational aspects of communication or "competence as to when to speak, when not [to], and as to what to talk about, with whom, when, where, in what manner" (Hymes, 1972, p. 277). For example, sociolinguistic skills include the abilities to 1) initiate, maintain, and terminate conversations; 2) give and take turns; 3) communicate a variety of functions (e.g., requesting, rejecting); and 4) engage in a variety of coherent and cohesive interactions. Light (1988) suggested that some sociorelational skills or attributes that are important for people who rely on AAC to develop include 1) a positive self-image, 2) an interest in others and a desire to communicate, 3) the ability to participate actively in conversation, 4) responsiveness to partners, and 5) the ability to put partners at ease.

Opportunities to practice social competence skills in natural contexts are critical for AAC communicators and facilitators. A number of facilitator training manuals and approaches have been developed for AAC communicators who have a variety of backgrounds and AAC system needs (e.g., Blackstone et al., 1988; Culp & Carlisle, 1988; Light & Binger, 1998; Light, Dattilo, English, Gutierrez, & Hartz, 1992; Light, McNaughton, & Parnes, 1986; MacDonald & Gillette, 1986; McNaughton & Light, 1989; Pepper & Weitzman, 2004; Reichle, York, & Sigafoos, 1991; Siegel-Causey & Guess, 1989). Both the number and the quality of such efforts are indicative of the importance of providing extensive training in social competence skills to AAC communicators and their facilitators.

Information, training, and support efforts related to social competence must often go beyond specific training. In many cases, it is also important for AAC teams to work directly with communication partners who encounter the person who uses AAC only on social occasions. For example, friends and peers may need information about how to adjust their interactions to accommodate the requirements of the AAC system (e.g., allowing sufficient pauses for message composition). The AAC team may need to explain how to interact with someone who uses a low-tech display (e.g., echoing messages as they are indicated, in order to provide feedback). Brief in-service training to an entire school class may help to demystify the AAC system, and in many cases the individual who uses AAC can participate in or conduct these sessions. Whatever the content and however brief, communication partner interventions such as these are often as critical as more extensive facilitator training endeavors.

Strategic Competence

Strategic competence involves the compensatory strategies used by people who rely on AAC to deal with functional limitations associated with AAC. These may include interacting with those unfamiliar with AAC, resolving communication breakdowns, and compensating for a slow speaking rate. Because even the most flexible AAC systems impose some interactive limitations on those who use them to communicate, people who rely on AAC need the knowledge, judgment, and skills that allow them to "communicate effectively within restrictions" (Light, 1989b, p. 141). Instruction in strategic competence involves teaching various adaptive or coping strategies to use when communication breakdowns occur. For example, the person who relies on AAC may learn to transmit the message PLEASE SLOW DOWN AND WAIT FOR ME TO FINISH or learn to use a gesture that means NO, YOU MISUNDERSTOOD. This is another area of training from which both facilitators and those who use AAC can benefit. For example, many times those who rely on AAC appreciate the increased efficiency that results if the communication partner helps to co-construct messages by guessing. In order for this to occur, however, a facilitator or the person who uses AAC must teach the partner how to guess accurately. Mirenda and Bopp (2003) published a summary of the research related to strategic competence in AAC.

The evolution toward expertise requires that key stakeholders be and remain competent in AAC strategies so that appropriate assessment, intervention, and mentoring can occur. It also assumes that the stakeholders are properly prepared and that the standards and guidelines of AAC practice are increasingly understood and implemented (ASHA, 2004, 2005). Unfortunately, this is not always the case. Yet, there are encouraging signs for the future. First, current research in AAC focuses on both the processes and the outcomes of AAC interventions (Schlosser, 2003b). It is hoped that the emphasis on evidence-based practice in AAC will increase the information base on which AAC practice guidelines can be developed. Such guidelines will clarify appropriate intervention practices to guide AAC service providers. The development of practice guidelines is an evolutionary process based on the best information available in the field at any given time. Second, there is a growing awareness of the need for mentoring (or coaching) of those who rely on AAC so that they can become increasingly competent communicators. People who rely on AAC strategies face a daunting challenge to become proficient communicators when those around them typically do not use AAC techniques. In other words, they simply cannot do what typically developing children do, which is to observe their parents, family members, and peers and learn from them. Usually, AAC intervention experts provide the only coaching and mentoring for someone new to AAC technology. Unfortunately, the quality and availability of such mentoring varies considerably. Several efforts that support mentor–protégé relationships among expert and novice AAC communicators have been described (Cohen & Light, 2000; Light, McNaughton, Krezman, Williams, & Gulens, 2000).

PREPARING FOR THE FUTURE

In late 2010, I attended an AAC research planning meeting in which Michael Williams (mentioned at the beginning of this chapter) also was a participant. One morning, I observed Michael at breakfast in the hotel where we were staying. He was seated at a table located close to the area where guests lined up for the breakfast buffet. On that weekend morning, we shared the hotel with a crowd of middle-school–age youth (and their families) who were participating in dance, swimming, and soccer competitions in the area. I watched Michael visit with them as they waited in line for breakfast. From a distance, I could see that Michael and the young people were having a great time—there was a lot of talking and laughing. For nearly an hour he interacted with different young people until it was their turn to move on and order breakfast. I also observed these young people as they sat down to eat with their families and friends. The prominent topic of conversation that morning was this guy who had talked to them using his "computer." Only later did I realize that a few months earlier, Michael had written the following to others who rely on AAC: "Every time you step out of your home, cruise down the street, catch the eye of a stranger, make a purchase, attend a ball game, or say 'hello' to a child, you are making a significant change in the expectations the world has of augmented communicators" (Williams, Krezman, & McNaughton, 2008, p. 203).

In addition to the efforts of people who rely on AAC themselves, the future success of the AAC effort depends on the preparation and development of competent AAC stakeholders. Beukelman, Ball, and Fager (2008) provided a personnel framework that clarifies various stakeholders' roles (see Chapter 5). The capability of universities to prepare graduates with competence in AAC is expanding. However, some universities still prepare professionals to assist people with disabilities but provide little or no systematic preparation in AAC. This book is written in the hope that university programs that educate special educators, physical therapists, occupational therapists, rehabilitation engineers, and speech-language pathologists will provide training in assistive technology and AAC to their students.

The need to provide continuing education to other AAC stakeholders so that they remain competent technology developers, researchers, interventionists, and public policy advocates is ongoing. Because people who rely on AAC are not limited to an age category, etiology, location, or situation and because they need ongoing support on at least at some level, the need for competent AAC personnel remains urgent. This text initiates the reader on a path toward competence and expertise in AAC to serve individuals with complex communication needs.

OVERVIEW OF CHAPTERS

The organization of this book reflects our experiences while teaching AAC classes together at the University of Nebraska–Lincoln as well as our solo experiences since that time. We realize that individuals from a wide range of disciplines will be introduced to AAC through this text; therefore, the chapters in Part I provide specific information about the concepts, strategies, and techniques that are unique to the AAC field. In Part II, we shift our focus to the AAC needs of people with developmental disabilities by emphasizing nonsymbolic and symbolic strategies for beginning communicators, language learning, literacy, and inclusion in school. In Part III, we deal with individuals who were at one time able to speak and write but now require AAC systems because of an acquired injury, disease, or condition.

QUESTIONS

1.1.   What type of individual should be considered for AAC support?
1.2.   In Chapter 1, five different communication purposes are described. What personal, social, and communication roles are associated with each of these purposes?
1.3.   From an AAC perspective, what is meant by linguistic competence?
1.4.   How do strategic and social competences differ?
1.5.   What are the various components of operational competence?
1.6.   If the parents of a child with communication difficulties asked you what it would be like to communicate using AAC supports, what would you tell them that you have learned from this chapter and from the webcasts listed in the chapter?

CHAPTER 2

Message Management
Vocabulary, Small Talk, and Narratives

Message management includes the formulation, storage, or retrieval of single words, codes, and messages to support face-to-face, written, and social media communication. People who rely on augmentative and alternative communication (AAC) have a wide range of capabilities and message formulation preferences. Some choose to formulate their messages using a letter-by-letter spelling strategy. For those who have the necessary spelling skills, this strategy allows them to formulate any message that they choose. Others augment their letter-by-letter spelling strategy by selecting individual words from core lists of words predicted by or stored in their AAC devices or applications. Most AAC technology contains language models that support word-by-word message formulation. Finally, some who rely on AAC communicate using full or partial messages stored by the manufacturer or programmed personally in their devices.

As AAC technology is designed with ever greater computing, storage, and display capacities, message sets (words, phrases, and sentences) are increasingly being programmed into technology by manufacturers and software developers who make the assumption that message type is uniform for people who rely on AAC at various ages or stages in life. Prestored vocabulary and messages reduce the workload of AAC facilitators (people who support an individual's AAC communication efforts) and, therefore, are attractive to them. In addition to prestored messages, some devices allow for more personalization of messages than others. The language content included in AAC devices by manufacturers is becoming ever more extensive and complex. While some messages are produced routinely within a culture, other messages are personal and unique. In this chapter, we review the knowledge base related to message management in AAC strategies and devices that comes from the communication patterns of those who rely on AAC as well as from typical speakers. Message-related content is provided throughout the book as we focus on communication support for children, youth, and adults in different communication settings. It is important for those who rely on AAC and those who assist them to carefully review the language content included within an AAC device to determine if it meets the cultural, social, care, and medical needs of the particular individual.

AAC is about helping people who cannot speak well enough to meet their daily communication needs to interact with others; therefore, the central goal of AAC is to provide individuals with the opportunity and capability 1) to communicate messages so that they can interact in conversations; 2) to participate in communication at home, in school, at work, and during recreational activities; 3) to learn their native language(s); 4) to establish and maintain their social roles (e.g., friend, student, spouse, mentor, and employee); 5) to meet their personal needs; and 6) to communicate accurately to guide their personal and medical care. This chapter introduces the factors that influence message selection in AAC in such contexts and roles. Because the message selection process in AAC is influenced by such a wide range of factors, this chapter provides an overview to supplement information provided in Chapters 8 through 18 that covers specific interventions.

The Barkley AAC Center's web site provides extensive vocabulary and message resources to support communication by individuals across the age span.

FACTORS THAT INFLUENCE AUGMENTATIVE AND ALTERNATIVE COMMUNICATION MESSAGE SELECTION

Because word selection and message formulation are such efficient processes for most typical speakers and writers, most of them usually enter communication situations without giving much consideration beforehand to the words, phrases, and stories they will use. Of course, there are times when they plan their messages and even rehearse them in advance, such as when they make marriage proposals, participate in employment interviews, testify in court, give a speech, or write a contractual agreement. However, message selection during natural speech interactions and written communication is usually so automatic that even most AAC specialists have little experience selecting vocabulary items in advance of the acts of speaking or writing. Even interventionists who have regular contact with individuals who experience communication conditions such as stuttering, voice problems, articulation problems, and cleft palate rarely need to preselect messages to support conversational or written communication.

In 2005, I assisted a close friend to communicate effectively in a range of situations. He had amyotrophic lateral sclerosis and used AAC technology. Each Monday evening, Tom and his wife invited members of their social and professional networks to drop by a local restaurant for "Time with Tom." They did not know who would attend or if they would visit with the usual 25 to 30 guests or the approximately 200 that appeared on his birthday. Of course, we had the usual small-talk messages entered into his talking AAC device. Each week we prepared for this event by predicting some of the messages Tom might use and then preprogramming them into his AAC device. The messages included pages of personal news, jokes, thoughts for the week, and comments on events in the local and national news and sports, as well as personal comments for specific individuals with special health, family, or personal issues who might attend. Tom formulated novel messages using letter-by-letter spelling and word prediction as well, but with the changing crowd of guests, he did not have much time to prepare complex, novel messages (Beukelman, 2005; Rutz, 2005).

In addition to the lack of experience with which most AAC facilitators approach message selection, a variety of other factors influence the types of messages used by different communicators. Differences in age, gender, social role, and medical conditions exert powerful influences on both natural speakers and those who rely on AAC. Children use different messages than adults. Older adults speak about different topics and use different small-talk phrases than younger adults. Men and women tend to talk about different topics. People with extensive medical and personal care needs communicate about different topics than those with less extensive needs. When those who rely on AAC and their facilitators represent different age, gender, and social cohorts, message selection becomes even more complicated.

In addition to generic differences in message use, individuals vary with regard to their message needs and preferences. The environments in which they live influence the ways in which they wish to communicate. Communication at home is different from that in nursing centers, nursing homes, community living facilities, schools, and hospitals. The type of disability or medical condition influences people's interactions with caregivers, medical staff, education personnel, and family. The messages included in AAC systems must reflect individual differences related to interests and to the names of family members, streets, stores, and pets. Finally, differing life experiences leave individuals with different stories to tell.

For a person who experiences a disabling event or condition, the transition from being an individual without disabilities to one with a chronic disability is an evolutionary journey (Beukelman, Garrett, & Yorkston, 2007). As one passes through the stages of awareness, loss, accommodation, and regaining of self, the specific vocabulary to express emotions related to these stages is necessary but is still poorly understood and represented in AAC systems. In time, individuals with chronic disabilities often go on to mentor others and teach others about their journey. These efforts also require specialized vocabulary different from that commonly available in most AAC systems.

Fortunately, the futures of people with lifelong disabilities hold much more freedom and promise than they once did (McNaughton & Beukelman, 2010). At one time, people with lifelong disabilities lived segregated lives at home or in institutions; thus, their communication needs were quite restricted and predictable. Since the 1970s, however, societal involvement of people with disabilities has increased dramatically. As people with disabilities participate more successfully in the educational, social, religious, recreational, volunteer, and vocational realms of our communities, their communication needs change dramatically (McNaughton, Light, & Arnold, 2002). Of course, the increase in electronic communication options also continues to change and expand communication needs.

Unfortunately, as people who rely on AAC become more involved in a variety of contexts and situations, they also face an increased risk of experiencing crime and abuse. Bryen, Carey, and Frantz (2003) reported that nearly half of the individuals (ages 18 to 39 years) who rely on AAC and participated in their survey experienced some type of crime during their lifetime. These results support the need for vocabulary that is necessary to report crimes for legal and counseling purposes. Collier, McGhie-Richmond, Odette, and Pyne (2006) concluded that the majority of the people who relied on AAC in their 3-year study had experienced a range of abuses, including sexual abuse, and they lacked information about abuse and supports that would help them to cope with the relationship difficulties associated with abuse and to access the services of the justice system. Bryen (2008) requested that people who rely on AAC and AAC professionals nominate the vocabulary needed to support communication related to six adult social contexts: college life, sexuality, crime reporting, management of personal assistants, health care, and transportation. She reported that an average of only 55% of the vocabulary nominated by the participants in the study was included in AAC symbol sets available at the time of the study.

Changes in technology have also had an extensive impact on the communication patterns of individuals with severe communication disorders. Early in the development of the AAC field, the memory and display capabilities of AAC systems were so limited that these devices could store only relatively small message sets. With new electronic designs and inexpensive computer memory, the storage and computing capacity of electronic communication devices has expanded dramatically; many now have a nearly limitless capacity for message storage. Thus, AAC devices can now include an almost unrestricted number of messages, including those related to small talk, scripts, and stories, which earlier systems could not manage. In addition, with the advent of dynamic display devices (computer screens that the individual can change as though turning the pages of a book and that use lights to signal available message options), AAC facilitators and manufacturers can organize and provide symbols for huge message pools using strategies that do not rely solely on the memory capabilities of those who rely on AAC (see Chapter 3). Finally, the voice output options available in modern AAC devices are intelligible and natural enough to allow AAC use in a wide range of social contexts. Together, these technological advances permit the use of message sets to support communication with strangers as well as with friends and in large or small groups as well as on a one-to-one basis.

Stuart, Lasker, and Beukelman (2000, pp. 25–26) observed the following about message management at the start of the 21st century:

> Debates over the "best" way to manage messages in AAC devices continue.... [D]iscussions regarding the relative merits of word-based versus phrase-based message formulation [are] recurrent themes....Those who [support] word-based strategies [stress] the generative flexibility of this approach as compared with the phrase-based approach. Those who [support] phrase-based strategies [cite] improved communication rate and timing as compared with the word-based approach. AAC device designers have responded to this debate by developing a range of AAC products that utilize a variety of message management strategies....Unfortunately, the debate focuses on the "best" way to design AAC devices rather than on approaches that adjust message management [strategies] in response to specific concerns influencing those who rely on AAC as they participate in all avenues of life.

These arguments have changed. Fortunately, most high-tech AAC devices now support a variety of different message management strategies so that individuals who rely on AAC can choose the strategy they prefer for specific communication situations.

THE MESSAGES OF CONVERSATION

Most conversations have a rather predictable structure. Usually, people initiate a conversation with greetings followed by a segment of small talk. Some conversations then progress to an information-sharing segment, whereas others do not. The shared information can take a variety of forms, including stories (i.e., narratives), procedural descriptions, or content-specific conversations. Most conversations close with some wrap-up remarks and a final farewell. To provide the messages needed to support conversation, it is useful to select and organize messages with this conversational contour in mind.

Greetings

Greetings are essential to initiating social interactions. Greetings can be rather generic in that they do not usually convey specific information. Rather, they signal awareness of someone's presence, communicate the speaker's intention to be friendly or interactive, and often include a bid to start a conversation. Despite the apparent simplicity of greetings, however, AAC teams must have some awareness of the culture, social status, and ages of the individuals involved when selecting appropriate greetings. This awareness is generally communicated by the degree of formality used for the greeting. Usually, a younger person does not greet an older person or a person of higher status (e.g., an employer, a teacher) with an excessively informal or familiar message. However, at least in middle-class North American culture, it is permissible to use informal messages that may contain personal references (e.g., "Hey! Big guy!") or even mild profanity (e.g., "How ya doing, you old *&#?") with close friends or peers. Although specific greeting conventions may change from culture to culture, there is always a need for variety in this type of message. Thus, greeting messages should include a range of culturally sensitive message options so that individuals are able to signal their awareness of social conventions. In addition, the availability of a range of different messages discourages the overuse of the same greetings.

This week, pay attention to how you greet others. Notice that you use a variety of different greetings. Analyze the social rules that you use. Pay careful attention to those around you, and note the age, familiarity, and gender of individuals who say things such as "Well, hello, dear!" "Hi there!" "Goodness gracious, it's been a long time!" "Good morning!" and "What's up?"

Small Talk

Small talk is a type of conversational exchange used for initiating and maintaining conversational interactions. Small-talk scripts provide for the incremental sequence of social engagement and disengagement messages that seem necessary when people attempt to interact in a social setting. Some conversations, such as those that occur at cocktail parties or large social gatherings, may never progress past the small-talk stage. Often, however, small talk is used as a transition between the greeting and the information-sharing stage, especially when the communication partners do not know each other well or do not possess much shared information.

Adults who rely on AAC frequently report that social situations are very difficult for them. The following are remarks we have collected through the years:

"Dinner parties with my spouse kill me. Eating, talking, smiling, and small talk— it is too much to handle."

"My fiancée told me that she wouldn't go to a party with me again until I learned something about small talk!"

"I didn't get serious about learning small talk until I was 45 years old. I thought it was a total waste of time. Why should I work so hard to say nothing of content? But I was wrong."

One type of small talk in particular can be quite effective for AAC use. Called *generic small talk,* it is small talk that people can use with a variety of different conversational partners because it does not refer to specific shared information. Table 2.1 contains some examples of generic and specific small talk.

In an effort to determine the relative frequency and types of generic small talk used by speakers of various ages without disabilities, several groups of researchers at the University of Nebraska–Lincoln recorded everyday conversations using portable, voice-activated voice recorders. Nearly half of the utterances of preschool children (3 to 5 years of age) in both home and school settings were classified as generic small talk. For young adults (20 to 30 years of age), 39% of all utterances were generic small talk (Ball, Marvin, Beukelman, Lasker, & Rupp, 1997; King, Spoeneman, Stuart, & Beukelman, 1995; Lasker, Ball, Bringewatt, Stuart, & Marvin, 1996). Older men and women used somewhat less small talk than the young adults; 31% of the utterances of 65- to 74-year-olds and 26% of the utterances of 75- to 85-year-olds were small talk. These results confirm the extensive role of small talk in everyday communicative interactions for individuals across the age range. To interact in integrated social contexts, access to small talk and the ability to use it are essential.

The messages used during small talk vary somewhat across the age span. Those who rely on AAC should have opportunities to select the messages that they prefer from detailed resource lists and other sources. Detailed information about small-talk use patterns is now available on the Barkley AAC Center's web site.

Narration: Storytelling and Public Speaking

For adults, storytelling is a common communication form. Older adults in particular use stories to entertain, teach, and establish social closeness with their peers. Storytelling remains an important communication form even for adults who are unable to speak. Storytelling is particularly important as older adults begin to focus more and more of their social time on acquaintances and friends rather than on families. As these individuals lose their spouses and move to retirement or care facilities, the need to socially connect with individuals their own age becomes important, and storytelling provides a vehicle for this.

In his book *Tell Me a Story: A New Look at Real and Artificial Memory,* Schank (1990) discussed story formulation, refinement, and storage in detail. He pointed out that we use stories from a variety of sources. *First-person stories* are those that have occurred to the speaker personally. *Second-person stories* are those that a speaker has learned from others through listening or reading. It is permissible to tell a second-person story as long as we give credit to the source. *Official stories* are those that are used to teach a lesson or explain a phenomenon and are frequently used by families, schools,

Table 2.1.   Examples of generic and specific small talk

Generic	Specific
How is your family?	How is your wife?
What's happening?	What are you doing?
Isn't that beautiful!	That is a beautiful flower!
Good story!	Good story about your vacation!
She is great.	She is a great teacher.

and religious groups. Finally, *fantasy stories* are those that are made up. Marvin and colleagues studied the communication patterns of typically developing preschool children and found that, on average, 9% of what they talked about at home and 11% of their conversations at school involved some type of fantasy (Marvin, Beukelman, & Bilyeu, 1994).

As the memory capacity of electronic AAC devices has increased and the intelligibility of speech synthesis has improved, storytelling with AAC systems has become much more practical. Many people who rely on AAC formulate and enter their own stories into AAC technology. For others, AAC facilitators play an important role in storytelling by assisting people who rely on AAC to capture stories for this type of communication. First, the facilitator must understand the story that the individual wishes to include in the AAC system. Understanding the story is critical because storytelling must be individualized to reflect personal experiences (e.g., through first-person stories), interests (e.g., through second-person stories), and affiliations (e.g., through official stories). Next, the facilitator can help to program the AAC device by dividing the story into segments (usually of sentence length) that the individual who uses AAC can release sequentially with synthetic speech to tell the story a sentence or two at a time. Finally, opportunities to practice telling the story should be provided. As the number of stories included in an AAC system increases, AAC facilitators also need to assist by indexing them according to the main topics, key participants, or major life events they represent so that stories can be retrieved efficiently. Of course, facilitators can also use nonelectronic AAC strategies to store and retrieve stories. For example, a man with aphasia due to stroke used to tell the story of how he got his unusual name, Roderick, by guiding his communication partner through his communication book one segment at a time, indicating the line of the story that the partner should read aloud (see Chapter 4 for a discussion of communication books). Other individuals may tell stories using line-drawing symbols arranged in sequential order with the written story underneath each symbol.

Many people use AAC technology to support their public speaking activities. Excellent examples that are available on the AAC-RERC (Rehabilitation Engineering Research Center on Communication Enhancement) web site include Michael Williams's talk about his AAC journey, *How Far We've Come, How Far We've Got to Go: Tales from the Trenches*; Colin Portnuff's presentation to a group of engineers and researchers, *AAC: A User's Perspective*; and Beth Anne Luciani's discussion of college life, *AAC and College Life: Just Do It!*

Procedural Descriptions

Procedural descriptions provide detailed information about processes or procedures. Usually, they 1) are rich in detail, 2) contain information that must be related sequentially, and 3) require communication that is both timely and efficient. Examples include giving someone directions to drive to your house for the first time or telling someone your recipe for a favorite cake. In addition to the kinds of procedures that most speakers may need to describe, many individuals with disabilities need to instruct family members and attendants about the procedures required for personal care and other specific needs. Typically, these descriptions are unique to the individual. Such descriptions are particularly important for people with complex medical or care needs because they need to instruct medical and care staff how they prefer to be treated or cared for. Collier and Self (2010) provide excellent information about barriers and accommodations related to communication effectiveness between those who rely on AAC and their personal assistants. It is important to remember that the communication needs of these individuals go beyond specific medical or care-based procedural communication. They must also maintain social relationships and share information with these caregivers.

Content-Specific Conversations

Content-specific conversations contain informational give and take. Typically, these conversations are not scripted, and the vocabulary in them varies widely depending on many different factors, including the communication partners themselves, the topic, the context, and so forth. To participate successfully in such conversations, individuals usually need to be able to formulate unique and novel messages. Most individuals do so by constructing messages on a letter-by-letter or word-by-word basis. However, vocabulary and message sets have been developed to support communication related to specific content. For example, Bryen (2008) provides vocabulary to support socially valued roles (see the Temple University Institute on Disabilities AAC Vocabulary web site). Balandin and Iacono (1999) documented break-time conversations in the workplace.

Wrap-Up Remarks and Farewell Statements

Most communicators use wrap-up remarks to signal their desire or intent to end an interaction. Then they terminate conversations with farewell statements. Phrases such as "Nice to talk with you," "We need to talk again some time," "I have to go now," "I have work to do," "The kids need me," and "The phone is ringing" are typical wrap-up remarks in conversations. Phrases such as "See ya," "Good-bye," "So long," and "See you later" are typically used as farewell statements, at least in North America.

The Barkley AAC Center's web site contains extensive information about wrap-up remarks and farewell statements used by people of different ages.

VOCABULARY NEEDS FOR DIFFERENT COMMUNICATION MODES AND CONTEXTS

The words with which people communicate are greatly influenced by different communication contexts and modalities. For example, individuals speak more colloquially and casually when conversing with friends than when presenting a formal report to a class, business meeting, or professional group. When adults speak to young children, they use different words and grammatical structures than when they speak to other adults. Furthermore, written communication is different from spoken communication. Conversational conventions utilized in social media vary considerably from those in face-to-face or traditional written communication. Abbreviations and codes are commonly used. Also, message length is reduced, especially while texting. It is important for the AAC team to have a general knowledge of these different vocabulary-use patterns when selecting vocabulary items for AAC systems.

Spoken and Written Communication

Although speaking and writing may seem to be different but equivalent ways of communicating, there are inherent differences between these two modes of communication that may not be immediately apparent (Barritt & Kroll, 1978). In general, spoken communication involves the use of more personal references and more first- and second-person pronouns (e.g., *I, we, you*) than written communication does. Less lexical (i.e., vocabulary) diversity is present in speech than in writing because speakers tend to repeat words more often. Speech also tends to contain shorter thought units, more monosyllabic and familiar words, and more subordinate ideas than writing.

In a study that compared spoken and written language in the classroom, McGinnis (1991) collected 1,000-word spoken and written samples from 34 third-grade students in a general education setting. She found that the students' written vocabulary was considerably more diverse than their spoken vocabulary. For example, the type-to-token ratio (TTR; the number of different words divided by the total number of words in a sample) was lower for spoken (TTR = 0.30) than for written language samples (TTR = 0.46). This result indicates that the children repeated more spoken words than written words because fewer spoken words represented a greater proportion of the total spoken language sample than a similar sample of written words did.

School Talk and Home Talk

Vocabulary use also varies for spoken communication depending on the communication context. For example, "school talk" can be quite different from "home talk." Children do not use language in school for the same purposes, such as to meet immediate needs and achieve social closeness with familiar partners, as they do at home. Instead, children talk primarily with relatively unfamiliar adults in school in order to build a theory of reality, share their understanding of actions and situations, and acquire knowledge (Westby, 1985). In doing so, they must "shift away from the expectation of shared assumptions (implicit meaning) to interpreting overtly lexicalized intentions (explicit meaning)" (p. 187).

Few investigations have documented in detail the vocabulary-use patterns of children or adults at home and in school. One exception is the work of Marvin and colleagues (1994), who recorded the vocabulary spoken by five typically developing preschool-age children at home and in school. Approximately one third of the words produced by these children were spoken only at school, one third were spoken only at home, and one third were spoken both at home and at school. Beukelman, Jones, and Rowan (1989) reported that 100 words accounted for 60% of those produced at school by six typically developing children (3–4 years of age) when 3,000-word samples from each child were analyzed. In addition, in a related study, Fried-Oken and More (1992) reported a vocabulary core list for preschoolers based on development and environmental language sources.

Differences across specific school environments might also be expected to have dramatic effects on the words that children use in classrooms. The content of elementary and secondary school curricula in various subject areas requires students to have access to vocabulary items that may change daily or weekly. For example, as the topics in a student's science unit shift from plants to planets to prehistoric animals to rocks, the extent to which the student can communicate successfully in the classroom will depend largely on the availability of appropriate vocabulary. The vocabulary set designed to support a student's conversational interactions, which are relatively stable and predictable, is unlikely to be useful in meeting frequently changing curricular communication needs. (For a more complete discussion of communication patterns in school settings, see Chapter 13.)

Age Variables

Research reports suggest that age, gender, and cultural (e.g., ethnic) differences may affect the topics and vocabulary words that an individual uses during interactions. For example, researchers have investigated the communication patterns of older adults from at least two different perspectives. One perspective has been to study and document the language differences between older adults and younger people in order to describe the language impairments that people experience as they grow older. Studies from this perspective have suggested that people produce fewer proper nouns, more general nouns, and more ambiguous references as they age. In addition, the lexical variety of their nominal and syntactic structures decreases (Kemper, 1988; Kynette & Kemper, 1986; Ulatowska, Cannito, Hayashi, & Fleming, 1985). Goodglass (1980) reported that the size of individuals' active expressive vocabularies decreases quite markedly during their 70s.

A second perspective has been to view aging in terms of a model of human cognitive development, in which the performance of older adults is seen as a legitimate, adaptive stage of development (Mergler & Goldstein, 1983). Viewed from this perspective, older adults appear to tailor their communicative interactions to the unique task of "telling," that is, information sharing. In their role as "tellers," older adults relate to the past as a resource for assigning meaning to the present (Boden & Bielby, 1983). For example, Stuart, Vanderhoof, and Beukelman (1993) examined the topical references that women ranging in age from 63 to 79 years made during conversational exchanges. The younger women made more present-oriented comments and referred much more frequently to topics related to family life than the older women did. In contrast, the older women referred to their social networks outside the family much more often than their younger counterparts did.

Balandin and Iacono (1998a, 1998b) studied vocabulary use by adults during meal-break conversations in an employment setting in Australia. Tonsing and Alant (2004) documented the topics of social conversation in the workplace in South Africa. These authors reported a relatively high degree of overlap among these studies.

Gender Variables

A number of researchers have written about the influence of gender on language and word use. For example, men and women appear to use parts of speech differently. Men use fewer pronouns and more adjectives, unusual adverbs, and prepositions than women do. Women use more auxiliary words and negations than men do (Gleser, Gottschalk, & John, 1959; Poole, 1979). Men also appear to speak about different topics than women. Gleser and colleagues (1959) found that women refer to motivations, feelings, emotions, and themselves more often than men do. Men tend to refer to time, space, quantity, and destructive actions more often than women do.

Stuart (1991, pp. 43–44) summarized the work of a number of different researchers who examined the differences between "male talk" and "female talk" as follows:

> The studies were conducted in a Spanish village; in a traditional working-class family in England; among !Kung bushmen in Africa; during sidewalk conversations in New York City; Columbus, Ohio; and London; among women working in a telephone company in Somerville, Massachusetts; between blue-collar couples in New York; and among participants in the draft resistance movement in the United States. The results were impressively similar and can be reported collectively. Female topics were found to be people (themselves, other women, men), personal lives/interpersonal matters (age, lifestyles, life's troubles), household needs, books, food, clothes, and decorations. Male topics were found to be work (land, crops, weather, animals, prices, business, money, wages, machinery, and carpentry), legal matters, taxes, army experience, and sports or amusements (baseball, motorcycles, sailing, hunting, mountain climbing, and cockfighting).

Information about the vocabulary-use patterns of those of different genders and ages who rely on AAC is still very limited. Until such information is available, AAC specialists must be sensitive to how these factors and others (e.g., cultural differences) may affect the vocabulary selection process. Peer informants are perhaps the best source of knowledge about an individual's specific vocabulary needs, and AAC teams should use their insights as a resource to select appropriate vocabulary.

The summary list provided on the Barkley AAC Center's web site provides excellent resource material from which personalized vocabulary lists can be developed.

VOCABULARY NEEDS OF PEOPLE WITH DIFFERENT COMMUNICATION CAPABILITIES

The overall communication capability of individuals who use an AAC system is another important factor that AAC teams should consider as they select vocabulary. This section discusses three types of individuals: 1) those who are preliterate, such as young children who have not yet learned to write and read; 2) those who are nonliterate, such as individuals who are not able to learn to read or write and people who have lost these abilities because of their impairments; and 3) those who are literate.

"They [people who use AAC] are unable to create spontaneously their own lexicon and must operate with a vocabulary selected by someone else or preselected, not spontaneously chosen by themselves" (Carlson, 1981, p. 140).

Vocabulary Selection for Preliterate Individuals

Individuals who are preliterate have not yet developed reading and writing skills. These individuals are often young children, but they may also be older individuals or even adults who never received the instruction needed to become literate. Thus, their AAC systems use one or more of the symbol or code sets discussed in Chapter 3 to represent vocabulary items. Generally, the vocabulary requirements of preliterate individuals can be divided into two categories: vocabulary that is needed to communicate essential messages and vocabulary that is needed to develop language skills.

Coverage Vocabulary

Vanderheiden and Kelso (1987) referred to vocabulary that is needed to communicate essential messages as coverage vocabulary because it contains messages that are necessary to cover an individual's basic communication needs. Because preliterate individuals are unable to spell out messages on a letter-by-letter basis, AAC teams must take care to include as many coverage vocabulary items as these individuals will require, regardless of how frequently they will use the messages. For example, a person may use a message such as I AM HAVING TROUBLE BREATHING very rarely, but if this could be even an occasional occurrence, the message should be included in the coverage vocabulary.

Coverage vocabulary is highly dependent on the communication needs of an individual. As noted previously, these needs are likely to change depending on the individual's age and the communicative context. For example, the coverage vocabulary needed at a birthday party would be very different from that required during a physical therapy session. Coverage vocabularies for preliterate individuals are selected through careful analyses of their environmental and communication needs. (The details of these processes are discussed later in this chapter.)

Coverage vocabularies for preliterate individuals are commonly organized by context (environment or activity) so that the words are available when needed. Thus, AAC teams may design separate communication activity displays to contain the vocabulary items that an individual needs while eating, dressing, bathing, playing a specific game, participating in specific school activities, and so forth. Team members or facilitators may situate these activity boards strategically in the environment in which a particular activity takes place, such as in the kitchen, bathroom, or specific classroom area, so that they are available when needed. At other times, the individual may store activity displays in a carrying case or notebook so that the appropriate board is available for a specific communication context. (Additional activity board strategies are discussed in detail in Chapters 8, 10, and 11.) Two excellent resources of coverage vocabulary are the AAC boards available on CD-ROM for adults with acquired medical conditions (Beukelman, Garrett, & Yorkston, 2007) and for those with acute medical needs (Hurtig & Downey, 2009). Alternatively, the AAC team may program vocabulary items into an electronic speech-generating device, using "themes" or "levels" that are contextually relevant to the individual.

Developmental Vocabulary

The vocabulary set for an AAC system may also include words that the individual does not yet know and that are selected not so much for functional purposes but to encourage language and vocabulary growth. At least some developmental vocabulary words should be provided to people across the age range because language growth is an ongoing process (Romski & Sevcik, 1996). For example, if a preliterate child is about to experience something for the first time, such as a circus, then the child's AAC team may include vocabulary items associated with the new context on the communication display even though the child has never used them before. During the circus, the child's parent or friend may point to various vocabulary items on the display that are associated with the circus events, such as CLOWN, LION, FUNNY, and SCARY. This gives the child opportunities to develop language and learn new vocabulary items through exposure, just as children who speak learn new words by hearing people say them over and over again.

For beginning communicators of any age, developmental vocabulary items should include words or messages that encourage them to use various language structures and combinations. For example, beginning communicators should have access to words such as MORE to indicate continuation, NO to indicate negation, and THERE to indicate location. AAC teams might include a variety of nouns, verbs, and adjectives to support the individual's use of word combinations (e.g., MORE CAR, NO EAT). As the person's language abilities expand, team members should select vocabulary to encourage the use of combinations of two, three, and four words or more. Lahey and Bloom (1977) suggested that developmental vocabulary should include words from at least the following semantic categories:

- Substantive words (i.e., people, places, things)
- Relational words (e.g., *big, little*)
- Generic verbs (e.g., *give, get, make*)
- Specific verbs (e.g., *eat, drink, sleep*)
- Emotional state words (e.g., *happy, scared*)
- Affirmation/negation words (e.g., *yes, no, not*)
- Recurrence/discontinuation words (e.g., *more, all gone*)
- Proper names for people first and personal pronouns later; initially, proper names can be used instead of pronouns for possessives (e.g., *Mike car* instead of *his car*) as well as object–agent relations (e.g., *Pat want* instead of *I want*)
- Single adjectives first (e.g., *hot, dirty*) and their polar opposites later (e.g., *cold, clean*); initially, *not* can be used with an adjective to indicate a polar opposite (e.g., *not + hot = cold*)
- Relevant colors
- Relevant prepositions

In one study, Banajee, Dicarlo, and Stricklin (2003) investigated the core vocabulary of 50 toddlers in preschool settings. They reported that all 50 children used nine common words (*I, no, yes/yeah, want, it, that, my, you, more*). Other commonly used words included *mine, the, is, on, in, here, out, off, a, go, who, some, help*, and *all done/finished*. These words represented different pragmatic functions such as requesting, affirming, and negating. No nouns were included in the list. Rescorla, Alley, and Christine (2001) studied the frequency of word use in the lexicons of toddlers. These authors provided extensive information about frequency of word use in the appendix of their article.

Vocabulary Selection for Nonliterate Individuals

Nonliterate individuals are unable to spell well enough to formulate their messages on a letter-by-letter basis and are not expected to develop or regain these spontaneous spelling skills. Most of these individuals are also unable to read, except perhaps for functional sight words that they have memorized. The vocabulary selection process for nonliterate individuals primarily aims to meet their daily, ongoing communication needs in a variety of environments. Nevertheless, the messages selected for these individuals may differ in a number of ways from those selected for preliterate individuals.

First, messages selected for nonliterate individuals are nearly always chosen from a functional rather than a developmental perspective. Single words or, more often, whole messages are selected to meet individual communication needs. These messages are represented by one or more types of symbols, as discussed in Chapter 3. Second, it is very important that the coverage vocabulary selected for nonliterate individuals be age and gender appropriate. Many of these individuals, especially those with intellectual or developmental disabilities, may be adolescents or adults; special care must be taken not to select words and messages for them that are appropriate only for infants or young children. For example, a symbol of a happy face may be used for a young child to represent HAPPY, whereas for an adolescent this same symbol might be translated to mean AWESOME. Even better, a thumbs-up symbol might be used to represent AWESOME or WAY TO GO on an adolescent's display.

It is also appropriate to include at least some developmental vocabulary in the AAC systems of nonliterate individuals. For example, new messages should be added whenever new environments or participation opportunities are encountered in the individual's life. However, the goal is to expand the number of words and concepts about which the individual can communicate rather than to increase the individual's use of complex syntactic forms. Again, efficient, functional communication in a variety of age-appropriate contexts is of paramount importance for these individuals.

Vocabulary Selection for Literate Individuals

Individuals who are able to read and spell have access to a greater variety of message preparation options. Literate individuals are able to formulate messages on a letter-by-letter and word-by-word basis and to retrieve complete messages, with appropriate AAC equipment, once they have been stored. Depending on the communication needs of an individual, AAC teams may prepare three different types of messages for quick retrieval: those related to timing enhancement, those related to message acceleration, and those related to fatigue reduction.

Timing Enhancement

Some messages require careful timing in order to be appropriate. Although a literate person may have the ability to spell time-sensitive messages, their meanings may be ineffective if the messages are not communicated quickly. For example, if the message PLEASE PICK UP MY FEET BEFORE YOU ROLL MY WHEELCHAIR FORWARD is not delivered in a timely manner, it loses its relevance when the wheelchair is moved while the person is formulating the message. Thus, messages that have important timing requirements are usually stored and retrieved in their entirety. Additional examples of such messages include WAIT JUST A MINUTE, I'M NOT FINISHED YET; BEFORE YOU GO, WOULD YOU HELP ME WITH THIS?; WHEN WILL WE MEET AGAIN?; DON'T LEAVE YET; MY IV IS LEAKING; and THAT REALLY HURTS, PLEASE STOP. Those who rely on AAC and their facilitators are the best sources for identifying unique messages related to timing enhancement.

Message Acceleration

In addition to timing enhancement, AAC teams often select vocabulary items to accelerate overall communication rate. Vanderheiden and Kelso (1987) introduced the term *acceleration vocabulary* to refer to words or messages that occur so frequently and are so lengthy that the use of an encoding strategy to retrieve them results in substantial keystroke savings (see Chapter 3 for a more complete discussion of message encoding and communication rate enhancement). Thus, the AAC team chooses words or messages for an acceleration vocabulary set not to allow an individual to communicate particular ideas but rather to speed up the rate at which the individual can communicate them.

Fatigue Reduction

The third type of vocabulary set that AAC teams typically select for people who are literate is one that will result in reduced fatigue. In many cases, words and phrases that compose the acceleration vocabulary set are the same as those that are encoded to reduce fatigue. In certain situations, however, selecting vocabulary to reduce fatigue requires a slightly different approach than that used when selecting other kinds of vocabulary. For example, fatigue is a cumulative problem for some individuals. Early in the morning, they may be able to use their AAC systems with more physical efficiency than later in the day or the evening. In such cases, AAC teams should select fatigue reduction vocabulary items to cover these individuals' communication needs during the portion of the day when their fatigue levels are highest (e.g., the evening). In this way, they can avoid having to spell out words when they are tired. Analyses of communication patterns during periods of high fatigue can guide the selection of words and messages that will be most helpful to reduce fatigue.

Social Media

During the past few years, the availability of social media, such as e-mail, texting, tweeting, and social network sites such as Facebook, Google+, and MySpace, has changed the communication options throughout the world. Some of those who rely on AAC have already gained access to social media. With the increasing use of mobile technology to support communication, undoubtedly social media options will increase considerably for those who rely on AAC during the next few years. The communication conventions used in social media differ considerably from face-to-face communication with extensive use of abbreviations and codes, grammatically incomplete messages, and limited punctuation to reduce the number of keystrokes required on the small screens or keyboards commonly incorporated into mobile technology. For those who rely on AAC, the use of social media will "connect them to the world" but will also introduce new conventions for message formulation, storage, and retrieval.

The AAC-RERC white paper *Mobile Devices and Communication Apps* discusses the use of mobile technology to support communication.

VOCABULARY RESOURCES

Rarely does one individual have enough knowledge and experience to select all the vocabulary items needed in a specific environment. Rather, it is necessary to obtain this vocabulary information from a variety of sources. This section summarizes the sources that AAC teams commonly use during vocabulary selection and includes indications of the situations in which particular sources are most useful.

Core Vocabulary

Core vocabulary refers to words and messages that are commonly used by a variety of individuals and occur very frequently. Empirical research or intervention reports that assess vocabulary-use patterns of a number of individuals generally identify core vocabulary items. AAC teams have used three sources to identify core vocabularies for specific individuals: 1) word lists based on the vocabulary-use patterns of other individuals who successfully use AAC systems, 2) word lists based on the use patterns of the specific individual, and 3) word lists based on the performance of natural speakers or writers in similar contexts.

Vocabulary-Use Patterns of People Who Communicate Through Augmentative and Alternative Communication

Of particular interest in developing core vocabulary lists is the performance of individuals who are operationally and socially competent with their AAC systems. Researchers collected communication samples from such individuals over extended periods of time and analyzed their word-use patterns. The first of these studies involved the entire body of words produced on a letter-by-letter basis over 14 days by five young adults with disabilities who used Canon Communicators (Beukelman, Yorkston, Poblete, & Naranjo, 1984). For a composite list that consisted of all of the words produced by all five individuals, see Vocabulary Resources on the Barkley AAC Center's web site. Approximately 80% of the words communicated by the five individuals were represented by the 500 most frequently occurring words.

In subsequent research, Yorkston, Smith, and Beukelman (1990) compared the vocabulary lists produced by people who used AAC strategies during communicative interactions with six different composite word lists selected from published vocabulary sources. The 10 individuals all used spelling to express their messages. The results indicated that the individuals actually used between 27% and 60% of the words included in the various published lists.

A manual entitled *See What We Say: Situational Vocabulary for Adults Who Use Augmentative and Alternative Communication* (Collier, 2000) was developed with input from 15 adults who rely on AAC. The manual contains suggested vocabulary items for numerous situations including directing personal care; interviewing service providers; communicating about one's AAC system; communicating about seating, transportation, advocacy, banking, and finances; eating out; using the telephone; participating at a conference; expressing one's sexuality; and facing situations of death and bereavement.

Hanson and Sundheimer (2009) acknowledge that telephone interaction is a challenging form of communication for those who rely on AAC. In their project they studied the impact of a floorholder message—PLEASE WAIT, I'M USING A COMPUTER TO TALK—and a delay when people using AAC technology attempted to complete a successful phone call. Calls with and without delays and with and without the floorholder message were placed to randomly selected businesses. Seventy-six percent of the calls were classified as unsuccessful. The majority of the successful calls occurred when the floorholder message was present and there was no delay.

In his AAC-RERC webcast, *AAC: A User's Perspective*, Colin Portnuff shares some of his personal strategies for communicating on the phone and face to face.

Vocabulary-Use Patterns of a Specific Individual

Individualized word lists, which are word lists compiled from the past performance of the specific individual for whom an AAC system is being developed, are even more efficient vocabulary sources than composite lists (Yorkston et al., 1990). This is not unexpected, because it could be assumed that an individual's past performance would be the best predictor of his or her future performance. In the past, it was difficult to obtain and analyze communication samples from an individual in order to develop an individualized word list. More recently, performance measurement and analysis technology is included in many AAC devices to help monitor vocabulary-use patterns of an individual. Privacy issues related to such technology have been a concern, so the person who uses AAC technology needs to be involved in any decision to monitor performance in this way (Blackstone, Williams, & Joyce, 2002). See Chapter 3 for more information.

Vocabulary-Use Patterns of Typically Developing Speakers or Writers

A considerable number of studies have examined vocabulary-use patterns of typical speakers and writers. These composite lists provide a rich source of core vocabulary information and can be useful when developing vocabulary lists for specific individuals. As noted previously, Yorkston and colleagues indicated that vocabulary selection for individuals who rely on AAC is complex because a composite vocabulary list contains only a fraction of the words that will be needed. These authors summarized their views about the role of core vocabularies in AAC applications in the following statement:

> Our data…suggest that [standard word lists] are an excellent source of potential words to be included in an AAC application. The inclusion of standard word lists in the memory of an AAC device is a great time savings for augmented communicators and their facilitators. However, these standard lists must not be taught without careful consideration. Systematic strategies are required to eliminate unnecessary or "costly" words from the standard vocabulary lists as an AAC device is individualized for a given client. (1990, p. 223)

Fringe Vocabulary

Fringe vocabulary refers to vocabulary words and messages that are specific or unique to the individual. For example, these might include names of specific people, locations, and activities as well as preferred expressions. Such words serve to personalize the vocabulary included in an AAC system and to allow expression of ideas and messages that do not appear in core vocabulary lists. By their very nature, fringe vocabulary items for those who rely on AAC must be recommended by informants who know them or their communicative situations quite well. Individuals who rely on AAC themselves are the most important potential informants. Their ability to serve as informants about their own vocabulary and message needs depends on numerous factors including age, cognitive and language abilities, and the level of facilitator support provided.

One type of fringe vocabulary relates to special interests of people who rely on AAC. Through face-to-face interaction and electronic mail, they have increasing opportunities to develop and maintain their interests and to communicate with others about them. Interests—such as pets, art, gardening, sports, politics, religion, advocacy, music, technology, and investments—are associated with specialized vocabulary. To effectively support communication about these topics, specialized vocabulary must be available in one's AAC system. Luo, Higginbotham, and Lesher (2007) described their Webcrawler project, which included strategies to obtain topic-relevant vocabulary from the Internet to be utilized in AAC technology. Such vocabulary might relate to specific topics or current events.

Informants

When selecting fringe vocabulary items, one or two AAC team members, often professionals, can have a tendency to select items without consulting a sufficient number of informants. A study by Yorkston, Fried-Oken, and Beukelman (1988) indicated that only about half of the top 100 fringe vocabulary words selected by two types of informants for those who rely on AAC were the same. Thus, AAC teams should consult multiple informants to obtain the best possible list of fringe words. The most obvious informants are spouses, parents, siblings, teachers, and other caregivers. Informants such as employers, co-workers, peers, and friends often offer valuable vocabulary suggestions as well. Of course, whenever possible, those who rely on AAC should identify potential informants as well as suggest words and messages to be included or retained in the vocabulary.

Little research has examined the performance or role of informants in vocabulary selection. Morrow, Beukelman, Mirenda, and Yorkston (1993) studied three types of informants—parents, speech-language pathologists, and teachers—who often select vocabulary. Their results indicated that each of the informants contributed an important number of fringe words to the composite vocabularies for the child participants and that none of the informants could be eliminated from the vocabulary selection process. Specifically, for three of the six children involved in the study, their mothers contributed the most fringe words. For the other three children, their speech-language pathologists offered the most fringe words. Fringe words contributed by teachers, although fewer in number, were particularly crucial to classroom participation. Fallon, Light, and Paige (2001) developed and field-tested a vocabulary selection questionnaire. A copy of the questionnaire is included in the appendix of their article.

Vocabulary Selection Processes

Although very little research has been done regarding how to select fringe vocabularies, important suggestions to guide this process have been made. Musselwhite and St. Louis (1988) suggested that initial vocabulary items should be of high interest to the individual, have potential for frequent use, denote a range of semantic notions and pragmatic functions, reflect the "here and now" for ease of learning, have potential for later multiword use, and provide ease of production or interpretation. In addition to the questionnaire by Fallon, Light, and Paige (2001), several other processes have been widely used in the AAC field to facilitate achievement of these criteria, including environmental or ecological inventories and communication diaries and checklists.

Environmental or Ecological Inventories   In an effort to personalize vocabulary, several authors presented environmental or ecological inventory processes that AAC teams can use to document how the individual participates in and observes various activities (Carlson, 1981; Mirenda, 1985; Reichle, York, & Sigafoos, 1991). Carlson stated, "By discriminating between observation and participation events, it is possible to gain a better picture of the [individual's] actual experiences within the area rather than the [facilitator's] perception of the experience" (1981, p. 142). During an environmental inventory, the AAC team observes and documents the vocabulary words used by peers both with and without disabilities during frequently occurring activities. The team then reduces this pool of vocabulary items to a list of the most critical words that the individual who uses AAC can manage.

"Parental vocabulary diaries…are invaluable supplements to professional observations. I find it is not possible to rely on such diaries for information about pronunciation or grammar, but most parents have little trouble learning how to keep a list of words used by the child during the day" (Crystal, 1987, p. 41).

Communication Diaries and Checklists   Vocabulary diaries are records of the words or phrases needed in a variety of contexts. Usually, communication diaries are kept by informants who simply record the needed vocabulary on a blank piece of paper throughout the day. Carefully constructed vocabulary checklists such as the MacArthur-Bates Communicative Development Inventory: Words and Sentences (Fenson et al., 2007) can also be useful as a shortcut to vocabulary selection because they provide informants with ideas about potential vocabulary words from which to choose. Morrow and colleagues (1993) studied informants' reactions to the communication diary, environmental inventory (after Carlson, 1981), and vocabulary checklist processes (Bristow & Fristoe, 1984). Parents, teachers, and speech-language pathologists all rated the communication diary and environmental inventory methods as being moderately easy to use and rated the vocabulary checklist as slightly more satisfactory.

Language Models in Augmentative and Alternative Communication Technology

AAC technology increasingly contains message content preprogrammed by the manufacturer. Differing language models have been developed based on the age and language ability of the people who are expected to use the device. Typically, these content systems contain a range of different vocabulary and messages that are beyond the scope of this chapter to review in detail.

VOCABULARY MAINTENANCE

Various aspects of the initial vocabulary selection process are discussed in this chapter. Vocabulary selection also involves the ongoing process of vocabulary maintenance. Individuals employ some words and phrases so commonly that it is easy for them and their AAC facilitators to decide to retain these words and phrases in the system. Other words and phrases may be used less frequently, either because they were poorly chosen in the first place or because they have outlived their usefulness. The latter applies particularly to vocabulary items that AAC teams selected for specific contexts, such as a particular unit of study in the classroom, or for special events, such as Thanksgiving or other holidays. Items for use in special contexts should be eliminated from the available lexicon once they are not needed, to make space for other, more important words and to reduce the cognitive load for the individuals, who must scan many items prior to selection.

QUESTIONS

2.1.   What is the central goal of AAC intervention?

2.2.   People who rely on AAC manage their message preparation in several different ways. How does word-by-word message preparation differ from letter-by-letter spelling?

2.3. What percentage of people who rely on AAC experience crime or abuse during their lives?

2.4. How can AAC systems be designed to deal with crime and abuse at the moment and later during legal and counseling activities?

2.5. How do the greeting, small-talk, information-sharing, and wrap-up stages in a conversation differ from each other?

2.6. How does AAC vocabulary and message selection differ for preliterate, literate, and nonliterate individuals who rely on AAC?

2.7. What are the differences between core vocabulary and fringe vocabulary in an AAC system?

2.8. Why would a person who can formulate messages through letter-by-letter spelling choose to store and retrieve whole messages with his or her AAC device?

2.9. What is the role of an informant in the message selection process for an individual who relies on AAC?

CHAPTER 3

Symbols and Rate Enhancement

> As I sit here at my breakfast table, my morning newspaper has printing on it; it has a graph telling me how the national budget will be spent, a map trying to tell me something about the weather; a table of baseball statistics, an engineering drawing with which I can build a garden chair, photographs of distant places and people, a caricature expressing what the editor thinks of a political figure....On the wall in front of me hangs...a calendar [and above it] is a clock. All this and more, and I haven't even turned on the TV or the computer. (Ittelson, 1996, p. 171)

Ittelson's account of the variety of visual media he viewed during breakfast reminds us that we are surrounded by symbols throughout the day. Some symbols represent concepts such as time (e.g., a calendar or a clock), others represent ideas (e.g., a graph or a caricature), and still others represent objects, actions, emotions, directives, and so forth. In many (but not all) cases, symbols are used to convey messages from one person to another. Indeed, without symbols, we would not be able to communicate in writing or send nonverbal messages conveying empathy, warmth, and approval. There would be no golden arches! No mouse ears! No labels, no warning signs, no newspapers, and no textbooks! Without the ability to send messages via gestures, body language, written words, and other symbols, communication as we now know it would be a vastly different—and much less rich—experience.

"Nothing so distinguishes humans from other species as the creative and flexible use of symbols" (DeLoache, Pierroutsakos, & Troseth, 1997, p. 38).

Much of the power of augmentative and alternative communication (AAC) lies in the vast array of symbols and signals, other than those used in speech, that people can employ to send messages. Especially for individuals who cannot read or write, the ability to represent messages and concepts in alternative ways is central to communication. Acknowledgment of the importance of symbols has prompted much of the research and clinical effort devoted to studying and developing comprehensive symbol systems that are easy to use and learn. In this chapter, we review many of the most commonly used types of symbols and discuss their usefulness for various individuals.

OVERVIEW OF SYMBOLS

A number of definitions and taxonomies have been used to describe symbols and their various forms (see Fuller, Lloyd, & Schlosser, 1992). Basically, a *symbol* is "something that stands for or represents something else" (Vanderheiden & Yoder, 1986, p. 15). This "something else" is termed its *referent*. Symbols can be described in terms of many characteristics, including realism, iconicity, ambiguity, complexity, figure–ground differential, perceptual distinctness, acceptability, efficiency, color, and size (see Fuller, Lloyd, & Stratton, 1997; Schlosser, 2003e; Schlosser & Sigafoos, 2002; Wilkinson & Jagaroo, 2004). Of these, iconicity has received the most attention from both AAC researchers and clinicians. The term *iconicity* refers to "any association that an individual forms between a symbol and its referent" (Schlosser, 2003e, p. 350). At one end of the iconicity continuum are *transparent* symbols, in which "the shape, motion, or function of the referent is depicted to such an extent that meaning of the symbol can be readily guessed in the absence of the referent" (Fuller & Lloyd, 1991, p. 217). At the other end are *opaque* symbols, "in which no [symbol–referent] relationship is perceived even when the meaning of the symbol is known" (Fuller & Lloyd, 1991, p. 217). For example, a color photograph of a shoe is transparent, whereas the written word *shoe* is opaque. Between the two extremes are *translucent* symbols, "in which the meaning of the referent may or may not be obvious but a relationship can be perceived between the symbol and the referent once the meaning is provided" (Fuller & Lloyd, 1991, p. 217). For example, one gesture commonly used in North America for "Stop!" involves moving a flat hand or finger quickly across the throat, often accompanied by a distressed facial expression. One needs to understand that this gesture of "cutting one's throat" refers to the Hollywood film-industry expression *Cut!* (which also means "Stop!"). Translucent symbols are often defined by numerical ratings of the amount of relationship to a referent perceived to be present in the symbol (Lloyd & Blischak, 1992).

Symbols can be divided into those that are *aided*, which require some type of external assistance such as a device for production, and those that are *unaided*, which require no external device for production (Lloyd & Fuller, 1986). Aided symbols include real objects and black-and-white line drawings, and unaided symbols include facial expressions, manual signs, and natural speech and vocalizations. In addition, some symbol sets incorporate the use of both aided and unaided elements; we refer to these as *combined symbol sets* (e.g., the Makaton Vocabulary; Grove & Walker, 1990).

THE DEVELOPMENT OF SYMBOL UNDERSTANDING

The meaning of any given symbol is mediated by various factors that are intrinsic to the viewer, including his or her motivation, neurological status, developmental age, sensory abilities, cognitive skills, communication/language abilities, and world experience (Mineo Mollica, 2003). For example, iconicity and symbol learning appear to be, to a large extent, "culture-bound, time-bound, and, in general, experience-bound" (Brown, 1977, p. 29). Thus, Dunham (1989) found that adults with intellectual disabilities differed in their ability to guess the meanings of manual signs that adults without disabilities deemed quite "guessable." The different cultural and experiential backgrounds of these two groups are among the factors likely to have influenced the results. In addition, the longitudinal work of Romski and Sevcik (1996, 2005) suggests that spoken language comprehension plays a critical role in the symbol learning process. In their work with youth with severe cognitive disabilities, these researchers found that those who understood the meanings of specific referents learned to recognize the referents' abstract symbols more readily than individuals without such comprehension skills did.

"In the past, it was believed that iconicity would assist early symbol learners and that different processes underlay learning of iconic symbols compared to arbitrary symbols, but this does not seem to be the case. Iconicity in communication symbols does not appear to provide an advantage for very young children, who map the meaning of a range of arbitrary and iconic symbols onto referents" (Stephenson, 2009a, p. 196).

Developmental age is another factor that influences symbol understanding, at least with regard to graphic (i.e., pictorial) symbols. Namy and colleagues (Namy, 2001; Namy, Campbell, & Tomasello, 2004) examined the symbolic development of young, typically developing children and found that the degree of iconicity does not facilitate meaning in 18-month-olds but does in 26-month-olds. This finding is congruent with the findings of other studies of children without disabilities indicating that the development of "pictorial competence"—the ability to perceive, interpret, understand, and use pictures communicatively—develops gradually over the first few years of life (DeLoache, Pierroutsakos, & Uttal, 2003, p. 114). Until the end of their second year, typically developing children respond to pictures as they would objects, by trying to grasp them (i.e., they perceive pictures to be the same as their referents; DeLoache, Pierroutsakos, & Troseth, 1997; Rochat & Callaghan, 2005). It is not until around age 3 that children begin to understand that 1) pictures are two-dimensional objects in their own right (i.e., "dual representation"); 2) pictures can stand for objects or concepts (i.e., they are symbols); and 3) referents can be depicted symbolically in multiple ways (e.g., a color photograph, a black-and-white line drawing). The ability to comprehend and use a variety of symbol types continues to develop until, at around age 5, children are able to consider attributes of the symbol producer as well—for example, they are able to match crudely drawn and sophisticated symbols with pictures of children and adults, respectively (Rochat & Callaghan, 2005).

"One can never assume that young children will detect a given symbol-referent relation, no matter how transparent that relation seems to adults or older children" (DeLoache, Miller, & Rosengren, 1997, p. 312).

Not surprisingly, pictorial competence does not emerge uniformly for all symbols and referents, even after age 3. Some linguistic concepts are more readily symbolized than others; for example, Visser, Alant, and Harty (2008) found that approximately one quarter of typically developing 4-year-olds struggled to recognize line-drawing symbols for the emotions *sad, angry,* and *scared/afraid,* but had little difficulty with *happy.* In general, nouns (e.g., people, objects, and places) are relatively easy to represent compared with verbs (e.g., *come, go, want*), descriptors (e.g., *big, more, all gone*) and *wh-* questions (e.g., *who, what;* Bloomberg, Karlan, & Lloyd, 1990; Lund, Millar, Herman, Hinds, & Light, 1998; Mizuko, 1987; Worah, 2008).

In this regard, Light and colleagues asked typically developing children (4–7 years old) to draw pictures (i.e., symbols) of abstract language concepts such as *all gone* and *who* (Lund et al., 1998; Light, Worah, et al., 2008). They found the children's drawings to be very different from those depicted in commercially available AAC symbol sets. For example, the children's drawings often included familiar people and embedded concepts within the contexts in which they occurred, rather than depicting them generically. Thus, their drawings for the word *who* typically included a small person standing with a larger person, with a third person depicted some distance away. When asked to explain their drawings, the children said that they were the small person, standing with their parent (the large person), asking, "Who's that?" when viewing someone they didn't know. This contrasts dramatically with the symbol for *who* that is featured in some AAC symbol sets, which consists of an outline of a person's head with a question mark in the middle. In a subsequent study, Worah (2008) used the children's drawings from Lund et al. (1998) and from Light, Worah, et al. (2008) to design a set of Developmentally Appropriate Symbols (DAS) for concepts that included *all gone, big, come, eat, more, open, up, want, what,* and *who* (see Figure 3.1 for examples). She found that typically developing 2- to 3-year-olds who received training in the DAS significantly outperformed children who were trained with Picture Communication Symbols (PCS; Mayer-Johnson LLC, 1981–2011). She concluded that initial symbol learning can be enhanced by representing early emerging concepts "that are congruent to children's conceptualizations and [that are] developed considering issues that are important to children's understanding" (p. 47).

To summarize, it appears that, although iconicity does affect symbol learning, "so does general experience with pictures, comprehension of the names of the referents in the pictures, [and] an understanding of the intent of the person using the symbol" (Stephenson, 2009a, p. 194). In addition, several researchers have suggested that the reinforcement value of a referent is also likely to affect its learnability (Schlosser & Sigafoos, 2002). Thus, a very abstract symbol representing a highly desired item such as a candy bar might be more readily learned than a highly guessable symbol for a less desired item such as water. Instructional factors such as the availability of voice output (Koul & Schlosser, 2004; Schlosser, Belfiore, Nigam, Blischak, & Hetzroni, 1995) and the teaching strategies used during instruction (Mineo Mollica, 2003; Stephenson, 2009a) are additional influences on both initial and generalized symbol learning. Finally, Worah (2008) noted that children's ability to identify and understand the meanings of symbols that depict abstract linguistic concepts (i.e., words other than nouns) can be affected by factors such as the following:

- *Concreteness.* Symbols that contain clearly depicted people and/or observable activities are more readily understood (Light, Worah, et al., 2008; Lund et al., 1998).
- *Familiarity.* Symbols that depict people, objects, and/or activities that children have often encountered or seen are more easily identified (Callaghan, 1999; Light, Worah, et al., 2008; Lund et al., 1998).
- *Context.* Symbols that depict familiar activities in context may reduce the learning demands (Drager, Light, Speltz, Fallon, & Jeffries, 2003; Light, Worah, et al., 2008; Lund et al., 1998).
- *Wholeness.* Symbols that depict complete people or objects rather than elements or body parts that are separated or disjoined are more readily identified (Light, Worah, et al., 2008; Lund et al., 1998).

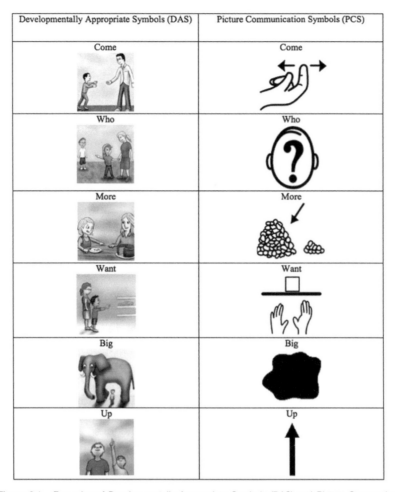

Figure 3.1. Examples of Developmentally Appropriate Symbols (DAS) and Picture Communication Symbols (PCS). (From Worah, S. [2008]. *The effects of redesigning the representations of early emerging concepts of identification and preference: A comparison of two approaches for representing vocabulary in augmentative and alternative communication [AAC] systems for young children* [Doctoral dissertation, Pennsylvania State University]. Retrieved from https://etda.libraries.psu.edu/paper/8622/. The Picture Communication Symbols ©1981–2012 by DynaVox Mayer-Johnson LLC. All Rights Reserved Worldwide. Used with permission.)

- *Color.* Symbols that use bright colors to highlight contrasts and details are more easily discriminated as well as more interesting to children (Light & Drager, 2002; Stephenson, 2007; Wilkinson, Carlin, & Jagaroo, 2006; Wilkinson & Jagaroo, 2004).
- *Focus.* Symbols that emphasize relevant characteristics via size and the position of characters or objects may be more easily recognized than those that use arrows or other markers to draw attention to relevant details (Blockberger & Sutton, 2003).

Many of these factors (e.g., concreteness, familiarity, context) can be addressed through the use of visual scene displays (VSDs) that use pictures to depict situations, places, or experiences. Clear images (digital pictures, color photographs, etc.) that are contextually rich and that depict people or objects in relation to one another, the natural environment, and the central action of a scene can be used to create personalized VSDs. When used in conjunction with a speech-generating device (SGD), language concepts are placed under "hot spots" on the picture that, when activated, speak the related message out loud. For example, Figure 3.2 depicts a photograph (originally

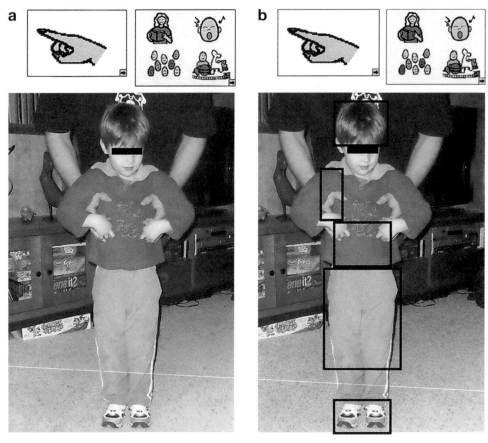

Figure 3.2. Example of a visual scene display for a "tickle" activity. The image is presented in color in the child's AAC system. a) The tickle display as the child views it; b) the tickle display with hot spots outlined that enable the child to choose where he wants to be tickled (the lines are invisible to the child). (From Drager, K., Light, J., & Finke, E. [2009]. Using AAC technologies to build social interaction in young children with autism spectrum disorders. In P. Mirenda & T. Iacono [Eds.], *Autism spectrum disorders and AAC* [pp. 247–278]. Baltimore: Paul H. Brookes Publishing Co.; reprinted by permission. The Picture Communication Symbols ©1981–2012 by DynaVox Mayer-Johnson LLC. All Rights Reserved Worldwide. Used with permission.)

in color) that was used by a boy with autism during a "tickle" activity. Figure 3.2a shows what he viewed, and Figure 3.2b shows hot spots related to various body parts that, when selected, produced spoken messages (e.g., TUMMY, LEG). VSDs will be discussed in more detail in Chapter 6.

In European countries, the term *sign* is used instead of *symbol* as a generic term for "linguistic forms that are not speech, [including] all kinds of manual and graphic forms" (von Tetzchner & Jensen, 1996, p. 10).

UNAIDED SYMBOLS: GESTURES AND VOCALIZATIONS

There's language in her eye, her cheek, her lip,
Nay, her foot speaks; her wanton spirits look out
At every joint and motive of her body.

(Shakespeare, *Troilus and Cressida,* Act IV, Scene 5)

Nonverbal behavior can repeat, contradict, substitute for, complement, accent, or regulate verbal behavior (Knapp, 1980). Nonverbal behavior includes gestures, vocalizations, and other paralinguistic elements; physical characteristics (e.g., physique, body and breath odor); proxemics (e.g., seating arrangements, personal space requirements); artifacts (e.g., clothes, perfume, makeup); and environmental factors that may influence impressions and interactions (e.g., the neatness or disorder of a room may affect how one interacts with the person who lives there). Although all of these elements are important, gestures and vocalizations are perhaps the most communicative forms of nonverbal behavior and are therefore discussed in more detail in the following sections.

"At 20 months, Amy conveyed the message 'You [one of several adults present in the room] give me that [a glass of water],' by orienting toward her potential partner, staring intently at her and then, once the communicative channel was open, pointing with one hand to the agent, the other to the object" (Adamson & Dunbar, 1991, p. 279, describing the communication of a young child with a tracheostomy).

Gestures

Gestural behavior includes fine and gross motor body movements, facial expressions, eye behaviors, and postures. Many years ago, Ekman and Friesen (1969) developed a classification system for describing these behaviors in terms of the communicative and adaptive purposes they generally serve. According to this system, emblems are gestural behaviors that can be translated, or defined, by a few words or a phrase and that can be used without speech to convey messages. There is usually a high level of agreement about the meaning of emblems among members of the same culture. For example, in North America, head shaking is generally understood as an emblem for "no," whereas head nodding is an emblem meaning "yes." People usually produce emblems with their hands, although they may use their entire bodies, as in pantomime. As is the case for verbal speech, people interpret emblems differently depending on circumstances; for example, a nose wrinkle may mean "I'm disgusted" or "Phew! That smells bad!" depending on the context.

Comprehension of some emblems may depend on a person's cognitive and language abilities. For example, individuals with Angelman syndrome, a genetic disorder that results in significant cognitive, communication, and motor impairments, often experience difficulty using even idiosyncratic (i.e., "natural") gestural emblems for communication (Jolleff & Ryan, 1993). In response to this dilemma, Calculator (2002) taught the families of 10 children with Angelman syndrome to encourage the children to use gestures that were already in their repertoires but were not used communicatively; he referred to these as "enhanced natural gestures."

"Ruth talks through her eyes, facial expressions, grunts and sighs and other sounds, and selects two or three words/messages/fragments/clues from her word board to germinate the conversation....Ruth's communication is, in the most fundamental sense, pure poetry" (Steve Kaplan, describing the communication skills of his coauthor for the book *I Raise My Eyes to Say Yes;* Sienkiewicz-Mercer & Kaplan, 1989, pp. xii–xiii).

Illustrators are nonverbal behaviors that accompany speech and illustrate what is being said (Knapp, 1980). Among other functions, illustrators 1) emphasize a word or a phrase (e.g., pointing emphatically to a chair while saying "Sit down"), 2) depict a referent or a spatial relationship (e.g., spreading the hands far apart while saying "You should have seen the size of the fish that got away"), 3) depict the pacing of an event (e.g., snapping the fingers rapidly while saying "It was over with before I knew it"), or 4) illustrate a verbal statement through repetition or substitution of a word or a phrase (e.g., miming the action of writing while saying "Where's my pencil?"). Knapp (1980) suggested that people use illustrators less consciously and less deliberately than emblems and that speakers use them most frequently in face-to-face interactions when they are excited, when the receiver is not paying attention or does not comprehend the message, or when the interaction is generally difficult.

Affect displays are facial expressions or body movements that display emotional states. Affect displays differ from emblems in that they are more subtle, less stylized, and less intentional (Knapp, 1980); in fact, in many cases, an affect display may contradict a concurrent verbal statement. The person using these subtle gestures may be largely unaware of them, although the gestures may be obvious to the receiver of the message. Affect displays that convey happiness, surprise, fear, sadness, anger, and disgust or contempt may occur cross-culturally, although their contextual appropriateness is governed by specific social rules regarding age, sex, and role position (Ekman & Friesen, 1969).

Saying "I agree completely" while shaking the head "no" and crossing the arms in front of the body is an example of an affect display that contradicts a concurrent verbal statement.

Regulators are nonverbal behaviors that maintain and regulate conversational speaking and listening between two or more people. Regulators may function to initiate or terminate interactions or to tell the speaker to continue, repeat, elaborate, hurry up, talk about something more interesting, or give the listener a chance to talk, among other functions (Ekman & Friesen, 1969). Similar to emblems, regulators tend to be quite culturally bound (Hetzroni & Harris, 1996). In North America, head nods and eye behaviors are the most common regulators of turn-taking interactions for most people. For example, when one wishes to terminate an interaction, the amount of eye contact often decreases markedly, whereas nodding accompanied by wide-eyed gazing can urge a speaker to continue. Like illustrators, regulators are thought to be learned from watching others interact, but, unlike illustrators, they are emitted almost involuntarily. However, people are usually aware of these behaviors when the behaviors are performed by those with whom they interact.

The final category of gestures, *adaptors*, are learned behaviors that a person generally uses more often when he or she is alone; adaptors are not intentionally used in communication. Nevertheless, their use may be triggered by verbal interactions that produce emotional responses, particularly those associated with anxiety of some sort (Knapp, 1980). Adaptors can be divided into three types: self-, object, and alter adaptors. *Self-adaptors* refer to manipulations of one's own body and include holding, rubbing, scratching, or pinching oneself. People often use self-adaptors with little conscious effort and with no intention to communicate, and these behaviors receive little external feedback from others; in fact, other people rarely wish to be caught looking at them. Rubbing one's nose when feeling stress and wiping around the corners of the eyes when feeling sad are two examples of this type of self-adaptor. *Object adaptors* involve the manipulation of objects, are often learned later in life, and have less social stigma associated with them. Often, the person producing these gestures is aware of them and may intend to communicate a message with them. Chewing on a pencil instead of smoking a cigarette when anxious is an example of an object adaptor. *Alter adaptors* are thought to be learned early in life in conjunction with interpersonal experiences such as giving and taking or protecting oneself against impending harm. Ekman (1976) distinguished these learned behaviors by their adaptability. For example, a child who has been physically abused may react to an adult's sudden advance by crouching and moving his or her hands toward his or her face in a protective motion. Later in life, this alter adaptor may be manifested as a step backward with a slight hand movement toward the body when a stranger approaches; this is an alteration of the initial self-protective behavior.

Some questions to ask during AAC assessment that acknowledge the differences across cultures with regard to nonverbal communication are as follows:

- Is eye contact expected when listening? when talking? for children? for adults? Does eye contact (or a lack thereof) have social significance—for example, is it seen as a sign of respect? disrespect? insincerity?
- Is touching or hand holding a norm? Are there gender differences? What are the norms related to personal space? related to displaying particular body parts?
- Is silence expected when listening? when learning? as a signal of respect? Does it indicate lack of interest? Is laughter used as a communication device, and if so, how?
- Are gestures acceptable? What do they mean?
- What types of nonverbal cues are used to assist communication? to commence and terminate communication? Is turn taking consecutive or coexisting? (Adapted from Harris, cited in Blackstone, 1993; and Hetzroni & Harris, 1996)

Vocalizations and Speech

People who have difficulty with speech often produce vocalizations that are communicative in nature. These may range from involuntary sounds, such as sneezing, coughing, hiccupping, and snoring, to voluntary vocalizations, such as yawning, laughing, crying, moaning, yelling, and belching, that often signify physical or emotional states. Some individuals are also able to produce vocalizations that substitute for speech, such as "uh-huh" for "yes" or "uh-uh" for "no." Such vocalizations may be idiosyncratic and may require interpretation by people who are familiar with these individuals' repertoires of vocal signals.

Communication partners may also use vocalizations and speech as all or part of a communication or message display. For example, auditory scanning, either unaided or aided, can be particularly appropriate for people with complex communication needs (CCN) who understand spoken language and have severe visual impairments (Kovach & Kenyon, 2003). Beukelman, Yorkston, and Dowden (1985) described the use of auditory scanning by a young man who sustained a traumatic brain injury in an automobile accident. Because of the resulting impairments, he was unable to speak and was cortically blind. He communicated by having his partner verbally recite numbers corresponding to "chunks" of the alphabet, for example, 1 = *abcdef* and 2 = *ghijkl*. When his partner gave the number of the chunk he desired, he indicated his choice by making a predetermined motor movement. His partner then began to recite individual letters in the chunk until he signaled that the letter he desired had been announced. This laborious process continued until he spelled out the entire message. Similarly, Shane and Cohen (1981) described a commonly used process they called "20 questions," in which the communication partner asks questions and the person with CCN responds with "yes" or "no" gestures or vocalizations. Many SGDs and software programs provide an aided form of this technique, in which the options are announced via digitized or synthesized speech (see Blackstone, 1994, for a review).

"Toni can say one word. She can raise her hand to say 'yes.' Kerry [her sister] will say, *Some juice please, Mom.* As soon as she says that, Toni will make loud noises. So I'll ask her if she wants some juice, and she'll raise her hand. A couple of months ago, we had supper and we got done eating and Kerry said, *More spaghetti, please.* As soon as Kerry said that, Toni, who was sitting between Dad and me, made loud noises. I said, *You want more spaghetti?* Then she shot up her hand. Now, when Toni gets off the school bus (or is taken off in her wheelchair), and the minute I pick up my teacup, she'll start with the noises. That's your cue to ask if she wants a drink. So she's figuring out ways to get her point across" (a mother describing the communication of her foster daughter, Toni, in Biklen, 1992, p. 56).

UNAIDED SYMBOLS: MANUAL SIGN SYSTEMS

A number of manual sign systems, the majority of which were originally designed for and used by people who are deaf, have also been used by people with CCN who are able to hear. Prior to 1990, manual signing, used alone or combined with speech, was the form of augmentative communication used most often with people diagnosed as having autism or intellectual disabilities in the United States (Matas, Mathy-Laikko, Beukelman, & Legresley, 1985), the United Kingdom (Kiernan, 1983; Kiernan, Reid, & Jones, 1982), and Australia (Iacono & Parsons, 1986). This approach has also been used to some extent in the remediation of childhood apraxia of speech (Cumley & Swanson, 1999). However, controlled research studies with people with intellectual disabilities have reported mixed success, with many reports indicating that spontaneous use of learned signs or structures often does not occur (see Bryen & Joyce, 1985, and Goldstein, 2002, for reviews).

Regardless of mixed results related to their effectiveness, manual signs continue to be useful for a wide variety of people with CCN. Lloyd and Karlan (1984) suggested six reasons why manual sign approaches might be appropriate alternatives to speech-only approaches. First, language input is simplified and the rate of presentation is slowed when manual signs are combined with speech (Wilbur & Peterson, 1998). Second, expressive responding is facilitated by reduction in the physical demands and psychological pressure for speech and by the enhancement of the interventionist's ability to shape gradual approximations and provide physical guidance. Third, vocabulary that is limited yet functional can be taught while maintaining the individual's attention. Fourth, manual signs allow simplified language input while minimizing auditory short-term memory and processing requirements. Fifth, stimulus processing is facilitated with the use of the visual mode, which has temporal and referential advantages over the speech mode. Finally, manual signs have the advantage over speech or symbolic representation because some signs are closer visually to their referents than spoken words are.

Considerations for Use

As noted previously, manual sign languages permit the coding of an essentially infinite number of messages; they also allow nuances of meaning to be added through accompanying body language. Some considerations relevant to the effective use of manual signs include intelligibility, the potential for combining signs and speech or other AAC techniques, motoric complexity, and other considerations, as discussed briefly in the sections that follow.

Intelligibility

Most manual signs cannot be guessed by unfamiliar individuals, such as those who might be encountered on buses or in stores, recreational facilities, and other community environments (Lloyd & Karlan, 1984). This concern was illustrated in a study of two adolescents with autism who were taught to use both manual signs and PCS to order food in a restaurant (Rotholz, Berkowitz, & Burberry, 1989). Almost none of the youths' manual sign requests were understood by the restaurant counterperson without assistance from a teacher. In contrast, successful request rates of 80%–100% were reported when the PCS system in the students' communication books was used. This study illustrated the intelligibility limitations of manual signing when it is used with untrained community members and suggested that multimodal systems (e.g., manual signing plus graphic symbols such as pictures) may be more appropriate.

Iconicity

Some research has shown that signs that are high in iconicity are both easier to learn and easier to recognize (e.g., Konstantareas, Oxman, & Webster, 1978; Kozleski, 1991b), although, as noted previously with reference to pictorial symbols, iconicity is not the only factor that affects manual sign acquisition (DePaul & Yoder, 1986). However, facilitators who are teaching single, functional signs to beginning communicators may find it advantageous to select individual vocabulary items from several different manual sign systems (e.g., American Sign Language, Signed English) to maximize iconicity and, therefore, learnability. Of course, if manual signing is being taught as a language system, such selective use of signs across systems is inadvisable.

Motoric Complexity and Other Considerations

Studies of manual sign acquisition have suggested that the signs generally acquired first by young children of deaf parents are those that 1) require contact between the hands (Bonvillian & Siedlecki, 1998); 2) are produced in the "neutral space" in front of the signer's body or against the chin, mouth, forehead, or trunk (Bonvillian & Siedlecki, 1996); 3) require a single, simple manual alphabet handshape, such as 5 (spread hand), G (index finger points), A (fist), or B (flat hand; Bonvillian & Siedlecki, 1998); and 4) require bidirectional movements (e.g., to and fro, up and down; Bonvillian & Siedlecki, 1998). Because signs with these characteristics are acquired earliest and produced most accurately by typically developing children, one can surmise that such signs are among the "easiest" to learn. In addition, Doherty (1985) noted that, ideally, signs taught in the same environment or time frame should be dissimilar from other signs being taught; for example, teaching the signs for both EAT and DRINK during lunch in the school cafeteria is probably not a good idea because these signs are both motorically and conceptually similar. Finally, and most important, manual signs selected for instruction should be motivating and functional.

Selecting signs for initial instruction that meet all of these requirements is a formidable task because it appears that functionality and learnability may be at least somewhat incompatible (Luftig, 1984).

Combining Signs and Speech or Other Augmentative and Alternative Communication Techniques

A number of research studies have found that a combined manual sign plus speech intervention is often more effective in establishing production and/or comprehension skills than either mode taught singly (e.g., Barrera, Lobato-Barrera, & Sulzer-Azaroff, 1980; Brady & Smouse, 1978). This combined approach is referred to as simultaneous or total communication and is often employed in the context of a telegraphic or key-word signing approach (see Bonvillian & Nelson, 1978; Casey, 1978; Konstantareas, 1984; Schaeffer, 1980). However, it is important to recognize that some individuals may be more apt to attend to the manual sign component than the speech component when the two modes are combined (Carr, Binkoff, Kologinsky, & Eddy, 1978). Furthermore, some research has suggested that the usefulness of total communication may depend on whether the individual has mastered generalized imitation at the point of intervention (Carr & Dores, 1981; Carr, Pridal, & Dores, 1984).

Interventions combining speech, manual signs, and other AAC techniques may also be useful for some individuals. For example, a series of studies by Iacono and colleagues demonstrated that instruction with manual signs plus line-drawing symbols on an SGD appeared to have advantages over sign-alone instruction in teaching the use of two-word utterances (Iacono & Duncum, 1995; Iacono, Mirenda, & Beukelman, 1993; Iacono & Waring, 1996). In addition, the use of a multimodal system has the advantage of "covering all the bases" in situations in which it is not clear which symbol system might be best (Reichle, York, & Sigafoos, 1991). Finally, for some individuals, such as children with childhood apraxia of speech, a multimodal AAC system might well be the system of choice (Cumley & Swanson, 1999).

The book *Let's Sign and Down Syndrome* (Smith & Uttley, 2008) was published in the United Kingdom to teach parents and others how to use British Sign Language to support language and communication development. It is available through DeafBooks.

At this time, there are no clear, empirically validated guidelines to use when making decisions about the appropriateness of manual signing, either alone or in combination with other techniques. However, Wendt (2009, p. 93) noted that, at least for individuals with autism spectrum disorders, "The available body of research on manual signs and gestures…reveals strong intervention effectiveness scores for symbol acquisition and production, as well as for related outcomes such as speech comprehension and production." Furthermore, the available evidence suggests that manual signing does not appear to reduce an individual's motivation to speak and may in fact enhance it (Millar, Light, & Schlosser, 2006).

Types of Manual Sign Systems

The term *manual sign system* actually refers to three main types of systems: 1) those that are alternatives to the spoken language of a particular country, 2) those that parallel the spoken language (e.g., manually coded English), and 3) those that interact with or supplement another means of transmitting a spoken language (e.g., fingerspelling). We review the primary manual sign systems used in North America in the sections that follow, with particular reference to their applicability to AAC interventions.

National Sign Languages

In most countries, national sign languages have been developed through use by the Deaf community for many years. In the United States and most of Canada, American Sign Language (ASL) is used within the Deaf community for face-to-face interactions. In Quebec, Canada, a distinctly different system, Langue des Signes Québécoises, is used by people who are deaf.

ASL is related neither to English nor to the sign languages of other countries. Deaf communities around the world have their own distinct languages (e.g., Auslan in Australia, Swedish Sign Language in Sweden). Relatively few teachers of people with hearing impairments in the United States appear to use pure-form ASL in the classroom; thus, it is not primarily a pedagogical language, although it is the predominant language of the Deaf community (Hoffmeister, 1990). Because ASL does not follow or approximate English word order, it is not used concurrently with speech.

The ASL Video Dictionary and Inflection Guide is an online resource available by subscription through the National Technical Institute for the Deaf. It has 2,700 ASL signs and English equivalents along with 2,000 signs linked to at least one of 650 sentences that illustrate how the signs change to show different meanings. All signs are performed by deaf native signers in high-quality QuickTime movies. Similarly, the Krown Sign Language Translator is a portable PDA-sized device containing videos of more than 3,500 signs that are accessed by typing the written equivalent. It is available from Krown Manufacturing, Inc.

Manually Coded English Sign Systems

In North America, a number of manual sign systems that code English word order, syntax, and grammar have been developed for educational use with individuals with hearing and other communicative impairments. We use the term *manually coded English* (MCE) to refer to these systems, in acknowledgment of its common use in the Deaf community (Stedt & Moores, 1990).

In North America, the United Kingdom, Australia, and New Zealand, the most common MCE system is called Contact Sign (sometimes referred to as Pidgin Signed English), a blend of a local Deaf sign language and English. Contact Sign is perhaps best described as ASL-like English when used by people who can hear and English-like ASL when used by people who have hearing impairments (Woodward, 1990). Contact Sign is used extensively in the education of students who have hearing impairments in a total communication context, in conjunction with speech or extensive mouthing of English words.

Many versions of Contact Sign have evolved from interactions between skilled Deaf and hearing signers. One of the most common varieties is Conceptually Accurate Signed English, which combines English grammatical order with ASL signs, invented signs, and fingerspelling. Another version is key-word signing (KWS; Grove & Walker, 1990; Windsor & Fristoe, 1989), in which spoken English is used simultaneously with manual signs for the critical words in a sentence, such as base nouns, base verbs, prepositions, adjectives, and adverbs. Thus, the sentence "Go get the cup and put it on the table" might involve the use of the signs GET, CUP, PUT, ON, and TABLE, while the entire sentence is spoken.

The American Sign Language Handshape Dictionary organizes more than 1,900 ASL signs by 40 basic handshapes and includes detailed descriptions and a DVD on how to form the signs (Tennant & Gluszak Brown, 2010). *Signs of the Times* (Shroyer, 2011) presents 1,300 ASL signs representing 3,500 English glosses in lessons that contain clear illustrations, equivalent words and synonyms, sample sentences to define vocabulary context, and practice sentences to display and reinforce ASL usage. Both are available from Gallaudet University Press.

Two additional MCE systems are Signed English (Bornstein, 1990) and Signing Exact English (Gustason & Zawolkow, 1993). Signed English was the first manual sign system reported to be successfully implemented with children with autism (Creedon, 1973). Signing Exact English is motorically and linguistically more complex than Signed English and may, therefore, be less useful for people with CCN not due primarily to hearing impairments. Neither system is widely used in North America.

Signing Exact English support materials, including articles, storybooks, DVDs, illustrated dictionaries, flash cards, songs, and posters and a web application are available for parents, teachers, and others through the Signing Exact English (S.E.E.) Center for the Advancement of Deaf Children and Modern Signs Press.

Tactile Signing

Tactile signing is commonly used by individuals with deaf-blindness who acquire their knowledge of sign language before becoming blind (Reed, Delhorne, Durlach, & Fischer, 1990). In this method, the deaf-blind person places one or two hands on the dominant hand of the signer and passively traces the motion of the signing hand. Thus, the various formational properties of signs are received tactually by the deaf-blind person, who then communicates expressively using conventional sign language. Tactile signing can be used in conjunction with ASL or any of the MCE systems. Research suggests that individuals with experience in the tactual reception of signing can receive approximately 1.5 signs per second; this compares favorably with typical signing rates of 2.5 signs per second for visual reception of signs by individuals who can see (Bellugi & Fischer, 1972; Reed, Delhorne, Durlach, & Fischer, 1995).

"We have to find out different ways to help the child to understand that communication is fun, communication can lead to fulfilling their necessities and not only speech, but using gestures, by using pictures, by using touch or alphabets or pointing, basically a way to make it easy" (AAC specialist from India, in Srinivasan, Mathew, & Lloyd, 2011, p. 240).

AIDED SYMBOLS: TANGIBLE SYMBOLS

Rowland and Schweigert (1989, 2000a) coined the term *tangible symbol* to refer to two- or three-dimensional aided symbols that are permanent, manipulable with a simple motor behavior, tactually discriminable, and highly iconic. We use the term in a more restricted sense to refer to symbols that can be discriminated based on tangible properties (e.g., shape, texture, consistency); thus, we do not include two-dimensional (i.e., pictorial) symbols in this category. Tangible symbols are typically used with individuals with visual or dual sensory impairments and severe cognitive disabilities, but they may also be appropriate for other populations (e.g., as beginning communication symbols for children with low vision; see Chen, 1999). Tangible symbols discussed in the following sections include real objects, miniature objects, partial objects, and artificially associated and textured symbols.

Real Objects

Real object symbols may be identical to, similar to, or associated with their referents. For example, an identical symbol for *brush your teeth* might be a toothbrush that is the same color and type as the individual's actual toothbrush. A similar symbol might be a toothbrush of a different color and type, whereas an associated symbol might be a tube of toothpaste or container of dental floss. Other examples of associated symbols include a sponge that represents *cleaning the kitchen counter* or a CD cover that represents *music time* in the preschool classroom. Associated symbols may also include remnants of activities—items such as a ticket stub from the movies or a hamburger wrapper from a fast-food restaurant.

Many people with intellectual disabilities are able to match identical and nonidentical (i.e., similar) object symbols with similar accuracy (Mirenda & Locke, 1989). This suggests that both types of object symbols may be equal in enabling recognition of their referent; however, it is important to be cautious in this assumption, especially with beginning communicators. It is also important to consider the individual sensory input needs of individuals with visual impairments when selecting real objects for them to use. Rowland and Schweigert (1989, 1990, 2000b) reported numerous examples of successful use of real object symbols with individuals who have visual and dual sensory impairments.

Miniature Objects

Miniature objects may be more practical than real objects in some situations but need to be selected carefully to maximize effectiveness (Vanderheiden & Lloyd, 1986). For example, miniatures that are much smaller than their referents may be more difficult for students with cognitive disabilities to recognize than some types of two-dimensional symbols (Mineo Mollica, 2003; Mirenda & Locke, 1989). Nevertheless, miniature objects have been used successfully with individuals with cerebral palsy (Landman & Schaeffler, 1986); dual sensory impairments (Rowland & Schweigert, 1989, 2000b); and a wide variety of intellectual, sensory, and/or motor impairments (Rowland & Schweigert, 2000b).

In addition to size, tactile similarity is also critical when using miniature objects with people who cannot see. For example, an individual with visual impairments may not readily recognize the relationship between a miniature plastic toilet and a real toilet because they feel different with respect to size, shape, and texture. In this case, a real object associated with the toilet (e.g., a small roll of toilet paper) might be more appropriate as a bathroom symbol.

People with visual impairments "see" with their fingers and hands, so the tangible symbols they use should be tactually similar to or associated with their referents. For example, Catherine, a woman with dual sensory impairments, wears a pair of leather half-gloves (i.e., gloves with the fingers cut off) whenever she goes horseback riding. She uses the same gloves as tangible symbols for horseback riding in her schedule system at home because they remind her of (and smell like!) this activity.

Partial Objects

In some situations, particularly those that involve large referents, partial objects may be useful symbols. For example, the top of a spray bottle of window cleaner may be used to represent *washing the windows* at a vocational site. Also included in this category are "symbols with one or two shared features" (Rowland & Schweigert, 1989, p. 229), such as plastic symbols that are the same size and shape as their referents. The use of partial objects may be a good alternative when tactile similarity cannot be met with miniature objects.

Artificially Associated and Textured Symbols

Tangible symbols may also be constructed by selecting shapes and textures that can be artificially associated with a referent. For example, if a wooden apple is attached to the door of the school cafeteria, a similar apple could be used to signify *lunchtime* (Rowland & Schweigert, 1989, 2000a). Textured symbols, a subtype of artificial symbols, may be either logically or arbitrarily associated with their referents. For example, a piece of spandex material would be a logically associated textured symbol to represent a bathing suit because many suits are made of this material. Alternatively, a square of velvet could be arbitrarily selected to represent a favorite snack. Several experimental or case studies have documented the successful use of textured symbols with individuals with one or more sensory impairments in addition to autism (Lund & Troha, 2008) or severe cognitive disabilities (Locke & Mirenda, 1988; Mathy-Laikko et al., 1989; Murray-Branch, Udvari-Solner, & Bailey, 1991; Turnell & Carter, 1994).

 Instructional materials and DVDs related to the use of tangible symbols are available through Design to Learn. A manual for using tangible symbols with individuals with autism (Vicker, 1996) is available from the the Indiana Institute on Disability and Community. A set of Tangible Symbol Cues that consist of portions of objects embedded on corrugated cards are available from Adaptive Design Association, Inc. Finally, a directory of tangible symbol suggestions, with illustrations, is available from the Texas School for the Blind and Visually Impaired.

AIDED SYMBOLS: PICTORIAL SYMBOLS

Many types of two-dimensional pictorial symbols, including photographs, line drawings, and abstract symbols, can be used to represent various concepts. This section reviews the major pictorial symbol types used in North America in terms of their relative iconicity, as well as in terms of the individuals with whom they have been used successfully.

Photographs

High-quality color or black-and-white photographs may be used to represent objects, verbs, people, places, and activities. Photographs may be produced with a camera or obtained from catalogs, magazines, coupons, product labels, or advertisements (Mirenda, 1985). A research study found that people with intellectual disabilities matched color photographs to their referents somewhat more accurately than they matched black-and-white photographs (Mirenda & Locke, 1989). Another study found that people with intellectual disabilities matched black-and-white photographs to their referents more accurately than they matched line drawings (Sevcik & Romski, 1986). Dixon (1981) found that students with severe disabilities were better able to associate objects with their color photographs when the photographic objects were cut out than when they were not. Reichle and colleagues (1991) suggested that the context in which a photograph appears might affect an individual's ability to recognize it; for example, a photograph of a watering can may become more recognizable when it appears next to a photograph of a plant.

Digital or printed sets of high-quality color or black-and-white photographs are available from companies such as DynaVox Mayer-Johnson; Silver Lining Multimedia, Inc.; and Speechmark Publishing.

Line-Drawing Symbols

Over the years, many sets of line-drawing symbols have been developed in North America and elsewhere to support communication and/or literacy development of individuals with complex communication needs. The primary sets that are used in North America (PCS, Widgit Symbols, Pictograms, and Blissymbols) are highlighted in this section and are illustrated in Figure 3.3.

Picture Communication Symbols

PCS is the most widely used line-drawing system for communication around the world. The PCS library consists of more than 18,000 pictorial graphics that represent words, phrases, and concepts on a range of topics. Both Windows- and Macintosh-based versions of the Boardmaker family of software products can generate communication displays of either black-and-white or color PCS in 44 languages. Animated PCS for many verbs (i.e., action words) are also available in several of these products. A recent research study suggested that animated PCS may be recognized more accurately by some children, especially when the animations are more realistic (Mineo, Peischl, & Pennington, 2008; see also Jagaroo & Wilkinson, 2008). Other studies suggested that clustering same-color PCS symbols may facilitate accurate selections by preschoolers and children with intellectual disabilities such as Down syndrome (Wilkinson et al., 2006; Wilkinson, Carlin, & Thistle, 2008).

Not surprisingly, PCS for concrete nouns (e.g., *apple*) appear to be learned more readily than those for abstract nouns (e.g., words such as *direction*), at least by children with cerebral palsy (Hochstein, McDaniel, Nettleton, & Neufeld, 2003). In addition, PCS have been found to be more transparent and more easily learned than Blissymbols. This finding applies to individuals both with and without disabilities for whom English is the primary language (Bloomberg et al., 1990; Huer, 2000; Mirenda & Locke, 1989; Mizuko, 1987; Mizuko & Reichle, 1989) and to those whose

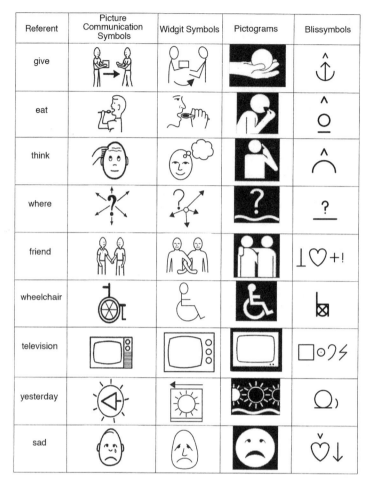

Figure 3.3. Examples of Picture Communication Symbols, Widgit Symbols, Pictograms, and Blissymbols. (The Picture Communication Symbols ©1981–2012 by DynaVox Mayer-Johnson LLC. All Rights Reserved Worldwide. Used with permission. WIDGIT SYMBOLS © WIDGIT SOFTWARE 2002-2012 www.widgit.com. Pictograms courtesy of Pictogram, http://www.pictogram.se. Blissymbols © Blissymbolics Communication International, www.blissymbolics.org)

first language is Chinese or Mexican Spanish (Huer, 2000). However, this is not to imply that the iconicity of PCS is identical for individuals across cultures (Nigam, 2003). For example, two South African studies reported a low to very low rate of accurate PCS identification by typically developing 6-year-old Afrikaans-speaking children and 10-year-old Zulu-speaking children (Basson & Alant, 2005; Haupt & Alant, 2002). This is a reminder that the cultural-linguistic background of people with CCN and their families is important to consider when using PCS or any other type of symbol.

An extensive catalog of Picture Communication Symbols and related products can be obtained from DynaVox Mayer-Johnson. In addition, PCS greeting cards, mugs, t-shirts, and other products are available from Giving Greetings.

Widgit Symbols

The Widgit Symbols set has been developed in the United States and the United Kingdom over the past 25 years and now contains more than 11,000 symbols that cover an English vocabulary of more than 40,000 words. Widgit Symbols are designed to conform to a set of standards and conventions (referred to as "schema") and can be used to support both communication and literacy. (See Figure 3.3.)

Literacy software products that utilize Widgit Symbols are available in the United Kingdom from Widgit Software. In North America, DynaVox Mayer-Johnson distributes a number of Widgit software products, including Communicate: SymWriter, a talking word processor that features more than 9,000 PCS and 8,000 Widgit Literacy Symbols. Apple iPad, iPhone, and iPod apps such as TapToTalk (Assistyx LLC) and Scene and Heard (TBox Apps) also use Widgit Symbols.

Pictograms

The Pictogram symbol set was originally developed in Canada and consists of 1,500 white-on-black "picto-images" that are designed to reduce figure–ground discrimination difficulties (Maharaj, 1980). Pictograms have been found to be less translucent than PCS but more translucent than Blissymbols (Bloomberg et al., 1990). Leonhart and Maharaj (1979) reported that adults with severe to profound intellectual disabilities learned Pictograms faster than Blissymbols. A recent study suggested that school-age participants with intellectual disabilities learned to recognize animated Pictograms of action words more readily than their static equivalents (Fujisawa, Inoue, Yamana, & Hayashi, 2011). (See Figure 3.3.)

Pictograms are available in 15 languages and are widely used in Scandinavia and many other Northern European countries (e.g., Iceland, Latvia, Lithuania). In 2005, Pictograms were adopted by the Japanese Ministry of Economy and Industry for use by the general public (Fujisawa et al., 2011). Symbols are available through the Pictogram web site.

Blissymbols

The history of Blissymbolics is both complex and fascinating (see Kates & McNaughton, 1975, for an in-depth explanation). Generally, the system was developed to function as an auxiliary language for international written communication. It consists of approximately 100 basic symbols that can be used singly or in combination to encode virtually any message (Silverman, 1995). The system is composed of approximately 4,500 symbols; new Blissymbols are added periodically by an international panel affiliated with Blissymbolics Communication International. Blissymbolics is used in more than 33 countries and has been translated into more than 15 languages. Numerous studies have indicated that Blissymbols are less transparent and more difficult to learn and retain than other types of line-drawing symbols (Bloomberg et al., 1990; Huer, 2000; Hurlbut, Iwata, & Green, 1982; Mirenda & Locke, 1989; Mizuko, 1987). (See Figure 3.3.)

BlissOnline is an online subscription-based service that provides a database of Blissymbolics Communication International–authorized Blissymbols in English and Swedish and a tool for simple Blissymbol chart creation. Additional supports can be obtained through Blissymbolics Communication International.

Other Pictorial Systems

Several additional representational symbol systems are also used widely in North America and elsewhere, although their relative iconicity and learnability have not been studied.

Pictographic Communication Resources   Pictographic Communication Resources (PCRs; Figure 3.4) were developed to assist health professionals and other conversation partners (e.g., family members) to communicate with adults who have aphasia and other acquired communication impairments. They include adult-oriented symbols designed to explain aphasia and to facilitate interactions between adults with disabilities and nurses, social workers, physical and occupational therapists, physicians, counselors, chaplains, and family members. PCRs are available through the Aphasia Institute in Toronto.

Gus Communication Symbols   Gus Communication Symbols (Figure 3.5) is a set that consists of more than 5,500 color line-drawing symbols representing standard vocabulary words as well as words related to entertainment, sports, current events, politics, and other common topics of conversation. The set was designed to appeal to adolescents and adults as well as children and is available via software called Overboard from Gus Communication Devices, Inc.

Pics for PECS   Pics for PECS (Figure 3.5) is a set of 2,800 color images that include vocabulary words for adolescents and adults as well as children (e.g., yoga, motor scooter). The set is available on CD-ROM in eight countries from Pyramid Educational Consultants.

Symbolstix   Symbolstix (Figure 3.5) include more than 12,000 color line-drawing symbols that depict activities and people as lively stick figures "with an attitude." Symbolstix are used in Proloquo2Go, which was the first large-scale communication app for the iPad, iPod, and iPhone. Symbolstix are available by subscription at Symbolstix Online.

Imagine Symbols   The Imagine Symbol Set (Figure 3.5) includes 3,600 realistic, colorful illustrations in 15 categories that include emotions, phrases, verbs, and computer devices. The symbols were designed to be appealing to adults and are available on a searchable DVD from Attainment Company.

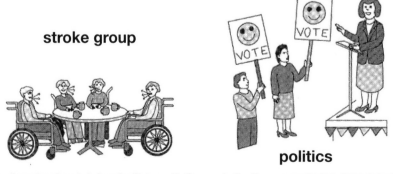

Figure 3.4.   Examples of symbols from the Pictographic Communication Resources collection. (From Aphasia Institute, Toronto, Ontario, Canada; reprinted with permission.)

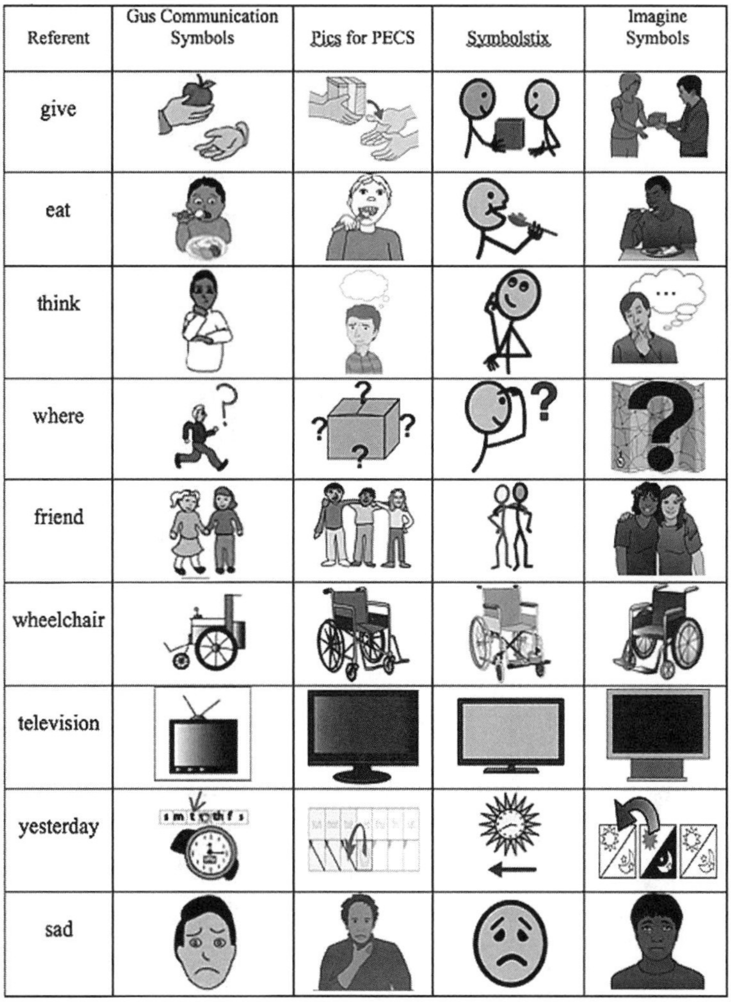

Referent	Gus Communication Symbols	Pics for PECS	Symbolstix	Imagine Symbols
give				
eat				
think				
where				
friend				
wheelchair				
television				
yesterday				
sad				

Figure 3.5. Examples of Gus Communication Symbols, Pics for PECS, Symbolstix, and Imagine Symbols. (Pics for PECS™ images used with permission from Pyramid Educational Consultants, Inc. [www.pecs.com] Pyramid Educational Consultants, Inc. reserves all rights to the Pics for PECS™ images.)

AIDED SYMBOLS: ORTHOGRAPHY AND ORTHOGRAPHIC SYMBOLS

Traditional orthography refers to the written characters used to transcribe a particular linguistic system (e.g., English letters, Chinese characters). Orthography is used in AAC systems in the form of single letters, words, syllables (e.g., prefixes, suffixes), sequences of commonly combined letters (e.g., *ty, ck, th*), and phrases or sentences. The term *orthographic symbol* is used to refer to aided techniques that represent traditional orthography, such as braille and fingerspelling. These are differentiated from orthographic codes, which use letters as message abbreviations and are discussed later in this chapter.

Braille

Braille is a tactile symbol system for reading and writing that is used by people with visual or dual sensory impairments. Braille characters are formed by combinations of six embossed dots arranged within a cell of two vertical columns of three dots each (see Figure 3.6). From top to bottom, the dots are numbered 1–3 on the left column and 4–6 on the right. The characters represent letters, parts of words, or entire words. Each character is formed according to a standard pattern within the six dots.

There are two methods of writing braille. One method uses one-to-one correspondence between each letter and braille cell; in this method, called *alphabetic braille* or *uncontracted braille,* all words are spelled out. The second method uses special symbols (called *contractions*) that stand for entire words or combinations of letters (such as *er, ch, ation*); this method, called *contracted braille,* is used to produce textbooks and trade books. The official rules for braille transcription in both Canada and the United States can be found in English Braille–American Edition (Braille Authority of North America, 2002). Updates to the braille code are governed by the Braille Authority of North America, and current rules can be found on their web site (see Holbrook, D'Andrea, & Sanford, 2011).

For more than a decade, there has been an international effort to develop a single braille code called Unified English Braille (UEB) that provides notation for mathematics, computer science, and other scientific and engineering disciplines as well as general English literature for use in all English-speaking countries. In April 2004, the International Council on English Braille declared that UEB was substantially complete, and in 2006, it was recognized as the international standard for English Braille. It has been adopted in Australia, Canada, New Zealand, Nigeria, and South Africa. The United States and United Kingdom are considering its adoption as well.

Fingerspelling (Visual and Tactile)

Sign language systems such as ASL use fingerspelling (Figure 3.7) to represent single letters of the alphabet that can be combined to spell words for which there are no conventional signs (e.g., proper names). Interest in literacy instruction for people who use AAC has drawn attention to this feature of sign language because of its potential to assist beginning readers to learn the phonological code needed for reading and writing (see Angermeier, Schooley, Harasymowycz, & Schlosser, 2010). Because many fingerspelled letters appear to be visually similar to their graphic counterparts,

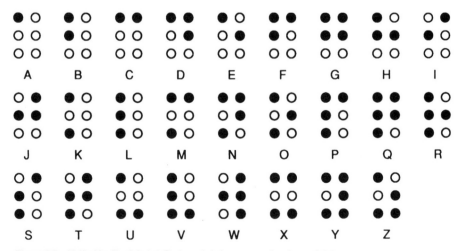

Figure 3.6.   Unified braille alphabet. Darkened circles represent embossed dots.

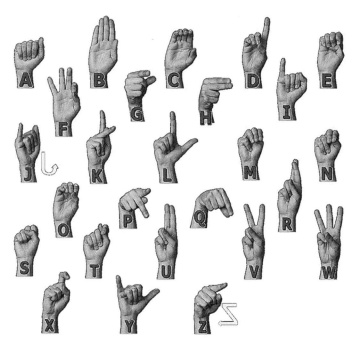

Figure 3.7.   American Sign Language manual alphabet. (From William Vicars, www. lifeprint.com; reprinted by permission.)

the learning of letter–sound relationships might be enhanced by pairing the two, at least during initial instruction (Koehler, Lloyd, & Swanson, 1994).

Tactile fingerspelling is commonly used by people with dual sensory impairments who are literate. For these individuals, information is transmitted in fingerspelling by placing the hand of the information receiver over the hand of the individual formulating the letters (Jensema, 1982; Mathy-Laikko, Ratcliff, Villarruel, & Yoder, 1987). Research has shown that, at communication rates of approximately two syllables per second (roughly half of the typical speaking rate), experienced deafblind individuals can receive key words in conversational sentences at roughly 80% accuracy using tactual reception of fingerspelling (Reed et al., 1990).

COMBINED SYMBOL SYSTEMS (AIDED AND UNAIDED)

Formal symbol systems that incorporate the use of at least manual signs with graphic symbols became popular in North America in the 1980s and have been used with people who do not speak. In general, use of such systems is based on the assumption that if a single AAC technique works, then using more than one technique should work even better. These combined systems differ from individualized communication systems that incorporate multiple modes (e.g., Hooper, Connell, & Flett, 1987) in that the symbols are combined in a standard intervention package. The combined symbol system that is used most widely in AAC is the Makaton Vocabulary.

Makaton Vocabulary

Makaton is a language program offering a structured, multimodal approach for the teaching of communication, language, and literacy skills. Devised for children and adults with a variety of communication and learning disabilities, Makaton is used extensively throughout the United Kingdom and has been adapted for use in many other countries as well. The approach combines speech, manual signs, and graphic symbols. The core vocabulary consists of approximately 450 concepts organized in a series of eight stages. For example, Stage 1 consists of concepts that meet immediate needs and can establish basic interactions, whereas Stage 5 consists of words that can be used in the general community as well as feelings and attributes. In addition, there is a large resource vocabulary of approximately 7,000 concepts for which there are manual signs and symbols.

The Makaton Charity, which oversees the use and development of Makaton worldwide, requires that signs from the sign language of a country's Deaf community be matched to the Makaton vocabularies. Thus, in the United Kingdom, British Sign Language signs are used; whereas in the United States, the signs are taken from American Sign Language. The Makaton Charity has produced a collection of Makaton signs and symbols that are related to the main core subject areas of the British National Curriculum, including information on developing literacy skills through Makaton.

The Makaton Vocabulary program has been adapted for use in more than 50 countries, including New Zealand, Australia, Canada, the United States, France, Germany, Spain, Portugal, Switzerland, Norway, Malta, Greece, Turkey, Kuwait and other countries in the Gulf region, Egypt, Sri Lanka, Pakistan, India, Nepal, Hong Kong, Japan, and several African countries. The Makaton Charity distributes a variety of Makaton resource and training materials and organizes training courses in the United Kingdom and other countries.

RATE ENHANCEMENT TECHNIQUES

The conversational speaking rates of speakers who do not have disabilities vary from 150 words per minute to 250 words per minute (Goldman-Eisler, 1986). These speaking rates allow for efficient communication of messages that are formulated and spoken virtually simultaneously. One has only to view the interaction patterns among a talkative, animated group of friends to realize the importance of efficiency in order for all speakers to take their conversational turns and communicate their messages before someone else claims the floor.

In addition to communicating efficiently, natural speakers formulate spoken messages to meet the needs of the particular communicative situation. During spoken interactions, much of the meaning of a message can be derived from the context and the timing of the message. For example, individuals frequently mumble greetings to friends or colleagues as they pass each other in the hallway at work. It is only because of the context that such poorly articulated messages can be understood. As people watch a sporting event with friends, someone may exclaim, "That's not fair!"—a message with no referent, which can be understood and appreciated only if it is produced in a timely fashion, not 3 minutes after someone has fumbled the ball. Unfortunately, communication inefficiencies and message-timing limitations interfere with the communication interactions of many individuals who rely on AAC to communicate. Communication rates associated with AAC range from 15 to 25 times slower than spoken speech rates. Clearly, such drastic reductions in communication rate are likely to interfere significantly with communication interactions, especially in educational and employment contexts with natural speakers who are accustomed to exchanging information at a much more rapid pace (McNaughton & Bryen, 2007).

One factor contributing to the slowed communication rates of individuals who use aided AAC is that they usually compose messages by selecting the component parts (e.g., pictures or other symbols, letters of the alphabet, words) from their communication displays, one item at a time. Obviously, this method requires considerable time and effort. A strategy that is often used to increase communication rates is to store complete words, phrases, or sentences in AAC systems and to assign a code of some type to the stored message. Then, rather than communicating messages incrementally, the individual is able to convey an entire message by using a single code.

A series of studies examined shopkeepers' attitudes toward adults who used SGDs to convey messages that varied with regard to speed (i.e., fast versus slow) and various message characteristics. Messages were characterized as containing repetitive, excessive, inadequate, or partly relevant information. In all cases, fast messages were responded to more favorably, quickly, and successfully than slow messages were. Repetitive messages were preferred over inadequate, excessive, or partly relevant messages (in that order; Hoag, Bedrosian, & McCoy, 2009).

AAC teams have developed and implemented a number of coding and retrieval strategies. The term *encoding* refers to any technique in which one gives multiple signals that together specify a desired message (Vanderheiden & Lloyd, 1986). How codes are represented is an individual decision that should be matched to a person's capabilities. Whether memory-based or display-based codes are used is also an individual decision. Memory-based codes require that the person have excellent long-term memory skills, whereas display-based codes (i.e., codes that are presented on a visual display or menu, or that are recited aloud so the person can choose) require either good visual skills or good auditory discrimination skills.

A display-based encoding system that might be used with eye pointing is illustrated in Figure 3.8. In this figure, the person with CCN looks at the numbers 5

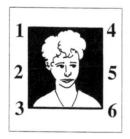 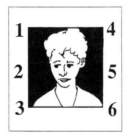

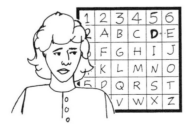

Figure 3.8. Display-based numeric encoding via eye pointing.

and 2 sequentially. The partner decodes this message, which represents the letter D, using her chart. The person with CCN then continues to spell a message or send an alphabetic code by indicating additional letters. Obviously, the rate of communication depends on how efficiently the AAC communicator and the partner can visually locate the desired code or message on the display.

Word Codes

Several types of codes can be used to represent single words. These include various letter, numeric, and alphanumeric techniques, as described in the sections that follow.

Alpha (Letter) Word Codes

Two types of letter codes are typically used for single words. *Truncation codes* abbreviate words according to the first few letters only (e.g., HAMB = HAMBURGER, COMM = COMMUNICATION), whereas *contraction codes* include only the most salient letters (e.g., HMBGR = HAMBURGER, COMUNCTN = COMMUNICATION). Truncation codes often have fewer letters and are thus easier to construct, but contraction codes may have the advantage of being more flexible. Both types of codes can be either memory based or display based.

Alphanumeric Word Codes

Alphanumeric codes use both letters and numbers for words. For example, COMM1 might mean COMMUNICATE, COMM2 = COMMUNICATION, COMM3 = COMMUNITY, and so forth. As can be seen from these examples, the advantage of this approach is that the same letters can be used repeatedly across words that are differentiated by number.

Letter-Category Word Codes

When letter-category codes are used for words, the initial letter is usually the superordinate category and the second letter is the first letter of the specific word. For example, if F = FRUIT and D = DRINKS, FA might mean APPLE, FB might mean BANANA, DC might mean COFFEE, DM might mean MILK, and so forth. Again, this encoding technique can be used in either memory- or display-based systems, depending on the ability of the person using the system.

Numeric Encoding

Occasionally, numeric codes alone are used to represent words or messages. For example, numeric codes may be used when a communication display must be small in order to accommodate a person's limited motor capabilities. In this case, it is advantageous if items in the small selection set can be combined in many ways to code words or messages. Usually, the relationship between the code and its corresponding word is completely arbitrary; thus, 13 might be the code for YESTERDAY and 24 might be the code for HELLO. Most systems that use numeric encoding display the codes and the associated words or messages on a chart or a menu as part of the selection display so that neither the person with CCN nor the communication partner must rely on memory for recall or translation. Extensive learning and instruction is necessary to memorize the codes if this option is not available.

Morse Code

Morse code is an international system that uses a series of dots and dashes to represent letters, punctuation, and numbers (see Figure 3.9). When used in AAC applications, the dots and dashes are transmitted via microswitches through a device or algorithm that translates them into orthographic letters and numbers.

In North America, Morse code emulators are available in a number of communication devices and communication software products, including E Z Keys (Words+, Inc.). In addition, computer access can be achieved through use of devices such as the Darci USB (WesTest Engineering Corp.).

Research on Learnability

An early AAC study investigated the learning curves of typical adults for five encoding strategies used to represent single words (Beukelman & Yorkston, 1984). The five strategies were 1) arbitrary numeric codes, 2) alphabetically organized numeric codes in which consecutive numbers were assigned to words based on their alphabetic order, 3) memory-based alphanumeric codes, 4) chart-based alphanumeric codes, and 5) letter-category codes. In this study, 10 literate adults without disabilities served as participants (2 per condition) and were introduced to 200 codes and their associated words during 10 sessions. The participants performed most accurately and retrieved the codes most quickly when using encoding approaches that grouped words according to a logical pattern—that is, the alphanumeric, alphabetically organized numeric, and letter-category codes. The participants' code selection was least effective

A	. _	V	... _	
B	_ ...	W	. _ _	
C	_ . _ .	X	_ .. _	
D	_ ..	Y	_ . _ _	
E	.	Z	_ _ ..	
F	.. _ .	1	. _ _ _ _	
G	_ _ .	2	.. _ _ _	
H	....	3	... _ _	
I	..	4	.... _	
J	. _ _ _	5	.....	
K	_ . _	6	_	
L	. _ ..	7	_ _ ...	
M	_ _	8	_ _ _ ..	
N	_ .	9	_ _ _ _ .	
O	_ _ _	0	_ _ _ _ _	
P	. _ _ .	period	. _ . _ . _	
Q	_ _ . _	comma	_ _ .. _ _	
R	. _ .	?	.. _ _ ..	
S	...	error	....	
T	_	wait	. _ ...	
U	.. _	end	. _ . _ .	

Figure 3.9. Morse code.

using arbitrary numeric codes. The learning curves for the arbitrary numeric codes and the memory-based alphanumeric codes did not improve as much over time as the learning curves for the other three encoding strategies did.

Three single-word encoding techniques were also investigated (Angelo, 1987), including truncation codes, contraction codes, and arbitrary letter codes. The 66 individuals without disabilities in this study attempted to learn 20 words during a series of 10 trials. The results indicated that the individuals recalled truncation codes most accurately, followed by contraction and arbitrary letter codes, in that order.

Studies investigating the learnability of Morse code by people with CCN are limited. One exception is a case study of a man with a spinal cord injury who wrote using Morse code at a rate of 25–30 words per minute. He learned to produce basic Morse code using a sip-and-puff switch within 2 weeks and became proficient in the use of the system within approximately 2 months (Beukelman, Yorkston, & Dowden, 1985). Hsieh and Luo (1999) also described the Morse code learning of a 14-year-old Taiwanese student with cerebral palsy who was able to read English at a Grade 2 (Taiwanese) level. He earned to type English words at approximately 90% accuracy over a 4-week period. In 2008 and 2009, researchers in Taiwan reported the successful use of Morse code for Internet and telephone communication by adolescents and adults with cerebral palsy or spinal cord injury after 2 months of practice (Yang, Huang, Chuang, & Yang, 2008; Yang, Cheng, Chuang, & Yang, 2009). It appears that 1–2 months of continuous use is required in order to become reasonably proficient with this technique.

Message Codes

Many of the strategies used to encode words can also be used for messages. In the sections that follow, we discuss the various message encoding options and the research related to the learning demands they place on the people who use them.

Alpha (Letter) Encoding

Letters of the alphabet are used to encode messages in a wide range of AAC systems. These codes are usually memory based and incorporate different strategies to assist the person using them to remember each code and its referent. In *salient letter encoding,* the initial letters of salient content words in the message are used to construct the code. For example, the message PLEASE OPEN THE DOOR FOR ME might be coded OD, because these are the initial letters of the primary words in the message OPEN DOOR. This technique attempts to establish a logical link between the code and how the message is spelled. Although the capability requirements for salient letter encoding have not been studied in detail, it seems that some familiarity with traditional orthography and the ability to spell at least the first letter of words are necessary. In addition, this technique is probably the most effective for those who are able to recall messages in their correct syntactic forms because the codes are often determined by the usual word order of the most salient items.

When *letter-category message encoding* is used, the initial letter of a code is determined by an organizational scheme that categorizes messages. For example, the messages HELLO, HOW ARE YOU?; IT'S NICE TO SEE YOU; SEE YOU LATER; and GOOD-BYE FOR NOW could be grouped in the category of greetings. The first letter of the code for each of these messages would then be the letter G, which represents the category. The second letter of the code would be the specifier within the category, which is based on the specific content of the message. Thus, the message HELLO, HOW ARE YOU? might be coded GH (for *hello*), and the message IT'S NICE TO SEE YOU might be coded GN (for *nice*).

Alphanumeric Encoding

Alphanumeric message encoding utilizes both letters and numbers. Generally, the alphabetic part of the code refers to the category of messages, such as G for greetings, T for transportation, and F for food. The number is used arbitrarily to specify an individual message within the category. Thus, G1 might refer to HELLO, HOW ARE YOU?; G2 might refer to I HAVEN'T SEEN YOU IN A LONG TIME!; and so forth. It is usually desirable to combine memory- and display-based strategies when this type of code is used.

Numeric Encoding

As noted previously, numeric codes can be used to represent messages as well as words. When numeric codes are used for messages, some type of system is often applied to organize the codes into categories. For example, Edgar is a man with multiple disabilities who uses a large repertoire of numeric codes, organized by the first number. Codes starting with 3 are about wants and needs, and codes starting with 6 are about people. Codes starting with 8 are used sparingly because they are four-letter words or sarcastic comments! Using partner-assisted auditory scanning, Edgar selects numbers up to three digits in length to communicate messages such as GET ME A CUP OF COFFEE (326), CAN YOU PHONE MY MOTHER AND TELL HER TO GET IN TOUCH WITH ME? (611), or EAT MY SOCKS! (825). Although Edgar has memorized more than 900 codes, this is a display-based system for his communication partners, who look up the codes in a codebook in order to translate their meanings. Obviously, such a system requires a good memory on the part of the person who uses it unless they, too, have access to a codebook for reference.

Iconic Encoding

Baker (1982, 1986) proposed an iconic encoding technique referred to as semantic compaction, or Minspeak. In this system, sequences of icons (i.e., pictorial symbols) are combined to store word, phrase, or sentence messages in one of the SGDs constructed to incorporate this technique. The icons used for this encoding are deliberately selected for their rich semantic associations.

Using iconic encoding, an apple icon might be associated with FOOD, FRUIT, SNACK, RED, and ROUND; a sun icon might be used to refer to WEATHER, YELLOW, HOT, SUMMER, and NOON; or a clock icon might represent time, numbers, and a daily schedule. Some of the codes that might by constructed from these three icons are depicted in Figure 3.10. As illustrated in this figure, the message LET'S HAVE A BARBECUE might be encoded with an apple icon (food) and a sun icon (summer, the time of year when many people in North America barbecue). Or, an apple icon might be combined with a clock icon to encode the message IT'S TIME TO HAVE A SNACK. Or a sun icon might be combined with a clock icon to signify IT'S TIME TO CATCH SOME RAYS! Of course, the concepts associated with each icon and the sequences in which multiple icons are combined will vary considerably, depending on an individual's age, prior learning, and cultural-linguistic background, among other factors (van der Merwe & Alant, 2004). Regardless, icon sequences and their corresponding messages are stored in an SGD that the person with CCN activates to produce synthetic speech for the message.

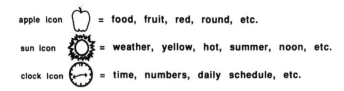

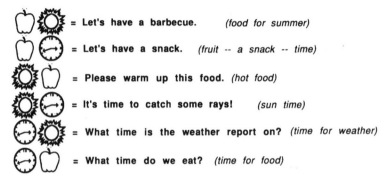

Figure 3.10. Examples of iconic codes. (The Picture Communication Symbols ©1981–2012 by DynaVox Mayer-Johnson LLC. All Rights Reserved Worldwide. Used with permission. Some symbols have been adapted.)

Using iconic encoding, messages can be semantically organized by activities, topics, locations, or other categories to enhance retrieval. The semantic associations with icons assist with retrieval, as do the icon prediction lights available on some SGDs (Beck, Thompson, & Clay, 2000).

Unity is the name of a Minspeak Application Program (MAP) widely used in most English-speaking countries. Other English-language MAPs, as well as MAPs in various languages (e.g., German, Spanish, Dutch, French, Danish, Swedish), are also available. More information about Minspeak, semantic compaction, and MAPs can be found on the Minspeak web site.

Color Encoding

Color has also been utilized to encode messages, usually in conjunction with specifiers such as numbers or symbols. In particular, color encoding is often used to formulate messages for eye-pointing communication systems (Goossens' & Crain, 1986a, 1986b, 1987). Imagine an eye-gaze display with color squares in eight locations, with letters of the alphabet assigned to each square (see Figure 3.11). The person who uses the display might have a series of color and alpha codes to represent various messages that are cataloged in a codebook for partners. For example, the message TURN ON THE MUSIC might be symbolized as BLUE M and the message CAN YOU SCRATCH MY FOOT? might be PURPLE F. In order to select the first message, the AAC communicator would gaze at the blue square on the display and then shift his or her gaze to the letter M. The communication partner would then find the message that corresponds with BLUE M in the decoding book and perform the requested action.

Color coding is often used with other types of access techniques as well, such as communication books and electronic displays. For example, all of the people symbols might be colored with yellow backgrounds, all of the food symbols might be

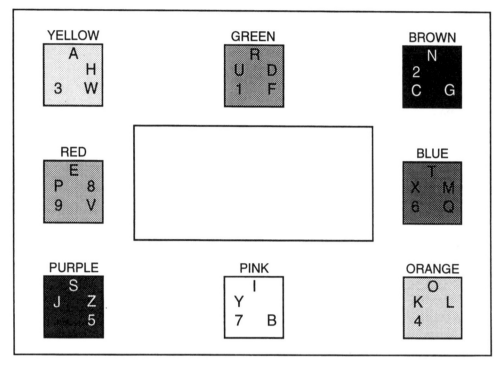

Figure 3.11.   Color eye-gaze display.

colored green, and all of the verbs might be colored blue. However, this practice was called into question in a 2009 study that involved typically developing children, ages 2–5. The results indicated that black-and-white line-drawing symbols on color-coded backgrounds were recognized *less rapidly* than internally colored symbols on white backgrounds were (Thistle & Wilkinson, 2009). This finding suggested that the common practice of using background color coding may interfere with symbol learning for some individuals.

Research on Learnability

Children and adults both with and without disabilities have been involved in studies comparing the learnability of different message encoding techniques after various amounts of training. In general, the results of these studies indicated that 1) both alpha and salient letter codes were recalled most accurately, whereas iconic codes were associated with the least accurate performance, regardless of the amount of training provided (Light & Lindsay, 1992; Light, Lindsay, Siegel, & Parnes, 1990); 2) regardless of the encoding technique, concrete messages (e.g., nouns or simple requests) were easier to learn than abstract ones (e.g., verbs or generic messages such as I DON'T AGREE; Beck & Fritz, 1998; Light, Drager, McCarthy, et al., 2004); 3) there was no apparent learning advantage of personalized codes—those selected by the person with CCN rather than by a researcher or a clinician—over nonpersonalized codes (Light & Lindsay, 1992); and 4) at least for some individuals, long iconic codes were more difficult to learn than short iconic codes (Beck & Fritz, 1998).

Among other things, this research suggests that the learning issues associated with iconic encoding in particular are particularly demanding. Light, Drager, McCarthy, and colleagues (2004) noted that, at the observed rate of learning for iconic encoding found in their study, 4-year-olds would require close to 1,000 instructional sessions and 5-year-olds would require approximately 400–500 sessions to learn even a 1,000-word vocabulary. This is not to say that iconic encoding is not a useful technique; however, it requires significant learning time and places considerable cognitive demand on those who use it, especially in the early stages of acquisition. AAC teams need to be aware of and consider these issues carefully when making decisions about when and with whom specific encoding techniques should be used.

Letter, Word, and Message Prediction

In addition to encoding, message prediction can also be used to enhance communication rates. Prediction involves a dynamic retrieval process in which the options offered to an individual with CCN change according to the portion of a word or message that has already been formulated. Prediction algorithms occur at one or more of three levels: single letter, word, or phrase/sentence.

Single-Letter Prediction

In virtually all languages that can be represented orthographically (i.e., with letter symbols), individual letters of the alphabet do not occur with equal probability. Some letters occur more frequently than others; for example, in English, the letters *e, t, a, o, i, n, s, r,* and *h* occur most frequently, and *z, q, u, x, k,* and *j* occur least frequently (as any frequent watcher of the television show *Wheel of Fortune* is well aware!). Furthermore, orthographic languages are organized so that the probability of the occurrence of a letter in a word is influenced by the previous letter. In English, the most obvious example of this is that the letter *q* is almost always followed by the letter *u*. Some letter combinations occur with more frequency than others. For example, *ch-, -ed, tr-, str-,* and *-tion* are frequent letter combinations in English, whereas combinations such as *sz, jq,* and *wv* occur rarely, if at all.

   Some AAC letter prediction systems use the probability of these individual letters and letter combination relationships so that when a letter is activated, a menu of the letters that are most likely to follow will be offered on a dynamic display. The overall letter display remains intact, but an additional, dynamic line of letter prediction is visible at the top or bottom of the display. Another letter prediction technique involves the use of "ambiguous keyboards" such as those used on modern telephones, in which each key is associated with several letters (e.g., 2 = *abc*, 3 = *def*). One of several available disambiguation algorithms is used so that a computer can predict which of the possible characters on each key was actually intended by the individual (Judge & Landeryou, 2007). Work in this area suggests that if the keyboard arrangement is optimized across a nine-key layout, keystroke efficiencies of up to 91% can be achieved (Lesher, Moulton, & Higginbotham, 1998a; see also Arnott & Javed, 1992, and Levine, Goodenough-Trepagnier, Getschow, & Minneman, 1987). For single-switch scanning, optimized layouts with character prediction can result in switch savings of approximately 37%, a 53% gain over a simple alphabetic matrix. This translates to substantial improvements in text production rates (Lesher, Moulton, & Higginbotham, 1998b). Work in this important area continues through the AAC-RERC (Rehabilitation Engineering Research Center on Communication Enhancement).

Word-Level Prediction

There are three basic types of prediction strategies that can occur at the word level: word prediction, word-pattern prediction, and linguistic prediction. These are discussed in the following sections.

Electronic *word prediction,* in its simplest form, involves a computer program that provides a set of likely words (e.g., words weighted for frequency of use) in response to one's keystrokes. As an example, a typical word prediction system with a dynamic menu display is illustrated in Figure 3.12. Words are displayed in a menu or "window" at the upper right of the screen. The letters selected by the typist determine the specific words that the computer program presents in the menu. For example, imagine that a person wants to type the word LETTER. When the letter L is typed, the six most frequently used words that begin with L appear on the menu. If the word of choice is not included in the listing, the person then types the next letter (E), and six frequently used words that begin with L-E are presented in the menu. This process continues until the desired word is displayed in the menu. When the desired word appears in the menu, the person simply types its associated number code (in this case, the number 3) to insert the word in the text; thus, this form of word prediction can also be thought of as a numeric encoding technique with dynamic displays. In this example, the person has "saved" three keystrokes by using the prediction feature.

The symbols or messages included in word prediction software can be selected in several ways. Some software contains preselected words that are determined by the manufacturer. Other products allow entry of specific words in the menus, and still other programs monitor the communication performance of the person using the system and update the menu content based on frequency of word use. More than one of these options may be available in the same software.

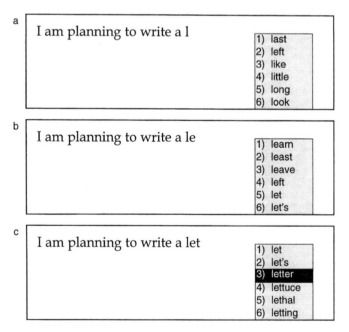

Figure 3.12. Dynamic menu display with word prediction (selecting the word LETTER). a) The screen displays the six most likely words that begin with L when that letter is typed; b) the screen changes to the six most likely words that begin with L-E when the letter E is added; c) the screen changes to the six most likely words that begin with L-E-T when the letter T is added. The number 3 is typed to select the word LETTER.

Some AAC systems predict words based on the *patterns of word combinations* likely to occur in conversational interactions. For example, the probability is high that in the English language, an article such as *a, an,* or *the* will follow a preposition in a prepositional phrase (e.g., *on **the** bed, under **a** tree*). Designers of AAC systems have translated this word-pattern information into prediction algorithms. These systems offer the typist a menu of words that are likely to follow each word that one selects. Thus, the words offered depend not on the letters typed (as with word prediction) but rather on the word patterns in the text. The person simply indicates in some way whether the predicted word is acceptable (e.g., by hitting the space bar) or unacceptable (e.g., by typing the next letter of the desired word).

In an effort to refine prediction strategies, some system designers have included *linguistic prediction* algorithms that contain extensive information about the syntactic organization of the language. The predictions offered to persons who use these systems are based on grammatical rules of the language. For example, if an individual selects a first-person singular noun as the subject of a sentence (e.g., CHRIS, MOM), only verbs that agree in subject and number will be presented as options (e.g., IS, LIKES, IS GOING). If the person selects an article (e.g., A, AN, or THE), the system will predict nouns rather than verbs as the next word, because it is unlikely that a verb will follow an article. Obviously, the algorithms that support linguistic prediction are complex. This type of message enhancement is becoming increasingly available, however, with the decreasing costs of computer processing. Not only does this type of prediction enhance communication rate, but it may also enhance the grammatical performance of some people who have language or learning disabilities.

Letter and/or word prediction is available in many AAC products, such as the WiViK 3 on-screen keyboard, ECO2, and Vanguard Plus (Prentke Romich Company); E Z Keys and Say-it! SAM software (Words+, Inc.); SpeechPRO software (Gus Communication Devices, Inc.); the Allora (ZYGO-USA); the Lightwriter (Toby Churchill Ltd.); and the V, Vmax, EyeMax and DynaWrite (DynaVox).

Phrase- or Sentence-Level Prediction

Several research teams have collaborated to develop computer programs that incorporate sophisticated algorithms for predicting language units longer than single words. Research at the University of Abertay Dundee and the University of Dundee in Scotland (File & Todman, 2002; Todman & Alm, 2003) resulted in development of TALK Boards (DynaVox Mayer-Johnson). This is a set of more than 700 phrase-based communication displays that can be individualized to assist literate individuals with CCN to engage in social conversations. Studies involving individuals with amyotrophic lateral sclerosis (Todman & Lewins, 1996) and cerebral palsy (File & Todman, 2002; Todman, 2000; Todman, Rankin, & File, 1999) suggested that communication rates of between 42 and 64 words per minute may be attained with the TALK software—rates that are 3–6 times faster than those attained with methods that rely on phrase construction during conversation. Meanwhile, researchers at the University at Buffalo and Enkidu Research, Inc., developed Frametalker, an utterance-based communication software program that was designed to support communication in structured situations that are highly sequential and predictable (Higginbotham & Wilkins, 2006). The keystroke savings achievable with Frametalker were far greater than that achievable with other commercially available word-level prediction software programs (Higginbotham, Moulton, Lesher, Wilkins, & Cornish, 2000).

Subsequently, the Scottish and American research teams joined forces to develop a prototype hybrid communication system called Contact that incorporated features of both word- and phrase-level prediction for social and structured conversation (Todman, Alm, Higginbotham, & File, 2008). Ultimately, this collaboration led to the development of a number of utterance-based devices (UBDs) that can be used to support social, transactional communication. UBDs can be used in conjunction with other types of rate enhancement techniques, such as letter and/or word prediction as well as iconic encoding, to enable people with complex communication needs to participate in educational, employment, and social contexts.

A set of more than 700 TALK Boards for conversational use can be used with Board-maker and Speaking Dynamically Pro software and are available from DynaVox Mayer-Johnson. The DynaVox Xpress incorporates UBD design features such as hundreds of preprogrammed phrases; short conversational messages (e.g., "Quickfires," such as YEAH and REALLY?); and sentence fillers called "Slots" that allow variation in intent and meaning without requiring construction of a new sentence word-by-word (e.g., in the sentence I FEEL SAD, the word *sad* is a slot that can be easily replaced with another emotion word). UBD elements have also been included in the DynaVox V and Vmax (J. Higginbotham, personal communication, May 6, 2010).

Prediction Research

Because a number of human factors affect various rate enhancement strategies, the extent to which these strategies actually enhance communication rates may not be as great as that implied by studies that have examined only one factor. As noted previously, the human factors associated with both encoding and predicting appear to vary depending on the interactions between visual monitoring and motor control. For example, in a study that involved six men with cervical spinal cord injuries, Koester and Levine (1996) found that the benefits of any keystroke savings for word prediction were generally offset or even exceeded by the keystroke cost of making each selection. The participants with cervical spinal cord injuries made selections 50% to 70% more slowly with the prediction system than when they used letter-by-letter typing. Much of the extra time was spent searching the word prediction menus, which may explain why participants rated the word prediction strategy as more difficult to use than the letter-only strategy.

Despite the complexity of this issue, there is no doubt that the rate and timing gains made possible by encoding and prediction strategies are potentially very important and can result in substantive interaction gains. In acknowledgment of the complexity of this issue, researchers have proposed several factors that should be considered when evaluating the effectiveness of various rate-enhancement strategies:

- The nature and goal of the communication task itself (Higginbotham, Bisantz, Sunm, Adams, & Yik, 2009)
- The extent to which the vocabulary and/or codes available in the AAC system are contextually relevant and easily accessed (Higginbotham et al., 2009; Venkatagiri, 1993)
- The cognitive processing time needed to decide which selections or motor acts are necessary (Light & Lindsay, 1992)
- The search time (i.e., the amount of time it takes to locate a letter, word, or phrase from a prediction menu; Koester & Levine, 1998)

- The key press time (i.e., the amount of time it takes to activate a key or switch; Koester & Levine, 1998; Venkatagiri, 1999)
- The motor act index (i.e., the number of keystrokes necessary to produce a message; Rosen & Goodenough-Trepagnier, 1981; Venkatagiri, 1993)
- The time or duration of message production (i.e., how long it takes to produce a message; Rosen & Goodenough-Trepagnier, 1981; Venkatagiri, 1993)

Currently, people who use AAC and their facilitators must weigh the relative benefits and costs of available strategies without much assistance from a research base. Research in message encoding and prediction continues to clarify the interactions among various human factors, while development efforts focus on innovative strategies that minimize costs to people with CCN.

QUESTIONS

3.1.   Define unaided symbols, and provide four examples.

3.2.   Define aided symbols, and provide four examples.

3.3.   What is iconicity, and how does it affect symbol learning?

3.4.   What are four factors in addition to iconicity that affect symbol learning, and how do they do so?

3.5.   What manual sign systems are currently used by people who rely on AAC in North America, and what are the advantages and disadvantages of each of them?

3.6.   What does research indicate about the relative learnability of Picture Communication Symbols, Pictograms, and Blissymbols?

3.7.   What are word codes, and what is known about their learnability? Provide three examples of word codes.

3.8.   What are message codes, and what is known about their learnability? Provide three examples of message codes.

3.9.   What is prediction, and how can it be used for rate enhancement?

3.10.   What factors affect the effectiveness of rate enhancement techniques?

CHAPTER 4

Alternative Access

In a middle school in Edmonds, Washington, I received an important lesson in alternative access. Kris, a middle school student with severe athetoid cerebral palsy, was interacting with her mother at the end of a school day. As I observed from across the room, they faced each other. Her mother stared intently at Kris's face and talked quietly throughout the interaction. Kris did not speak at all; however, after watching for a while, it was clear to me that she was communicating a great deal. At the time, I was impressed with the magic of the interaction. Her mother was "reading" Kris's face, as they discussed her homework assignments. I was observing an authentic interaction in which both individuals were contributing, adding their opinions, and even arguing a bit.

My curiosity led me to move behind Kris's mother, where I observed a series of very rapid eye movements that were somehow being translated into letters, words, and eventually messages. As I came to know Kris and her mother better, they let me know the nature of their code. When Kris directed her eyes at her mother's feet, she was communicating the letter F. When she directed her eyes toward her mother's elbow, she signaled an L. When she looked at her mother's nose, she signaled the letter N. After they explained these codes to me, most seemed quite logical. Then, they told me that when Kris raised her eyes and looked slightly to the left, she was signaling the letter Y, referring to the "yellow curtains in the living room," the location where Kris and her father had developed this eye code. Although Kris spelled some words completely, she and her mother were actually co-constructing messages. Kris would begin to spell, and her mother would predict the word or phrase that Kris has started. Kris would accept the prediction with a slight head nod or negate the prediction by shaking her head slightly from side to side. In time, her mother would predict subsequent words in the message before Kris even spelled the first letter. Of course, Kris would confirm or negate her mother's predictions. In addition to eye pointing and word prediction, messages were enhanced with facial expressions and at times vocalizations to add emphasis. We often think of communication as involving a sender (speaker) and a receiver (listener), and while [interactions supported by augmentative and alternative communication (AAC)] may resemble this type of interaction, with familiar communication partners, interaction is more of a "duet" with both people co-constructing the message.

At one point, I attempted to communicate with Kris using her system and quickly found that, although the system was technically inexpensive, it required extensive learning and ability on the part of a communication partner. I didn't have the training and practice to be an effective communication partner for Kris, so her mother and her speech-language pathologist patiently interpreted for me. Kris and I knew the same language, English. She communicated through spelling letter-by-letter, which was the same strategy that I used every day. I knew the words that she spelled, but I was not proficient with the form of alternative access (eye pointing) that she used so efficiently, and I did not know her and her world well enough to contribute much to the co-construction of messages using this strategy. Over the years, Kris learned to use other forms of alternative access so that she could efficiently control electronic AAC communication and computer technology. (D. Beukelman, personal communication, February 2004)

People who speak learn verbal communication skills at an early age. These skills and processes become so automatic that the individual usually has little awareness or understanding of them. Only when beginning to translate spoken language into written form do people realize that messages are coded by combining and recombining a relatively small set of elements. In the English language, people who are literate are able to write nearly anything they wish by combining and recombining a set of 26 letters. A child's task in learning to write is to select the appropriate letters from the set of 26 and to formulate them in a way that meets certain standards of accuracy, intelligibility, and aesthetics. Similarly, people who speak are able to say every word in spoken English by combining approximately 45 sounds. Only those who have difficulty learning to speak need to know that words are made up of sounds and that certain sounds require special attention in order to be spoken correctly.

Communication is based on the selection of one or more types of symbols used alone or in combination to express messages. In natural speech, a person produces messages by combining specific sounds. In writing, a person forms orthographic symbols (i.e., letters) and places them in a systematic order. People who are unable to speak or write through traditional means need alternative strategies in order to communicate. The task of learning alternative access methods is easier to understand when the organization of natural language is first considered. For a person with complex communication needs, learning alternative access methods involves the selection of messages or codes from a relatively small set of possibilities. The person then uses these elements alone or combines them in ways that allow for the communication of a variety of messages. Obviously, the person must present the message to the listener in a way that the listener can understand.

In the past, many people with complex communication needs operated standard communication devices such as typewriters or computers by using headsticks and special keyguards. If the individuals were unable to use these devices, interventionists considered the individuals to be inappropriate candidates for electronic communication options. However, beginning in the 1970s, alternative access options for people who are unable to use standard devices have expanded dramatically. In order to adequately cover the influx of new technology without making this book outdated before it is published, we offer readers only limited examples of communication devices that represent specific access techniques or features. This is in no way meant to imply that the products mentioned in this chapter are the only examples or even the "best" examples of the concepts they illustrate. It is not our intention to offer a comprehensive overview of the latest technology. The resource list included in this book contains the names and addresses of many of the major communication device manufacturers and distributors. In addition, the Barkley AAC Center's web site contains links to most of the commercial companies associated with the AAC field. Readers are also directed to the AAC TechConnect web site, which highlights the features of nearly all commercially available AAC options.

THE SELECTION SET

The *selection set* of an AAC system includes the visual, auditory, or tactile presentation of all messages, symbols, and codes that are available at one time to a person who relies on AAC (see Chapter 3). Most AAC techniques utilize visual displays of items in the selection set. For example, electronic AAC technology is often used by people who have difficulty writing by hand. The displays of such computer devices contain a finite set of symbols that make up the selection set. On standard computer keyboards, for example, these symbols include individual letters of the alphabet; punctuation characters; numbers; and control commands for the device, such as Enter, Control, Tab, and Return. Other individuals use visual displays that consist of pictorial symbols or codes. When visual displays are inappropriate because of an individual's visual impairments, the selection set may be displayed auditorily or tactually. Auditory displays usually involve presentation of the selection set through spoken words or messages. Tactile displays are composed of tactile representations of items in the selection set using real or partial objects, textures, shapes, or raised dots (braille).

The items in a selection set are determined in a number of ways. In the case of standard computer keyboards, the manufacturer assigns the symbols (numbers, letters, punctuation symbols, and commands) to specific locations. It is the task of the individual who relies on this technology to learn what the various symbols mean and how to use them. For many people who use AAC systems, however, symbols and codes may be preprogrammed by the device or application developer or are selected on an individual basis, after the device has been delivered, so that relevant messages can be represented in a way that enables them to be understood and used efficiently.

In 2008 we provided communication support to a man with amyotrophic lateral sclerosis who relied on AAC technology. The upcoming Olympic Games were of particular interest to him because he was a sports enthusiast and, more importantly, because he and his wife had a very close relationship with a woman who was one of the participants on the national volleyball team. Months earlier, this athlete had requested permission from the Olympic Committee to change the number on her jersey from 18 to 12 in honor of this man, who had worn the number 12 throughout years of athletic performance.

During the Olympics he and his wife invited friends to come to their home and join them to watch the coverage on television. In preparation for these evenings, he programmed his AAC device to support his communication. He selected specific messages for a number of different reasons. He needed to communicate some messages immediately if they were to have meaning. For example, the message WHAT A GREAT PLAY! would be meaningful only if he could produce it at exactly the right moment during a fast-moving volleyball game. If he had to spell the message letter by letter, he would not meet this timing requirement, and the message—completed long after the play that elicited the comment—would lose its meaning. He chose to include other phrases (such as greetings, comments, and questions) because he anticipated that they would be used frequently and because he needed to be able to retrieve them in a timely manner that also allowed him to conserve energy. Examples of some of these messages included HI, THANKS FOR COMING, WHAT DID YOU THINK OF THAT?, I THINK THAT THEY WILL PLAY AGAIN ON _____, WOULD YOU LIKE SOMETHING TO EAT (OR DRINK)?, and SEE YOU LATER. He also prepared several pages of jokes, news, and specific thoughts that he wanted to communicate to his friends. In addition, he programmed names of family members, friends, and athletes to enhance communication speed. Finally, alphabet and word prediction functions were available to him so that he could prepare unique messages on a letter-by-letter and word-by-word basis. Obviously, choosing messages to be included in this selection set required cooperative effort by this individual and his facilitators. As is always the case, the symbolization and coding of the messages on his display depended on his unique linguistic and learning abilities as well as on personal preferences.

Types of Selection Set Displays

The display of a selection set depends on the technique and device employed in the AAC application. Displays are generally one of three main types—fixed, dynamic, and hybrid; a fourth type is visual scene displays.

Fixed Displays

The term *fixed display* refers to any display in which the symbols and items are "fixed" in a particular location. Fixed displays (also known as *static displays;* Hochstein, McDaniel, Nettleton, & Neufeld, 2003) are typically used in low-tech communication boards as well as in some digitized speech-generating technology. The number of symbols that a fixed display can include is limited and depends on a person's visual, tactile, cognitive, and motor capabilities. Often, individuals who rely on AAC use a number of different fixed displays in order to accommodate all of their needed vocabulary items. For example, if a person wishes to change the topic of discussion from the Olympic Games to plans for an upcoming holiday, he or she might need to change from the display with sports-related images to one with travel and family vocabulary items.

Because of the obvious limitations imposed by the use of multiple fixed displays (e.g., difficulty with portability, inefficiency), interventionists have made extensive efforts to compensate for the limited symbols or images that a fixed display can contain. One compensatory technique is to organize displays into levels. For example, a communication book in which symbols are arranged topically on pages is an example of a fixed display with several levels (in this case, each page is a different level). Other AAC technology contains visual or auditory selection sets that incorporate levels in their design and operation. Another compensatory technique involves various encoding strategies by which an individual can construct multiple messages by combining one, two, three, or more items (symbols) on a fixed display. Obviously, by coding messages this way, the number of messages a person can communicate can greatly exceed the number of items on the display (see Chapter 3). Most commercial AAC companies sell some technology with fixed displays. Readers are referred to the resource list to review these options.

Dynamic Displays

The term *dynamic display* refers to computer screen displays with electronically produced visual symbols that, when activated, automatically change the selection set on the screen to a new set of programmed symbols. For example, if an individual has access to a dynamic display, he or she might first see a screen displaying symbols related to a number of different conversational topics, such as volleyball, jokes, personal care, news, or family. By touching the volleyball symbol, he or she can activate the screen to display messages related to volleyball. When a break occurs during the volleyball game, he or she can return to the initial screen by touching an appropriate symbol, select a new topic (e.g., jokes, personal care), and have access to a new screen with related vocabulary. A wide variety of commercial AAC products offer dynamic displays. Figure 4.1 provides an example of how a dynamic display operates.

Hybrid Displays

The term *hybrid display* refers to electronic fixed displays with a dynamic component, such as indicator lights that inform the individual which items in the selection set are available for activation. When one activates the first icon in a sequence, indicators on the display screen light up next to each icon that could be chosen next. After a selection is made from one of these options, the lights change to indicate the icons that could come next in the sequence. AAC specialists designed this technique as a memory aid, particularly for individuals who use numerous icon sequences to communicate. In a study that examined this issue, college students without disabilities recalled significantly more codes when icon predictor lights were used compared with when they were not (Beck, Thompson, & Clay, 2000).

Displays containing the letters of the alphabet plus word prediction features can also be viewed as hybrid displays. Typically, the display of the letters of the alphabet is fixed, in that the letters do not change locations. However, the content in the word prediction buttons changes with each keystroke as the language model in the AAC device attempts to predict the words (usually four to eight words) needed to formulate a message. Figure 4.2 illustrates the changes in the word prediction buttons as a message is formulated.

Visual Scene Displays

A *visual scene display* (VSD) is a picture, photograph, or virtual environment that depicts and represents a situation, a place, or an experience. Individual elements such as people, actions, and objects appear within the visual scene (Blackstone, 2004). For example, in a photograph of a birthday party, the people, food, and gifts all appear in a single picture. Messages such as the names of the guests or the food items that are served can then be accessed from the picture. Additional displays, such as those that contain more information about the person having the birthday and his or her family, may also be accessed. While VSDs usually employ dynamic display technology, the concept can also be applied to fixed displays, at least in a limited way; they can also be implemented as a hybrid display. Figure 4.3 illustrates a hybrid version of a VSD with a series of photographs of a vacation. An extended family is shown engaged in actual and implied activities in a variety of settings. In addition to representing individuals and objects, these photographs provide topical information that can guide and support conversational interactions. These pictures function as a dynamic display in that different pictures and associated messages can be displayed. The miniature photographs located along the top, bottom, and right sides of the screen allow navigation to content that represents other communication themes, such as food, shopping, personal care, maps, extended family, and so forth. In many VSD applications these

a

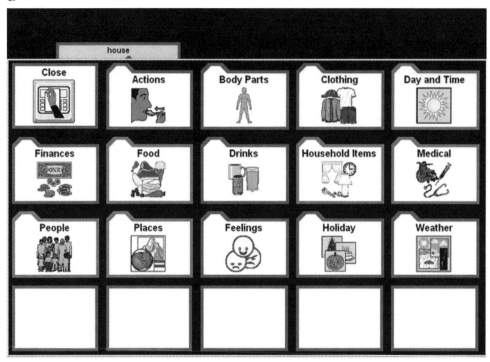

b

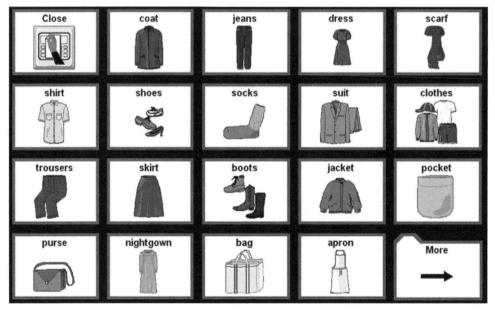

Figure 4.1. Examples of dynamic display screens using DynaVox Vmax. (The Picture Communication Symbols ©1981–2012 by DynaVox Mayer-Johnson LLC. All Rights Reserved Worldwide. Used with permission.)

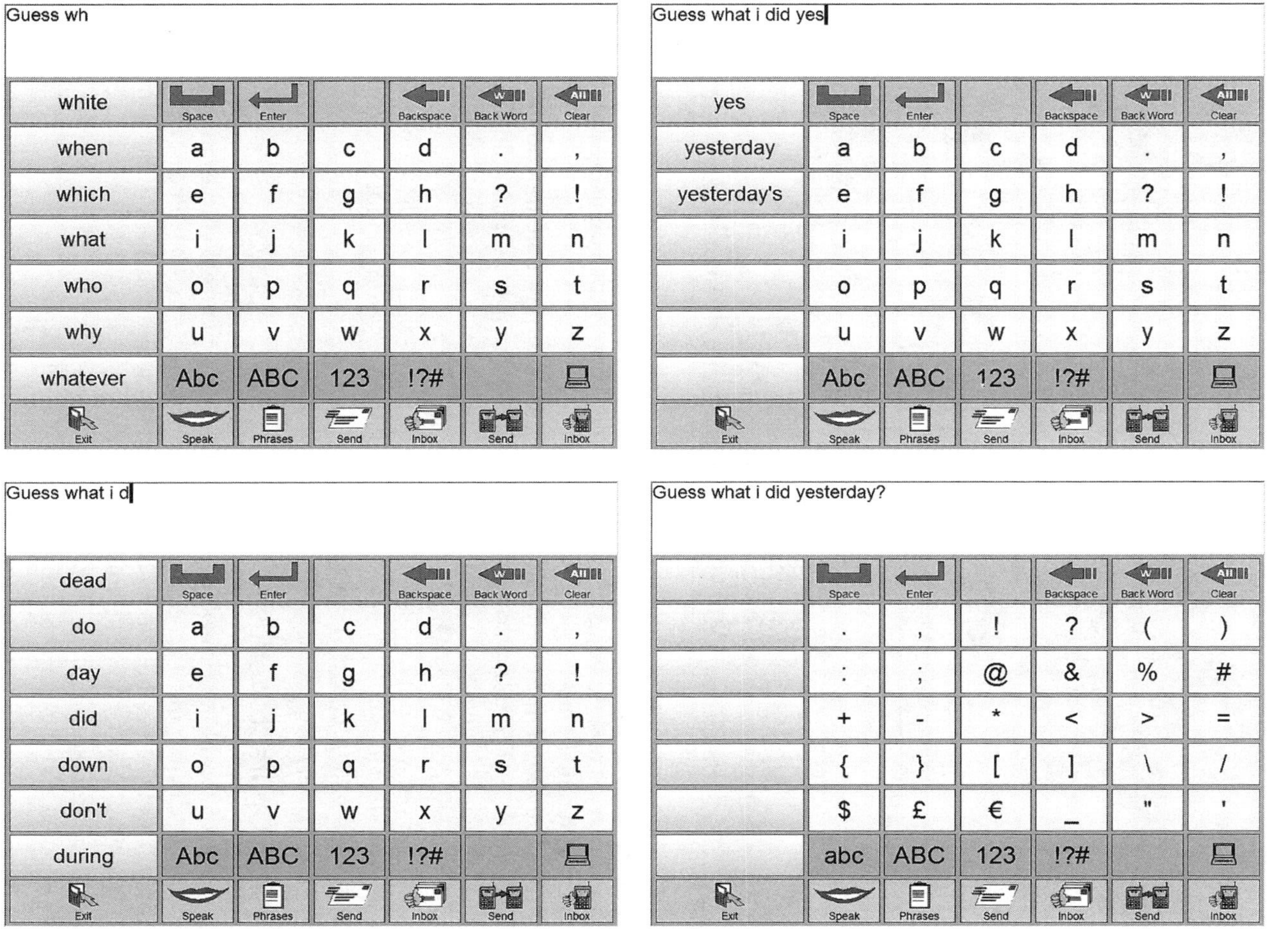

Guess wh

Prediction: white, when, which, what, who, why, whatever

Space	Enter		Backspace	Back Word	Clear
a	b	c	d	.	,
e	f	g	h	?	.
i	j	k	l	m	!
o	p	q	r	s	n
u	v	w	x	y	t
Abc	ABC	123	!?#		z
Speak	Phrases	Send	Inbox	Send	Inbox

Exit

Guess what i did yes|

Prediction: yes, yesterday, yesterday's

Space	Enter		Backspace	Back Word	Clear
a	b	c	d	.	,
e	f	g	h	?	.
i	j	k	l	m	!
o	p	q	r	s	n
u	v	w	x	y	t
Abc	ABC	123	!?#		z
Speak	Phrases	Send	Inbox	Send	Inbox

Exit

Guess what i d|

Prediction: dead, do, day, did, down, don't, during

Space	Enter		Backspace	Back Word	Clear
a	b	c	d	.	,
e	f	g	h	?	.
i	j	k	l	m	!
o	p	q	r	s	n
u	v	w	x	y	t
Abc	ABC	123	!?#		z
Speak	Phrases	Send	Inbox	Send	Inbox

Exit

Guess what i did yesterday?

Space	Enter		Backspace	Back Word	Clear
.	,	!	?	(	)
.	:	&	&	%	#
+	-	*	v	^	=
{	}	[	]	/	/
$	£	€	–	"	'
abc	ABC	123	!?#		
Speak	Phrases	Send	Inbox	Send	Inbox

Exit

Figure 4.2. Alphabet keyboard with word prediction. (The Picture Communication Symbols ©1981–2012 by DynaVox Mayer-Johnson LLC. All Rights Reserved Worldwide. Used with permission.)

79

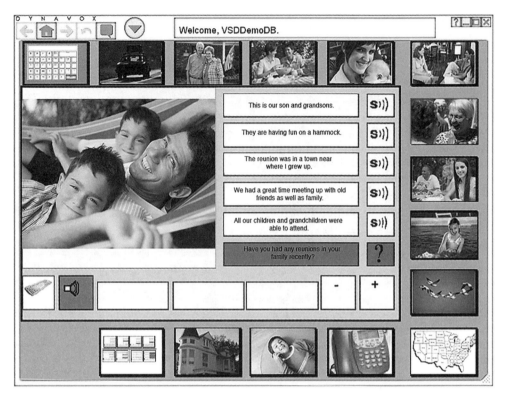

Figure 4.3. Visual scene display.

pictures are fixed and do not change, thereby allowing the person using the displays to access different themes.

VSDs are different from the more typical grid displays that are widely used in AAC technology. The visual scene depicts a set of elements (people, actions, objects) within a coherent, integrated visual image, whereas a grid or matrix display arranges elements in separate boxes usually organized in rows and columns; the elements in the grids may or may not be related. Currently, VSD research and development work is ongoing with children with developmental disabilities, young adults with multiple disabilities, and adults with aphasia.

Physical Characteristics of Selection Set Displays

Regardless of the type of display employed, several physical characteristics of the selection set display must be considered after the messages have been chosen (see Chapter 2) and the symbolization or encoding strategies for the various items have been identified (see Chapter 3). Intervention decisions should be based on a match among the cognitive, language, sensory, and motor capabilities of the individual who relies on AAC and the characteristics of the AAC technique.

Number of Items

Whether a display is visually, auditorily, or tactually based, the actual number of items in the selection set is a compromise involving many factors. The most important factor is the number of messages, symbols, codes, and commands that the individual requires. When symbols other than those representing letters or codes are used exclusively, the size of the selection set increases with the number of messages because there is a one-to-one correspondence between messages and symbols. Thus, 500 symbols are typically required for 500 messages. When VSDs are used, more than one message may be integrated into a single photograph or picture, but multiple pictures will still be needed to represent various situations or topics. In contrast, the number of items in the selection set may be greatly reduced when encoding strategies are used, depending on the number of codes used. Thus, if a large number of codes are used, the display may contain fewer items than if a small number of codes are used. This is because each item can be used in multiple ways to make up numerous codes; for example, hundreds of two-letter codes can be constructed by combining each of the 26 letters in the alphabet with the other 25.

Size

Intervention teams should consider two issues related to size when making selection set decisions: individual item size and overall display size. For visual displays, the actual size of the symbols or messages on the display is determined by an individual's visual capabilities, the motor access technique employed, the type of symbol, and the number of items to be displayed. For many individuals, visual capabilities determine individual item size; this factor is discussed in more detail in Chapter 6. For others, motor control is the critical variable because items need to be sufficiently large to allow accurate and efficient selection.

The overall size of the visual display also involves compromises among the number of items that must be displayed, the size of individual items, the spacing of items, mounting and portability factors, and the physical capabilities of the person using AAC. For example, if the technology is to be carried around by the individual, its shape and weight must be manageable and nonfatiguing, and its exact dimensions will depend on the person's physical capabilities. If the individual uses a wheelchair, the AAC display must not be so large that it obscures vision for guiding the chair. If the individual selects items using finger pointing, head tracking, or eye tracking, the overall size of the display must accommodate the individual's range of movement or some items will be inaccessible.

The physical size of AAC technology varies considerably. During the past few years more and more AAC options have been developed for mobile technology originally designed to support communication, games, calendars, music, and even global positioning applications. These technologies have been attractive to a range of people with AAC needs because the technology is small, lightweight, and "typical" in that it is used by most people without disabilities. For some with AAC needs, such technology is functional, but for others, the size makes it inadequate for them.

For auditory displays, used primarily by people with visual conditions, the size of the display is determined by the individual's memory and ability to retain the organizational scheme of the display. When large auditory displays are employed, individuals need to remember that a particular item will eventually be displayed (i.e., announced) if they wait long enough. When multilevel displays are available in electronic auditory scanners, the person must be able to remember the categorical scheme used for organization. For example, if messages are organized by main topic (e.g., food, drinks, places, people), the person must remember that COKE is a message under DRINK, whereas SHOPPPING MALL is stored under PLACES. If the display contains more than two levels, this categorical scheme can become even more complex, and COKE might be a message under SODA POP, which is a subcategory of DRINKS.

For tactile displays, the size of the selection set depends on tactile recognition capabilities. Some individuals, such as those who use braille, require very little information to recognize options presented tactually, whereas others with less cognitive or tactile ability may require larger tactile symbols or actual objects.

Spacing and Arrangement of Items

Spacing and arrangement of items on a visual or tactile selection display is determined largely by the visual and motor control capabilities of the individual. For example, some individuals are better able to discriminate among items on the display if the items are widely separated and surrounded by a large empty area. For others, performance may be improved if the space surrounding the items is colored to contrast with the rest of the communication board. Still other individuals may have field cuts (loss of vision on one side caused by brain injury) or blind spots that require irregular spacing arrangements to match their visual capabilities. Assessors need to make determinations such as these on an individual basis (see Chapters 6, 15, and 17).

The motor control profile of each person also influences the spacing arrangement. Many people with physical disabilities who use AAC systems have better control of one hand than the other. The items on the display should be positioned accordingly to enhance access. For example, Figure 4.4 illustrates a communication board in which frequently used items are displayed to be most accessible to the individual's right hand, which has better motor control. In addition, the size of the items in the area in which this person has the best motor control (i.e., the right side of the board) is smaller than in areas of reduced motor control (i.e., the left side of the board).

Another example of a communication board display, a curved array, is provided in Figure 4.5. This arrangement is designed to accommodate the motor control capabilities of a person using a headstick. By positioning the items in an arch, the forward and backward movements of the head and neck are minimized, compared with the

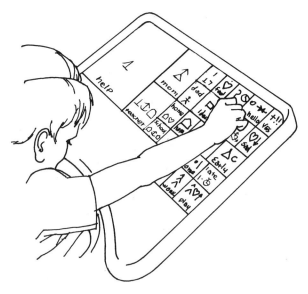

Figure 4.4. Communication board with frequently used items displayed to be most accessible to the individual's dominant hand.

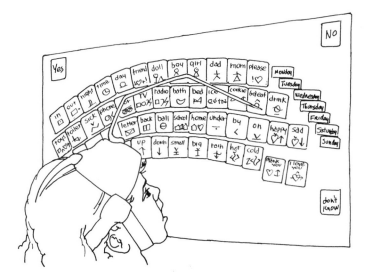

Figure 4.5. Communication board display designed to accommodate the use of a headstick.

movements that would be needed to reach items in a square or rectangular display. With the availability of head- and eye-tracking strategies, the use of headsticks to access AAC technology has decreased. However, some people who rely on AAC continue to use this method.

Orientation of the Display

Orientation refers to the position of the display relative to the floor. The orientation of a visual or tactile display is dependent on a person's postural, visual, and motor control capabilities. Visual and motor capabilities are the most critical in a direct selection display, in which one needs to be able to point in some way to items on the display. If a scanning approach is used, visual and postural factors will probably determine the orientation because these are critical skills for the switch activation required by this technique. These issues are detailed later in this chapter.

A visual or tactile display mounted on a table or wheelchair tray that is horizontal to the floor provides considerable arm and hand support, as well as stabilization, which can be helpful if weakness, tremor, or extraneous movements are present. This display orientation requires that the person maintain upright posture (either independently or with adaptive equipment) while viewing and using the display. Alternatively, a display positioned at a 30°–45° angle to the floor provides a compromise for many people with physical disabilities. This orientation allows an individual to see the display clearly but avoids the neck flexion required by the horizontal display, while still providing some degree of hand and arm support and stability. Many people with very limited motor control due to weakness or extraneous movements may experience difficulty using a display that is oriented in this way. For these individuals, mobile arm supports may be used to elevate their arms and hands so that they can access a slanted display. Finally, displays that are used in combination with light or optical pointers are usually oriented at a 45°–90° angle to the floor, again depending on the individual's vision, motor control, and posture. When a display is positioned at a 45°–90° angle, care must be taken not to obstruct the person's vision of other people or for other activities, such as operating a wheelchair or viewing instructional materials. For those who rely on head- or eye-tracking strategies, the display is usually positioned at nearly a 90° angle.

SELECTION TECHNIQUES

The term *selection technique* refers to the way an individual who relies on an AAC system selects or identifies items from the selection set. People who use AAC technology may choose from two principal approaches to item selection: direct selection and scanning.

Direct Selection

With *direct selection* techniques, the person who relies on AAC indicates the desired item directly from the selection set. Most people have experienced several types of direct selection. When typing, individuals are able to directly choose or activate any item on the typewriter or computer keyboard by depressing a key. Even those who are single-finger typists have the option to select any key that they wish. In addition, most people have used natural speech and gestures, and many have either observed or used manual signing. These modes are direct selection techniques because gestures or signs are directly selected to communicate specific messages from a large set of options.

Direct Selection Options

Direct selection via finger pointing or touching is the most common selection method. Some individuals employ an optical pointer, light pointer, head tracker, or eye tracker to select items; point their gaze in order to indicate choices (see Kris's story at the beginning of this chapter); or even use speech recognition (Fager, Beukelman, Jakobs, & Hossum, 2010). Options for direct selection are reviewed briefly in the following sections.

Physical Contact   With many nonelectronic AAC options, individuals select items with physical contact rather than pressure or depression. For example, when a person uses a communication board (or book), items are identified from the selection set by touching them. Because electronic activation is not involved, pressure is not required. New mobile technology and tablet computers, such as the iPad, are activated by touch of a particular duration or gestural movement.

Physical Pressure or Depression   Individuals may activate many AAC devices by depressing a key or a pressure-sensitive surface. A standard keyboard requires this activation mode, as does the touch pad (i.e., membrane switch) on many microwave ovens and AAC technology. If a device requires pressure for activation, an individual usually generates the pressure with a body part, such as a finger or a toe, or with some device that is attached to the body, such as a headstick or a splint mounted on the hand or arm. The movement of the body part or body-part extension (e.g., a headstick) must be sufficiently controllable so that only a single item is activated with each depression. Facilitators can usually help individuals set pressure-sensitive keys and touch pads to a variety of pressure thresholds that enhance accurate activation.

Pointing (No Contact)   A person does not always need to make actual physical contact when selecting an item from the selection set. For example, with eye pointing, tracking, or gazing, one looks at an item long enough for the communication partner to identify the direction of the gaze and confirm the selected item. Many people who are unable to speak as a result of physical impairments employ eye pointing because these individuals often retain relatively accurate eye movements. In addition, eye pointing is often employed by young children who have not yet learned other communication techniques, as well as by those with poor positioning, chronic fatigue, or ongoing medical conditions that prevent them from utilizing more physically demanding options. Some nonelectronic eye-gaze communication techniques are quite advanced and incorporate complex encoding strategies (Goossens' & Crain, 1987). Figures 4.6 and 4.7 illustrate an eye-linking display and an eye-gaze communication vest, respectively.

A number of eye-tracking technologies have been developed to access AAC technology. EyeMax (DynaVox), ECOpoint (Prentke Romich Company), My Tobii (Tobii ATI), and EyeTech's vision tracking devices and Quick Glance software (EyeTech Digital Systems) are examples of this technology. In general, these products provide cursor control in response to eye movement. The AAC-RERC (Rehabilitation Engineering Research Center on Communication Enhancement) webcast *Supporting Communication of Individuals with Minimal Movement* demonstrates the use of eye-tracking AAC technology. Additional information about these technologies can be accessed at the web sites included in the resource list in this book.

Those who use AAC strategies can also use pointing without contact with an optical or light-generating (or laser-generating) technology that is mounted on the head in some way (e.g., on a headband, attached to eyeglasses or a cap; see Figure 4.8) or held in the hand. This technique can be used with both high- and low-tech AAC options. For example, an individual who uses a communication board can indicate a choice by directing a light or laser beam toward the desired item. Individuals can

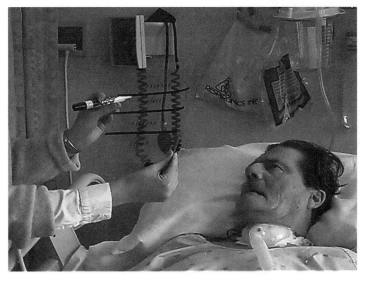

Figure 4.6.   Eye-linking display.

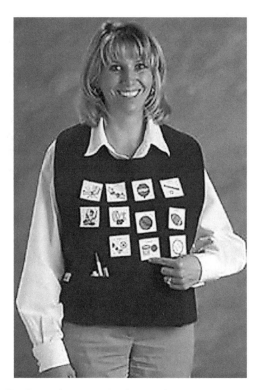

Figure 4.7. Eye-gaze vest. (The Picture Communication Symbols ©1981–2012 by DynaVox Mayer-Johnson LLC. All Rights Reserved Worldwide. Used with permission.)

also activate electronic AAC technology with optical or light pointing. Technology that incorporates this selection technique electronically monitors the position of the light beam or optical sensor and selects an item if the beam or sensor remains in a specific location for a period of time. The two primary motor requirements for use of this technique are the ability to direct the light beam to a desired item and the ability to maintain the direction for a prescribed period of time. Because light pointers and optical sensors are usually mounted on the head, individuals must have head control without excessive tremor or extraneous movements for accurate and efficient use of these options.

Individuals can also make selections with sonar or infrared technology instead of direct physical contact. A receiving unit positioned near a computer screen displays infrared signals that are imperceptible to human senses. The person using AAC wears a sensor (usually referred to as a head tracker) that is mounted on the forehead or eyeglasses and is directed to symbols on the screen through fine head movements. These movements control the cursor on the computer screen to indicate items from the selection set. The motor control requirements for infrared technology are similar to those for light pointing and optical technology.

The HeadMouse Extreme (Origin Instruments), SmartNav (NaturalPoint), and AccuPoint (InvoTek, Inc.) are examples of sonar or infrared technologies for direct selection typically controlled by head movement. Fitzgerald, Sposato, Politano, Hetling, and O'Neill (2009) compared the performance of three head-controlled mouse emulators under three different lighting conditions. They report that, in general, each mouse emulator performed consistently across lighting conditions; however, under one of the lighting conditions there was some difference in performance accuracy.

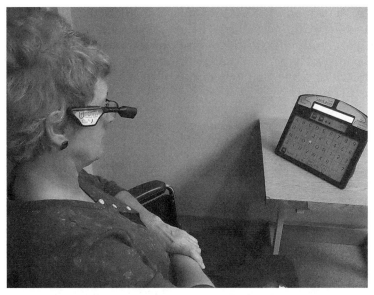

Figure 4.8.   Head-mounted laser pointer. (GEWA Laser Pointer sold by ZYGO-USA; http://www.zygo-usa.com.)

Speech Recognition   In the past, individuals who were typical speakers but were unable to write or control a conventional computer keyboard (e.g., because of spinal cord injury) opted primarily for voice recognition strategies. AAC researchers and developers continue to focus on voice recognition as an alternative access selection mode for people who can produce consistent speech patterns even though their speech is mildly or moderately distorted. At the time this book was written, the use of speech recognition strategies by people with speech impairments has received considerable research attention but has not achieved routine acceptance to support those who rely on AAC technology (Fager et al., 2010); therefore, we do not discuss speech recognition strategies in this edition.

Direct Selection Activation Strategies

When an individual uses direct selection to choose an item from an electronic display, he or she must then activate the item so that the AAC technology recognizes and translates it into usable output. Because many people who rely on AAC have limited motor control capabilities, they must employ alternative activation strategies. For example, some individuals may be unable to isolate a pressure key on a selection display without dragging their fingers across the display, inadvertently activating other items. Several electronic options can compensate for these difficulties.

Timed Activation   Most electronic technology that allows for direct selection offers the option of timed activation. This access strategy requires one to identify an item on the display in some way (e.g., through physical contact, by shining a light or a laser beam, or by directing one's eye gaze) and then sustain the contact (or dwell on a location) for a predetermined period of time in order for the selection to be recognized by the device. Timed activation allows individuals to move their fingers, headsticks, light beams, or cursors across the display surface without activating each item that they encounter. The length of the "dwell time" can be adjusted to accommodate individual abilities and situations. The clear advantage of this strategy is that it reduces both inadvertent activations and motor control demands.

Release Activation   Release activation is another activation strategy available in some electronic AAC technology. The individual can use release activation only with displays controlled by direct physical contact, either with a body part or with an extension of some type. The strategy requires the person to contact the display, for example, with a finger, and then retain contact until the desired item is located. The individual can move his or her finger anywhere on the display without making a selection as long as direct contact with the display is maintained. To select an item, the person releases contact from an image (symbol) on the display. Again, the contact time can be adjusted to accommodate individual abilities and needs. The advantages of this strategy are that it allows an individual to use the display for hand stability and that it minimizes errors for those who move too slowly or inefficiently to benefit from timed activation.

Filtered or Averaged Activation   Some people who rely on AAC are able to select a general area on the display but have difficulty maintaining adequately steady contact with a specific item for selection. In other words, it is impossible to set a sufficiently low activation time to accommodate their selection ability. Often, these individuals are able to use head-mounted light or optical pointers but do not have the precise and controlled head movements needed for accurate selection. Technology with filtered or averaged activation "forgives" (i.e., ignores) brief movements away from a specific item by sensing the amount of time the pointer spends on each item in the general area of an item. The device averages this accumulated information over a short period of time and activates the item to which the light or optical device was pointed the longest. To personalize the system, facilitators can set the amount of time that elapses prior to activation.

When selecting an access method for a person who requires AAC, care must be taken to match the access features with the capability of the individual. Some AAC applications for mobile technology support the access options discussed above, whereas others do not.

Scanning

Some individuals who require AAC technology are unable to choose items directly from the selection set. Although this inability can occur for many reasons, the most common reason is lack of motor control. In such situations, the items in the selection set are displayed either by a facilitator (i.e., a trained communication partner) or by electronic technology in a predetermined configuration. The individual must wait while the facilitator or electronic device scans through undesired items before reaching the item of choice. At this point, the person who relies on AAC indicates in some way that the desired item has been presented. This type of item selection is called *scanning*. Typically, those who rely on scanning access involving an AAC device accept the preferred item by activating a switch. Beukelman, Garrett, and Yorkston (2007, Form 4.3) describe and illustrate a range of different switches.

In 2010, Ball and colleagues noted the impression that people who rely on AAC are choosing scanning access much less frequently than they did a decade ago, as the head- and eye-tracking access strategies are chosen more frequently. The cognitive load associated with scanning of AAC displays is considerable, and the learning requirements are extensive. Nevertheless, we discuss various aspects of scanning selection in the following sections.

Scanning Patterns

The configuration in which items in the selection set are presented is one important feature of scanning. It is important that items in the selection set be identified systematically and predictably so that the intention of the individual who uses AAC and the actions of the facilitator or device are coordinated. Three primary selection set patterns are *circular, linear,* and *group–item scanning* techniques.

Circular Scanning   Circular scanning is the least complicated pattern that electronic devices use to present items in the selection set (see Figure 4.9). The technology displays individual items in a circle and scans them electronically, one at a time, until the individual stops the scanner and selects an item. The scanner is usually a sweeping hand like the big hand on a clock or takes the form of individual lights near each item in the selection set. Although circular scanning is visually demanding, it is relatively easy to master cognitively and for this reason may be introduced first to children or beginning AAC communicators. Horn and Jones (1996) provided a case report of a 4-year-old child involving circular scanning. They found that, for this child, scanning was more difficult than direct selection via headlight pointing, even though assessment information suggested that scanning would be the more appropriate option.

Linear Scanning   In visual linear scanning, a cursor light or an arrow moves across each item in the first row, each item in the second row, and each item in the

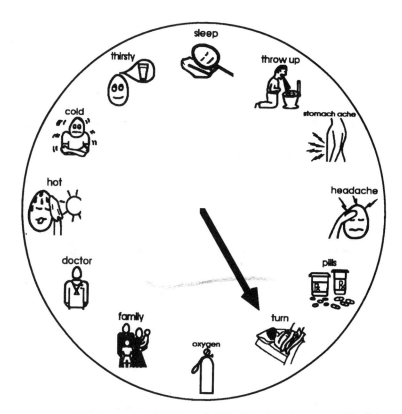

Figure 4.9.   A circular scanning display for an individual in an intensive care unit. (The Picture Communication Symbols ©1981–2012 by DynaVox Mayer-Johnson LLC. All Rights Reserved Worldwide. Used with permission.)

subsequent row, until an item is selected. Figure 4.10 illustrates a visual display in which items in the selection set are arranged in three lines or rows. In auditory linear scanning, a synthetic voice or a human facilitator announces items one at a time until a section is made. For example, the facilitator might ask, "Which shirt do you want to wear today? the red one? the blue one? the striped one? the purple and green one?" until the individual indicates that the desired choice has been named. Linear scanning, although more demanding than circular scanning, is straightforward and easy to learn. Nevertheless, because items are presented one at a time in a particular order, it may be inefficient if the selection set contains many items.

Light (1993) reported a case study documenting a developmentally based instructional protocol to teach automatic linear scanning to a 5-year-old child with severe physical and communication disabilities. Previously, the child had not learned scanning from instruction focused primarily on the motor control process. Analyses of the performances of individuals who used scanning suggested that the task of automatic linear scanning involves coordination of the relation of the cursor (light) to the target symbol in the array and the relation of the switch to the selection process. Instruction was effective in providing the conceptual bridge that enabled this child to progress from a partial representation of the task (relation of the switch to the selection process) to the representation that allowed her to use the scanning technique.

Group–Item Scanning   AAC technology designers have developed a number of group–item scanning approaches in an effort to enhance scanning efficiency. Basically, group–item scanning involves identifying a group of items and then eliminating options gradually until a final selection is made. For example, in auditory group–item scanning, the device or facilitator might ask, "Do you want food items? drink items? personal care items?" and continue until the individual identifies the group or topic. Then, the device or facilitator recites a predetermined list of options within that group. For example, if the individual selects DRINK ITEMS, the facilitator might ask, "Water? Pop? Tea? Beer?" until a choice is made. Clearly, this would be more efficient than if the facilitator first went through a list of food items and then repeated the process for drink items before the selection could be made.

One of the most common visual group–item strategies is row–column scanning (see Figure 4.11). Each row on the visual display is a group. The rows are each elec-

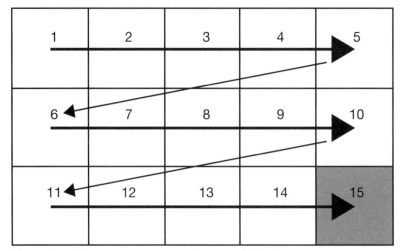

Figure 4.10. A linear scanning display with three rows of symbols.

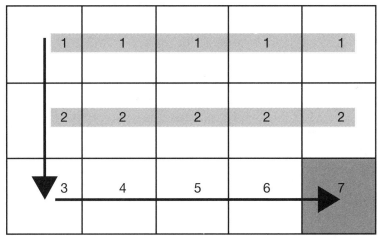

Figure 4.11. A row–column scanning display.

tronically highlighted in presentation until the target item is selected. Then individual items in that row are highlighted one at a time until the scanning is stopped at the specific item desired.

There are also a number of row–column scanning variations. To increase efficiency, sophisticated AAC technologies that contain many items in the selection set often employ group–row–column scanning, a common variation of row–column scanning. Group–row–column scanning requires one to make three selections. First, the entire display is highlighted in two or three groups. When the person identifies a group—for example, the group at the top of the screen—each row in that group is scanned. When the individual selects a specific row, the scanning pattern changes to highlight each item in that row. Finally, the person identifies the desired item within a row.

Scanning Timing and Speed

In addition to customizing the scanning pattern, the speed and timing of scanning must be personalized according to each individual's physical, visual, and cognitive capabilities. When nonelectronic scanning is used, a facilitator can announce the items audibly or point to them on a communication display (e.g., an alphabet or communication board) as quickly or as slowly as the individual requires. The facilitator can usually observe the individual's response patterns and adjust the speed of scanning accordingly. When electronic equipment is used, however, scanning speed must be individualized for or by the person because a facilitator is not involved in the scanning presentation. Most electronic AAC technology has sufficient scanning speed options to meet individual needs.

Selection Control Techniques

People who use auditory scanning or electronic visual scanning must be able to select an item while a device systematically scans items in a display. Generally, three selection control techniques are used: directed (inverse) scanning, automatic (regular or interrupted) scanning, and step scanning.

Directed (Inverse) Scanning   In directed scanning, the indicator or cursor begins to move when the person activates (e.g., holds down) a switch of some type. As long as the switch is activated, the indicator moves through the preset scanning pattern (e.g., circular, linear, row–column). The selection is made when the switch is released. Directed scanning is particularly useful for people who have difficulty activating switches but who can sustain activation once it occurs and can release the switch accurately.

Automatic (Regular or Interrupted) Scanning   In this type of scanning, the movement of the indicator or cursor is automatic and continuous, according to a preset pattern (e.g., circular, linear, row–column). The person activates a switch to stop the indicator at the group or item of choice in order to make a selection. This type of scanning is particularly useful for people who are able to activate a switch accurately but who have difficulty sustaining activation or releasing the switch. This type of scanning is also employed when the display presentation is auditory. A facilitator might recite names of movies, for example, until the individual stops (or interrupts) the recitation at the one he or she wishes to see.

Step Scanning   In step scanning, the indicator or cursor moves through a preset selection pattern, one step (i.e., one group or item) at a time for each activation of the switch. In other words, there is a one-to-one correspondence between cursor movement and switch activation. In order to select a specific item, the individual simply stops activating the switch for an extended period of time or activates a second switch that indicates that the displayed item is the desired selection. Step scanning is often used by individuals who have severe motor control or cognitive restrictions or who are just beginning to learn to operate electronic scanners. Because step scanning requires repeated, frequent switch activations, it is often fatiguing for complex AAC applications.

FEEDBACK

The two primary purposes of feedback from communication technology are 1) to let the individual using AAC know that an item has been selected from the selection display (activation feedback) and 2) to provide the individual with information about the message that has been formulated or selected (message feedback). Some communication devices provide neither type of feedback, some provide one but not the other, and some provide both. Feedback can be visual, auditory, tactile, or proprioceptive.

Activation Feedback

Lee and Thomas defined activation feedback as "the information sent back to the person, upon activation of the input device" (1990, p. 255). Activation feedback differs from message feedback in that it informs the individual that activation has occurred but usually does not provide information about which symbol or message has been selected. It differs from output in that it provides information that is useful to the person operating the technology but not, generally, to the communication partner.

Activation feedback must occur in a sensory modality that is within the person's capabilities. Auditory activation feedback may be a beep, click, or other generic sound produced by an electronic communication device. Nonelectronic displays do not provide auditory activation feedback. Visual activation feedback on an electronic communication device may be provided via a light flash after a switch has been activated or via an area or symbol flash on a backlit display. Visual activation feedback on a nonelectronic display may consist of seeing one's body part contact the device.

Contact with the textured surface of symbols on either electronic or nonelectronic devices provides tactile activation feedback. Finally, proprioceptive activation feedback is obtained when the individual applies pressure against a resistant surface (a switch or key) that moves when the pressure threshold is exceeded. Persons who produce manual signs and gestures also get proprioceptive and kinesthetic feedback from the position and movement of their hands in space.

Message Feedback

Message feedback provides information about the symbol or message itself after it has been formulated. Unlike activation feedback, message feedback may be useful to the communication partner as well, although this is of secondary importance. For example, when an individual interacts with a keyboard that echoes each letter as it is typed via synthetic speech, the echo provides message feedback. The echo may also serve as output for the communication partner, if he or she can hear the echo and chooses to listen, but this output is not its primary purpose. Similarly, most dynamic display devices provide the person using AAC technology with message feedback in the form of a screen display of symbols as they are activated in a sequence.

Message feedback, like activation feedback, is available through auditory, visual, tactile, or proprioceptive modalities. Auditory message feedback may be provided on an electronic device as either a key echo (e.g., a speech synthesizer announces each alphabet letter as it is activated when using orthographic symbols) or a word/phrase echo (e.g., a speech synthesizer says individual words or phrases in a message as they are produced). With nonelectronic displays (both aided and unaided), the communication partner often provides auditory message feedback (sometimes referred to as "partner reauditorization"; Bedrosian, Hoag, Calculator, & Molineux, 1992) by echoing each letter, word, or phrase as it is produced or selected.

Visual message feedback may be provided on electronic devices as computer screen displays of letters, words, or phrases as they are selected. Many communication devices and software products provide message feedback in screen displays of symbol sequences as each symbol is selected. Visual message feedback from aided and unaided nonelectronic devices is generally identical to activation feedback—the individual sees the symbol he or she produces. AAC applications do not provide tactile and proprioceptive message feedback, with the exception of writing aids used by people with visual impairments.

MESSAGE OUTPUT AND INPUT

Those who rely on AAC, like all people who communicate, are both the senders and the receivers of messages during communicative interactions. In this section, the term *message output* refers to the information that they send to their communication partners. Examples of message output modes include synthetic speech, print, gestures, manual signs, and nonelectronic aided symbols. Conversely, the term *message input* refers to the information that people who rely on AAC receive from others. Message input usually takes the form of natural speech, gestures, and vocalizations (assuming that most partners do not have disabilities), although input may also take the form of written or printed materials (e.g., letters, notes) or manual signs (see Chapters 15 and 16).

It is important to distinguish message input and output from *feedback*, which is primarily provided during rather than at the end of message construction and was discussed in the previous section. Feedback lets the individual know that an item has been selected and, in some cases, also provides him or her with information about the selected item.

For some individuals, the input mode through which they receive messages may be as much of an intervention concern as the output mode by which they send messages. For example, Beukelman and Garrett noted that "the incidence of auditory reception problems among the adult population with aphasia is large" (1988, p. 119), and these individuals may need augmented input in the form of gestures, pictures, or writing in addition to natural speech. People with impairments that affect cognitive, sensory, and linguistic processing (e.g., intellectual disability, traumatic brain injury) may also require and benefit from augmented input techniques. The following sections review the major types of message output and input used in AAC applications in terms of general characteristics and the learning and performance abilities that they require.

Synthesized Speech

Synthetic speech technology continues to improve. People who once had no choice but to use devices that produced robotic, barely intelligible voices are now able to choose from an array of natural-sounding male, female, and childlike voices in dozens of languages! At this time, minimal public information about the intelligibility or acceptability of these new voices is available. Readers are encouraged to follow research reports to learn about the characteristics of these new voices. Commercial companies provide web access to samples of their synthesized speech products. The main types of synthesized speech are described in the following sections.

 Speech technology research can be found in journals such as *Augmentative and Alternative Communication, Assistive Technology,* and the *International Journal of Speech Technology.*

Types of Synthesized Speech and Speech Communication

Text-to-Speech   A common method used to generate synthetic speech in AAC devices is text-to-speech synthesis. The approach generally involves three steps. First, text (words or sentences) that has been entered into an AAC device or retrieved from its memory as codes is transformed into phonemes and allophones. Second, the device uses the stored speech data to generate digital speech signals that correspond to phonetic representations of the text. Finally, the device converts the digital signals to analog speech waveforms that listeners can interpret and understand.

Rule-generated speech involves a flexible mathematical algorithm representing the rules for pronunciation, pronunciation exceptions, voice inflections, and accents. In standard text-to-speech synthesis applications, the algorithms generate speech sounds that reflect the phonetic representation of the text. The device does not store speech itself in digitized form; rather, the device generates speech for each utterance by the rule-based algorithm. A complete discussion of the algorithms used for these applications is beyond the scope of this text (see Venkatagiri & Ramabadran, 1995, for additional information).

A second type of text-to-speech synthesis uses diphone-based strategies to produce speech. Because the diphones are extracted from carrier words recorded by natural speakers, the resulting speech is intended to be more natural sounding than conventional text-to-speech synthesis. New diphonic voices continue to be introduced regularly, but these developments are beyond the scope of this book.

There is growing interest in personalizing text-to-speech voices by recording the speech of an individual while he or she can still speak and then building a speech synthesis model using that speech sample. In this way, the speech produced by the synthesizer would sound somewhat like the voice of the individual. Whether or not this strategy becomes commonplace in AAC technology remains to be seen.

Digitized Speech   Digitized speech, also called waveform coding, is another type of electronic speech used in AAC technology. This method consists primarily of natural speech that has been recorded, stored, and reproduced. In digitized speech, natural speech is recorded with a microphone and passed through a series of filters and a digital-to-analog converter (Cohen & Palin, 1986). When reproduced, the speech is a close replica of the original speech entry. Digitized speech is stored in word or message form and must be retrieved as a word or message. Therefore, it cannot be used to convert text into speech.

For those with a particular interest in the role of speech output in AAC, the March 2003 issue of *Augmentative and Alternative Communication* contains some excellent summary articles by Blischak, Lombardino, and Dyson (2003); Koul (2003); Schepis and Reid (2003); and Schlosser (2003d).

Only a few studies have been conducted regarding the intelligibility of digitized speech. Because it is a digital recording of natural speech, the assumption has been that the intelligibility of digital voices rivals those of natural speech. However, in practice, researchers and clinicians are realizing that that is not always true. Differences may occur in the quality of the digital-to-analog converters, playback mechanisms, or other components that produce better speech in some systems than in others. This evaluation awaits future comparative research.

Advantages and Disadvantages of Synthesized Speech

The major advantages of intelligible synthesized speech are that it 1) may significantly reduce the communication partner's burden in the interaction because interpretation of the output requires only the ability to understand spoken language, 2) provides information in a mode that is relatively familiar and nonthreatening to communication partners, 3) allows communication even with communication partners who are not literate (as long as they understand spoken language) and with those who have visual impairments, 4) allows the person using AAC to send messages without first obtaining his or her partner's attention through some other mode, and 5) allows communication to occur at a distance. Telephone interactions can also be enhanced by the use of synthetic speech. For example, Drager, Hustad, and Gable (2004) reported that synthetic voices were more understandable over typical audio speakers and over the telephone than the speech (which was 85% intelligible) of a 45-year-old woman with cerebral palsy was.

To illustrate the advantages of high-quality synthetic speech output, consider Ahmad, a boy with severe disabilities who is included in a general kindergarten classroom of 30 children, has limited receptive language skills, and does not speak. If he uses an unaided AAC technique such as manual signing or a low-tech aided system such as a communication board, his teacher and his classmates must also learn to use and understand the symbols in that system. In fact, if Ahmad uses a communication board, his communication partners must be near him when he communicates so that they can see the symbols on the display. Now, imagine Ahmad using an AAC device that produces high-quality synthetic speech output when he touches a symbol on the display. His teacher and classmates now face fewer learning demands regarding reception and comprehension of the output, and Ahmad can communicate from anywhere in the classroom assuming that he can adjust the volume on the device sufficiently.

Speech output has several disadvantages as well. Even when synthetic or digitized speech is fairly intelligible in optimal listening situations, some voices can be difficult to hear and understand in noisy environments, by people with hearing impairments, or by nonnative language speakers. AAC teams must consider such limitations individually before deciding whether a specific speech output option is appropriate for a particular individual. Generally, limitations of particular synthesized speech options are revealed during a device trial completed before a final recommendation for purchase is made. Fortunately, speech synthesis is steadily improving in intelligibility and quality.

Visual Output

As the quality of synthetic speech has improved over the years, visual output has changed from being a primary output method in AAC to being a supportive one. Generally speaking, visual output serves to clarify messages when the listener does not understand synthetic or natural speech. When an AAC device has a computer output screen, the listener may request clarification or message reformulation less frequently (Higginbotham, 1989). Visual output is particularly important for communication partners who have hearing impairments, who are unfamiliar with the person using AAC and his or her system, or who communicate in noisy environments in which synthetic speech may not be intelligible. In addition to employing visual output to supplement synthetic speech output, many individuals who use AAC utilize printed output in similar ways as individuals without disabilities do—to write letters, complete assignments, leave notes, make lists, and keep personal journals.

AAC teams have often considered the type of visual display that electronic devices provide to be secondary to selection of the symbol set, access mode, and encoding technique. Nevertheless, as an increasing number of options have become available, and as stationary AAC computer displays have become increasingly common in schools and vocational settings, information concerning visual display options has become more relevant to device selection. A detailed discussion of the visual technology used in AAC devices, however, is beyond the scope of this book (see Cook & Polgar, 2008, for a discussion of visual screens).

Hard Copy

A printer that may be part of a communication device or an adjunct to it produces permanent, "hard copy" output on paper. Many communication devices can be connected to standard peripheral printers or interfaced with small, portable printers. The printer may produce full-page, wide-column, or strip output in many paper and font sizes. Some software/hardware combinations can also print messages with nonorthographic symbols. For example, computers can display and print PCS symbols using software programs such as Boardmaker and Speaking Dynamically Pro (Mayer-Johnson, Inc.), and Blissymbols can be printed using programs such as AccessBliss (McNaughton, 1990a, 1990b).

Computer Screen Messages

Computer-generated messages are widely used in AAC technology as feedback and output. This technology can manage both orthographic and specialized symbols. A variety of technologies help display computer-generated symbols on screens (see Cook & Polgar, 2008, for detailed information).

Unaided Symbols

Nonelectronic forms of output such as gestures or manual signs impose memory requirements on both of the participants in the communicative exchange. Because no permanent display is available, all of the gestures or manual signs must be produced from memory by the sender and processed in memory by the receiver. These tasks may be very difficult for people who have memory impairments (e.g., people with traumatic brain injury) or who have difficulty processing transitory information (e.g., people with autism; see Mirenda, 2003b). Many researchers and clinicians have encouraged the use of aided technology with permanent displays as a solution for people with memory impairments.

Another major concern regarding unaided symbol output is that relatively few people without disabilities are likely to understand it. For example, it appears that only 10%–30% of American Sign Language (ASL) signs and 50%–60% of Amer-Ind gestures are guessable by typical adults (Daniloff, Lloyd, & Fristoe, 1983; Doherty, Daniloff, & Lloyd, 1985). Thus, if an individual produces unaided symbols as the sole output to unfamiliar partners, he or she will almost always require a translator. Again, multimodal systems that incorporate both aided and unaided symbols often serve to resolve this dilemma.

Aided Symbol Displays

In nonelectronic applications that use aided symbols, communication partners interact directly with the symbol set itself. As the person who uses AAC identifies the symbols of choice, the partner formulates the message, often speaking it aloud as feedback. Whenever unfamiliar (i.e., translucent or opaque) symbols are used to form messages in communication systems, constraints may be placed on the range of communication partners who will comprehend the message. Potentially problematic aided symbols include textured symbols with arbitrarily assigned meanings, selected symbols from all of the pictorial line-drawing sets discussed in Chapter 3, Blissymbols, orthographic symbols, abstract lexigrams, and other symbols such as braille and Morse code. To maximize aided output intelligibility in such situations, AAC teams often choose systems that provide simultaneous written translations of aided messages for literate communication partners. To facilitate interactions with nonliterate partners, AAC teams may opt for a multimodal AAC system with at least one component that provides synthetic speech output for the communication partner(s).

Another difficulty with the output provided by nonelectronic AAC options has to do with partner attention to the display. When people communicate with books, boards, or other low-tech displays, they must first get their partner's attention. Then, the partner must be able to turn or move toward the individual using AAC in order to see the board, book, or device that displays the message symbols. Finally, the communication partner must possess sufficient sensory acuity to see the output. There are many situations in which one or more of these requirements is difficult or impossible to fulfill. Such situations include communicative interactions in which a partner has a visual impairment and interactions in busy, crowded, or dimly lit environments or places that allow limited mobility (e.g., classrooms, factories, movie theaters, football games). The best solution in these situations may be for AAC teams to introduce one or more forms of speech or print output as part of a multimodal, individualized communication system.

"The role and potential impact of communicative [input]...has been underutilized in intervention approaches to date....Research focus should be directed to the influence of the partner's communication [input] in [AAC] system exchanges" (Romski & Sevcik, 1988b, p. 89).

Visual Input

The availability of visual input appears to facilitate receptive language comprehension for some individuals. People with autism spectrum disorders, for instance, have been found to process concrete visuospatial information more readily than temporal or visuotemporal information such as speech or manual signs (Biklen, 1990; Mirenda & Schuler, 1989). Providing visual input models also appears to enhance their communication and language abilities or literacy skills, as exemplified by the work of Romski and Sevcik (1996; see Chapter 12 for additional information). Some individuals with aphasia may also benefit from augmented input, as discussed in Chapter 15.

Unaided Symbols

Gestures and signs are convenient types of input because they require no additional paraphernalia (e.g., books, boards, computers) and are always available for use because they do not have to be switched on as electronic devices do. Teachers and family members of people with developmental disabilities often use manually signed input within a total (or simultaneous) communication paradigm, in which the communication partner accompanies spoken words with their corresponding signs (Carr, 1982). Some evidence suggests that communication partners who use total communication slow their rates of both speaking and signing and insert more pauses than when they use speech alone (Wilbur & Peterson, 1998; Windsor & Fristoe, 1989, 1991). This may account, at least in part, for the expressive and receptive language gains that some people with autism and other developmental delays display when using this approach (Kiernan, 1983). The type and amount of input that partners should provide to the individual are, however, major considerations. Should manually signed input accompany all or most spoken words, or should communication partners opt for a telegraphic or key-word approach instead? Should the individual employ a total communication approach throughout the day or only during designated instructional periods? Unfortunately, existing research does not supply the answers to these important questions, so clinicians must use their best judgment to make individualized decisions in these areas.

Aided Symbols

Communication partners can also provide input to people who rely on AAC by using aided symbols of many types. For example, a facilitator may draw simple pictures or write letters and words while speaking to a person with receptive aphasia to help him or her to comprehend messages (see Chapter 15). The two most prevalent input methods that utilize aided symbols are aided language stimulation (Elder & Goossens', 1994; Goossens', Crain, & Elder, 1992) and the System for Augmenting Language (Romski & Sevcik, 1996). In both methods, a facilitator points to key symbols while speaking, in a manner parallel to that used in total communication. In order to accomplish this, facilitators must have the necessary symbols available for transmission and must organize the environment in order to apply the symbols appropriately. For aided language stimulation, facilitators must prepare activity boards with the necessary symbols in advance and have them available when needed (Goossens', 1989). Unfortunately, the logistical demands of aided symbol input often prevent facilitators from using the technique extensively, despite research evidence that it can have positive effects on both speech and language development over time (Romski & Sevcik, 1996; see Chapter 12 for additional information about these techniques).

QUESTIONS

4.1. How do fixed and dynamic displays differ?

4.2. How do a grid display and a visual scene display differ?

4.3. In direct selection access, what is meant by the word *dwell*, and what capabilities does the successful use of dwelling require of an individual who relies on AAC?

4.4. What type of individual might wish to use activation on release?

4.5. What are the differences between synthesized and digitized speech?

4.6. How do feedback and output differ?

4.7. The parent of a child with severe physical limitations who cannot use direct selection wishes to know the difference between directed scanning and automatic scanning. What would you tell this parent?

4.8. What is the difference between the *sender-receiver* and the *co-construction* models of communication?

4.9. What are the similarities and differences between aided and unaided AAC strategies?

CHAPTER 5

Principles of Assessment

In the broadest sense, the goals of augmentative and alternative communication (AAC) interventions are 1) to assist individuals to meet their current communication needs and 2) to prepare them to meet their future communication needs. AAC assessment involves gathering and analyzing information so that people with complex communication needs (CCN) and those who support them can make informed decisions about 1) the adequacy of current communication, 2) the individual's current and future communication needs, 3) the AAC techniques that appear to be most appropriate, 4) how to provide instruction regarding use of these techniques, and 5) how to evaluate the outcomes. This chapter presents some of the general principles and procedures of AAC assessment. (See Chapter 6 for information about assessment of specific capabilities related to selection of an AAC system.)

PERSONNEL INVOLVED IN AUGMENTATIVE AND ALTERNATIVE COMMUNICATION INTERVENTIONS

AAC teams that serve individuals with CCN are usually composed of a group of people who guide the AAC intervention decision-making process and implement communication supports. Typically, these individuals include people with CCN themselves, their family members and/or caregivers, and professionals who play a variety of roles. We begin this section by considering all of the people who have important roles in achieving positive outcomes for people who rely on AAC, as summarized in Table 5.1 (Beukelman, Ball, & Fager, 2008; Beukelman & Ray, 2010).

People with Complex Communication Needs

Individuals who rely on AAC are always important members of the team. The role of these individuals may change in response to their maturation, restoration of capability, or decrease in capability. To the extent possible, they should participate in decisions regarding personal and medical care, life choices and goals, social

Table 5.1.   Roles of individuals involved in augmentative and alternative communication interventions

Personnel	Potential roles
People with complex communication needs (CCN)	Provide input related to communication needs and decisions about personal and medical care, life choices and goals, social relationships, and augmentative and alternative communication (AAC) system and intervention preferences
AAC facilitators	Provide everyday assistance to people with CCN; support implementation of multimodal interventions; support unfamiliar communicative partners; maintain AAC technology; prepare low-technology materials; assist people with CCN to select and program words and messages in their AAC devices; serve as a liaison with other AAC personnel and device manufacturers
AAC finders	Identify persons with CCN; be aware of current, appropriate communication options for individuals with CCN; prepare potential decision makers; organize decision-making process to seek AAC assessment; refer to appropriate AAC intervention provider(s); certify AAC prescription(s) (when appropriate)
General practice clinicians or educators	Implement multimodal interventions; integrate low-tech AAC materials in restorative/developmental and compensatory interventions; implement appropriate low-tech AAC options; implement routine high-tech AAC options; monitor impact of individual AAC interventions; prepare and support AAC facilitators; instruct communication partners
AAC specialists	Implement multimodal interventions; integrate low-tech AAC materials in restorative/developmental and compensatory interventions; implement appropriate low-tech AAC options; implement complex or unique high-tech AAC options; monitor impact of individual AAC interventions; obtain funding for intervention technology; prepare and support AAC facilitators; support general practice clinicians; instruct communication partners; provide continuing education to AAC facilitators; collaborate to support technology transfer; collaborate to support AAC research; support AAC professional organizations and activities; provide expert testimony for legal and policy proceedings
AAC experts	Promote, sustain, and enhance AAC services at program or agency level; provide preprofessional preparation of AAC finders, intervention specialists, and experts; provide continuing education for AAC finders; provide continuing education for general practice clinicians, AAC intervention specialists, and experts; develop AAC policies; execute AAC research; collaborate to support technology transfer; prepare AAC educational materials; participate in the leadership and management of AAC professional organizations; support AAC professional organizations and activities; provide expert testimony for legal and policy proceedings

From Beukelman, D., Ball, L., & Fager, S. (2008). An AAC personnel framework: Adults with acquired complex communication needs. *Augmentative and Alternative Communication, 24*, 255–267; adapted by permission of Informa Healthcare.

relationships, and support options, including those that are related to the AAC system and interventions.

Augmentative and Alternative Communication Facilitators

Here (and throughout this book), we use the term *facilitator* to refer to family members, friends, professionals, and frequent communication partners who, in various ways, assume some responsibility for keeping the AAC system current and operational and/or for supporting the person with CCN to use it effectively (Beukelman et al., 2008). Facilitators support communication interactions with new or less familiar communication partners by coaching the partners, co-constructing messages, serving as interpreters, and resolving communication breakdowns. In addition, facilitators often monitor AAC equipment to make sure it is working properly and, when necessary, assist the person with CCN to select and program messages into the AAC device. It is important to remember that the role of the facilitator is to support the individual with CCN to communicate as independently as possible, not to communicate *for* the person (Beukelman & Ray, 2010).

In 2007–2008, Augmentative Communication Community Partnerships Canada (ACCPC) developed and evaluated a project to train "communication assistants" to act as facilitators for people with CCN who use AAC. Results indicated that the provision of trained communication assistants significantly increased participants' ability to communicate and participate in their communities and their feelings of dignity, empowerment, autonomy, and privacy (Collier, McGhie-Richmond, & Self, 2010).

Augmentative and Alternative Communication Finders

AAC finders are people who identify children, youth, and adults with actual or potential unmet communication needs and recommend AAC interventions. Although usually not AAC experts or specialists, they need to be generally aware of AAC strategies that might benefit those with CCN. A range of people can fill the finder role, including family physicians, pediatricians, neurologists, nurses, speech-language pathologists, social workers, physiatrists (i.e., rehabilitation physicians), and teachers. AAC finders often prepare families to seek appropriate AAC services in a timely manner. Some AAC finders support funding applications for AAC technology purchases or intervention services by certifying medical diagnoses, confirming communication needs, and signing appropriate prescriptions or intervention plans.

General Practice Clinicians and Educators

Generalists may include speech-language pathologists, occupational therapists, teachers, education paraprofessionals, and others who work in educational, health care, and assisted living settings. They provide a range of clinical and education services as part of their daily workloads. Although they do not specialize in AAC, they support and implement AAC services and interventions, often in collaboration with an AAC specialist. Typically, they are aware of low-technology AAC options and have some operational competence with the AAC strategies typically used in a specific setting (e.g., a rehabilitation center or long-term care facility) or with the type of people they tend to serve (e.g., people with aphasia). They are often involved in providing support to facilitators and other communication partners as well (e.g., classmates, new staff in a group home).

"[The AAC specialists] would come out about every year to meet and talk to his new teachers and try to explain what they were trying to do…and then that kind of opened a door so that there could be a direct communication between someone at the center and the teachers" (mother of Carson, a young man with cerebral palsy, in Lund & Light, 2007, p. 330).

Augmentative and Alternative Communication Specialists

AAC specialists regularly provide direct AAC intervention services to people with CCN. They instruct and educate others about AAC, and they design and implement unique or complex AAC interventions that generalists cannot provide without consultation. Some AAC specialists take on additional responsibilities that are usually associated with AAC experts, such as providing continuing education to generalists and other specialists, participating in AAC-related research, and preparing preprofessional students enrolled in university programs.

Augmentative and Alternative Communication Experts

AAC experts such as researchers, university faculty, policy makers, master clinician specialists, and administrators focus on developing the knowledge, technical, policy, and service bases of the AAC field. They may be responsible for promoting, sustaining, and enhancing AAC services at a program or agency level, and they often provide preprofessional and/or continuing education courses or workshops on a regular basis. AAC experts may also assume leadership roles in professional organizations and provide expert testimony for legal and policy proceedings related to AAC.

BUILDING INTERVENTION TEAMS TO SERVE SPECIFIC INDIVIDUALS WITH AUGMENTATIVE AND ALTERNATIVE COMMUNICATION NEEDS

The AAC field has developed and continues to develop in the context of a broad-based international community of people who rely on AAC, family members, professionals, researchers, developers, and manufacturers (see Zangari, Lloyd, & Vicker, 1994, for a detailed chronology of the development of the AAC field). Although the models used to deliver AAC services vary widely from country to country, one common goal unites these efforts: to enable people to communicate effectively. And, although the policies, legislation, and organizations that affect AAC continue to change, the efforts of teams of people, including individuals with CCN and their families, are essential during the assessment and intervention process. Because a team approach is so important to the success of any AAC intervention, this section introduces some features of AAC team development. For a much more detailed discussion of intervention teaming, readers are referred to the work of Robinson and Solomon-Rice (2009), who described strategies to support collaborative teams and families involved in AAC interventions.

Team Development

Why work within a team structure, anyway? Wouldn't it be easier for professionals to "do their own thing" in each specialty area and write reports or have occasional meetings to share information? The answer is "yes, it would be easier for professionals, but it usually is not better for those who rely on AAC and their families!" Effective communication is essential to successful participation in social relationships, education, community activities, employment, and volunteering. Therefore, the AAC team must include not only the individual who relies on AAC, key family members, and AAC specialists but also experts and facilitators who can support AAC use in the activities and settings in which the person with CCN is involved. As the individual transitions from home to preschool, to school, to postsecondary education, to employment or volunteering, and to supported or independent living, the configuration of the team must change accordingly (McNaughton & Beukelman, 2010).

It is essential to involve people with CCN as well as other significant individuals as members of the AAC team from the outset of intervention. Furthermore, AAC teams should base intervention decisions on a broad range of information. For example, teams need information regarding the cognitive, language, sensory, and motor capabilities of the individual, as well as information regarding the operational, linguistic, social, and strategic competence of the individual's current communication strategies. Teams also need to know about current and future communicative contexts and about the support systems available to the individual. Intervention teams must also identify and respect the preferences of those with CCN, their families or guardians, and their personal advisers. Few individual AAC specialists are capable of assessing and intervening in all of these areas; therefore, it is nearly always necessary to involve a team of individuals to provide appropriate AAC services. When it comes to AAC, the old adage that "two heads are better than one" holds true—collaborative efforts are integral to the success of most interventions (Utley & Rapport, 2002).

"In the early years, we had about 40 people involved with [Josh] from physicians to school personnel and they wouldn't talk to each other....There are lots of good skills around the table and lots of good problem solving skills, but because of professional ideology and people not knowing how to work together, the whole process is diminished" (mother of Josh, a young man with cerebral palsy, in Lund & Light, 2007, p. 328).

Team Membership and Participation

It is important to make thoughtful decisions about who should be on an AAC intervention team. The following three questions should be asked when formulating any team:

1. *Who has the expertise needed by the team to make the best decisions?* The days when "the more, the merrier" was the predominant approach to AAC team membership are long past. Funding, time, and other constraints often make it necessary to economize for the sake of efficiency, but smaller teams can also be more effective. The literature on this issue suggests that a team of four to six members is ideal to ensure diversity of viewpoints while supporting effective communication (Johnson & Johnson, 1987). However, at any given time, team membership might change as the consumer's needs dictate. For example, during the initial assessment for an AAC system or device, the involvement of one or two team members might be sufficient if the issues are quite clear. Later on, teams might invite additional members to consult about specific motor, sensory, or other concerns that arise. This concept of utilizing a small "core team" of people who are most immediately and directly involved with a specific individual with CCN plus an "expanded team" of people with additional expertise as needed is likely to enhance both team effectiveness and team efficiency (Swengel & Marquette, 1997; Thousand & Villa, 2000).

2. *Who is affected by the decisions?* In almost all cases, the answer to this question is simple: the person with CCN and his or her family. Ironically, these are often the individuals who are least involved and least consulted during the AAC assessment and intervention process (McNaughton, Rackensperger, Benedek-Wood, Williams, & Light, 2008). As a result, the outcomes desired by the consumer may take a "back seat" to the goals identified as important by the professionals on the team. As Michael Williams, a man with cerebral palsy who has relied on AAC for more than 70 years, reminded us, "Whose outcome is it anyway?" (1995, p. 1).

3. *Who has an interest in participating?* This question is meant to encourage the team to think beyond the obvious. In every community, there are people who might be interested in helping to solve particular problems or in lending their expertise. For example, we know of a high school computer science teacher who acts as an informal "technology consultant" to his daughter's elementary school. In this capacity, he has made numerous suggestions for simple adaptations that have resulted in better computer access for students with physical disabilities. Although unusual, his membership on the team has been a critical factor in those students' successful use of technology. Thinking broadly about team membership will often reveal such opportunities to "build bridges" into the larger community.

"People should get together and sort of brainstorm, people from various walks of life, not only parents, not only people who are in this field, because each one of us holds enormous amount of observation, about real life in general, it doesn't need to be something that is very highly specialized, somebody is already making use of that we don't know of, probably each one of us in our own little fields we do know about certain things, as a resource pool we could put this together" (AAC specialist from India, in Srinivasan, Mathew, & Lloyd, 2011, p. 241).

As an individual with CCN approaches a life transition related to education, work, or a living setting, it is necessary to adjust the team to include expertise about the anticipated transition (McNaughton & Beukelman, 2010). Team membership during transition planning often needs to be quite broad and must include the person who relies on AAC and family members as integral—not just "token"—members. Several negative outcomes can result if these individuals are not incorporated into the team throughout the assessment and intervention-planning processes. First, the team will lack information that pertains to subsequent intervention efforts. Second, the individual with CCN and his or her family may not be able to assume "ownership" of interventions that are formulated by others on the team without their input and agreement. Third, distrust of the agency delivering AAC services may develop if the family is not permitted to participate, regardless of the quality of the evaluation or interventions. Fourth, family members may not learn to participate as team members if they are excluded when team dynamics and interaction styles are established.

Negative consequences are also likely to result if key professionals, especially those who manage the natural environments in which the people with CCN participate, are excluded or ignored as team members. For example, general and/or special education teachers usually manage a child's educational environment, speech-language pathologists often manage the communication-conversation environment, employers may manage the work environment, and family members or residential staff may manage the living environment. One or more of these individuals is likely to be affected by each of the AAC team's decisions. Therefore, their involvement is absolutely critical in order to avoid later problems that are related to a lack of collaboration or a failure to follow through with team decisions. Once the initial AAC team has been assembled, members can proceed to assess an individual's communication needs and participation goals, existing barriers to participation, and capabilities.

ASSESSMENT MODELS

Several models have been developed over the years to guide the AAC assessment process. These include candidacy models (which are no longer considered best practice and should not be used, but are included here because of their historical significance) and the Participation Model, on which this book is based. We describe both of these briefly in the following sections.

Candidacy Models

A primary goal of an AAC assessment is to determine whether an individual requires AAC assistance. This might appear to be an easy task because it seems obvious that all people who are unable to meet their daily communication needs through natural speech require AAC interventions. Nevertheless, in the 1970s and 1980s in particular, considerable controversy was generated about "candidacy" or "eligibility" criteria for AAC services. In some cases, individuals were considered to be "too something" to qualify for AAC services—for example, too young, too old, or too cognitively (or motorically or linguistically) impaired. Ironically, some individuals were also excluded from AAC services because they were perceived as having "too many" skills, especially with regard to natural speech. For example, AAC supports were often withheld from children with childhood apraxia of speech in the hopes that their speech abilities might improve and/or out of concern that if they received AAC systems they might not exert the effort required to become natural speakers. Similarly, adults with aphasia and individuals with traumatic brain injury were often considered to be inappropriate candidates for AAC interventions until it became clear—sometimes months or even years after their injuries—that speech recovery had failed to occur. Consequently, these individuals were deprived of the ability to communicate their wants, needs, preferences, and feelings, often during the very period of time when they were attempting to restructure their lives in order to live with their severe communication limitations and other disabilities.

In other cases, "not ready for" criteria were used as a result of misguided interpretations of research examining communication and language development in typical children (see Kangas & Lloyd, 1988; Reichle & Karlan, 1985; and Romski & Sevcik, 1988a, for refutations of this practice). In particular, people with CCN secondary to intellectual impairments, autism spectrum disorders, congenital deaf-blindness, or multiple disabilities were frequently viewed as "not ready for" AAC. This thinking predominated so much that the service delivery guidelines of educational agencies often imposed specific requirements for cognitive or linguistic performance before interventionists would consider an individual to be an appropriate AAC candidate. In order to "become ready," these individuals were often expected to work on a variety of activities that were hypothetically designed to teach them the "prerequisite" skills that they lacked. Most of these activities, such as learning about object permanence by finding toys hidden under towels or learning about visual tracking by following stuffed animals moved across the line of visual regard, were nonfunctional and often age inappropriate, and usually failed to lead to the "readiness" they were intended to promote.

Finally, many individuals were excluded from AAC services because there was an "insufficient" amount of discrepancy between their cognitive and language/communication functioning on formal tests; because they had a specific medical condition or diagnosis that was thought not to be amenable to AAC supports (e.g., a degenerative disorder such as dementia, Huntington disease, or Rett syndrome); or because they had not benefited from previous communication services. External factors such as restrictive interpretations of educational, vocational, and/or medical necessity with regard to insurance regulations; lack of appropriately trained personnel; and lack of adequate funds or other resources have also been used—alone or in combination—to restrict access to AAC services.

In response to these practices, the National Joint Committee for the Communication Needs of Persons with Severe Disabilities (NJC) issued a position statement on eligibility for communication services and support in 2003. The statement emphasized that

> decisions regarding…types, amounts, and duration of services provided, intervention setting, and service delivery models should be based on the individual's communication needs and preferences. Eligibility determinations based on a priori criteria violate recommended practice principles by precluding consideration of individual needs. These a priori criteria include, but are not limited to: (a) discrepancies between cognitive and communication functioning; (b) chronological age; (c) diagnosis; (d) absence of cognitive or other skills purported to be prerequisites; (e) failure to benefit from previous communication services and supports; (f) restrictive interpretations of educational, vocational, and/or medical necessity; (g) lack of appropriately trained personnel; and (h) lack of adequate funds or other resources. (NJC, 2003a, 2003b; the complete position statement and supporting materials are posted on the NJC web site)

Largely because of this position statement and subsequent advocacy efforts, the candidacy model is no longer used in most developed countries.

Participation Model

In a 2004 technical report, the American Speech-Language-Hearing Association (2004) endorsed the Participation Model as a framework for carrying out AAC assessments and interventions. The Participation Model was first presented by Beukelman and Mirenda (1988), who expanded on concepts that were initially described by Rosenberg and Beukelman (1987) to guide AAC decision making and intervention. Over the years, minor modifications to the model have been suggested by several authors, based on research in which the model was implemented (Light, Roberts, Dimarco, & Greiner, 1998; Schlosser et al., 2000). The revised Participation Model, shown in Figure 5.1, provides a systematic process for conducting AAC assessments and designing interventions based on the functional participation requirements of peers without disabilities of the same chronological age as the person with CCN. This is similar to the Human Activity Assistive Technology model described by Cook and Polgar (2008), in which interventionists consider the interactions of the individual who relies on assistive technology, the activity to be completed, and the context in which the activity is performed.

PHASES OF ASSESSMENT

AAC interventions are usually ongoing, long-term processes because the individuals who require them usually are unable to speak and/or write due to physical, cognitive, language, and/or sensory impairments that persist over time. Nevertheless, as people who rely on AAC mature and age, their communication needs and capabilities often change. Some people experience an expanding world with increased opportunities, whereas others become less able to participate as they age or as their impairments become more severe. Thus, AAC assessment and intervention is a dynamic process and usually consists of four general phases.

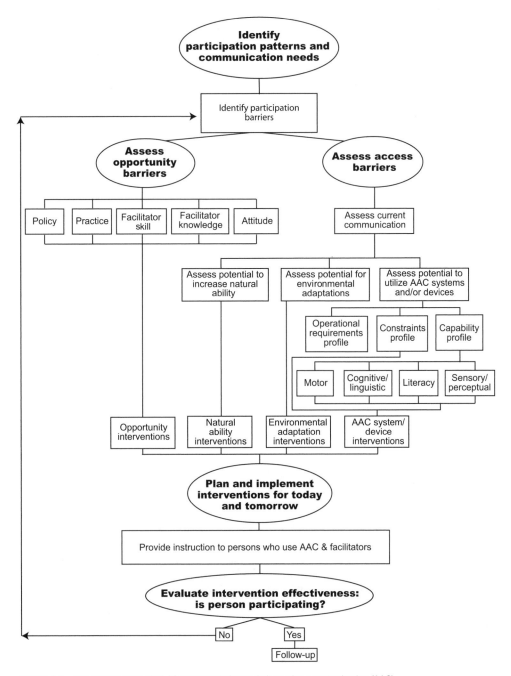

Figure 5.1.   The Participation Model for augmentative and alternative communication (AAC).

Phase 1: Referral for Augmentative and Alternative Communication Assessment

During this phase—which may be either brief or prolonged, depending on the resources available—the person with CCN or (more often) an AAC finder (see previous section) initiates a referral for an AAC assessment. During this phase, finders play several important roles: 1) they recognize both that an individual has a complex communication need and that an AAC intervention may be an appropriate solution, 2) they assist the person who will use AAC and his or her family to initiate a referral to an appropriate resource, and 3) they may support an AAC funding application by certifying a medical diagnosis and/or signing a prescription for the recommended service. Although the role of the finder is often short-term or episodic, this individual plays a key role in the AAC assessment process and requires adequate information in order to fulfill his or her responsibilities.

Phase 2: Initial Assessment and Intervention for Today

During this phase, a team composed of one or more AAC specialists assesses the individual's current communication interaction needs and his or her physical, cognitive, language, and sensory capabilities so that efforts to support interaction and communication can begin as soon as possible after the time of referral. Thus, the goal of this phase is to gather information to design an initial intervention to match the individual's existing needs and capabilities. The initial AAC intervention typically focuses on enabling communicative interactions between the person with CCN and familiar AAC facilitators. The AAC intervention usually undergoes continuous refinements over time as the individual learns about the operational requirements of the AAC system and as the AAC team gathers additional information.

"[We all need to be] looking at what she needs now and how she's likely to progress and what she's likely to need in the future so that you can see where things are going and you can plan accordingly and school can do the same so that everyone's working down the same path" (parent of a child who relies on AAC, in Goldbart & Marshall, 2004, p. 202).

Phase 3: Detailed Assessment for Tomorrow

The goal of assessing for tomorrow is to develop a robust communication system that will support the individual with CCN in a variety of environments beyond those that are familiar, both now and in the future. These environments will reflect the individual's lifestyle and thus may include school, employment, residential (independent, assisted, retirement), recreational, and leisure environments. Such settings require basic conversational communication as well as specialized communication that matches the participation requirements of each setting. For example, a child in a classroom must have access to a system that allows educational as well as social participation. Similarly, an adult at work might need to write and talk on the telephone as well as to converse with co-workers during break times. An older adult may anticipate transitioning into a retirement or supported care facility after living in a family home for years, and will require a communication system that enables participation in this new environment. Thus, this phase requires careful assessment of the individual's current participation patterns as well as assessments to refine the AAC system to accommodate future participation. This phase will also require the involvement of additional AAC facilitators, such as teachers, communication assistants (Collier et al., 2010), personal care attendants, and residential/vocational agency support staff (Beukelman et al., 2008).

Phase 4: Follow-Up Assessment

Follow-up, in general, involves maintaining a comprehensive AAC system that accommodates the individual's changing capabilities and lifestyle. Assessment in this phase may involve periodically examining communication equipment to detect replacement and repair needs, assessing the needs and abilities of new communication partners and facilitators, and reassessing an individual's capabilities if they change. For individuals whose lifestyles and capabilities are relatively stable, follow-up assessment may occur irregularly and infrequently; for others, such as those with degenerative illnesses, follow-up assessments are likely to be a major part of intervention planning.

IDENTIFY PARTICIPATION
PATTERNS AND COMMUNICATION NEEDS

The remainder of this chapter follows the Participation Model flowchart depicted in Figure 5.1. The top part of the model depicts the process for describing the participation patterns and communication needs of the individual, referenced against the participation requirements of same-age peers without disabilities. The sections that follow describe this process.

Conduct a Participation Inventory

The assessment of participation patterns begins with a Participation Inventory (see Figure 5.2), which can be completed for each of the regularly occurring activities in which the individual with CCN participates at home, at school, at work, or in other settings. In addition to an inventory of activities, it is also helpful to identify those individuals with whom the person with CCN is likely to communicate. In their description of the Social Networks framework, Blackstone and Hunt Berg (2003a, 2003b) identified and provided an assessment tool to document five "circles of communication partners" who might constitute an individual's social network: family members/life partners, friends, acquaintances, paid professionals, and unfamiliar people. We discuss the Social Networks approach in more detail in Chapter 9.

Obviously, an individual's specific activities and communication partners will depend on numerous social, vocational, and educational factors. In any case, it is important at this stage of assessment for AAC team members to reach a consensus regarding the environments and activities to be assessed with the Participation Inventory because this list will influence the subsequent assessment process and intervention program. Furthermore, if the team cannot reach a consensus about the key activities in a person's life, it will be very difficult to determine whether or not the AAC intervention has been effective and has achieved the desired outcomes.

Identify Participation Patterns of Peers

The first step in completing a Participation Inventory for a specific activity is to determine how peers participate in it, by recording the critical steps required for successful completion. The team should select as a model a peer of approximately the same age as the individual (and the same gender if gender is relevant to the activity), one whose participation is representative of the desired performance in a given situation. As team members observe and document the peer's participation

Person's name: _____   Date: _____   Completed by: _____

Setting and activity: _____   Goal of activity: _____

Critical steps to meeting the activity goal	Level of independence (*P:* peer; *CCN:* person with CCN)					Opportunity barriers				Access barriers			
	Independent	Independent with setup	Requires verbal assistance	Requires physical assistance	Policy	Practice	Knowledge	Skill	Physical/ motor	Cognitive	Literacy	Visual/ auditory
1.												
2.												
3.												
4.												
5.												
6.												
7. etc.												

Figure 5.2.   Participation Inventory. (Source: Blackstien-Adler, 2003.) (Key: CCN, complex communication needs.)

Augmentative & Alternative Communication, Fourth Edition, by David R. Beukelman & Pat Mirenda
Copyright © 2013 by Paul H. Brookes Publishing Co., Inc. All rights reserved.

112

in each delineated activity, they base peer performance standards on the following criteria and record them in the Participation Inventory (Figure 5.2, in the section titled "Level of independence").

- *Independent:* The peer is able to participate in the activity without assistance.
- *Independent with setup:* The peer is able to participate independently once assistance has been provided to set up the activity (e.g., art materials are laid out for a student in school, the raw data for an engineering report are compiled for an employee).
- *Requires verbal or physical assistance:* The peer is able to complete an activity if provided with verbal or physical prompts or instruction (e.g., a trainer prompts an employee verbally as he or she learns to operate a new piece of equipment, a parent or a teacher provides physical guidance while a student completes an activity).

Accurately determining the critical steps required to complete an activity is an important step in the AAC assessment process. People with CCN and/or their teachers, co-workers, caregivers, or family members may at times set unrealistic goals for an activity. For example, a junior high school social studies teacher once indicated to us that a student in her class who had severe cerebral palsy should be prepared to discuss the assigned readings during every class. However, an assessment of peer participation patterns in the classroom revealed that few, if any, of the other students were prepared to discuss the readings daily, and, in fact, some of them were almost never prepared to do so. If the AAC team had accepted the teacher's standard as its goal, they would have placed excessively high expectations on the student with CCN. Instead, the teacher, who was a member of the team, agreed to alter her expectations of this student once she received the results of the peer participation analysis.

Assess Participation Effectiveness of the Person with Complex Communication Needs

Once team members have identified the critical steps and participation patterns required of peers to complete an activity, they can use the same criteria to assess and document how the person with CCN participates. The individual may be able to participate in some steps at a level similar to the peer, and in such situations, no participation gap exists. For other steps, however, discrepancies between the participation of the peer and that of the individual will be evident. These can be indicated on the Participation Inventory (Figure 5.2) in the section titled "Level of independence."

Identify Participation Barriers

According to the Participation Model, two types of barriers may affect an individual's participation—those related to opportunity and those related to access. Opportunity barriers refer to those that are imposed by people other than the individual with CCN and that cannot be eliminated simply by providing an AAC system or intervention. For example, an individual may be unable to participate at the desired level because facilitators do not have the skills that are required for support, even though an appropriate AAC system has been provided. Access barriers, on the other hand, are present primarily because of limitations in the current capabilities of the individual or his or her current communication system. For example, an access barrier might occur because an individual's AAC device does not have sufficient memory for the specialized vocabulary needed for a specific activity. Assessments aimed at identifying the source of barriers to participation are needed in order to formulate effective assessment and intervention strategies for each barrier. In the sections that follow, we describe the specific issues related to assessment of opportunity and access barriers in more detail.

"When my son went to school so many opportunities were missed....The teachers knew nothing of the AAC, and wanted to know nothing. There is no acceptable reason that he was not expected, encouraged, or allowed to use the device in school. So many missed opportunities" (Barbara, mother of a 20-year-old man with cerebral palsy, in McNaughton et al., 2008, p. 49).

OPPORTUNITY BARRIERS

The Participation Inventory (Figure 5.2) contains a section in which the AAC team can record four types of opportunity barriers that may exist: policy, practice, knowledge, and skill barriers. We discuss each of these briefly in the sections that follow.

Policy Barriers

Policy barriers are the result of legislative or regulatory decisions that govern the situations in which many individuals with CCN find themselves. In schools, vocational environments, residential centers, hospitals, rehabilitation centers, and nursing homes, policies are usually outlined in the written documents that govern the agency. In less formal situations, such as family homes, policies may not be written but are nonetheless set by the decision makers (e.g., parents, guardians) in the environment.

A wide variety of policies can act as barriers to participation. For example, many educational agencies and school districts still have policies that place students with disabilities into classrooms that separate them from their peers without disabilities. In such situations, by policy, students with disabilities cannot be included in general education classrooms, participate in the school district's general education curriculum, or communicate regularly with peers who do not have disabilities. Furthermore, because many school districts with such policies offer educational programs only in certain schools, students may be bused to facilities far away from their neighborhoods. This not only limits these students' access to peers without disabilities during the school day but also greatly reduces these students' opportunities to make friends in their neighborhoods. The combination of these restrictions severely limits the communication opportunities afforded to students with CCN. Similar situations can occur in sheltered workshops, in group homes or institutions, and in other settings intended only for people with disabilities.

Another example is the "limited-use" policy that exists in many acute medical settings and intensive care units that contain complicated and expensive equipment. To prevent mechanical or electronic interference with this equipment, some hospitals have stringent policies regarding other types of equipment that patients can bring with them. People with electronic AAC devices may face opportunity barriers in these medical settings due to such policies. This situation may also exist in agencies or nursing homes that serve adults who use AAC.

Practice Barriers

Whereas policy barriers are legislated or regulated procedures, practice barriers refer to procedures or conventions that have become common in a family, school, or workplace but are not actual policies. The staff of an agency may think that long-standing practices are formal policies, but a review of written documents often reveals that this is not the case. For example, it is a matter of practice in some school districts to restrict the use of district-funded AAC equipment outside of school. We know of several cases in which teachers or administrators have told families that the "district policy" prevents students with CCN from taking their AAC devices home with them when, in fact, no such policy exists. Professional practices may also limit participation opportunities. Until the 1990s, for example, some speech-language pathologists made it their practice not to work with individuals who were unable to speak, believing that this would be inappropriate because they were trained to assist people with speech problems. Now, speech-language pathologists have largely abandoned this practice, although it may still exist in isolated situations.

"Unfortunately, no one helped [my son] learn signs but me, and he had little support in this until about sixth grade when they hired a classroom aide that knew sign language. To have AAC not be integrated into a child's life until middle school is sad and [makes it] very difficult for them to adjust" (Rosie, mother of a 17-year-old man with cerebral palsy, in McNaughton et al., 2008, p. 49).

Knowledge Barriers

A knowledge barrier refers to a lack of information on the part of a facilitator or another person that results in limited opportunities for participation. Lack of knowledge about AAC intervention options, technologies, and instructional strategies often presents tremendous barriers to effective participation by individuals with CCN. Knowledge barriers on the part of some members of the intervention team are likely to exist at some point during nearly every AAC intervention. One purpose of assessment is to identify these barriers in advance so that information can be provided in order to eliminate or minimize them.

Skill Barriers

A skill barrier occurs when, despite even extensive knowledge, facilitators have difficulty with the actual implementation of an AAC technique or strategy. For example, consider the experience of attending a class, conference, or workshop that was full of good ideas and information and then encountering difficulty putting the newly acquired knowledge into practice at work on Monday morning! Numerous technical and interaction skills are often necessary to assist someone to become a competent communicator. It is important to assess the "hands-on" skill level of individuals who will be responsible for various aspects of the AAC intervention, in order to identify skill deficiencies and design interventions to reduce these barriers to communicative competence.

Attitude Barriers

A fifth type of barrier, in which the attitudes and beliefs held by an individual present a barrier to participation, can also exist. We did not include the barrier related to attitude in the assessment form provided in Figure 5.2 because, if it is present in one or more members of the AAC team, it is probably not helpful to identify it publicly. Telling someone "You have an attitude problem"—either implicitly or explicitly—is unlikely to solve the problem! Nonetheless, it is important to be aware of the potential for attitude barriers that may occur for a variety of reasons and may be manifested in a number of ways. Parents, relatives, co-workers, supervisors, professionals, peers, and the general public all may hold negative or restrictive attitudes.

Some time ago, we were involved in a situation in which a university professor did not want to permit a student who relied on AAC to enroll in his course. The *policy* of the university was clear: People with disabilities who had been admitted to the university were entitled to enroll in all courses. It was also the *practice* of the university to comply with this policy, even if this meant moving classes to more accessible locations. In addition, the university's Disability Resource Center had staff with the *knowledge* and the *skills* that were needed to support both the student and the faculty members who taught the courses in which she was enrolled. Nevertheless, an individual professor, because of his negative *attitude* about students with disabilities, attempted to set up a barrier. Of course, he was not permitted to maintain this barrier in the face of the policies and practices of the institution, and the student was granted access to (and support within) his course.

At times, attitude barriers are quite blatant, but more often they are subtle and insidious because most people realize the social unacceptability of such views. The result of most attitude barriers is that one or more members of the AAC team have reduced expectations of the person with CCN, which in turn results in limited communication opportunities. It is outside the scope of this book to discuss the wide range of attitude barriers that exist. However, assessors should be sensitive to restrictive attitudes that may prevent an individual with CCN from participating in activities with same-age peers who do not have disabilities.

Even though people who rely on AAC are receiving increasingly better elementary, secondary, and postsecondary educational opportunities, opportunities for employment remain severely restricted. For example, the Americans with Disabilities Act was passed in the United States in 1990, yet people who use AAC are still routinely screened out at the initial interview stage when they seek employment. As two men with cerebral palsy who rely on AAC noted: "The REAL barrier…[is] people's stagnant and outdated attitudes toward…people with speech disabilities.…When people see me, they do not see me. They just see a person in a wheelchair" (McNaughton, Light, & Arnold, 2002, p. 66).

ACCESS BARRIERS

In the Participation Model (see Figure 5.1), access barriers pertain to the capabilities, attitudes, and resource limitations of individuals who communicate through AAC, rather than to societal or support system limitations. Many types of access barriers can interfere with an individual's participation. Although access barriers related to communication are of primary importance in this book, it is important to remember that access barriers might also be related to lack of mobility or difficulty with manipulation and management of objects, problems with cognitive functions and decision making, literacy problems, and/or sensory-perceptual impairments (i.e., vision or hearing impairments). The Participation Inventory (Figure 5.2) contains a section in which the AAC team can record their general impressions about the types of access barriers that appear to affect participation. However, it is important to identify the nature and extent of an individual's capabilities as they relate to communication in particular. An individual's current communication, potential to use and/or increase the ability to use natural speech, and potential to use environmental adaptations should all be assessed.

Assess Current Communication

It is important to remember that everyone communicates in some fashion. Thus, the initial step in assessing communication access is to determine the effectiveness and the nature of the individual's current communication system. In general, the assessment of current communication focuses on two aspects of communicative competence: operational and social. Some individuals have a very difficult time using a specific communication technique. For example, a child may be unable to use eye gaze consistently, or an adult with aphasia may be unable to write messages with a standard pen or pencil. Some individuals, however, may be operationally competent but not socially competent with a specific technique. For example, an individual might be able to operate an electronic communication device but might never use it to initiate interactions. Therefore, when assessing the current communication system, it is necessary to examine both the individual's operational and social competence for each technique currently used. Figure 5.3, a survey of current communication techniques, can be used in this regard. In addition, a number of excellent observation and/or interview instruments are available to assist the AAC team to identify both the forms and the functions of a person's current communication. Table 5.2 summarizes some of the instruments that can be used in a variety of environments to assess current communication behaviors, primarily in beginning communicators (e.g., those with developmental disabilities). Beukelman, Garrett, and Yorkston (2007) provided a CD-ROM with a number of additional instruments for use with adults with acute or chronic medical conditions.

Available from the American Speech-Language-Hearing Association (ASHA), the Functional Assessment of Communication Skills for Adults (ASHA FACS; Frattali, Holland, Thompson, Wohl, & Ferketic, 2003) and the Quality of Communication Life Scale (ASHA QCL; Paul et al., 2004) are both reliable and valid measures that can be used to assess communication participation in adults with neurogenic communication disorders. They can be used to assist with treatment planning and documentation of outcomes.

Once the AAC team has assessed a person's current communication system and how it is used, they can then begin to examine the potential of various solutions to existing communication barriers. One solution might be to help increase the person's speech communication abilities, as discussed briefly in the next section.

Assess Potential to Use and/or Increase Speech

One of the most contentious issues in AAC assessment, especially with children, is whether AAC is necessary to augment existing but insufficient speech or (much less commonly) to serve as a replacement for speech altogether. Understandably, parents often worry that the use of AAC will discourage speech development, reasoning that children might be less inclined to speak if they have access to an "easier" alternative such as a manual sign, picture, or speech-generating device (SGD). Family members of adults affected by an acquired brain injury as a result of trauma or stroke are often

Current Communication Techniques

1. List all of the various **techniques** the person with complex communication needs currently uses to communicate.
   Examples: natural speech, vocalizations, gestures, body language, manual signs, pointing to a communication board with pictures, eye gaze to photographs, scanning with _____ device, typing on a typewriter, head mouse, and so forth.

2. Describe the **body part** used for each technique listed (e.g., both eyes, right hand, left thumb, right side of head).

3. Describe any **unique adaptations** needed for each technique (e.g., must sit on mom's lap, uses keyguard, needs to have eye gaze chart held 6 inches from face).

4. After observing the person's use of the technique, **rate** the person's **operational competence** (1 = poor, 5 = excellent). Operational competence is the person's ability to use the technique *accurately and efficiently* over time, without getting fatigued.

5. After observing and interacting with the person, **rate** his or her **social competence** (1 = poor; 5 = excellent). Social competence is the person's ability to use the technique in an interactive, socially appropriate manner.

Technique	Body part	Adaptations	Operational competence					Social competence				
			Poor 1	2	3	4	Excellent 5	Poor 1	2	3	4	Excellent 5
1.												
2.												
3.												
4.												
5.												
6.												
7.												

Figure 5.3. Survey of current communication techniques.

Table 5.2. Selected instruments for documenting current communication behaviors and/or functions

Instrument	Items assessed	Population	Source
Communication Matrix (Rowland, 1996, 2004)	Communication behaviors and functions	Individuals who use any form of communication, including presymbolic communication or augmentative and alternative communication (AAC)	Design to Learn
Interaction Checklist for Augmentative Communication–Revised Edition (Bolton & Dashiell, 1991)	Communication behaviors and functions	Individuals who use any form of communication, including presymbolic communication or AAC	PRO-ED, Inc.
Inventory of Potential Communicative Acts (IPCA) (Sigafoos, Arthur-Kelly, & Butterfield, 2006, Appendix A)	Prelinguistic communication behaviors and functions	Presymbolic communicators with developmental and/or physical disabilities	Paul H. Brookes Publishing Co.
SCERTS® Model Assessment forms (Prizant, Wetherby, Rubin, Laurent, & Rydell, 2006a)	Behaviors used for communication and emotional regulation	Children at the social partner, language partner, and conversational stages of development	Paul H. Brookes Publishing Co.
Social Networks: A Communication Inventory for Individuals with Complex Communication Needs and Their Communication Partners (Blackstone & Hunt Berg, 2003a, 2003b)	Communication skills and abilities, communication partners, modes of expression, representational strategies, selection techniques, strategies that support interaction, topics of conversation, and types of communication	Individuals who use AAC across the range of age and ability	Augmentative Communication, Inc.

concerned about this issue as well, reasoning that their loved one may be less motivated to participate in the (often arduous) therapy needed for speech recovery if an alternative is provided.

These concerns must be addressed with sensitivity and objectivity as part of an AAC assessment. Fortunately, a growing number of research studies have provided evidence that the use of AAC techniques does not inhibit speech production and may, in fact, facilitate it. For example, Millar, Light, and Schlosser noted that their extensive review of research on AAC for people with developmental disabilities provided

> empirical evidence to support the…argument that AAC intervention facilitates the production of natural speech. This evidence, coupled with the existing evidence that AAC interventions support the development of communicative competence and language skills, provides a strong case for implementing AAC with individuals with developmental disabilities who are unable to meet their communication needs through natural speech. (2006, p. 258)

Subsequently, Millar, in a review of AAC research specific to individuals with autism spectrum disorders, noted that "no data were found to support the suggestion that AAC implementation negatively affected the speech production of individuals with

ASD. In fact, most of the existing research suggests that AAC may enhance speech development in these individuals" (2009, p. 187).

Most individuals with CCN demonstrate at least some ability to communicate using speech—that is, they are not 100% unable to vocalize or speak. Functionally, the effectiveness of speech for communicative interaction can be divided into 10 levels, according to the Meaningful Use of Speech Scale (MUSS; Robbins & Osberger, 1992):

1. In communicative exchanges, makes vocal sounds
2. Gets another person's attention using speech
3. Uses various vocal sounds depending on the intention and content of messages
4. Uses speech primarily for communication about known topics with familiar people
5. Uses speech for communication about known topics with unfamiliar people
6. Uses speech primarily for communication about new topics or situations with familiar people
7. Uses speech primarily for communication about new topics or situations with unfamiliar people
8. Uses speech to produce messages that are understood by familiar people
9. Uses speech to produce messages that are understood by unfamiliar people
10. Clarifies or recasts messages as needed when communication breakdowns occur

The AAC team can assess speech usage by interviewing family members using the MUSS to get an estimate of typical speech usage. Each item is scored on a scale of 0–4, with 0 indicating that the behavior never occurs and 4 indicating that it always occurs. Although the MUSS was designed for use with children with severe hearing impairments, Kent, Miolo, and Bloedel (1994) suggested that it can also be used appropriately with children who produce speech with reduced intelligibility of any kind. More specific information related to speech intelligibility in children and adults can be obtained through the use of standardized measures such as those that are listed on the American Speech-Language-Hearing Association's web site.

It is important to note that intelligibility, which refers to the adequacy of the acoustic signal to convey information, is affected by many intrinsic factors such as articulation, respiration, phonation, rate of speech, positioning, utterance length, and so forth (Kent et al., 1994; Yorkston, Strand, & Kennedy, 1996). Typically, intelligibility scores for someone who communicates through AAC will either be extremely low or will fluctuate widely because of the combined influence of these factors. A second measure, supplemented intelligibility, refers to the extent to which a listener can understand an individual's speech when he or she is provided with contextual information, such as the topic, first letters of words, and gestures. Hanson, Yorkston, and Beukelman (2004) completed a meta-analysis and developed practice guidelines for the use of such supplemented speech techniques. In response to the need to assess supplemented intelligibility, specialists have also begun to develop assessment tools for clinical use. For example, The Index of Augmented Speech Comprehensibility in Children (I-ASCC) was developed for use with children as young as 30 months of age (Dowden, 1997). First, target words from common categories are identified (e.g., foods you can eat at breakfast, things you might see at a birthday party, a number between 1 and 10). Next, the target words are elicited via speech in the following order: 1) only a picture cue (e.g., *Can you tell me what this is?*), 2) a picture plus a context cue (e.g., *It's something you see at a birthday party. Can you tell me what it is?*), and 3) a picture plus an embedded model (e.g., *It's a cake. Can you say it?*). Assessors make an audio recording of the speech productions of the individual being assessed, and then familiar and unfamiliar listeners review the recordings with and without supporting contexts. In the no-context listening task, assessors ask listeners to play the recording of each word twice and then write down what they hear. In the context condition, listeners receive a context cue phrase (e.g., *something a person might eat for dinner*) related to each word and are asked to listen and then write down the word they hear that best fits the context. Tools such as the I-ASCC can be useful for understanding the extent to which speech is comprehensible *under different conditions* rather than the degree to which speech is simply intelligible without context.

Cress (1997) and Cress and Marvin (2003) provided an excellent resource for parents of young children considering AAC and the teams that support them. The authors summarized much of the research related to common questions often asked by parents, including "Will the use of AAC interfere with my child's vocal development?" and "Will my child talk?" A summary of Cress (1997) is available on the Barkley Augmentative and Alternative Communication (AAC) Center web site.

Assess Potential for Environmental Adaptations

Environmental adaptations that involve altering physical spaces, locations, or structures may be relatively simple solutions to communication opportunity and/or access barriers. For example, in the classroom, school staff can raise or lower desks and tables, create a vertical work surface with a slanted board, or cut out countertops to accommodate wheelchairs or AAC devices. In a family home, furniture rearrangements and/or renovations to widen door frames or lower countertops may be necessary to accommodate the needs of a resident with newly acquired disabilities. Assessment of the need for such adaptations is a common-sense process, and teams can almost always conduct such assessments by observing problematic situations.

Assess Potential to Utilize Augmentative and Alternative Communication Systems or Devices

In the Participation Model (see Figure 5.1), three assessments determine an individual's ability to use AAC systems or devices in order to reduce access barriers. These include an operational requirements profile, a constraints profile, and a capability profile. We discuss the first two of these profiles in the following section; the capability profile is discussed at length in Chapter 6.

Operational Requirements Profile

Often, AAC teams will need to institute a combination of nonelectronic and electronic AAC techniques to reduce existing access barriers to communication. Thus, it is necessary to identify which of the many AAC options may be appropriate. The first step is for the assessment team to become familiar with the operational requirements of various AAC techniques. For example, there may be display requirements regarding the number of total items in the selection set as well as the size and layout of the array. There are always alternative-access system requirements regarding the motor and sensory interface between the individual and the device so that the individual can operate the device accurately and efficiently. In addition, the output provided by the device may require the individual to have certain skills or abilities. (See Chapters 3 and 4 for descriptions of the operational and learning requirements of many AAC options.)

"In order to obtain accurate [information], the *right person* must ask the *right questions* of the *right people* in the *right way* at the *right place* and *time* (the six R's)" (Bevan-Brown, 2001, p. 139).

Constraints Profile

Practical issues aside from those directly related to individuals and AAC techniques may also influence the selection of an AAC system and the strategies for instruction. The AAC team should identify such constraints early in the assessment process so that subsequent decisions do not conflict with the constraints and so that team members can make efforts to reduce them whenever possible. The most common constraints are those related to individual and family preferences, the preferences and attitudes of other communication partners, communication partner and facilitator skills and abilities, and funding.

Druin (1999, p. xviii) noted that "technology for kids has to have *high smile* value. If the smile value is low, it is just no good." Druin et al. noted that "children care what something looks like as much as how it works or what it does" (1999, p. 67) and that they "are empowered...when they feel they 'own' the environment" (p. 65).

Preferences and Attitudes of People with Complex Communication Needs and Their Families   Undoubtedly, the most important constraints that AAC teams must assess are those related to the preferences of the person with CCN and his or her family. These may include concerns about 1) system portability, durability, and appearance (i.e., cosmetic appeal); 2) the quality and intelligibility of speech output in SGDs; and 3) the "naturalness" of the communication exchange achieved through the system. In particular, children with CCN and their family members may be especially sensitive to these issues out of concern that the AAC device not make the child look or sound any more different from typically developing peers than necessary. To examine this issue, Light, Page, Curran, and Pitkin (2007) asked children without disabilities to "invent" communication devices, using drawing and craft materials, for a fictitious boy who used a wheelchair and was unable to talk. The five resulting AAC "device prototypes" incorporated some features of existing AAC devices (e.g., voice output, multiple levels of vocabulary, protection from messy activities, bright colors) but also included many additional elements (e.g., cartoon characters, humor, the ability to engage in amazing feats, lights, and popular themes). These results suggest that children may value aspects of AAC devices that are not considered to be of high priority by professionals or other adults. In fact, a number of studies have provided evidence that children and adolescents with severe intellectual disabilities or autism are able to demonstrate preferences about the AAC system they use, and have provided strategies for assessing them (Canella-Malone, DeBar, & Sigafoos, 2009; Sigafoos, O'Reilly, Ganz, Lancioni, & Schlosser, 2005; Son, Sigafoos, O'Reilly, & Lancioni, 2006).

In an interesting Canadian study, O'Keefe, Brown, and Schuller (1998) asked 94 people with CCN, their communication partners, AAC service providers, AAC device manufacturers, and people unfamiliar with AAC to rate the importance of 186 possible features of AAC devices. People who used AAC rated items related to situational flexibility, reliability, learning ease, and intelligibility of speech output significantly higher than people in the other four groups did. In addition, people with CCN made several suggestions about a number of desirable features not included in the survey, including the need for devices that 1) provide speech output in languages other than English, 2) enable private conversations when necessary, 3) can be used in bed, and 4) are easy for partners to program. What is clear from this study and the ones by Light, Page, et al. (2007) is that people with CCN may be considerably "more demanding than those who work with them clinically or who are responsible for the design, manufacture, and distribution of AAC communication aids" (O'Keefe et al., 1998, p. 47) and that their preferences are of paramount importance when making AAC device decisions.

Many factors can account for the wide variability in individual and family preferences related to AAC. One of the most salient has to do with the impact of ethnicity and culture on peoples' perceptions of disability in general and communication or AAC in particular (Bridges, 2004). In both North America and elsewhere, AAC assessment and intervention approaches based on Anglo-European ideals and values tend to predominate, even though they may conflict with the values embraced by families from other cultural groups (Hetzroni, 2002; Judge & Parette, 1998). For example, in the dominant Anglo-European culture in North America, there tends to be an emphasis on individualism and privacy, equality, informality, planning for the future, efficient use of time, work and achievement, directness, and assertiveness (Judge & Parette, 1998). Children in Anglo-European cultures are often encouraged to be independent, self-reliant, hardworking, and competitive. Disability is often viewed as having multiple causes; disability "labeling" is widely accepted as a necessary step to obtaining services; and technology in the form of drugs, surgeries, adaptive equipment, and so forth is generally valued as a potential solution to disability-related obstacles.

These values may be in sharp contrast to the values of many other cultural groups that place a high value on attributes such as collectivism and cooperation, interdependence, hierarchical family structures, politeness, living in the here and now, a fluid understanding of time, indirect communication, and/or respect and agreement of elders and authority figures. Although children from other cultures are often raised to value education and hard work, they may also be taught to assume a relatively passive role in social interactions and encouraged to place family loyalty above all other alliances. Views of disability may also vary widely and may emphasize both natural and supernatural causes; a view that "labeling" is both stigmatizing and unnecessary; and a reluctance to employ modern technologies to the exclusion of folk, spiritual, and/or natural remedies.

Communities and countries that are economically and socially disadvantaged present unique circumstances that must be taken into account when planning and implementing AAC interventions. An edited book entitled *Augmentative and Alternative Communication: Beyond Poverty* (Alant & Lloyd, 2005) explores the challenges faced by AAC providers who support individuals from around the world who live in poverty and offers a wide range of potential solutions.

Of course, it is inappropriate to apply "across the board" generalizations to families from diverse backgrounds because many factors (e.g., culture, socioeconomic status, spoken and written language proficiency, educational background) are likely to affect their perceptions of AAC use (Parette, Huer, & Scherer, 2004). Fortunately, since the late 1990s, a number of researchers have examined many of these issues as they relate to specific ethnic/cultural groups that are prevalent in North America. For example, a number of researchers have written extensively about the attitudes and preferences of families from the following backgrounds with regard to educational and AAC assessment practices, devices, and/or instruction:

- African American (Huer & Wyatt, 1999; Parette, Huer, & Wyatt, 2002)
- Mexican American (Huer, Parette, & Saenz, 2001)
- Latino (Binger, Kent-Walsh, Berens, del Campo, & Rivera, 2008; Rosa-Lugo & Kent-Walsh, 2008)
- Asian American (Parette & Huer, 2002)
- Vietnamese American (Huer, Saenz, & Doan, 2001)
- Chinese American (Parette, Chuang, & Huer, 2004)

Other authors have summarized research related to the communication styles, practices, and/or preferences of families from the following backgrounds:

- American Indian (Bridges, 2000; Inglebret, Jones, & Pavel, 2008)
- Hispanic American and Mexican American (Harrison-Harris, 2002; McCord & Soto, 2004)
- Filipino American (Roseberry-McKibbin, 2000)
- Southeast Asian (Hwa-Froelich & Westby, 2003)
- South Indian (Srinivasan et al., 2011)
- Chinese Canadian (Johnston & Wong, 2002)
- Indo-Canadian (Simmons & Johnston, 2004)

From studies such as these, AAC teams can learn much about the importance of truly understanding the values, expectations, historical contexts, child-rearing and communication styles, and perceptions of families from diverse backgrounds. Team members can also appreciate the importance of evaluating their own knowledge, awareness, attitudes, and skills both prior to and during the AAC assessment and intervention processes. Huer (1997) provided a protocol for culturally inclusive assessment of AAC, including the self-evaluation component presented in Figure 5.4.

In addition, team members must appreciate the complexities of conducting AAC assessments with individuals who are bilingual, who represent an increasingly large proportion of the population. The American Community Survey report issued in 2010 indicated that, of the more than 59 million Americans who speak a language other than English, 42% are able to speak English "less than very well" and will probably require English assistance in at least some situations (U.S. Census Bureau, 2010). Because very little research exists to guide AAC practices for individuals who are bilingual, team members must work closely with families to accommodate individual situations and needs. Fortunately, an increasing number of assessment tools are available in languages other than English and can be accessed by searching the web sites of the major test distributors (see the Resources and Web Links section).

Factors other than language and culture also influence people's attitudes and preferences with regard to disability and intervention in general and AAC in particular. One such factor has to do with people's experiences with and attitudes toward technology (see Goldbart & Marshall, 2004; McNaughton et al., 2008; Saito & Turnbull, 2007). For example, one parent of a child with a communication disorder

The Protocol for Culturally Inclusive Assessment of AAC
Self-Assessment: Extent of Multicultural Competencies
©Mary Blake Huer, Ph.D.

Criteria: During self assessment, read the 20 statements below. Next to each statement place a "yes" if you feel you possess the competence and a "no" if you feel you do not. Participate in AAC service delivery when you have acquired at least 70% (14 of 20) of the competencies.

Knowledge base

_____ I have extensive knowledge regarding AAC components, techniques, strategies, symbols, and assistive technology.

_____ I have studied the characteristics of several different disabling conditions.

_____ I have knowledge regarding the history of and attitudes toward multiculturalism.

_____ I can identify cross-cultural similarities and differences in the communicative behaviors of my own culture as well as among culturally/linguistically diverse populations.

_____ I have knowledge regarding policy and laws impacting AAC and multiculturalism.

_____ I have knowledge of community and professional resources for all clients.

_____ I can define terms such as ethnicity, world view, and acculturation.

Awareness of own cultural biases and beliefs

_____ I enjoy interacting with persons from other cultures as much as when interacting with persons from my own culture.

_____ I feel comfortable interacting with families from cultural backgrounds different from my own.

_____ I am sure of what to expect from families.

Awareness of culturally appropriate assessment strategies

_____ I am confident in my ability to evaluate linguistically diverse persons needing AAC services.

_____ I use all family members, as appropriate, during the collection of information, e.g., parent(s), grandparent(s), aunt(s)/uncle(s), cousin(s), friends, elders, and folk healers.

_____ I am confident in my ability to utilize comprehensive evaluation instruments.

_____ I have experience conducting a culturally sensitive interview and a nonbiased assessment.

_____ I use different methods for collecting information, i.e., observations, interviews, open-ended questions, and secondary sources.

_____ I can conduct an effective interview with a family from a cultural background different from my own.

_____ I monitor and correct my own errors, defensiveness, anxiety, and misunderstandings when communicating with persons form cultures other than my own.

Relationships with culturally/linguistically diverse families

_____ I believe that I am perceived by most families to have the quality of trustworthiness.

_____ I believe that families feel comfortable when interacting with me over time.

_____ I believe that most persons do not perceive me as having biases or using stereotypes.

Total self score:_____ Date:_____ Action:_____

Figure 5.4. Self-assessment of multicultural competence. (From Huer, M.B. [1997]. Culturally inclusive assessments for children using augmentative and alternative communication [AAC]. *Journal of Children's Communication Development, 19,* 27; reprinted by permission. Copyright © Mary Blake Huer, Ph.D. All rights reserved.)

may be very interested in an electronic AAC option, whereas the other parent may strongly prefer a low-tech approach. The basis for such disagreements may come from a variety of sources. One individual may have had more positive experiences with technology than the other, or one of the parties involved may be lured by the magic of technology, regardless of its appropriateness in a given situation.

"I had to bear the whole burden of getting [my son's] device up and running....And I thought I had to be the person who took what his school needs were and to put that into the [AAC device]....I felt for a long time very stressed like, okay, this is difficult. I really don't have any understanding of it, but it's been put on my shoulders. I felt no help from the district or his local school at all in programming the device. So, yeah it was extremely stressful in fitting it into my busy schedule" (Bob, father of Joe, a junior high school student with moderate-to-severe disability, in Bailey, Parette, Stoner, Angell, & Carroll, 2006, p. 56).

There may also be a general consensus against the use of any type of AAC—either low tech or high tech—in some situations. As noted previously, it is not uncommon for the parents of young children to be biased against AAC because they are worried that natural speech will not develop if an alternative option is available. Family members of an individual who has experienced an acquired brain injury may also reject AAC options either because they have a strong desire that their child, spouse, or parent regain the use of natural speech or because they just cannot imagine their relative operating a system that produces artificial speech. Individuals may also reject AAC options when they are overwhelmed with a medical situation. For example, some individuals do not wish to attempt alternative forms of communication in an intensive care unit even if they cannot communicate important information because of a temporary absence of speech. It often seems that such individuals simply do not have the cognitive or emotional resources that are needed to acquire basic operational skills in the midst of high levels of existing stress.

In an assessment of constraints, it is important to help individuals who are considering the use of AAC and their families to identify their preferences and attitudes so that AAC teams can consider these during subsequent decision making. Sensitivity and attention through consensus building are critical in an assessment of constraints, even if this means that the final assistive device decision is "less than perfect" from the perspective of the AAC professionals on the team. After all, it is the person with CCN and his or her family who will have to live with whatever decision is made. Failure to consider individual and family preferences will almost certainly result in "abandonment" of the AAC strategy (see Johnson, Inglebret, Jones, & Ray, 2006) and the widespread lament: "The individual has this great system/device but hardly ever uses it!" (Creech, Kissick, Koski, & Musselwhite, 1988).

The Family Center on Technology and Disability web site offers a wide range of resources on assistive and instructional technologies, including the *Family Information Guide to Assistive Technology* (available in both English and Spanish) that can be downloaded at no cost.

Preferences and Attitudes of Other Communication Partners   Less important than the preferences of people with CCN and their family members, but still of concern, are the preferences and attitudes of other individuals with whom the person who relies on AAC interacts, either regularly or occasionally. A number of studies have sought to empirically measure the influence of various communication techniques on the perceptions of unfamiliar communication partners. Individuals without disabilities in these studies typically watch video recordings of interactions between a person relying on AAC and a natural speaker and then rate their perceptions or attitudes along a number of dimensions.

In studies involving school-age children, it appears that those who are already familiar with peers with disabilities have more positive attitudes toward AAC than those who are not familiar (Beck & Dennis, 1996; Beck, Kingsbury, Neff, & Dennis, 2000; Blockberger, Armstrong, & O'Connor, 1993). In several studies, girls have been found to have more positive attitudes toward AAC than boys (e.g., Beck, Bock, Thompson, & Kosuwan, 2002; Beck, Kingsbury, et al., 2000; Beck, Thompson, Kosuwan, & Prochnow, 2010; Blockberger et al., 1993; Lilienfeld & Alant, 2002). With regard to specific AAC techniques, several studies have found no differences with regard to grade-school children's attitudes after they viewed videotapes of peers using electronic, aided nonelectronic (e.g., alphabet board), and/or unaided (i.e., manual sign) systems (Beck et al., 2002; Beck & Dennis, 1996; Beck, Fritz, Keller, & Dennis, 2000; Blockberger et al., 1993; Dudek, Beck, & Thompson, 2006). However, studies with adolescent and adult raters have found more positive attitudes toward individuals with cerebral palsy or aphasia when they used SGDs rather than low-tech displays (Gorenflo & Gorenflo, 1991; Lasker & Beukelman, 1999; Lilienfeld & Alant, 2002). Finally, there is some evidence that, regardless of the type of AAC device (i.e., low-tech versus electronic) or the age of the individual using the device, more positive attitudes are associated with communication displays that employ phrase- or sentence-length messages rather than just single-word messages (Beck, Kingsbury, et al., 2000; Raney & Silverman, 1992; Richter, Ball, Beukelman, Lasker, & Ullman, 2003).

Given that AAC devices are selected primarily to meet the communication needs of the people who will use them rather than unfamiliar communication partners, what can we make of these results? First, it appears that children are less influenced by the type of AAC system than by positive past experiences with children with disabilities in general. This finding suggests that children in schools that include students with disabilities in regular classrooms may be relatively open to AAC techniques in general and may require only basic orientation when encountering classmates who use AAC for the first time. Males may require somewhat more support than females, but this need will vary depending on age. Supports that may result in more positive attitudes include providing adults with information about AAC (Gorenflo & Gorenflo, 1991) and providing children with opportunities to role-play using AAC techniques (Beck & Fritz-Verticchio, 2003).

Second, although there is some evidence that electronic devices are perceived more positively than low-tech displays by adolescents and adults, there is also evidence to suggest that either AAC option is strongly preferred over poorly intelligible speech (Richter et al., 2003). Finally, this research shows that efficiency with regard to the rate of communication is an important consideration for unfamiliar communication partners regardless of age, and that strategies in this regard are critical, regardless of the type of AAC device that is used. Unfortunately, information about the attitudes of communication partners from various cultural, ethnic, and socioeconomic backgrounds is sorely lacking, and research is needed in this area (McCarthy & Light, 2005).

Skills and Abilities of Communication Partners and Facilitators   Beyond the complex issues related to attitudes and preferences are those related to the skills and abilities of potential communication partners and facilitators. It is imperative that potential communication partners be able to understand the messages conveyed through a communication system and/or provide the necessary supports to optimize its use (Kent-Walsh & McNaughton, 2005). For example, if unfamiliar listeners cannot readily understand the AAC system output, as may be the case with manual signs or low-quality synthetic speech, frequent communication breakdowns will occur (see Chapter 4). If communication partners do not know how to interact appropriately with the person using AAC—for example, if they dominate interactions by asking many directive questions and failing to provide sufficient time for message construction—the quality of communication interactions will suffer as a result (Müller & Soto, 2002). Other constraints that may influence the selection of one system over another are the ages and literacy skills of potential partners and other display-related issues. At present, common-sense considerations such as these guide the assessment of partner abilities because the field has accumulated little empirical research investigating the impact of such issues on AAC system use.

Facilitator skills also affect communication system use in a number of ways. If facilitators do not have the skills or the commitment required to provide supports for AAC system use, abandonment of the system is likely (Galvin & Donnell, 2002). For example, facilitators need to be operationally competent in the programming, use, and maintenance of electronic AAC devices. They often need to know how to operate various technologies (e.g., software programs, digital cameras) that are used to create communication displays on an ongoing basis. They may need to provide extensive instruction to individuals who are learning to use iconic encoding or other learning-intensive communication techniques, or who are working to improve their grammar, social interaction, or other skills (e.g., Light & Binger, 1998; Lund & Light, 2003). They must also demonstrate social and strategic competence with AAC techniques in order to provide good models and instruction to the individuals they support. A lack of adequate facilitator skills may place constraints on the intervention selected, simply because the necessary, ongoing expertise is unavailable. Failure to specifically consider the adequacy of facilitator skills during the assessment process will almost always result in implementation failure later on; this is especially true for more demanding electronic devices. Unfortunately, few training or assessment tools for evaluating the capabilities of potential facilitators are available (Beukelman et al., 2008). In the absence of additional assessment instruments, the AAC team must rely on informal methods for evaluating partner and facilitator expertise (Kent-Walsh & McNaughton, 2005).

Funding   The funding of AAC technology and services varies considerably from country to country. Even within countries, funding patterns often change from region to region as well as over time. Thus, a detailed discussion of AAC funding will not be provided here. Readers in the United States are referred to the AAC Funding Help web site for information about current funding regulations and requirements. Readers in other countries should consult their state or provincial AAC center for funding information.

QUESTIONS

5.1.   What are the main roles that are typically assumed by AAC finders, facilitators, specialists, and experts?

5.2.   What are the roles of a person with complex communication needs and his or her family in the AAC assessment process?

5.3. What are three essential questions to ask when deciding who should be on an AAC team?

5.4. What is the AAC candidacy model, and why is it no longer in widespread use?

5.5. What are the phases of AAC assessment, and what issues are addressed in each phase?

5.6. Why is it important to assess the participation patterns and needs of an individual with complex communication needs, and how can this be accomplished?

5.7. What are the five types of opportunity barriers? For each type, give an example that is not provided in the chapter.

5.8. What does research tell us about the effect of AAC interventions on speech development and production?

5.9. In general, how does culture affect the AAC assessment and intervention process?

5.10. What does research tell us about the relationship between various AAC techniques and the attitudes of potential communication partners?

CHAPTER 6

Assessment of
Specific Capabilities

Capability assessment is the process of gathering information about an individual's capabilities in a variety of areas in order to determine appropriate augmentative and alternative communication (AAC) options. In this chapter, we present some general principles and procedures for constructing a capability profile. In Chapters 8 to 18, we review additional capability assessment considerations for people with specific disabilities and needs. First, however, we discuss some of the approaches that can be used for capability assessment in general.

OVERVIEW OF APPROACHES TO CAPABILITY ASSESSMENT

Capability assessment involves identifying an individual's level of performance in critical areas that pertain to AAC intervention, such as motor control, cognition, language, and literacy (Yorkston & Karlan, 1986). The assessment should result in a profile of the individual's capabilities that can be matched to the operational requirements of various AAC options. One of the characteristics of a capability profile is that it emphasizes an individual's strengths and skills rather than his or her impairments. A strengths-based approach is critical to the endeavor because the assessor will match these strengths to one or more AAC techniques.

Several assessment approaches can be used to assess a person's skills with regard to AAC use. Two of these, criterion-referenced assessment and feature matching, are used in combination and predominate in current practice, whereas the third, norm-referenced assessment, must be used with considerable caution. We begin by discussing the limitations of norm-referenced assessment.

Limitations of Norm-Referenced Assessment

Many professionals in fields such as psychology, education, and speech-language pathology have been taught to use a norm-referenced approach to assessment. In this approach, formal or standardized tests are administered to compare an individual's abilities with those of same-age peers. Professionals are often frustrated when they attempt to use norm-referenced assessment tools to evaluate people with complex communication needs (CCN) because it is difficult to administer these tests in a standardized manner. For example, an assessor cannot use a test that requires verbal responses if the individual is unable to speak. A test that requires object manipulation may be useless for assessing an individual with upper-extremity impairments. Even instruments that incorporate "AAC-friendly formats" such as multiple-choice questions can present difficulties if they are timed or if they require advanced literacy skills.

Fortunately, AAC assessment almost never requires that professionals administer norm-referenced tests in a standardized manner, because the purpose of such an assessment is not to compare the individual with peers of the same age. Thus, many professionals use norm-referenced tests that contain appropriate content during an AAC assessment, with test modifications as needed. For example, some individuals may require response options to be presented in a yes/no format instead of an open-ended format or a multiple-choice array. Many formal language assessment instruments can be adapted for use with people who have upper-extremity impairments and need to use eye gaze or alternative techniques to respond. Literacy limitations can be overcome if the assessor reads questions (and answer choices, in a multiple-choice test) out loud to the person being tested. When norm-referenced tests are administered with modifications, they can be useful for obtaining general information related to the person's capabilities. It is inappropriate to use such tests, however, to compare individuals with CCN to peers of the same chronological age without disabilities, or to determine an individual's "eligibility" for AAC services (Snell et al., 2003).

Criterion-Referenced Assessment and Feature Matching

Most AAC specialists use a feature-matching approach for AAC assessment (Costello & Shane, 1994; Glennen, 1997; Yorkston & Karlan, 1986). In this approach, the team first administers a number of carefully selected, criterion-referenced tasks that are designed to answer relevant questions. For example, in order to identify the most appropriate AAC selection technique, one of the first questions often asked is, "Can this individual access the device in a direct selection mode?" If the answer is no, then a number of scanning options are usually explored in more detail. However, if the answer is yes, scanning options are eliminated from consideration, and attention can be focused on selecting the most appropriate direct selection option. This iterative process can also be used to answer specific questions about the person's cognitive, language, literacy, and sensory capabilities.

Basing their predictions on the results of this assessment, a knowledgeable AAC team should be able to predict with reasonable accuracy one or more AAC devices or techniques that are likely to be appropriate for a specific individual with CCN. The team then uses the predictions to set up a "trial" of the selected AAC components for a designated period of time (from a few weeks to several months, depending on the techniques involved). Obviously, feature matching requires that AAC team members be knowledgeable about the operational and learning requirements of a wide variety of AAC options. Otherwise, it may be necessary to have many AAC options available at the time of the assessment or afterward so that the person with CCN can complete successive trials with each device. In many settings, such equipment availability is simply impossible.

AAC TechConnect offers a feature-matching tool called Device Assistant that provides information on almost 100 AAC devices from major manufacturers. It is meant to help identify devices that have the specific features identified during the assessment process as part of a comprehensive evaluation. Numerous free resources and assessment forms are also available on the AAC TechConnect web site.

In the United States, in response to the requirements of the Assistive Technology Act Amendments of 2004 (PL 108-364), all 50 states and U.S. territories have established assistive technology (AT) centers whose mandate is to increase the availability and utilization of AT devices and services for individuals with disabilities. Through these centers, a variety of AT assessment protocols and information-gathering tools have been developed, many of which are relevant to AAC assessment. In addition, a variety of AAC assessment guides are available to facilitate the capability assessment process, provide guidance to clinicians with regard to feature matching, or both. Table 6.1 provides information about some of the most widely available tools and software products that pertain to AAC assessment.

ASSESSMENT DOMAINS

Several domains usually require investigation as part of an AAC assessment. These domains include assessment of positioning and seating; motor capabilities for direction selection and/or scanning; cognitive/linguistic capabilities; literacy skills; and sensory/perceptual skills.

Assess Positioning and Seating

Assessment of positioning and seating is critical for individuals with a range of motor impairments. People who have disabilities that severely restrict movement (e.g., cerebral palsy, spinal cord injury, amyotrophic lateral sclerosis) may spend the majority of the day in a seated position; therefore, they need to be able to do so safely and without sacrificing functional communication effectiveness. Other individuals may have more subtle motor impairments that affect their concentration, range of movement, and ability to use AAC functionally in a variety of positions. Consequently, it is important to consult with clinicians such as occupational and physical therapists, who specialize in motor control and can aid in assessing seating and positioning, as an initial step toward capability assessment in general. In that spirit, we welcome the contributions of Donna Drynan, an occupational therapist and Academic Fieldwork Coordinator in the Department of Occupational Science and Occupational Therapy at the University of British Columbia, who assisted us with developing the section on seating and positioning.

Neuromotor Impairments

Several types of neurological and motor impairments can affect positioning and movement. Some individuals have increased or decreased muscle tone; too much tone makes voluntary movement difficult, whereas too little tone creates problems with maintaining posture, balance, and strength. Many individuals have high tone or spasticity in their extremities and low tone in their trunk area and therefore may experience all of the above problems, depending on the task at hand. Efficient use of

Table 6.1. Tools for assessment of assistive technology (AT) and augmentative and alternative communication (AAC) strategies

Assessment tool or protocol	Purpose	Features	Target population	Source
ACES Low-to-Lite Tech Evaluation Toolkit and High-Tech Evaluation Toolkit (McBride, 2008a, 2008b)	To determine an appropriate AAC technique	Low-to-Lite Tech Evaluation Toolkit provides assessment resources for beginning AAC devices; High-Tech Evaluation Toolkit provides resources for electronic devices.	All ages	AAC TechConnect
The Source for Augmentative Alternative Communication (Reichert Hoge & Newsome, 2002)	To identify key components of the assessment process	Provides tools to assess purposeful responses and fine motor abilities, a communication checklist, and an assistive technology checklist.	Ages 3 to adult	LinguiSystems
Medicare Funding of AAC Technology, Assessment/ Application Protocol (2004)	To document the need for a speech-generating device (SGD) for AAC	Protocol includes directions for documenting the nature of the communication impairment, assessment results (hearing, vision, physical, language, and cognitive skills), daily communication needs, functional communication goals, and features of the recommended SGD and accessories. Protocol is required for Medicare funding of SGDs in the United States.	Adults with acquired communication disorders	AAC-RERC
Protocol for Culturally Inclusive Assessment of AAC (Huer, 1997)	To document AAC-related assessment information	Protocol includes a cultural self-assessment for professionals as well as an assessment of communication partners, communication needs, capabilities related to AAC use, and technology use.	Children from diverse cultural and/or linguistic backgrounds	Huer (1997)
University of Kentucky Assistive Technology (UKAT) Toolkit (University of Kentucky Assistive Technology Project, 2002)	To guide professionals through the AT service delivery process	Includes printed forms for information gathering, observational assessment and data collection, summarizing assessment data, documenting the results of equipment/device trials, planning implementation, monitoring student progress, and professional self-assessment of AT knowledge and skills.	School-age	University of Kentucky Assistive Technology Project
Assessing Students' Needs for Assistive Technology (ASNAT; Gierach, 2009)	To evaluate a student's need for AT in his or her customary environment	Provides printed forms to guide the assessment team in gathering information related to a student's abilities and difficulties, identifying relevant environments and tasks, setting priorities, generating potential solutions, making decisions, implementing equipment/device trials, and monitoring trial results and long-term outcomes.	School-age	Wisconsin Assistive Technology Initiative

Assessment tool or protocol	Purpose	Features	Target population	Source
Functional Evaluation for Assistive Technology (FEAT; Raskind & Bryant, 2002)	To facilitate an ecological assessment of AT needs	Protocol consists of five scales: Contextual Matching Inventory, Checklist of Strengths and Limitations, Checklist of Technology Experiences, Technology Characteristics Inventory, and an Individual-Technology Evaluation Scale, plus a Summary and Recommendations Booklet.	All ages	National Professional Resources
Augmentative and Alternative Communication Profile (Kovach, 2009)	To assess communicative competence and design AAC interventions	Profile measures areas of strength and areas that may need intervention and instruction.	Ages 2 to 21	LinguiSystems

AAC devices necessitates providing external support or adapting the environment to compensate for these difficulties.

Other problems can result from the presence of primitive reflexes, involuntary muscle responses that are present in typically developing infants but disappear as they grow and mature. For example, if an infant's cheek is stroked, the child will turn his or her head and open his or her mouth to that side. This response is the rooting reflex, which usually disappears within the first few months of life. If the reflex persists, it can interfere with voluntary head control (Orelove & Sobsey, 1996). Care must be taken not to position an access switch such that this reflex is elicited.

Other reflex patterns, such as the asymmetrical tonic neck reflex (ATNR), can also affect the motor control needed for the use of switches or other adaptive devices. ATNR usually disappears by the time an infant is 6 months of age. It is activated when the infant's head is turned to the side, causing the infant to extend the arm and leg on the same side to which his or her face is turned and also prompting the flexion of the infant's arm and leg on the opposite side (see Figure 6.1a). Once the reflex has been activated, many individuals become "stuck" in the atypical motor pattern and are unable to resume a midline position without assistance. Therefore, AAC systems for individuals who exhibit ATNR should be designed to prevent the need for head rotation to scan a display, because once the person's head is turned, he or she will be unable to use the arm on that side for direct selection (see Figure 6.1b and Figure 6.1c). The AAC team should conduct a thorough motor assessment to ensure appropriate switch placement for each individual (see Figure 6.1d and Figure 6.1e).

Another common reflex pattern is the symmetrical tonic neck reflex (STNR), which occurs in response to either extension or flexion of the neck. When the individual's neck flexes (i.e., bends forward), STNR prompts flexion of the arms at the elbows and extension of the hips (see Figure 6.2a). The opposite occurs when his or her neck extends (i.e., moves backward): The individual's arms extend outward and his or her hips flex (see Figure 6.2b). Again, the individual often becomes "stuck" in the reflex position and requires assistance to resume a functional position. Because STNR interferes with the individual's functional use of his or her arms, its presence affects AAC motor access. One technique to avoid triggering STNR is to position displays or switches that are oriented vertically rather than horizontally (e.g., on a

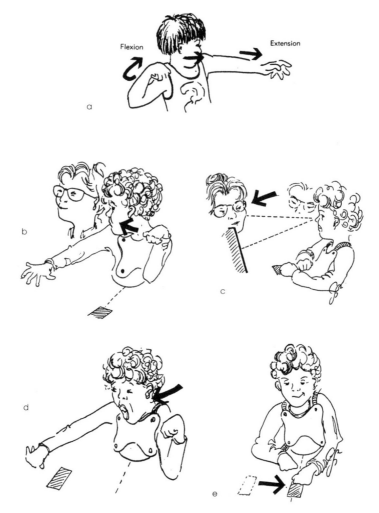

Figure 6.1. a) Asymmetrical tonic neck reflex (ATNR); b) facilitator and/or augmentative and alternative communication (AAC) display should not be placed to the side; c) midline placement of facilitator and//or AAC display is preferred; d) switches should not be placed to the side; e) midline placement of switches is preferred. (From Goossens', C., & Crain, S. [1992]. *Utilizing switch interfaces with children who are severely physically challenged* [p. 40]. Austin, TX: PRO-ED; copyright © Carol Goossens'; reprinted by permission.)

desk; see Figure 6.2c and Figure 6.2d). Similarly, people interacting with the individuals should not approach them from above (see Figure 6.2e) but should approach them at eye level (see Figure 6.2f).

Some individuals also have skeletal deformities that affect various aspects of positioning. Two common examples include scoliosis (lateral curvature of the spine), which can affect upright posture as well as comfort; and the windswept position of the hip (i.e., hip dislocation, pelvic rotation, and scoliosis), which affects sitting balance and posture. Prevention of such conditions is of primary importance, but if they have already developed in the individual and are fixed, the motor experts on the AAC team will need to compensate for the resulting difficulties.

Finally, movement disorders such as athetosis, which is characterized by involuntary movements of the face and limbs during muscle activation, are common in people with certain types of brain lesions. These individuals may not have sufficient control of their upper extremities to be able to write or point to symbols on a display, and as a result they may need to use switches to activate AAC devices.

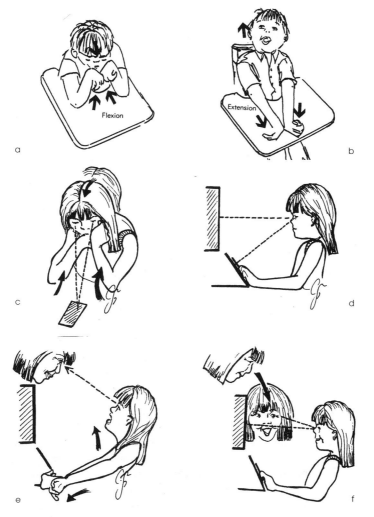

Figure 6.2. a) Symmetrical tonic neck reflex (STNR) in response to neck flexion; b) STNR in response to neck extension; c) horizontal placement of augmentative and alternative communication (AAC) display and/or switches may activate STNR; d) AAC display should be placed at eye level and switches should be aligned vertically; e) approaching from above may activate STNR; f) facilitator should approach at eye level. (From Goossens', C., & Crain, S. [1992]. *Utilizing switch interfaces with children who are severely physically challenged* [p. 43]. Austin, TX: PRO-ED; copyright © Carol Goossens'; reprinted by permission.)

An engaging and informative webcast entitled *Seating and Positioning for Individuals Who Use AT* by Aileen Costigan, an occupational therapist at the Pennsylvania State University, is available on the web site of the AAC-RERC (Rehabilitation Engineering Research Center on Communication Enhancement).

Principles and Techniques

Most individuals with neuromotor impairments are likely to use their AAC devices while in a seated position in a wheelchair, at a school or work desk, or at home. It is possible to grossly underestimate an individual's capabilities if he or she is not properly positioned and supported in a seated position. Improper positioning and inadequate physical support can affect a person's fatigue and comfort levels, emotional state, and ability to move and attend to a task. Therefore, the first step in an assessment should involve optimizing the individual's positioning so that the AAC team can accurately assess cognitive, language, and motor capabilities. This does not mean that the team should delay all other AAC assessments until the optimum wheelchair or seating insert has been developed to improve an individual's posture. Rather, it means that the team members who are experts at evaluating physical posture and control should be prepared to at least temporarily position the individual so that he or she can complete an appropriate assessment. Over time, a comprehensive assessment of the individual's seating and positioning needs should be completed so that more permanent solutions for the individual's postural and movement difficulties can be implemented as part of the AAC intervention.

Ideally, a symmetrical seated position should be the goal; however, this will not be possible for many individuals with severe neuromotor impairments, especially those with fixed deformities. A number of principles should guide the assessment of (and the later design of supports for) positioning and seating. These principles, adapted from Radell (1997) and York and Weimann (1991), include the following.

1. *Use yourself as a reference.* Almost automatically, people without disabilities position themselves for comfort, stability, and functional movement during tasks. Therefore, in evaluating the position of a person with motor impairments, using yourself as a reference is usually a good idea. The process involves engaging in a task (e.g., activating a switch, using a keyboard) and asking yourself questions such as "How would I position myself for this task?," "How would I align my trunk?," and "How would I position my head, arms, and legs?" The answers can then be used as guidelines to optimize positioning for the individual whose AAC needs are being assessed.

2. *Ensure a stable base of support.* It is impossible for a person to move in functional ways if his or her trunk and extremities are not sufficiently stable. For instance, if you place a piece of paper on a table and try writing without resting your forearms on the table surface, you will probably find the task fairly difficult. This is because the forearms stabilize the arms, shoulders, upper trunk, and wrists, so in order to use any of those body parts, the forearms must be supported. Similarly, the feet stabilize the lower part of the body and the trunk, which is why it is difficult to sit for long periods of time without resting your feet on the floor. For the individual undergoing AAC assessment, this stability can be achieved through the use of seat belts, bars, harnesses, lap trays, and other adaptive devices designed for static positioning (see Figures 6.3–6.5).

3. *Decrease the influence of atypical muscle tone.* An individual with low muscle tone often requires external supports to achieve a proper seated position for AAC assessment. For example, a person who cannot keep his or her head in an upright position may need a headrest or neckrest, either temporarily or permanently. Individuals with high muscle tone (i.e., spasticity) require the careful positioning of AAC displays, switches, and other assistive devices to avoid triggering reflex patterns and to maximize their ease of movement. Often, professionals use a trial-and-error approach to identify the position(s) that allows the individual to have the most functional movement.

4. *Accommodate fixed deformities and correct flexible deformities.* As noted previously, the ideal seated position is one that is symmetrical and stable. By applying the first principle ("use yourself as a reference"), AAC team members can correct most flexible deformities through the appropriate use of positioning devices. In many cases, fixed deformities may prevent the attainment of symmetry, and the individual may require accommodations to maintain residual movement, maximize comfort, decrease

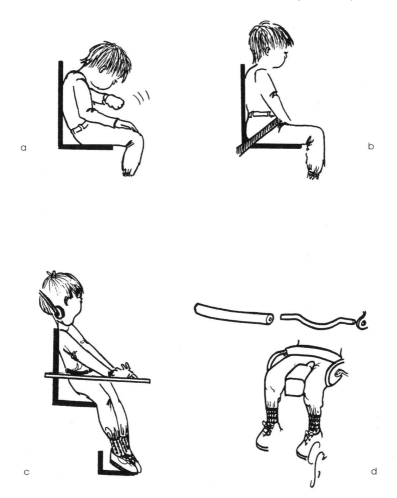

Figure 6.3.   a) Poor positioning in a chair; b) good positioning with the pelvis back in the chair and stabilized with a seat belt at a 45° angle across the hips; c) extensor thrust with hips extended and buttocks raised across the seat; d) subasis bar (rigid pelvic restraint used to stabilize the pelvis and prevent extensor thrust) in place, with two variations shown. (From Goossens', C., & Crain, S. [1992]. *Utilizing switch interfaces with children who are severely physically challenged* [p. 26]. Austin, TX: PRO-ED; copyright © Carol Goossens'; reprinted by permission.)

fatigue, and minimize the effort required for movement. For example, an individual with severe scoliosis or other deformities may be unable to sit in an upright position, and the team will need to utilize either temporary or permanent supports to achieve alignment in as functional a position as possible (McEwen & Lloyd, 1990).

5. *Provide the least amount of intervention needed to achieve the greatest level of function.* It is important that the individual not be so rigidly supported in a seated position that he or she is unable to move. As the person's center of gravity changes with upper-body shifting (e.g., leaning forward, reaching, leaning back), his or her feet and arms must be free to move and compensate. In addition, most people both enjoy and need to assume a variety of positions throughout the day.

6. *Provide support for resting.* It is important to ensure that people who become fatigued while using their AAC systems can rest with appropriate physical support. For example, individuals with weakness due to a degenerative disease such as amyotrophic lateral sclerosis need to be able to rest when they are not actively using their AAC technology (see Chapter 14).

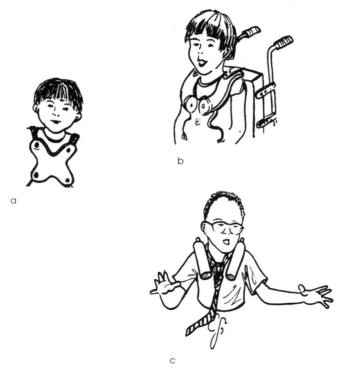

Figure 6.4. Devices used for trunk and shoulder stability. a) Butterfly harness; b) Danmar harness; c) shoulder retractors. (From Goossens', C., & Crain, S. [1992]. *Utilizing switch interfaces with children who are severely physically challenged* [p. 32]. Austin, TX: PRO-ED; copyright © Carol Goossens'; reprinted by permission.)

Several general procedures are usually involved in the assessment of positioning and seating that is related to AAC use (Cook & Polgar, 2008; McEwen & Lloyd, 1990; Radell, 1997). First, the AAC team should observe the individual in his or her wheelchair or while he or she is seated in a standard chair. If the person's hips have slid down in the chair, the team should lift the individual so that his or her pelvis is centered on the back edge of the seat or on a custom insert. The person's feet and arms should be supported as needed for proper alignment and movement. If the person is likely to use an AAC device frequently in other positions, the team should observe the individual in these other situations as well. Second, if the person cannot assume or maintain a proper seated position independently, the AAC team should provide assistance in this regard while allowing as much participation by the individual as possible. The assessor(s) should provide firm support to allow the person to achieve a stable and well-aligned position on his or her chair, beginning with his or her pelvis, which provides the base of support and therefore must be stable. Next, the AAC team should position the individual's lower extremities, followed by his or her trunk, upper extremities, head, and neck. In effect, the support provided by the hands of the team members simulates the type of support that might be sought through the use of assistive equipment. Third, the team should help the person with CCN move out of the chair (if possible) so that team members can take note of the seat, back angles, and any adaptations already in place (e.g., a contoured seat back). Fourth, the team should assess the individual while he or she is out of the chair, looking for any deformities, pressure sores, contractures (i.e., shortening of certain muscle groups), and other physical problems.

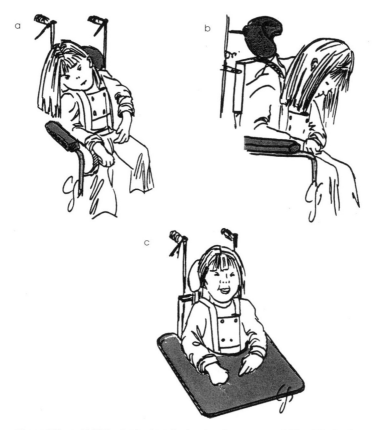

Figure 6.5. a, b) Without a lap tray, the head and arms are unstable; c) the lap tray provides trunk, shoulder, neck, and head stability. (From Goossens', C., & Crain, S. [1992]. *Utilizing switch interfaces with children who are severely physically challenged* [p. 36]. Austin, TX: PRO-ED; copyright © Carol Goossens'; reprinted by permission.)

Once the AAC team has completed its observations, temporary changes can be implemented to improve the individual's positioning. Table 6.2 summarizes the elements of an optimal seated position, although not all of these elements may be attainable for every individual. After the team has properly positioned the person's pelvis, hips, and thighs and secured them to create a stable base, the individual's trunk, upper extremities, lower extremities, head, and neck can also be supported. Rolled towels, foam inserts, heavy cardboard supports, temporary splints, Velcro straps, blocks, and other nonpermanent materials can serve as "mock-ups" for any supports that will eventually need to be custom made. The goal at this stage is simply to optimize positioning so that assessment of the motor skills necessary for AAC use can proceed. Over time, a variety of permanent supports may be needed to ensure that the individual has the efficiency and accuracy of movement needed for communication in a seated position. These permanent supports may be relatively simple in nature, such as floor sitters or seating orthoses that support children while they are seated on the floor, in the bathtub, or on other horizontal surfaces. The supports can also be quite sophisticated, including those used to stabilize and align the pelvis, trunk, hips, thighs, legs, shoulders, and/or head. Figures 6.6 and 6.7 depict some of the most common permanent components used to support seating and positioning.

Table 6.2.   Elements of an optimal seated position

Ideally, the **pelvis, hips, and thighs** should be positioned so that

- The sitting bones (i.e., ischial tuberosities) bear equal weight
- The pelvis is tilted slightly forward or in a neutral position
- The pelvis is centered in the back edge of seat
- The pelvis is not rotated forward on one side
- The hips are flexed to 90°
- The pelvis is secured to the chair with a belt at a 45° angle across the hips (not across the abdomen)
- The thighs are equal in length
- The thighs are slightly abducted (apart)

Ideally, the **trunk** should be positioned so that it is

- Symmetrical, not curved to the side
- Curved slightly at the low back
- Upright or leaning forward slightly

Ideally, the **shoulders, arms, and hands** should be positioned so that

- The shoulders are in a relaxed, neutral position (not hunched up or hanging low)
- The upper arms are flexed slightly forward
- The elbows are flexed in midrange (about 90°)
- The forearms rest on a tray for support, if necessary to maintain alignment
- The forearms are neutral or rotated downward slightly
- The wrists are neutral or slightly extended
- The hands are relaxed, with fingers and thumbs opened

Ideally, the **legs, feet, and ankles** should be positioned so that

- The knees are flexed to 90°
- The feet are aligned directly below or posterior to the knees
- The ankles are flexed to 90°
- The feet are supported on a footrest
- The heels and balls of the feet bear weight
- The feet and toes face forward
- The feet can be moved backward behind the knees when the upper body moves forward (i.e., no straps or other restrictive devices unless needed)

Ideally, the **head and neck** should be positioned so that

- They are oriented toward the midline of the body
- The chin is slightly tucked (i.e., the back of the neck is elongated)

From York, J., & Weimann, G. (1991). Accommodating severe physical disabilities. In J. Reichle, J. York, & J. Sigafoos (Eds.), Implementing augmentative and alternative communication: Strategies for learners with severe disabilities (p. 247). Baltimore: Paul H. Brookes Publishing Co.; adapted by permission.

Assess Motor Capabilities

As is the case with assessment of seating and positioning, the involvement of physical and/or occupational therapists in the assessment of motor access is critical for individuals with severe motor impairments. There are two related motor assessment concerns: identifying a motor technique that the individual can use during the assess-

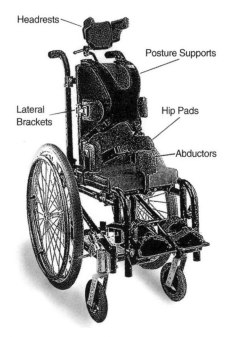

Headrests

Posture Supports

Lateral
Brackets

Hip Pads

Abductors

Figure 6.6.   Seating system with positioning components. This article was published in *Cook & Hussey's assistive technologies: Principles and practice* (3rd ed.), p. 204, by A.M. Cook and J.M. Polgar. Copyright Elsevier (2008).

ment process and identifying a technique that the individual can use for alternative access in the long term. (At this point, readers might wish to review the alternative access options presented in Chapter 4.) The AAC team might select the same motor technique for both the assessment and for long-term access, or the team might choose two techniques that are quite different, depending on the individual with CCN. Regardless, it is important to remember that the goal of an AAC motor assessment is to discover motor capabilities, not to describe motor problems.

Identification of Motor Skills for Assessment

The AAC assessment process requires identification of a number of cognitive, symbolic, language, literacy, and other skills related to communication. Therefore, whoever is involved in the assessment must ensure that the individual has a reliable and reasonably efficient way to answer questions and provide other information during the assessment process itself. The means of communication will need to be a direct selection technique because scanning adds considerable cognitive demand to a task (McCarthy et al., 2006; Mizuko, Reichle, Ratcliff, & Esser, 1994; Ratcliff, 1994). In addition, Glennen (1997) noted that, when a team uses scanning for initial assessment, it is difficult to determine the source of any errors that occur—the individual may not understand how scanning works, may not be able to access the switch in time to select a desired response, may have forgotten the question while waiting for the scanning cursor to move to a desired response, or simply may not know the answer to the question! For these reasons, choosing one of the direct selection options is important, at least during assessment.

Identification of a short-term direct selection technique can be quite straightforward and usually begins by determining whether the person can answer yes/ no questions accurately because this question format can then be used productively

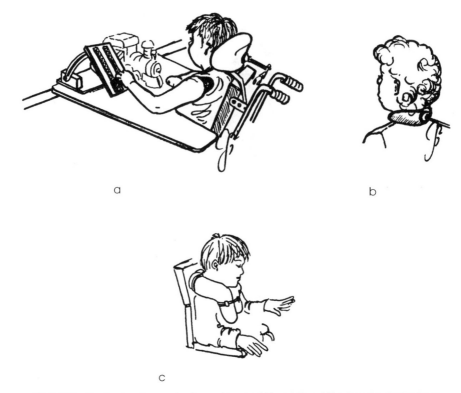

a   b

c

Figure 6.7.   Head and neck supports. a) curved headrest; b) neck ring; c) Hensinger head collar. (From Goossens', C., & Crain, S. [1992]. *Utilizing switch interfaces with children who are severely physically challenged* [p. 40]. Austin, TX: PRO-ED. Copyright © 1992 Carol Goossens'; reprinted by permission.)

throughout the assessment. It is important to ask questions that are developmentally appropriate, such as asking a child *Is your name Santa Claus?* or *Is this a car?* (while holding up a toy car or another item), asking an adult *Did you get here today in an airplane?*, and so forth. Many individuals will be able to respond to such questions quite accurately with vocalizations; eye blinks; facial expressions; head shakes, turns, or nods; and other gestures. If the team plans to use a yes/no format during the remainder of the assessment, it is critical that the individual's responses be highly accurate and unambiguous. If the person's responses are vague, the team usually proceeds to examine finger/hand use as a second option. To do this, the assessor may place a variety of food items, toys, or other motivating items on a table or lap tray. He or she can then encourage or ask the person with CCN to reach for, pick up, or point to the objects while the assessor notes accuracy, range, and movement patterns (e.g., ability to cross the midline of the body). If the individual's hand and arm use is limited, the assessor can hold up items in front of the person at various distances and locations in the visual field in order to assess his or her eye gaze in a similar manner.

It is important to allow adequate time for responses during a preliminary direct selection assessment because individuals who do not regularly use these techniques may require considerable processing time before they can execute the necessary motor actions. For example, one woman we know had been deemed "unassessable" by two consecutive AAC teams because she could not demonstrate a reliable motor behavior during the initial screening. In reality, she could point to pictures and objects with her hand quite accurately—as long as assessors were willing to wait for up to 2 minutes so that she could slowly drag her hand across the lap tray to select an answer! Although this method was too slow to be useful as a permanent access technique, it was used successfully during the initial assessment to identify this woman's language, symbol, and literacy skills, which were considerable.

Identification of Long-Term Motor Skills

Once the team has identified a temporary response technique, the assessment may proceed to determining the best long-term technique. As we have seen, there are two approaches to indicating items in the selection display: direct selection and scanning. Because, in general, direct selection can be more efficient for individuals with sufficient motor control and is generally preferred to scanning techniques, motor assessment usually focuses first on direct selection (Dowden & Cook, 2002). If direct selection techniques prove to be inaccurate, very slow, or fatiguing for the individual being assessed, the team will then initiate a scanning assessment. Of course, there are exceptions to this rule: consider, for example, a person who can communicate using direct selection in the morning but needs to change to scanning in the afternoon or evening as fatigue sets in. Or consider an individual who can use a direct selection technique when properly positioned in a wheelchair but must control a communication system or computer through scanning when seated in other types of chairs, when lying in bed, or when participating in personal care activities. In such cases, assessment will need to examine both direct selection and scanning abilities. Fortunately, because many electronic AAC devices are manufactured with both scanning and direct selection options, individuals can incorporate both selection techniques into their systems as needed, while using the same or similar symbol representation, message formulation, and output strategies for both.

Direct Selection   An assessment of direct selection capabilities generally occurs in the following stages: 1) assessment of hand and arm control, 2) assessment of head and orofacial control, and 3) assessment of foot and leg control. The individual's upper limbs are assessed first because the hand potentially provides the most discrete control and has the greatest social acceptance as an alternative access site (Dowden & Cook, 2002). Second, head, neck, and orofacial movements (e.g., eye pointing, head pointing) may be used. Third, the team usually assesses the individual's foot and leg control last because few people with physical impairments have the fine motor control of their lower extremities needed for direct selection techniques.

The direct selection survey in Figure 6.8 has been developed to collect and summarize the information from a direct selection assessment. Some of the techniques that teams may use to gather this information are summarized in the sections that follow. Additional forms for direct selection assessment can also be found in Cook and Polgar (2008).

Assess Range and Accuracy of Movement   A team usually begins an assessment of direct selection capabilities by observing the individual for a time to determine the types of movements he or she makes during communication or other routine activities. Interviews with the individual, family members, caregivers, and others also provide information about current movement patterns and activities. For example, some individuals may already point with their hands or their eyes to indicate items of choice. Such information is useful in guiding the assessment.

Next, the assessment generally involves testing the individual's range and accuracy of finger, hand, head, and eye movements without using adaptations. The AAC team usually assesses hand control (e.g., for pointing) by using a horizontal

Direct Selection Survey

Site	Direct selection device	Adaptations used (e.g., splint, keyguard)	Target (size, number, spacing, orientation to body)	Times hit/ missed	Negative impact (e.g., increased muscle tone, reflex activation, posture, fatigue)	Comments
Right hand/arm						
Left hand/arm						
Head	Head mouse					
Head	Safe-laser					
Head (other)						
Eyes	Gaze/point					
Eyes	Tracking					
Other						

Figure 6.8. Direct selection survey.

grid surface, whereas head control (e.g., for mouse control or laser pointing) and eye movement control (e.g., for eye tracking or pointing) is assessed using a vertical surface, often on a computer screen. Of course, the person with CCN must understand the task requirements in order for the results to be valid; therefore, the team should make every effort to minimize the cognitive, linguistic, and technical aspects of the assessment so that motor control can be isolated and studied. For this reason, the team usually does not use AAC symbols or ask people to formulate messages during the initial screening process. Rather, team members begin by placing various types of targets on a display surface and indicating that the individual is to select each target using one or more direct selection techniques. For adults with acquired conditions, individual numbers or letters might be used to mark locations to which they are asked to point. Coins or small candies often make excellent targets for children, especially when they are told they can keep each coin or candy that they touch or hit with a finger or hand. We have found that even children with severe cognitive impairments often understand this task almost immediately. Alternatively, the team can use small toys or other motivating pictures or items as targets. In some cases, individuals with CCN may be able to reach for items with their hands but lack the ability to point accurately and efficiently. If this is the case, AAC assessors can provide a variety of manual supports or devices to facilitate pointing during assessment. These aids include temporary finger or wrist splints, handheld pointers (e.g., a pencil, a small flashlight), and mobile arm supports such as slings or hinged arm positioners.

To assess head control, the AAC team can mount a low-cost laser pointer on an eyeglass frame and ask the person with CCN to direct the beam toward specific targets of different sizes that are fastened to a wall or another display surface. Of course, laser pointer use must be monitored carefully during the assessment to insure that the beam is not directed at another person. Both children and adults may be willing to play "tag" with a laser pointer by chasing targets (e.g., large pictures) moved slowly across a solid background in order to demonstrate the range and accuracy of their head control. Of course, if a head mouse and computer are available, numerous computer games can be used to assess head control as well.

Computer games for head mouse assessment are available through the GameBase web site.

Many of the same techniques used to assess head control can also be used to examine nonelectronic eye-gaze or eye-pointing capabilities as well. Assessment for eye tracking on a computer screen or AAC device requires specific eye-tracking software and the related equipment.

Optimizing Control   For motor techniques with which the individual was somewhat successful during screening, additional assessment can help to further define capabilities in areas such as 1) the degree of accuracy with which the person can use the technique to access targets of various sizes; 2) the maximum range and number of targets that he or she can access; and 3) the extent to which adaptations such as keyguards, various display surface angles, various textured surfaces (e.g., slick versus rough), head supports, and trunk supports can optimize his or her accuracy, efficiency, and range of motion. Because people with CCN may have had little experience with the access options used in the assessment, AAC team members should be quite conservative in their judgments about motor control. During an initial evaluation, an individual may demonstrate little of the ability that instruction and practice might produce. This is particularly true for techniques that involve the use of a head mouse or optical pointer because few individuals are likely to have had any experience with these methods of alternative access prior to an evaluation. Therefore, the team should reassess options that appear even marginally viable—if possible, after the individual has practiced for a few weeks.

Assess Negative Impact   Throughout the motor control assessment, the AAC team should also focus on the overall impact each access technique has on the individual with CCN. For example, some direct selection control techniques can lead to unwanted consequences such as persistent atypical reflexes, excessive muscle tone, atypical postures, or excessive fatigue. In the assessment, AAC team members must determine the extent to which they can minimize the negative impact of various alternative access options while preserving the potential benefits. Often, a compromise may be reached; however, the negative consequences associated with a particular alternative access option occasionally can be so detrimental that the team must abandon the option for the moment. Such techniques often can be considered later with additional instruction, practice, or adaptations.

Manual Signing   Perhaps surprisingly, no widely accepted assessment measures are available to determine the appropriateness of manual signing for individuals with CCN. Some studies have suggested that the ability to imitate hand and finger positions/movements is related to manual sign acquisition (Gregory, DeLeon, & Richman, 2009; Seal & Bonvillian, 1997; Tincani, 2004); however, an unambiguous causal relationship between fine motor ability and sign learning has not yet been established (Ogletree, 2010). Thus, AAC teams considering the use of manual signs should first attempt to teach a few signs that are highly motivating and functional for the person of concern. The team can then monitor, as indicators of manual sign appropriateness, both the accuracy of sign formation and the length of time it takes for the person to begin to use the signs accurately and independently. Manual signs are unlikely to be truly functional if they cannot be acquired at a reasonable rate and if they cannot readily be understood by both familiar and unfamiliar partners (Mirenda, 2003b).

Switch Assessment for Scanning   The AAC team will need to complete a switch assessment for scanning if an individual is unable to directly select items from a display. Fortunately, technologies such as those used for eye tracking (a direct selection technique) have been developed over the past several years and have considerably reduced the need for scanning, which is much slower than direct selection. Nonetheless, switch assessment may be necessary in some cases and involves identification of one or more body sites that the individual can use to activate one or more switches, as well as assessment of the individual's ability to use various scanning strategies and arrangements (see Chapter 4).

Screening for a switch activation site on the body is the first step of a scanning assessment. A note of caution: AAC teams have a tendency to utilize tasks that are too complex when identifying switch activation sites that are appropriate for an individual. The team should attempt to minimize the cognitive, visual, and communicative demands in a switch control assessment; for this reason, we rarely use AAC equipment to gather this information. We have found that asking an individual to control a simple computer game (or to turn on a battery-operated toy) is an effective way to provide a consequence during the scanning assessment. The team can then try different switches while assessing various motor control sites, such as fingers, hands, head, and feet.

Accessible computer games that can be used during assessment to identify a switch site for scanning are available for people of all ages through the Nanogames, One Switch, RJ Cooper & Associates, Inc., Shiny Learning, and Inclusive Technology Ltd. web sites. The latter site also offers a free *Switch Progression Road Map* booklet that describes how to attach one or more switches to a computer and how to teach scanning using computer games and other digital media.

Generally, a criterion-based assessment approach should be used to identify a switch activation site. To this end, a switch assessment should begin with the most socially appropriate body site for switch control: the hands. If hand or finger control of a switch allows accurate, efficient, and nonfatiguing alternative access, the assessment is not continued with other body parts. If hand control seems insufficient, the head should be assessed next, followed by the feet, legs, and knees.

Components of Switch Control   There are essentially six components of switch control. To operate an electronic scanner, the individual must first be able to *wait* for the right moment in order to avoid inadvertently activating the switch. Some individuals have difficulty waiting because of cognitive or motor control problems. The second step in controlling a switch is *activation,* or closing the switch. During assessment, the team should determine whether the individual can activate a variety of switches, note the approximate length of time it takes for each activation to occur, and observe the efficiency with which the person completes activation movements. The third step in controlling a switch is to *hold* it in an activated position for the required time. Some individuals who are able to activate the switch accurately and promptly are not able to hold or maintain switch closure. The fourth step in switch control is the ability to *release* the switch accurately and efficiently, a step that may be problematic for some people. Finally, the fifth and sixth steps involve the individual *waiting* and then *reactivating* the switch at the appropriate times.

The AAC team can assess each of these components by using the computer game or toy strategy described previously. For example, the team may ask the person with CCN to turn an mp3 player on and off according to directions designed to assess each component, such as *Wait, don't hit it yet; Okay, hit it now; Stop;* and *Hit it again.* Alternatively, if an individual is unable to follow verbal directions because of cognitive or other limitations, the AAC team may need to observe the individual while he or she uses a switch to control a toy, a computer game, or an appliance (e.g., a blender) in the natural environment. Regardless, this assessment should give the team an overall indication of the individual's ability to activate switches at various motor control sites. We provide a form to record the results of assessment of motor (switch) control for scanning in Figure 6.9. Again, we remind readers that, although many body parts are listed on this form, it is often unnecessary to evaluate all of them.

Cursor Control Techniques and Switch Control Capabilities   The choice of cursor control technique for scanning (e.g., automatic, directed, or step scanning; see Chapter 4) is influenced by an individual's motor control capabilities. The match between techniques and capabilities is illustrated in Tables 6.3 and 6.4. The types of scanning are found as the column headings in Table 6.3, and the six components of switch control described previously are listed in the first column. The table includes the motor component skill-accuracy requirements for each type of scanning. Therefore, in the case of automatic scanning, in which the cursor moves automatically across the selection set and the person with CCN is required to stop it at a desired item, there is a high skill-accuracy requirement for the individual to wait until

Voluntary motor control (single switch)

	Is able to wait		Is able to activate		Is able to hold		Is able to release		Is able to wait		Is able to reactivate		Accuracy*
	Yes	No	Yes	No	Yes	No	Yes	No	Yes	No	Yes	No	
Fingers on left hand													
Fingers on right hand													
Left hand (palm? back?)													
Right hand (palm? back?)													
Left shoulder													
Right shoulder													
Head rotation (R? L?)													
Head flexion													
Head–side flexion (R? L?)													
Head extension													
Vertical eye motions													
Horizontal eye motions													
Tongue or chin													
Left outer leg/knee													
Right outer leg/knee													
Left Inner leg/knee													
Right inner leg/knee													
Left foot (up? down?)													
Right foot (up? down?)													

*Accuracy = rate of overall accuracy on a 0–4 scale in which 0 = never and 4 = always.

Figure 6.9. Assessment of motor (switch) control for scanning.

Table 6.3. Skill-accuracy requirements of cursor control techniques for scanning

Motor component	Cursor control technique		
	Automatic scanning	Directed scanning	Step scanning
Wait	High	Medium	Low
Activate	High	Low	Medium
Hold	Low	High	Low
Release	Low	High	Low
Wait	High	Medium	Medium
Reactivate	High	Medium	Medium
Fatigue value	Low	Medium	High

the cursor is in the correct location. There is also a high skill-accuracy requirement for the individual to activate the switch to stop the cursor. Because the item is selected at the moment of switch activation, it does not matter how long the person holds the switch closed; thus the skill-accuracy requirement for holding is low. The release phase also has a low skill-accuracy requirement because nothing is required during this phase of automatic scanning. Finally, this technique requires high skill-accuracy for waiting and reactivating the switch. Automatic scanning relies on timing rather than on repeated movements or endurance, so it produces a low level of fatigue.

In directed scanning, the cursor moves to the desired item only when the switch is activated, and the individual must release the switch to make a selection. Table 6.3 indicates that waiting prior to activation has a medium skill-accuracy requirement for this type of scanning. Although waiting does not affect accurate item selection directly, inadvertent activation at this point will initiate cursor movement before the individual is ready to begin. Switch activation has a low skill-accuracy requirement in directed scanning because activation does not involve precise timing. Holding has a high skill-accuracy requirement in directed scanning because the individual must hold the switch closed until the cursor is positioned at the desired item; therefore, inability to adequately hold the switch closed will result in a selection error. During directed scanning the individual makes a selection in the switch release phase, requiring a high skill-accuracy level, whereas waiting and reactivation have medium skill-accuracy requirements. The fatigue value in directed scanning is medium because the individual must have some motor endurance to hold the switch closed for a period of time.

In step scanning, the cursor moves one step with each activation of the switch. Therefore, the individual's ability to wait has a low skill-accuracy requirement because waiting is not involved in item selection. Switch activation has a medium skill requirement because, although the activation does not have to be rapid, accurate, or well timed, it may be quite fatiguing. Holding in step scanning requires only low skill-accuracy because the cursor moves one step with each activation and therefore holding is not part of the selection process. For the same reason, releasing is also a low skill-accuracy requirement. Waiting and reactivation require medium motor control abilities because inadvertent switch activation at these phases will result in erroneous selections. Fatigue is high in step scanning because of the multiple, repeated switch activations.

Clinical Illustrations   The preceding discussion is based on clinical experience, not research. Nonetheless, professionals with whom we have worked tell us that generally applying these guidelines helps them achieve effective matching between an individual's motor control capabilities and a cursor control pattern for scanning. We illustrate clinical applications of these guidelines in the following case studies by discussing three people who rely on scanning for alternative access. We remind the reader that the clinical interpretations made in these case studies are illustrations only. In no sense do we mean to suggest that all individuals who experience athetosis, spasticity, or weakness will have switch activation profiles similar to those in these case studies. We simply present these examples to illustrate the process of matching an individual's capabilities with the motor control requirements for scanning. Readers should also note that the goal of the type of motor assessment described here is to screen an individual's motor capabilities so that intervention can begin. In addition to this initial process, the AAC team should continually assess an individual's motor control after an intervention is in place in order to further refine the alternative access technique and ensure that the person's performance becomes increasingly more accurate and efficient and less fatiguing.

The results of a switch assessment for Francesca, a child with athetoid cerebral palsy, are illustrated in Table 6.4, which indicates the ease or difficulty with which Francesca was able to accomplish the various components of switch activation. As is the case for many individuals with athetosis, accurate waiting was difficult for her. Because of involuntary motor movements ("overflow") associated with her athetosis, Francesca inadvertently activated the switch during the waiting phase. Similarly, accurate and efficient switch activation was also difficult because Francesca's overflow movements were accentuated in times of stress or anticipation. Therefore, she was unable to activate the switch quickly on command. The holding phase was of medium ease for Francesca because she was able to maintain contact with the switch once she managed to activate it. In contrast to the difficulties associated with switch activation, the release phase was easy for her; she was able to release the switch efficiently and accurately. Finally, Francesca found that waiting and reactivation were again difficult because of her extraneous motor movements.

A comparison of Francesca's switch control profile with the requirements of cursor control in Table 6.3 suggests that directed scanning might be an alternative access mode for her. Directed scanning has high skill-accuracy requirements for holding and releasing, which match her capabilities. Conversely, automatic scanning has high skill requirements for waiting and activating, the two phases of switch activation that Francesca found most difficult. Step scanning would probably exacerbate her involuntary motor movements because it requires the greatest amount of actual motor activity and is fatiguing.

Isaac is a young man with severe spasticity resulting from a traumatic brain injury. We provide a summary of his switch activation profile in Table 6.4. The assessment showed that Isaac had medium ease with waiting and switch activation, and that his activations were rather deliberate and slow. He found it easy to hold the switch closed briefly but difficult to release it in a timely and accurate manner. Release was difficult for Isaac because the spasticity prevented him from relaxing his contact with the switch when he wanted. He experienced medium ease with waiting and reactivation.

A review of the requirements of cursor control patterns suggests that Isaac's difficulty with switch release would probably make it difficult for him to use directed

Table 6.4.   Clinical illustrations of ease of motor control and capabilities for scanning

Motor component	Ease of motor control		
	Francesca (athetosis)	Isaac (spasticity)	Jin (weakness)
Wait	Difficult	Medium	Easy
Activate	Difficult	Medium	Medium
Hold	Medium	Easy	Difficult
Release	Easy	Difficult	Easy
Wait	Difficult	Medium	Easy
Reactivate	Difficult	Medium	Medium
Fatigue value	Medium	Medium	Difficult

scanning successfully. Instead, automatic scanning might be a more appropriate choice for him because it has high waiting and activation requirements, activities that Isaac found moderately easy. Automatic scanning also has low skill-accuracy requirements for switch releasing, the phase with which Isaac had the most difficulty.

Jin, a woman with amyotrophic lateral sclerosis that causes severe weakness throughout her body, could operate a very sensitive switch affixed just above her eyebrow by raising her forehead slightly. Jin found waiting quite easy and was able to activate the switch with moderate ease when asked. She experienced difficulty holding the switch closed because of her weakness, but she could easily release it. She then had no difficulty waiting and could reactivate the switch with medium ease. As can be seen by consulting Tables 6.3 and 6.4, the optimal cursor control pattern for Jin appears to be automatic scanning because this option requires the greatest amount of waiting and causes the least fatigue, a major concern for someone such as Jin who has little motor stamina.

Assess Cognitive/Linguistic Capabilities

In the Participation Model, assessment of an individual's current communication skills occurs at an earlier phase of assessment (see Chapter 5). At this point in the assessment process, we can use additional assessments to gather relevant information about specific cognitive, language, and related skills.

Cognitive/Communication Assessment

The purpose of cognitive/communication assessment in AAC is to determine how the individual understands the world and how the AAC team can best facilitate communication within this understanding. Rowland and Schweigert (2003) suggested six aspects of cognitive/communication development that are highly relevant to AAC: awareness, communicative intent, world knowledge, memory, symbolic representation, and metacognition. In addition, Wilkinson and Jagaroo (2004) suggested that a variety of visual perceptual skills are important to consider when making decisions about AAC devices or techniques.

Awareness involves a number of increasingly sophisticated understandings: 1) that one is separate and different from one's surroundings; 2) that specific behaviors one performs (e.g., kicking, smiling at a familiar face) have specific consequences (e.g., a mobile moves, a person smiles and vocalizes back); and 3) that other people have thoughts, desires, and perceptions that may differ from one's own (i.e., theory of mind).

Communicative intent, an extension of social contingency awareness, involves behavior that is "purposefully directed toward another person with intended meaning…[and that] requires dual orientation—orientation to both the communication partner and the topic or referent" (Rowland & Schweigert, 2003, p. 251). Of course, communicative intentionality does not simply "happen" overnight; rather, it develops as caregivers respond positively to preintentional behaviors that become increasingly purposeful over time as a result.

World knowledge includes general experience in the world that results in 1) expectations about how both people and inanimate objects should work, and (even more important) 2) the motivation to repeat pleasant experiences and avoid unpleasant ones. Motivation may be compromised in individuals who have repeatedly experienced unsuccessful attempts to communicate using conventional but nonsymbolic modes; this effect has been referred to as "learned helplessness" (Seligman, 1975).

Memory involves a complex set of skills that are needed for all learning and that have profound implications for a person's ability to attend to, categorize, retrieve, select, and sequence messages that are represented through both unaided and aided symbols or codes (Light & Lindsay, 1991; Mirenda, 2003b; Oxley & Norris, 2000). Memory is also an important factor to consider when making decisions about many electronic communication devices, especially those that utilize dynamic displays or auditory scanning (Kovach & Kenyon, 2003).

Symbolic representation involves an understanding of the relationship between symbols (e.g., manual signs, photographs, line drawings) and their referents. As noted in Chapter 3, a number of studies have demonstrated that the meanings of symbols that more closely resemble their referents are easier to learn and to deduce.

Metacognitive skills allow people to consider their own cognitive experiences with regard to language use and learning (metalinguistics), memory strategies (metamemory), and self-regulation (executive functions). These more advanced cognitive skills are especially important for individuals who use electronic scanning as a selection technique (Light & Lindsay, 1991) and/or who use either low- or high-technology AAC devices with large vocabulary capacities organized in levels or categories (Oxley & Norris, 2000).

Unfortunately, no empirically validated assessment tools are available to assess an individual's capabilities across all six of these areas. However, some instruments are available to assess at least basic cognitive and communication skills such as contingency awareness, communicative intentionality, symbolic representation, and basic concepts related to world knowledge, using either observational, interview, or direct assessment methods. Table 6.5 presents a summary of some instruments and resources that might be useful in this regard, including both those designed for general assessment and those specifically designed for individuals who rely on AAC. Although several of these instruments may be useful for assessing the skills of individuals who are primarily nonsymbolic communicators, it is important to note that adaptations may be needed to accommodate motor or sensory impairments. For example, Iacono, Carter, and Hook (1998) modified the "communicative temptations" from the Communication and Symbolic Behavior Scales™ (CSBS™; Wetherby & Prizant, 1993) for individuals with cerebral palsy by providing repeated activity exposures to allow time for orientation and by adding a microswitch to facilitate self-activation of a toy or music activity. Several authors have emphasized that formal

Table 6.5. Selected instruments and resources for assessment of basic cognitive/communication skills related to augmentative and alternative communication (AAC) use

Instrument or resource	Designed for AAC?	Skills assessed	Type(s) of assessment	Appropriate participants	Source
Augmentative Communication Strategies for Adults with Acute or Chronic Medical Conditions (Beukelman, Garrett, & Yorkston, 2007)	Yes	Comprehension, expression, cognition, motor/ perceptual skills, partner needs, and others	Direct assessment, interviews, observations	Adults with a wide range of acute and chronic medical conditions	Paul H. Brookes Publishing Co.
Augmentative and Alternative Communication in Acute and Critical Care Settings (Hurtig & Downey, 2009)	Yes	Comprehension, expression, cognition, motor/ perceptual skills, partner needs, and others	Direct assessment, interviews, observations	Adults in intensive care and other medical settings	Plural Publishing
Bracken Basic Concept Scale–Revised (Bracken, 1998)	No	Basic concepts and receptive language skills	Direct assessment with verbal directions and responses via pointing	Individuals ages 2 years 6 months through 7 years who are unable to speak, read, or write English	Harcourt Assessment
Child-Guided Strategies: The van Dijk Approach to Assessment (Nelson, van Dijk, Oster, & McDonnell, 2009)	No	Behavioral state, orienting response, learning channels, approach-withdrawal, memory, social interactions, communication, problem solving	Observations, interactive elicitation	Individuals with multiple disabilities and/or deaf-blindness across the age range	American Printing House for the Blind
Communication and Symbolic Behavior Scales™ (CSBS™; Wetherby & Prizant, 1993)	No	Communicative functions; gestural, vocal, and verbal communicative means; reciprocity; social-affective signaling; symbolic behavior	Caregiver questionnaire, interactive behavior sample with parent present	Individuals with developmental ages between 6 and 72 months, if cognitive delays are present	Paul H. Brookes Publishing Co.
Communication and Symbolic Behavior Scales Developmental Profile™ (CSBS DP™; Wetherby & Prizant, 2002)	No	Emotion and eye gaze, communication, gestures, sounds, words, understanding, and object use	Screening checklist, caregiver questionnaire, interactive behavior sample with parent present	Individuals with developmental ages between 6 and 72 months, if cognitive delays are present	Paul H. Brookes Publishing Co.

(continued)

Table 6.5. *(continued)*

Instrument or resource	Designed for AAC?	Skills assessed	Type(s) of assessment	Appropriate participants	Source
Communication Matrix (Rowland, 1996, 2004)	Yes	Symbolic abilities related to four functional categories of communication	Observations, interviews, or direct elicitation	Individuals who are functioning at the earliest stages of communication	Design to Learn
School Inventory of Problem-Solving Skills (SIPSS) and Home Inventory of Problem-Solving Skills (HIPSS; Rowland & Schweigert, 2002)	Yes	Basic object skills (e.g., using simple actions, transferring), gaining access to objects (e.g., object permanence, tool use), object use (e.g., functional use, matching)	Rating scale for each skill: mastered, mastered with limitations, emerging, not present	Nonverbal children with multiple disabilities (e.g., severe intellectual disabilities or sensory impairments, including deaf-blindness)	Design to Learn
Test of Early Communication and Emerging Language (TECEL; Huer & Miller, 2011)	Yes	Receptive and expressive communication/ language abilities of infants and toddlers	Interview, observation, or both; multiple response modalities	Individuals of all ages who have moderate to severe language delays	PRO-ED
The Triple C: Checklist of Communication Competencies–Revised (Bloomberg, West, Johnson, & Iacono, 2009)	Yes	Reflexivity and reactivity, contingency awareness, object use, imitation, object permanence, cause and effect, communicative intentionality, symbolic representation	Observational checklist and accompanying videotape	Adolescents or adults with severe or multiple disabilities	Scope Communication Resource Centre

measures are not appropriate for many nonsymbolic communicators because of the idiosyncratic forms of their communication, and have described the use of a dynamic assessment process that is designed to accommodate individual needs in terms of tasks, materials, procedures, and assessors (Iacono & Caithness, 2009; Snell, 2002). Although dynamic assessments usually require more time than static (i.e., formal) assessments, they also provide much richer information about an individual's communication skills, the contexts and interaction methods that are most likely to facilitate communication, and the types and amount of intervention that will be needed.

In addition, there may be situations—aside from those in which the goal is to achieve a good match between an individual and an AAC technique—in which formal assessment of an individual's cognitive abilities may be necessary or useful. For example, we are frequently asked to suggest instruments that can be used in educational settings for cognitive assessment related to individual education planning, especially for individuals with developmental disabilities. In the past few years, several reasonably reliable and valid standardized tests of cognitive ability have been used with children, adolescents, or adults who are unable to speak, as presented in Table 6.6. Many of these tests require no motor responses other than pointing. Alternatively, they can be adapted by, for example, cutting up test pages with pictures into separate items that can then be arranged on an eye-gaze display or individualized array for pointing; limiting the number of choices from which the individual is asked to choose; enlarging test stimuli (i.e., pictures) for individuals with visual impairments; and using a yes/no or multiple-choice format instead of asking open-ended questions (Glennen, 1997). For example, if the original test question is *How are an orange and an apple the same?*, the assessor might ask the question and then

Table 6.6.   Selected instruments for nonverbal assessment of cognitive ability

Instrument	Skills assessed	Direction and response modes	Appropriate participants	Source
Comprehensive Test of Nonverbal Intelligence– Second Edition (CTONI-2; Hammill, Pearson, & Wiederholt, 2009)	Nonverbal reasoning abilities	Directions given via gestures; responses via pointing	Individuals ages 6 through 90 who are unable to speak and who may not read or write in English	PRO-ED
Leiter International Performance Scale–Revised (Roid & Miller, 1997)	Visualization and reasoning (intellectual ability), attention, and memory	Directions given via pointing, gesture, and pantomime; responses via pointing, card match, or manipulatives	Individuals ages 2 through 20 who are unable to speak and who may not read or write in English	Stoelting
Naglieri Nonverbal Ability Test– Individual Administration (Naglieri, 2003)	Nonverbal reasoning and general problem-solving ability	Directions given via gestures; responses via pointing	Individuals ages 5 through 17 who are unable to speak and who may not read or write in English	Pearson Assessments
Pictorial Test of Intelligence– Second Edition (PTI-2; French, 2001)	General cognitive ability	Directions given verbally; responses via pointing	Individuals age 3 to 9 who are unable to speak	PRO-ED
Stoelting Brief Intelligence Test (S-BIT; Roid & Miller, 1999)	Nonverbal cognitive ability	Directions given in pantomime; responses via pointing or card matching	Individuals ages 6 through 21 who are unable to speak and who may not read or write in English	Stoelting
Test of Nonverbal Intelligence– Fourth Edition (TONI-4; Brown, Sherbenou, & Johnsen, 2010)	Nonverbal intelligence, aptitude, abstract reasoning, and problem solving	Directions given in pantomime; responses via pointing, nodding, or symbolic gestures	Individuals ages 6 through 90 who are unable to speak and who may not read or write in English	Pearson Assessments
Universal Nonverbal Intelligence Test (UNIT; Bracken & McCallum, 1998)	Memory, problem solving, symbolic reasoning, nonsymbolic reasoning, overall intellectual ability	Directions given in pantomime and gestures; responses via pointing, paper-and-pencil tasks, or manipulatives	Individuals ages 5 to 18 who are unable to speak and who may not read or write in English	Riverside

present a series of yes/no options in random order: *Are they both red?*, *Are they both round?*, *Are they both fruit?*, *Are they both toys?*, and so forth. Although such modifications technically invalidate the results of standardized cognitive assessments, they may have practical value in that they allow the team to assess the cognitive skills that are measured by the test items.

The article "A Guide to Child Nonverbal IQ Measures" (DeThorne & Schaefer, 2004) provides a useful summary of the psychometric properties (e.g., reliability, validity) of the most commonly used tests of this type in North America. It also contains descriptive tables summarizing the motor requirements and subtests contained in each test.

Although various AAC techniques require different types and degrees of cognitive ability, these requirements have been described only minimally in the clinical and research literature. Thus, in most cases, the AAC team must analyze the cognitive requirements of a particular approach, estimate the extent to which each individual will be able to meet these requirements, and then conduct intervention trials with one or more AAC techniques or devices to determine the optimal match. It is important to realize that thousands of successful AAC interventions have been instituted without formal documentation of cognitive abilities.

Symbol Assessment

Symbols or codes represent a majority of the messages included in AAC systems (see Chapter 3). It is not uncommon to see people who rely on AAC successfully employ a variety of symbol types. Thus, the goal of symbol assessment is not to identify a single symbol set to represent all messages. Instead, the goal of assessment is to select the types of symbols that will meet the individual's current communication needs and match his or her current abilities, as well as to identify symbol options that might be used in the future.

Assessment of an individual's ability to use symbols usually involves several steps. Before starting, the team members responsible for the symbol assessment should identify approximately 10 functional items with which the individual is familiar, basing their selections on the recommendations of the individual's family members, teachers, or frequent communication partners. These functional items might include a cup, a brush, a washcloth, a spoon, and so forth. Next, team members should reach a consensus about the individual's familiarity with the selected items because one of the most common errors is to attempt a symbol assessment using items with which an individual is unfamiliar. When the team reaches consensus on the items, they should compile symbols that represent each of them. These symbols might include both color and black-and-white photographs, miniature objects, various types of line-drawing symbols (see Chapter 3), and written words.

Tangible Symbol Systems (2nd ed.; Rowland & Schweigert, 2000b) presents a protocol for conducting a basic symbol assessment, along with relevant recording forms. It can be downloaded at no cost from the Ideas That Work web site of the Office of Special Education Programs.

Functional Use Format   At the most basic level of symbol understanding is the ability to understand the functional use of objects (Glennen, 1997). An AAC team can assess a child's level of functional understanding in a play context by giving him or her the items selected for the assessment and observing whether the child uses them functionally (e.g., trying to drink when presented with a cup). With older individuals, the team can make direct requests related to the uses of functional objects, such as *Show me what you do with this* or *Which one do you (eat with, comb your hair with, etc.)?* Often, interviewing family members, teachers, or others reveals useful information in this regard; for example, a child's mother might report that the child gets excited and looks at the door of his house whenever she gets out his "going to the park" jacket, indicating that he recognizes its function. Individuals with severe motor impairments that prevent them from manipulating objects can be assessed for functional understanding of object use if the assessor is willing to act as a "demonstrator." In this case, the demonstrator mimes both correct and incorrect uses of each object and observes the individual's reactions. For example, the assessor might brush his or her own hair with a spoon or use a cup as a hat, and then wait for the individual to give gestural or other indications that the demonstrated action is wrong. The individual's responses should be different from those elicited by a correct mime (e.g., eating from a spoon, drinking from a cup). Success in one or more of these formats would suggest that the person recognizes that the test objects have specific uses. Figure 6.10 provides a form for assessing functional object use.

Receptive Labeling and Yes/No Formats   Observing an individual's receptive labeling ability is often the next step in symbol assessment because this is the most straightforward way to establish whether an individual can recognize a symbol as representing its referent. The person conducting the assessment presents the individual with two or more items or symbols of a particular type and asks him or her to give to the assessor, point to, or look at one of the items. Alternatively, the assessor can use a yes/no format in which he or she holds up one item or symbol at a time and asks, *Is this a _____?* The assessor should arrange the trials so that yes/no questions are presented randomly for all target items. This testing format is appropriate only if the individual understands the concept of yes/no and has a clear and accurate way of answering yes/no questions. The team can assess several types of symbols, one type at a time, using either of these formats. The assessor records on a form (see Figure 6.11) whether the individual can identify target items from the various symbol sets.

Alternative Visual-Matching Format   In some cases, AAC team members cannot use the receptive labeling or yes/no formats because the person undergoing the symbol assessment does not understand either the task expectations or the verbal labels presented. However, there is empirical evidence that a visual-matching format produces results similar to those elicited with the receptive labeling format (Franklin, Mirenda, & Phillips, 1996). Thus, a visual-matching format similar to the one provided in Figure 6.12 may serve as a useful alternative to the receptive labeling option. In a standard matching assessment, the team provides the individual with a single object and places two or more symbols, one of which matches the object, on the table (see Figure 6.13a). The assessor then asks the individual to match the object, using eye gaze, pointing, or another direct selection option, to the corresponding symbol. Alternatively, the team may give a single symbol to the individual, who then attempts to match the symbol to the correct object in an array (see Figure 6.13b). A study examining alternative symbol assessment strategies found these formats to be equivalent in difficulty (Franklin et al., 1996). The AAC team can also adjust the configuration, spacing, and number of items in the array in order to meet the needs of specific individuals. The goal is to make systematic adjustments that facilitate the acquisition of accurate and useful information about the person's ability to associate objects with their referents on the basis of perceptual characteristics.

Format used: Direct request ("Show me what you do with this") _____   Caregiver interview _____

Assessor demonstration of correct usage _____

Instructions used _____

Response accepted as correct _____

List objects used	Confirmation of item knowledge by informant?

Indicate whether trial is correct or incorrect in appropriate column and describe responses

Trial no.	Object	Function correct? (describe)	Function incorrect? (describe)
1			
2			
3			
4			
5			
6			
7			
8			
9			
10			
11			
12			

Figure 6.10.   Symbol assessment: Functional object use format.

Format used: Receptive labeling _____   Yes/no _____

Number of items in array _____

Instructions used _____

Response accepted as correct _____

List items used   Confirmation of item knowledge by team?

_____

_____

_____

_____

_____

_____

_____

_____

_____

_____

Indicate whether trial is correct (+) or incorrect (−) in appropriate column

Trial no.	Target item	Real objects	Color photographs	Line drawings	Other (specify)
1					
2					
3					
4					
5					
6					
7					
8					
9					
10					
11					
12					

Figure 6.11.   Symbol assessment: Receptive labeling and yes/no formats.

Format used: Standard matching _____   Sorting _____

Number of items in array _____

Instructions used _____

Response accepted as correct _____

List items used   Confirmation of item knowledge by team?

_____

_____

_____

_____

_____

_____

_____

_____

_____

_____

Indicate whether trial is correct (+) or incorrect (−) in appropriate column

Trial no.	Target item	Real objects	Color photographs	Line drawings	Other (specify)
1					
2					
3					
4					
5					
6					
7					
8					
9					
10					
11					
12					

Figure 6.12.   Symbol assessment: Visual-matching format.

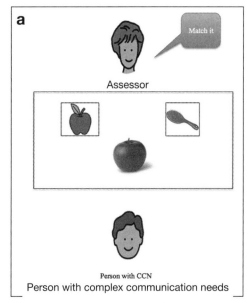 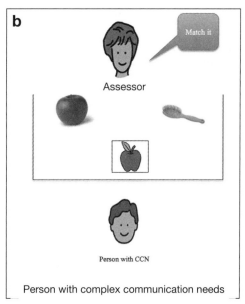

Figure 6.13. a) Single-object-to-multiple-symbol matching format; b) single-symbol-to-multiple-object matching format. (The Picture Communication Symbols ©1981–2012 by DynaVox Mayer-Johnson LLC. All Rights Reserved Worldwide. Used with permission. Pics for PECS™ images used with permission from Pyramid Educational Consultants, Inc. [www. pecs.com]. Pyramid Educational Consultants, Inc. reserves all rights to the Pics for PECS™ images.)

Several cautions are in order with regard to the matching format. First, it is not essential for an individual to be able to match objects and symbols in order to learn to use symbols successfully (Romski & Sevcik, 1996). If a person can do this, it is clear that he or she understands the visual relationship between symbols and their referents; but if an individual lacks this understanding, it does not mean that he or she cannot learn to use symbols. Second, the matching assessment is not a standardized testing protocol; rather, it is a flexible format that the team can alter to suit the individual's abilities and interests. For example, many people with limited cognitive abilities may need to be taught to match items and symbols before actual assessment. The team can usually accomplish this instruction in a short time using a "teach-then-test" approach and discrete trial teaching (Lovaas, 2003). During the "teach" phase, team members first introduce and gradually fade physical or other prompts in order to teach the person with CCN to match identical real objects. Once the person can do this independently and accurately, the team can test symbol understanding by presenting various object-symbol matching tasks, as described previously (see Mirenda & Locke, 1989, for a more complete description of this approach).

Analyzing Results of Basic Symbol Assessment   By this point in the symbol assessment, two things should be clear: 1) whether the individual understands the functional use of selected, familiar objects and 2) whether the person can either recognize the verbal labels for a variety of symbols or match them to their referents. If one or both of the latter skills is not evident, this may indicate that the person will be best served by several "beginning communicator" strategies designed to build communicative skills while teaching symbol-referent associations. These strategies include visual schedule systems and "talking switch" techniques, as described in Chapter 9. The individual's ability to perform the assessment tasks successfully can be used to predict the type(s) of symbols with which he or she is most likely to be successful, at least initially. The initial symbol set(s) selected should enable accurate, efficient, and nonfatiguing communication, with minimal instruction required. Over time, the individual can learn and use more sophisticated types of symbols, if needed. Symbol sets that require extensive learning and practice may be excellent choices for the future but may not be appropriate for initial use.

Because real communication rarely involves either receptive language labeling or symbol matching, it is important to extend the assessment beyond these basic tasks to determine whether an individual can use symbols in a more communicative manner. The AAC team should include the following portion of the assessment process regardless of whether the individual is successful during the initial symbol tasks because some individuals may find it easier to demonstrate symbolic understanding during natural interactions. AAC team members can use one or both of the following formats to assess symbol use in context.

Question-and-Answer Format   Figure 6.14 contains a form with which a team can assess whether an individual can use symbols to answer verbal questions. As in the basic assessment, the assessor should first identify items or concepts that are known to the individual by interviewing familiar communication partners and listing items on the form. The assessor should present two or more symbols of a specific type—such as objects, photographs, or line drawings—and then ask a question that the individual can answer correctly by indicating one of the symbols. Receptive labeling questions such as *Can you show me the car?* or *Where is the picture of your dog?* should not be used in this situation. Instead, the assessor should ask simple knowledge-based questions such as *What did you eat for breakfast?* while presenting symbol choices such as the person's favorite breakfast food, a car, and a dog. This format can also be used in the context of a book activity in which the assessor first reads a story to a child with CCN and then asks simple questions based on the story, while providing correct and incorrect symbols for answers.

In order to complete this task successfully, the individual must understand the task expectations, the questions, and the symbol options presented, and he or she must be motivated and cooperative during the evaluation. If the individual performs poorly in the assessment, it is important for the team to try to determine which of these aspects of the question-and-answer task is responsible for the individual's difficulties. Alternative formats, such as question-and-answer assessments in natural contexts, may be useful to counteract some factors contributing to poor performance, especially with people who have severe cognitive impairments. For example, many individuals may be able to answer the question *What did you have for breakfast?* if they are seated in the kitchen in which they usually eat rather than in a classroom in which meals never take place. Figure 6.14, the symbol assessment in question-and-answer format, allows the assessor to provide relevant information related to context.

Requesting Format   Individuals with severe communication and cognitive limitations may be able to match symbols to objects and even answer simple questions using symbols, yet they may still be unable to use symbols to make requests. In Figure 6.15, we provide a form to guide the team's assessment of symbol use in a requesting format. An AAC team usually conducts this assessment in an appropriate natural context, such as during snack time, a play or craft activity, or the performance of some domestic task (e.g., washing the dishes), or in any other context that is of interest to the person being assessed. As before, the team lists and confirms items that the person knows and that are available in the context. Then, the assessor provides symbols representing two or more of the available options, trying one type of symbol at a time. The

Number of items in array _____

Instructions used _____

Context: Out of context _____   In context (specify) _____

Response accepted as correct _____

List items used   Confirmation of item knowledge by informant?

_____

_____

_____

_____

_____

_____

_____

_____

_____

_____

Indicate whether trial is correct (+) or incorrect (−) in appropriate column

Trial no.	Question asked	Real objects	Color photographs	Line drawings	Other (specify)
1					
2					
3					
4					
5					
6					
7					
8					
9					
10					
11					
12					

Figure 6.14.   Symbol assessment: Question-and-answer format.

Number of items in array _____

Instructions used _____

Were options: Visible? _____   Out of sight? _____

Context: Out of context _____   In context (specify) _____

Response accepted as correct _____

List items used   Confirmation of item knowledge by informant?

_____

_____

_____

_____

_____

_____

_____

_____

_____

_____

_____

Indicate whether trial is correct (+) or incorrect (−) in appropriate column

Trial no.	Items available	Real objects	Color photographs	Line drawings	Other (specify)
1					
2					
3					
4					
5					
6					
7					
8					
9					
10					
11					
12					

Figure 6.15.   Symbol assessment: Requesting format.

structure of the interaction provides opportunities for the person to request objects or actions by selecting one of the available symbols without the assessor instructing him or her to do so. Indirect cues such as *I don't know what you want. Can you help me out?* may be used to elicit requests. Direct instructions such as *Touch the picture to tell me what you want* should be avoided because the purpose of this assessment is to determine whether the individual can make spontaneous, unprompted requests.

Analyzing Results of Symbol Assessment in Question-and-Answer and Requesting Formats   The question-and-answer and requesting formats provide basic information about how the person can communicate with symbols; they do not indicate which symbols he or she recognizes linguistically or perceptually. Individuals who can do only one or neither task will need instruction in functional contexts to be able to use the symbols that were identified during the basic assessment. The strategies described in Chapter 10 for teaching requesting, rejecting, and so forth may be useful in this regard. Individuals who are able to answer questions or make requests using symbols may have the skills needed for more advanced symbol use, as assessed through the next two formats.

The Test of Aided-Communication Symbol Performance (TASP; Bruno, 2005) can be used with children and adults to determine the optimal size and number of symbols for an array and to assess grammatical encoding, categorization, and syntactic performance. The TASP uses Picture Communication Symbols, requires only an eye gaze or pointing response, and is available from DynaVox Mayer-Johnson.

Advanced Symbol Use   Individuals who are adept at single-symbol use in communicative contexts may be able to use symbols for words other than nouns and/or chain two or more symbols together to construct messages. The team can assess both of these abilities through the use of an activity display with symbols that represent various syntactic elements—nouns, verbs, adjectives, and so forth. For example, we often use dual Go Fish displays with symbols representing the various elements of this simple card game because it is appropriate for individuals across the age range (see Figure 6.16). While playing the game, the assessor produces multiple one- and two-symbol messages using his or her display, thus providing models for advanced symbol use (e.g., DO YOU HAVE + KING). If the person being assessed learns how to use the display quickly, the assessor can then observe whether he or she uses any symbols that are not nouns or makes a sequence of two symbols when provided with opportunities to do so. For example, at appropriate times, the assessor can create opportunities for the individual to communicate two-symbol messages such as YOU + LOSE, I + WIN, and so forth. Of course, an individual with motor impairments that limit hand use will need to play the game with a partner who manages the cards, and he or she may need to use an eye-gaze display with the appropriate messages as well. Alternative activities, such as pretend play, book reading, or board games, can also be used during such assessments.

Symbol Categorization Assessments   Some individuals might be able to use a communication system that is organized categorically. For example, symbols in communication books or boards may be organized in semantic or activity category sections. Similarly, dynamic display devices require the ability to use categorization techniques to locate symbols located in hidden levels. Teams can assess existing categorization skills with symbols of various items placed in two or more semantic categories, such as

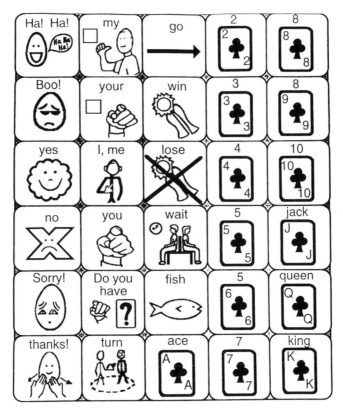

Figure 6.16. Go Fish display for assessment of advanced symbol use. (The Picture Communication Symbols ©1981–2012 by DynaVox Mayer-Johnson LLC. All Rights Reserved Worldwide. Used with permission.)

vehicles, foods, clothing, and animals. The individual is asked to sort the symbols into categories *(Put all of the animals in this box and all of the vehicles in that box)* or is helped to do so using eye gaze *(Which box should I put this one in?)*. Alternatively, a team can assess categorization abilities by asking the person to sort symbols for two very different activities, such as going to the beach and going to a birthday party *(Put the ones you'd use at the beach in this box and the ones you'd need at a birthday party in that box)*. The results of this type of assessment can be useful to determine whether the person can use a category-based system right away or whether facilitator scaffolding, modeling, and instruction will be required first. Porter (2007) offered suggestions for teaching people with CCN to use AAC symbol displays that are organized categorically.

The use of iconic encoding techniques such as Minspeak requires the ability to associate multiple meanings with pictures. *A Protocol for Assessing Metaphoric Use of Pictures* (Van Tatenhove, 2005), along with associated pictorial templates and data collection forms, is available at no cost from Gail Van Tatenhove's web site.

Language Assessment

Language assessment should include an evaluation of the individual's single-word vocabulary capabilities as well as his or her use of common language structures (i.e., morphemes, syntactic structures; Roth & Cassatt-James, 1989). Basic strategies for assessment in these areas are discussed in the sections that follow.

Single-Word Vocabulary Two types of language assessment typically are completed for AAC purposes. In the first type of assessment, the AAC team makes an attempt to measure vocabulary comprehension in relation to the individual's overall level of functioning. Assessment instruments such as the Peabody Picture Vocabulary Test–Fourth Edition (PPVT-4; Dunn & Dunn, 2007) or the Receptive One-Word Picture Vocabulary Test–Fourth Edition (ROWPVT-4; Martin & Brownell, 2010) are often used in AAC evaluations to assess an individual's knowledge of nonrelational words (e.g., nouns) because they can be easily modified to meet the needs of individuals with motor limitations, without sacrificing validity. Using a previous version of the PPVT (the Peabody Picture Vocabulary Test–Revised; Dunn & Dunn, 1981), Bristow and Fristoe (1987) compared scores that were obtained using the standard protocol with those obtained using six alternative response modes, including eye gaze, scanning, and headlight pointing. The results indicated that, with few exceptions, scores obtained under the modified conditions correlated highly with those obtained using standard test protocols. For young children, the MacArthur-Bates Communicative Development Inventories (Fenson et al., 2007) can also be used to estimate single-word vocabulary comprehension by parent report (Romski & Sevcik, 1999).

In addition to assessing nonrelational words, it is important to assess the individual's comprehension of action words and relational words (i.e., those that do not have concrete referents, such as *in, out, hot,* and *cold* (Roth & Cassatt-James, 1989). The Bracken Basic Concept Scale–Revised (Bracken, 1998) and portions of both the Test for Auditory Comprehension of Language–Third Edition (TACL-3; Carrow-Woolfolk, 1999) and the Sequenced Inventory of Communication Development–Revised (Hedrick, Prather, & Tobin, 1984) can be used in this regard. For individuals who are unable to complete formal tests, a team can often obtain an estimate of vocabulary comprehension by having family members, caregivers, and school personnel develop a diary of the words and concepts that the individual appears to understand.

Morphosyntactic and Grammatical Knowledge In the past decade, AAC researchers have increasingly noted the importance of assessing morphosyntactic and grammatical knowledge of individuals who rely on AAC because those who have not mastered skills in these areas are likely to have difficulty conveying ideas, fulfilling academic requirements, and securing or maintaining employment (Binger, 2008b; Binger & Light, 2008; Blockberger & Johnston, 2003; Blockberger & Sutton, 2003; Fey, 2008). For people who can participate in formal testing, a number of standardized instruments that are based on simple multiple-choice or pointing formats and require no verbal output are available. These include selected subtests from one of the Clinical Evaluation of Language Fundamentals (CELF) instruments (Semel, Wiig, & Secord, 2003, 2004), the TACL-3 (Carrow-Woolfolk, 1999), and the Test for Reception of Grammar–Version 2 (TROG-2; Bishop, 2003). Although some adaptations may need to be made to accommodate the needs of specific individuals, such tests offer the advantage of empirical support related to reliability and validity.

In addition, a number of informal assessment techniques have been developed for language assessment of individuals who rely on AAC. For example, Blockberger and Johnston (2003) developed two assessment tasks to examine children's acquisition of morphemes, including the past tense *-ed* (e.g., *walk/walked*), plural *-s* (e.g., *boy/boys*), and third-person regular *-s* (e.g., *I drink/he drinks*). In the first task, picture selection, the person with CCN is presented with three similar pictures (e.g., pictures of a baby with a dirty toy pig, a baby with a dirty shirt, and a dirty baby pig with a mother pig) and is asked to select the one that best matches a verbal utterance (e.g., *The baby's* *pig is dirty*). The task can be adapted to a yes/no format for children who are unable to select a picture by pointing or via eye gaze. In the second task, structured writing, the assessor reads out loud a short, illustrated story that will be of interest to the person with CCN. The individual is then asked to print or type single words to fill in blanks in sentences from the story. For example, in a story about a girl named Kate, one part of the story might read as follows: "Yesterday Kate woke up. She ate breakfast. Then she pl_____ with her teddy bears."

In addition, several authors have used grammaticality judgment tasks for AAC assessment. In a study with adults who used AAC, Lund and Light (2003) presented correct and incorrect sentences verbally and in print, and then asked participants to indicate via a gesture whether or not each followed a specific grammatical rule (e.g., *Please give me the blue book* versus *Please give me the book blue* or *Please give me blue the book*). In a study with children who used AAC (Blockberger & Johnston, 2003), children with CCN were introduced to a dog puppet that was described by the examiner as just learning to talk, and were asked to help the puppet practice saying some sentences. Two buckets were placed in front of a child, one containing dog biscuits and one containing rocks. The child was instructed to listen to a sentence that was "spoken" out loud by the puppet and, if it was correct, to give the dog a biscuit; if the sentence was wrong, the dog was to be given a rock. For example, for the third person regular -*s*, an example of a correct sentence was *Hockey players wear helmets* and an example of an incorrect sentence was *The cows eats the grass*. Children who were unable to pick up a biscuit or a rock used eye gaze or gestures to indicate which one the examiner should give to the puppet. A similar task was used by Redmond and Johnston (2001) with adolescents with CCN, except that the dog puppet was replaced by two action figures called "moon guys." The adolescents were told that the action figures were from outer space and were just learning to speak English, so they needed help to know when they talked "right" and "not so good."

Several more complex tasks have also been used to assess understanding and use of specific language forms in adults with CCN. For example, Sutton and colleagues (Sutton, Gallagher, Morford, & Shahnaz, 2000; Sutton & Morford, 1998; Trudeau, Morford, & Sutton, 2010) developed tasks using photographs of plastic figurines to assess both comprehension and production of relative clauses, such as *The girl pushes the clown who wears a hat* versus *The girl who pushes the clown wears a hat*. The comprehension task requires the person being assessed to indicate a photograph corresponding to a graphic symbol utterance, whereas the production task requires the person to use graphic symbols to construct a sentence describing the photograph (Figure 6.17).

Finally, assessors may use symbolic and written language sampling in dyadic play or conversational contexts to examine the morphosyntactic abilities of individuals with CCN (Kelford Smith, Thurston, Light, Parnes, & O'Keefe, 1989; Lund & Light, 2003; Sutton & Gallagher, 1995). Because language sampling require transcription and/or coding of utterances to be useful, it is more time intensive than other tasks. However, it is also likely to yield richer and more broad-based information (Binger & Light, 2008; Sutton, Soto, & Blockberger, 2002).

 The Universal Language Activity Monitor (U-LAM; Hill, 2004) facilitates the collection and analysis of language samples that are produced using speech-generating devices (SGDs). The U-LAM is available through the AAC Institute.

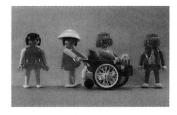
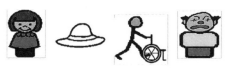

The girl who pushes the clown wears a hat.

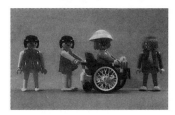
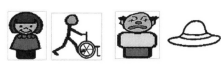

The girl pushes the clown who wears a hat.

Figure 6.17.   Sample tasks that can be used to assess comprehension and production of relative clauses. (Photos courtesy of Ann Sutton. The Picture Communication Symbols ©1981–2012 by DynaVox Mayer-Johnson LLC. All Rights Reserved Worldwide. Used with permission.)

Analyzing Results of Language Assessment   Once again, it must be emphasized that the purpose of language assessment, both formal and informal, is not to assign a score or developmental age to the individual, but rather to gather information that is needed for intervention planning. The goal is to develop a functional profile of the person's current language capabilities so that appropriate symbols, vocabulary items, and instructional procedures can be selected. There is no recipe for matching specific AAC strategies and techniques with the characteristics of the individual's language profile because this information must be considered in its totality along with information about the individual's motor, sensory, and other capabilities. For example, imagine a language profile for an individual with no motor or vision impairments indicating that he or she has a one-word vocabulary of 300 line-drawing symbols, produces no two- or three-word combinations, and is able to initiate simple requests and answer questions with symbols. It is likely that the initial AAC intervention would involve a system with a large vocabulary capability that can be expanded easily and that includes techniques aimed at encouraging multiword combinations and increasing communicative competence in conversational and other interactive contexts. Contrast this with the profile of an individual with severe motor and vision impairments who has a vocabulary of 10 manual signs, cannot make choices, and initiates no interactions. Clearly, the recommended intervention would be much different for the second individual than for the first one—not just because of differences in language ability, but because of a combination of many factors. These two examples illustrate the importance of considering language assessment information as part of the "big picture" of all intervention information.

Assess Literacy Skills

Literacy encompasses a multitude of skills that, cumulatively, result in a person's ability to read, spell, and write (see Chapter 12). Literacy assessment is particularly important for people who rely on AAC because the development of literacy skills is often an important goal. The ability to use the 26 letters of the English alphabet to construct messages enables a person with CCN to say anything he or she wants! Unfortunately, many individuals who rely on AAC receive very irregular instruction in this area when they are in school and may have scattered profiles of ability as a result. It is important to assess both strengths and weaknesses across a number of basic skill areas that form the foundation for literacy. Many of these assessment strategies are from the *Accessible Literacy Learning (ALL)* curriculum (Light & McNaughton, 2009a), which was specifically developed to teach literacy skills to individuals who rely on AAC as a result of autism spectrum disorders, Down syndrome, cerebral palsy, and other developmental disabilities.

Letter–Sound Correspondence

Assessing the ability to associate letters with their *sounds* (not their *names*) is a useful beginning step in an overall literacy assessment. The letter–sound relationship (e.g., *r* sounds like /rrr/) is more important than the letter–name relationship (e.g., the name of the letter *r* is *ar*) because it is the former skill—not the latter—that is used for decoding and sound blending. AAC teams can conduct this assessment quite easily using simple letter boards, eye-gaze displays, or keyboards, by asking the individual to point to, look at, print, or type specific letters by sound. Light and McNaughton (2009a) suggested that, for each letter sound, four letter cards (including the target letter) should be placed in front of the learner, insuring that the target letter is not always in the same location. The assessor can then give an instruction such as *I am going to say a sound. Listen, and then show me the letter that makes that sound.* Letter sounds should be presented in random order, and those that are identified incorrectly should be presented at least twice to insure that the results are reliable. Figure 6.18 provides an example of a data sheet that can be used for this assessment, from the *ALL* curriculum. Sounds that are identified incorrectly should be targeted for instruction.

Sound-Blending Skills

Since the mid-1990s, an increasing number of AAC researchers have emphasized the importance of the skills involved in phonological processing, which is known to be critical for reading achievement of both people without disabilities (Adams, 1990; Wagner & Torgeson, 1987) and those with severe speech and physical impairments (Dahlgren Sandberg, 2001; Dahlgren Sandberg & Hjelmquist, 1996a, 1996b; Foley & Pollatsek, 1999; Iacono & Cupples, 2004; Vandervelden & Siegel, 1999, 2001). Sound-blending skills are one of the most important components of phonological processing and can be assessed in a variety of ways.

In the *ALL* curriculum (Light & McNaughton, 2009a), sound blending is assessed using a number of response plates that each depict four Picture Communication Symbols (PCS; see Figure 6.19). The assessor first labels each of the pictures and then gives an instruction such as *I am going to say a word slowly. Listen, and then blend the sounds together in your head and show me the picture of the word.* For example, if the target symbol is CUT, the assessor says /c-u-t/ slowly and then gives the person with CCN time to respond by pointing to or looking at the corresponding picture. The *ALL* authors suggest a criteria of at least 80% accuracy for sound blending; if this is not achieved over several assessment sessions (repeated to insure consistent performance), focused instruction in sound blending will be required.

Data Collection Form

Assessment and instruction in Sound Blending, Phoneme Segmentation, Letter-Sound Correspondence, Single Word Decoding, and Sight Words

Learner's Name: _JILL_   Circle one: (Assessment)

Date: _10 – 12_   Baseline

Instructor: _ANN_   Instruction Guided Practice

Target Skill: _LETTER-SOUND_   Instruction Indep. Practice
CORRESPONDENCES
_p. 1 of 3_

Trial	Target	Choices provided				+/–
		Choice 1	Choice 2	Choice 3	Choice 4	
1.	e	e	m	(i)	p	–
2.	k	h	a	k	(l)	–
3.	g	d	(t)	o	g	–
4.	r	(b)	r	c	u	–
5.	t	(i)	e	c	t	–
6.	m	p	(m)	g	l	+
7.	v	k	(p)	v	e	–
8.	a	a	r	(f)	l	–
9.	g	g	v	m	(g)	–
10.	x	(c)	d	g	x	–

Summary of learner performance   _see p. 3_

Number correct / 10 trials _____

% accuracy _____

Error analysis

Comments

Figure 6.18.   Data sheet for assessment of letter–sound correspondences. (From Light, J., & McNaughton, D. [2009a]. *Accessible Literacy Learning [ALL]: Evidence-based reading instruction for individuals with autism, cerebral palsy, Down syndrome, and other disabilities* [p. 49]. Pittsburgh: DynaVox Mayer-Johnson; reprinted by permission.)

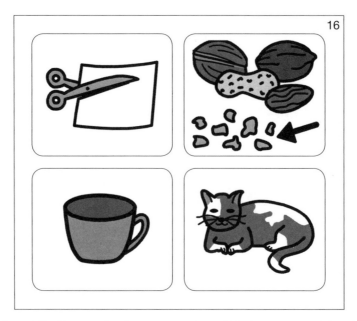

Figure 6.19. Response plate for assessment of sound blending, with symbols for CUT, NUT, CUP, and CAT. (From Light, J., & McNaughton, D. [2009a]. *Accessible Literacy Learning [ALL]: Evidence-based reading instruction for individuals with autism, cerebral palsy, Down syndrome, and other disabilities* [p. 38]. Pittsburgh: DynaVox Mayer-Johnson; reprinted by permission. The Picture Communication Symbols ©1981–2012 by DynaVox Mayer-Johnson LLC. All Rights Reserved Worldwide. Used with permission.)

 The Assessment of Phonological Awareness and Reading (APAR; Iacono & Cupples, 2004) can be used to assess a wide range of beginning literacy skills. It was designed for adults with CCN who are unable to speak and/or write, but it can be used with people of all ages. The APAR can be administered online or using printed stimuli to assess sound blending, single-word vocabulary, sentence comprehension, and text listening comprehension. Directions, stimulus cards, and scoring sheets for the APAR are available at no cost online. The APAR was designed to teach beginning reading skills when used with the Accessible Word Reading Intervention program, which is available from the Monash University Centre for Developmental Disability Health Victoria web site.

Phoneme Segmentation

Phoneme segmentation is, in many ways, the opposite of sound blending. It involves the ability to break words down into individual sounds (e.g., breaking the word *run* into the sounds /r/, /u/ [short u], and /n/). In the *ALL* curriculum, an individual's ability to identify the initial phoneme sound in a word is assessed using response plates with four PCS symbols, each beginning with a different sound (see Figure 6.20). First, the assessor presents a plate of four symbols and labels each of them. This is followed with an instruction such as *I am going to say a sound. Listen, and then show me a word that starts with that sound.* The assessor then models a sound (e.g., /m/) and says, *Which one starts with /m/?,* allowing the learner to point to or look at one of the pictured options. As with sound blending, the *ALL* authors suggest that learners who do not achieve at least 80% accuracy across all initial sounds will require instruction in initial phoneme segmentation as part of an overall literacy curriculum. A similar assessment procedure can also be used to assess final and medial phoneme segmentation skills; stimulus cards for these skills are also available in the APAR.

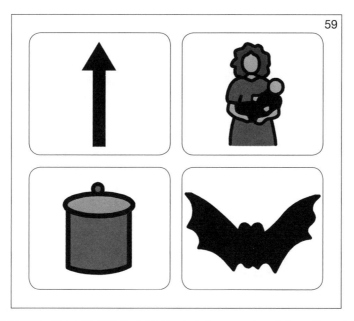

Figure 6.20. Response plate for assessment of phoneme segmentation, with symbols for UP, MOM, POT, and BAT. (From Light, J., & McNaughton, D. [2009a]. *Accessible Literacy Learning [ALL]: Evidence-based reading instruction for individuals with autism, cerebral palsy, Down syndrome, and other disabilities* [p. 43]. Pittsburgh: DynaVox Mayer-Johnson; reprinted by permission. The Picture Communication Symbols ©1981–2012 by DynaVox Mayer-Johnson LLC. All Rights Reserved Worldwide. Used with permission.)

Word Decoding

Decoding (i.e., reading new words) requires a combination of letter–sound correspondence and sound-blending skills; thus, assessment of this component is required only for learners who demonstrate competence in both of these areas. In the *ALL* curriculum, response plates with a printed word (e.g., *bed*) and four symbol options (e.g., RED, BEG, BAD, and BED) are provided for this task (see Figure 6.21). The assessor first provides practice trials to show the learner what is required, by modeling and describing each step in the task. Then, the person with CCN is provided with a response plate, and the assessor labels each of the pictures. The assessor gives an instruction such as *Here is a word* (pointing to the word). *Look at the word and say the sounds for each of the letters in your head. Blend the sounds together and say the word in your head. Then, show me the picture of the word.* The person whose skills are being assessed can then look at or point to one of the pictures in response; if appropriate, he or she can also use a manual sign, communication display, or SGD to respond. Less than 80% accuracy across all of the target response plates is an indicator that decoding instruction will be required.

Sight Word Recognition

It is advisable to conduct a sight word recognition assessment as well, even when an individual demonstrates limited skills in other components of literacy. Sight word recognition often emerges spontaneously because words are paired with symbols on many AAC displays (Romski & Sevcik, 1996). In addition, some individuals with CCN may have been taught to recognize familiar words such as their names, names of family members, or words for highly motivating edible items or high-interest activities. Words that a person is able to recognize by sight can be incorporated into motivating shared literacy activities that are focused on topics of interest.

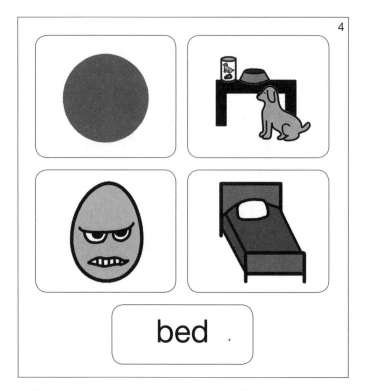

Figure 6.21.   Response plate for assessment of word decoding, with symbols for RED (colored), BEG, BAD, and BED. (From Light, J., & McNaughton, D. [2009a]. *Accessible Literacy Learning [ALL]: Evidence-based reading instruction for individuals with autism, cerebral palsy, Down syndrome, and other disabilities* [p. 53]. Pittsburgh: DynaVox Mayer-Johnson; reprinted by permission. The Picture Communication Symbols ©1981–2012 by DynaVox Mayer-Johnson LLC. All Rights Reserved Worldwide. Used with permission.)

AAC teams can conduct informal assessments using words to which the individual has been exposed either formally or informally on a regular basis, by first consulting with family members and teachers to compile a list of such words. Individual cards can then be created for each of the words and presented to the individual, four at a time. The assessor gives an instruction such as *I am going to say a word. Listen, and then show me the word I say,* providing an opportunity for the person being assessed to point to or look at a word. Alternatively, the assessor can use a multiple-choice format that places target sight words in context. For example, for the target word *pizza*, a sentence such as *I like to eat (pizza, chair, dog, shoe)* can be presented and read out loud to the person with CCN, who is then asked to select the correct word from four options. Figure 6.22 provides an example of a data sheet that can be used for this assessment, from the *ALL* curriculum. It is important to remember that sight word recognition is a useful skill that can be incorporated into literacy instructional activities, but sight word "drill and practice" activities should not be conducted for their own sake or in isolation.

Reading Comprehension

Assessment of reading comprehension typically involves asking an individual to read a passage of text and then answer explicit questions about the content of the text. This type of assessment is most appropriate for individuals who have demonstrated basic reading skills and are able to use graphic symbols on a communication display or SGD. Subtests in several literacy assessment instruments that are commonly

Data Collection Form

Assessment and instruction in Sound Blending, Phoneme Segmentation, Letter-Sound Correspondence, Single Word Decoding and Sight Words

Learner's Name: _Emily_   Circle one: (Assessment)

Date: _9 - 20_   Baseline

Instructor: _Mrs. B._   Instruction Guided Practice

Target Skill: _sight word recognition_   Instruction Indep. Practice

Mom reports that Emily recognizes the following words: Emily, Zack, McDonalds

Trial	Target	Choices provided				+/−
		Choice 1	Choice 2	Choice 3	Choice 4	
1.	Emily	Zack	(Emily)	Sally	Edith	+
2.	McDonalds	(McDonalds)	mom	Target	Mary	+
3.	Zack	Zoo	Jack	(Zack)	Emily	+
4.	McDonalds	Monday	Mary	Wendy's	(McDonalds)	+
5.	Emily	Family	Zack	(Emily)	Edith	+
6.	Zack	Zap	Zoo	Jack	(Zack)	+
7.						
8.						
9.						
10.						

Summary of learner performance

Number correct / 10 trials   _6/6_

% accuracy   _100%_

Error analysis

Comments   Use these words in personalized books for shared reading. Teach sight word recognition of new, high interest, motivating words.

Figure 6.22. Data sheet for assessment of sight-word recognition. (From Light, J., & McNaughton, D. [2009a]. *Accessible Literacy Learning [ALL]: Evidence-based reading instruction for individuals with autism, cerebral palsy, Down syndrome, and other disabilities* [p. 60]. Pittsburgh: DynaVox Mayer-Johnson; reprinted by permission.)

used in North America have been constructed to examine reading comprehension and require only a yes/no response or simple pointing response and/or can be easily adapted for use with alternative response modes. A selection of tests and subtests available in this area are summarized in Table 6.7.

The SEDL web site provides a searchable database of both criterion- and norm-referenced assessment instruments for beginning readers (prekindergarten to Grade 3), many of which can be adapted for use for individuals who rely on AAC.

Spelling Assessment

Spelling abilities are also important targets during AAC assessment. Because various AAC techniques require different types of spelling skills, a nontraditional language or spelling evaluation may be necessary. Overall, three components of spelling ability should be assessed: spontaneous spelling, first-letter-of-word spelling, and, if necessary, recognition spelling.

Spontaneous Spelling   In spontaneous spelling, the person with CCN is asked to spell words letter by letter. Estimates of spontaneous spelling ability can be assessed either informally or by using the spelling subtests from measures such as the Wide Range Achievement Test (Wilkinson & Robertson, 2006) or the Woodcock-Johnson III (Woodcock, McGrew, & Mather, 2006). Individuals who can spell, at least phonetically (e.g., *f-o-n for phone*), can use these skills when operating dedicated or computer-based AAC devices that rely on orthography.

First-Letter-of-Word Spelling   Most word prediction techniques require first-letter-of-word spelling so that the individual can use word menus for each of the letters of the alphabet. Thus, it is important to evaluate the extent to which individuals can spontaneously indicate the first letters of words, even if their other spelling skills are minimal. This can be assessed by using the initial letter subtest from a measure such as the Gates-MacGinitie Reading Tests–Fourth Edition (MacGinitie, MacGinitie, Maria, Dreyer, & Hughes, 2006). This skill is also quite easy to assess informally, using one of two procedures. The first (and more difficult) procedure involves showing the person pictures of common items and asking *What's the first letter of this word?* without saying the word out loud. The second procedure is to say the word while asking the question, such as *What's the first letter in cat?* In order to use first-letter-of-word spelling for AAC, individuals without speech need to be able to do the first of these tasks; however, it is also important to identify skills in the easier assessment task so that they can be built on and expanded, if necessary.

Recognition Spelling   Many individuals who acquire literacy skills without appropriate writing systems may have learned to spell on a recognition basis—that is, they can recognize words that are spelled correctly but cannot spontaneously produce either those words or their first letters. They have, in effect, a "sight word vocabulary" in that they have memorized the configurations of certain words. Assessment of recognition spelling is only necessary if the individual can produce neither the first letters of words nor their correct spellings spontaneously. To assess recognition spelling, the individual is asked to recognize either the correct or the incorrect word from a series of options. For example, assessors might present the words *esarar, eraser,* and *erisir* with a picture of an eraser, and the individual's task is to identify the word that is spelled correctly. A subtest from the Peabody Individual Achievement Test–Revised–Normative Update (Markwardt, 1998) also measures recognition spelling ability.

Table 6.7. Selected instruments that do not require verbal responding for assessment of literacy skills

Instrument	Skills assessed	Response mode	Appropriate participants	Source
Gates-MacGinitie Reading Tests–Fourth Edition (MacGinitie, MacGinitie, Maria, Dreyer, & Hughes, 2006)	Subtests for basic literacy concepts, phonological awareness, letter and letter/sound correspondences, initial/final consonants and consonant clusters, vowels, word decoding, reading comprehension, vocabulary	Pointing (multiple choice)	Kindergarten through adulthood; different tests available for different age ranges	Riverside
Group Reading Assessment and Diagnostic Evaluation (GRADE; Williams, 2001)	Subtests for phonological awareness; visual skills; concepts; early literacy skills; phoneme-grapheme understanding; word reading/meaning abilities; listening, sentence, and passage comprehension; vocabulary	Mark on paper; can be adapted easily to pointing for individual administration	Prekindergarten through adulthood, English and Spanish	Pearson Assessments
Peabody Individual Achievement Test–Revised–Normative Update (PIAT-R/NU; Markwardt, 1998)	Subtests for recognition of printed letters, reading comprehension, correct spelling comprehension	Pointing (multiple-choice)	Kindergarten through adulthood	Pearson Assessments
Test of Phonological Awareness–Second Edition (Torgeson & Bryant, 2004)	Phonological awareness (initial and final sounds); pseudoword spelling	Pointing (multiple choice)	Kindergarten, Grades 1–3 (ages 5 through 8)	PRO-ED
Test of Reading Comprehension–Third Edition (TORC-3; Brown, Hammill, & Wiederholt, 1995)	Subtests for general vocabulary, syntactic similarities, paragraph comprehension, sentence sequencing, reading directions for schoolwork	Marking or pointing (multiple choice)	Ages 7 through 17	PRO-ED
Woodcock-Johnson III Complete Battery (Woodcock, McGrew, & Mather, 2006; selected subtests)	Subtests for sound blending, sound awareness, incomplete words, visual matching, reading fluency, listening comprehension, spelling, writing speed and ability	Pointing, yes/no; some subtests require writing	Preschool through adulthood	Nelson

Analyzing Results of Literacy Assessment   AAC teams should incorporate any reading skills that are identified during assessment into the overall design of the AAC system at an appropriate level of difficulty. At the most basic level, words that the person with CCN can recognize by sight can be used as symbols instead of or in addition to pictorial symbols. Otherwise, displays using single-word options in a multiple-choice format can be provided, as reported for adults with aphasia in Chapter 15. In addition, reading assessment information can be used to design an appropriate program of literacy instruction. We discuss the importance of literacy instruction for individuals who rely on AAC in detail in Chapter 12 and provide numerous suggestions for literacy instruction based on the assessments reviewed in this chapter.

It is not at all unusual for individuals with CCN to have very uneven spelling and reading profiles; for example, individuals with fairly good reading skills are often unable to spell at the same level. Assessors should not overestimate the spelling skills of these individuals because the implications for each type of spelling skill with regard to AAC intervention differ considerably. For example, in order to learn Morse code, it appears that people need spontaneous spelling skills at a Grade 2 level, at least (Marriner, Beukelman, Wilson, & Ross, 1989). Nevertheless, individuals who are not this proficient but who have first-letter-of-word spelling abilities and adequate reading abilities may be able to use a word prediction or word menu selection technique. As with other types of assessments, it is important that the AAC team be aware of the available intervention options and the operational requirements to ensure a good match between the system and the individual.

Assess Sensory/Perceptual Skills

Because vision impairments accompany many of the developmental and acquired disabilities that are common in people who rely on AAC, an accurate vision assessment is quite important. Decisions about the type, size, placement, spacing, and colors of symbols will often be guided by the results of such an assessment. Assessment of hearing capabilities, although less critical, will also allow the AAC team to make decisions about output options (e.g., types of synthetic or digitized speech the person can hear) as well as options related to language input (e.g., whether to supplement speech with manual signs or symbols). Assessment in both of these areas is discussed in the sections that follow.

Vision Assessment

Vision is a three-stage system that involves 1) the reception of sensory stimulation through the eye (i.e., sight), 2) transmission of an image along the optic nerve, and 3) interpretation of the image in the visual cortex of the brain. During interpretation, images are transformed into meaningful information. The interpretation of an image is a result of all that an individual brings to the task, including motivation, experience, and self-image, which are the tools of functional vision. How an individual actually uses and enhances his or her existing vision through various means is at least as important from a functional perspective as is the nature or severity of the visual impairment itself. This certainly applies to AAC system considerations; thus, it is important for intervention teams to consider the individual's impairment as well as perceptions of his or her visual abilities and disabilities.

Assessment of an individual's visual status involves evaluation of a number of components, including visual acuity, visual field magnitude, oculomotor functioning, light and color sensitivity, visual stability, and functional visual competence. Each element contributes to an individual's functional vision skills. Most of these components will require assessment by ophthalmologists, optometrists, or vision specialists either before or during the AAC evaluation process.

Visual Acuity   Visual acuity, or clarity of vision, allows an individual to discriminate details. Visual acuity is expressed by notations that describe the size of a visual target and the distance at which the target is identified. Fractional notation is most commonly used, with the numerator indicating the testing distance and the denominator indicating the size of the test item that can be identified on an eye chart (see Figure 6.23). The designation for normal vision is 20/20 (Cline, Hofstetter, &

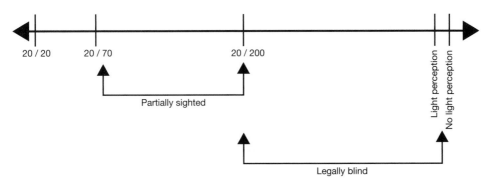

Figure 6.23. Continuum depicting the range of visual impairments.

Griffin, 1980). People with acuities of 20/70 to 20/200 are considered to be partially sighted, and those with less than 20/200 vision are labeled legally blind. When vision decreases to awareness of light only, visual level is referred to as light perception, and a person is considered to be totally blind in the absence of light perception.

Visual acuities should be measured close up and at a distance because visual performance may differ depending on the task, as well as on the person's overall abilities and the visual condition causing the impairment. Indirect tests, forced-choice preferential looking (FPL) procedures, and visual evoked potential tests can all be used to examine visual acuity in individuals with whom standard "eye chart" exams cannot be used (Orel-Bixler, 1999). Sobsey and Wolf-Schein (1996) described a simple FPL procedure that utilizes either two computer screens with the same illumination or one large split screen. Two images, one of which contains no pattern and the other of which is boldly striped, is checkered, or has wavy lines, are displayed on the screen(s) in alternating order during several trials (see Figure 6.24). Because most individuals will consistently look at the patterned screen, vision assessors can determine the person's ability to see at all. If the person orients toward the bold pattern, repeated pairings can then be presented with increasingly finer patterns until the stage at which the person is unable to make a discrimination is reached. Assessors can also vary the size of the squares systematically to approximate the size of potential communication symbols (e.g., 4" × 4", 2" × 2"). In addition, the distance from the screen can be varied to determine the minimal and maximal distances within which the person demonstrates pattern preferences. Although the FPL procedure provides only an informal estimate of visual acuity, it can be useful in the absence of alternative tests.

AAC teams need information about visual acuity in order to decide whether to use aided symbols or unaided symbols (e.g., manual signs for someone with vision) and, if aided symbols are chosen, the type(s) of symbols to use, their size, their distance from the eyes of the person with CCN, and so forth. Even individuals who are considered legally blind often have some residual vision that they can use for communication. Utley (2002) described a number of simple procedures that can be used to assess distance and angle (e.g., horizontal, vertical) for optimal presentation of visual displays in AAC.

The Technology Assessment Checklist for Students with Visual Impairments and other forms for assessment are available online through the Texas School for the Blind and Visually Impaired.

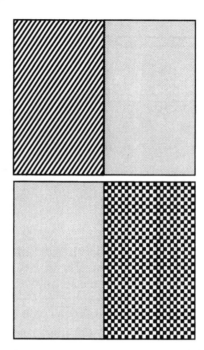

Figure 6.24. Examples of computer screens used for the forced-choice preferential looking (FPL) procedure for assessing functional vision acuity.

Visual Field   Visual field refers to the area in which objects are visible to the eye without a shift in gaze, normally extending in arcs of 150 degrees horizontally and 120 degrees vertically (Jose, 1983). The central visual field corresponds to the foveal and macular areas of the retina, which contain the cells most adapted to yield high visual acuity. Stimulation of these areas by visual impulses produces vision of the greatest clarity. Normal acuity decreases in proportion to the distance of the target from the fovea and macula. Thus, vision in the peripheral visual field is less clear than in the central visual field. The peripheral visual field detects movement and assists with vision in conditions of decreased illumination (Cline et al., 1980).

There are many impairments associated with the visual field, including 1) decreased vision in either the central or the peripheral field; 2) depressed visual sensitivity in specific areas; 3) blind spots (also referred to as opacities or scotomas) of varying shapes and sizes; 4) hemispheric losses; and 5) field losses that may occur subsequent to acquired brain injury, stroke, or other causes, in which entire segments of the visual field are missing. These losses can occur in one or both eyes. An individual with a central visual field loss has difficulty seeing a visual target presented at the midline of the body. This person must shift his or her focus off center to bring a target into view, generally by moving the head or eye horizontally or vertically. Individuals with peripheral visual field losses tend to experience difficulties when moving because they may be unable to detect movement or locate objects to their sides or beneath them. Depressed visual sensitivity results in areas of decreased acuity, which affect functional vision depending on the location of the affected areas and their shape and size. Similarly, blind spots or hemispheric losses in the visual field can create a variety of problems that require adjustment of the point of visual fixation, head position, and the placement of materials. Such adjustments are often difficult to achieve for individuals with visual impairments who rely on AAC if they also experience additional physical impairments that interfere with their ability to move, maintain head control, or precisely direct their eye gaze. A qualified professional should make a careful assessment of visual field impairments in order to ensure proper placement and arrangement of communication symbols and devices for such individuals.

Oculomotor Functioning   Oculomotor functioning refers to the operation of the eye muscles that enable the eyes to move together smoothly in all directions. These muscles allow the eyes to move into position and to place and maintain the image of an object on the optimal area of the retina. Oculomotor functioning includes movements that allow the eyes to establish and maintain visual fixation, locate and scan for objects, and follow moving objects. Problems with oculomotor functioning impair an individual's ability to direct his or her gaze precisely and may result in double vision or other problems. For example, a person with strabismus is unable to maintain the eyes in a position of binocular fixation because of weak eye muscles; thus, the eyes either converge (i.e., cross) or diverge. Nystagmus, another oculomotor disorder, is characterized by various involuntary movements of the eye and results in significantly reduced visual acuity. Individuals with this oculomotor disorder often attempt to compensate for it by repositioning their eyes, their head, and/or the materials they are examining. The detection of oculomotor disorders is of particular importance when an intervention team designs an AAC system for an individual with physical disabilities because the individual may lack the ability to freely adjust his or her body position in order to compensate for the oculomotor disorder. Decisions regarding the positioning of an AAC device, the configuration of a symbol array, and the spacing of items on the display are all affected by the person's ocular motility and coordination. In addition, an individual with oculomotor problems may have great difficulty using scanning devices that require him or her to track moving lights on a display (see Utley, 2002; Wilkinson & Jagaroo, 2004).

Light and Color Sensitivity   Light sensitivity must also be considered when evaluating an individual's visual status. Some disorders necessitate reduction or intensification of ambient light in order to achieve optimal visual functioning. For example, individuals with retinal problems may demonstrate atypical sensitivity to light and require low light conditions for maximum performance. Individuals with conditions such as degenerative myopia (nearsightedness) require significantly increased levels of illumination in order to see. In addition to various disorders affecting light sensitivity, glare is a consideration for all individuals except those with the most severe visual impairments. Glare is the dazzling sensation that is caused by bright light or the reflection of bright light, and it produces discomfort and interferes with optimal vision (Cline et al., 1980). Glare is a concern for individuals who communicate by using displays that are laminated or are otherwise covered by plastic because such coverings heighten the reflection of light off the surface of the page. In addition, glare may be a problem for people who rely on AAC devices with computer screen displays, especially ones that are highly reflective. Attention to ambient light sources used for illumination, as well as to the positioning of displays with reflective surfaces, is important in order to minimize glare.

Color perception occurs when certain eye structures are stimulated by specific wavelengths of light and may be impaired in ways that affect accurate visual discrimination of contrast and detail. Generally, color perception problems occur in the ability of the eyes to interpret particular (but not all) wavelength frequencies, so total color blindness is quite rare. People can learn to accommodate color vision problems, but the problems may be difficult to identify in very young children or in those who have difficulty labeling or matching. Nonetheless, AAC teams need to identify color impairments accurately to ensure that functional implications are minimized. For example, color codes using color wavelengths involved in an individual's particular impairment may serve only to reduce communication accuracy and increase frustration. Colors used on AAC displays for organizational or coding purposes must be discriminable and helpful to the person using the display and must be used in ways that enhance communication accuracy rather than detract from it (Bailey & Downing, 1994; Wilkinson & Jagaroo, 2004).

Visual Stability   Another visual component affecting AAC use is visual stability. Some individuals have eye conditions that are stable and relatively unchanging over time. Others have conditions that fluctuate, sometimes daily, depending on the individual's physical status or on environmental factors. In addition, some conditions deteriorate over time, with variability in both the rate of deterioration and the final visual outcome. For example, individuals with retinitis pigmentosa (a progressive genetic visual impairment) experience a gradual reduction in the size of their visual field, along with night blindness, abnormal sensitivity to light, and color impairments. They may retain some vision throughout life, or they may eventually lose most or all vision. Because the condition is progressive and unpredictable and because it cannot be treated, these individuals must consider their current and potential visual status when making long-term decisions. Teams should consider AAC techniques for both current and future use even at the point of initial assessment.

Functional Visual Competence   Functional visual competence refers to how an individual actually uses and enhances his or her existing vision through various means. It is at least as important, in a practical sense, as the nature or severity of any visual impairments that may exist. For example, consider two individuals with the same eye condition that results in identical visual acuities of 20/200 (the point at which one is considered legally blind). One person lives a typical life: She uses adaptations to perform certain tasks but continues to work, raise a family, and generally function independently in society. Her counterpart functions much less independently and is unable to perform basic tasks, including those necessary for employment. The major difference between these two individuals is in the functional use of the vision they have, not in their impairments. This variation in functional use of vision certainly affects AAC system considerations because it is important to consider not only the individual's impairments but also his or her perceptions and ability to compensate for them.

Numerous practical assessment strategies and assessment forms for functional vision assessment of young children, school-age individuals, and adults—including those with multiple disabilities—are available (see Lueck, 2004). The work of Roman-Lantzy (2007) and a free, downloadable resource entitled *A Team Approach to Cortical Visual Impairment (CVI) in Schools* (Shaman, 2009) provide specialized strategies for assessing individuals with cortical visual impairments. Finally, an excellent DVD called *Functional Vision: A Bridge to Learning and Living: Functional Vision Assessment* is available from the American Printing House for the Blind. The American Printing House for the Blind also publishes braille versions of many popular tests that measure overall cognitive ability and academic achievement.

Analyzing Results of Visual Assessment   Throughout this section, we have suggested how information in each area might be useful in the overall design of an AAC system. In our experience, it is not at all uncommon for inadequate vision assessment or inadequate application of assessment information to cause individuals to abandon using their systems. Information about a person's visual *abilities* is far more important for AAC applications than is information about his or her visual *impairments*. Some of the most important questions to ask include the following: What can the person see accurately? How close to the person and how large do stimuli need to be? How far apart should they be arranged? Would colored or dark backgrounds help accommodate for problems of contrast? Are there blind spots or areas of reduced vision, and, if so, where in the visual field is vision most accurate? How should displays be positioned to allow maximal visual efficiency? If oculomotor problems are present, how are they best minimized or accommodated? Which colors can be seen? What lighting is required for optimal vision? If additional visual losses will occur over time, what is the time line and predicted progression? The answers to such questions are often implicit in formal vision assessments but may not be addressed explicitly by an examiner without prompting from other team members. It is up to the AAC team to ensure that information needed for system design is made explicit to the person conducting a vision assessment, and we have found that most vision specialists are able and willing to provide such information if it is requested.

Hearing Assessment

AAC teams often recommend auditory scanning systems for people with severe visual impairments. Auditory scanning requires that the person with CCN be able to hear and understand the items in the selection set as they are announced, either by a partner or via an SGD. If the latter vehicle for auditory scanning is an option, a hearing assessment should serve to determine the individual's ability to comprehend the synthesized or digitized speech used in potential devices. In many SGDs, activation feedback is also provided to indicate that an item has been selected, either in the form of a beep or a spoken echo. The person's ability to hear these sounds should also be assessed in advance. Finally, many SGDs provide spoken output, primarily for the benefit of the communication partner. Nonetheless, it is generally desirable that the person with CCN be able to hear and understand the spoken output.

Assessment of hearing capabilities is usually straightforward and can be conducted by a qualified audiologist, even if he or she does not have experience with AAC. If needed, evaluation of a person's ability to understand synthetic or digitized speech may be requested as an additional service. The American Speech-Language-Hearing Association (2004) provided a document entitled *Guidelines for the Audiologic Assessment of Children from Birth to Five Years of Age* that suggests strategies for individuals who are unable to participate in conventional hearing assessments.

GOAL AND AMOUNT OF CAPABILITY ASSESSMENT

The goal of capability assessment is to gather a sufficient amount of information for the AAC team—which is composed of the person with CCN, family members, professionals, and other facilitators—to make intervention decisions that meet the individual's current and future communication needs. Because of the complex issues that must be considered in such assessments, there is a widespread tendency to overassess capabilities. Too much testing of an individual's motor, cognitive, linguistic, and sensory performance can actually interfere with AAC intervention because it takes so much time and places many undue demands on the family and the person who will rely on AAC to communicate. In this chapter, we have provided a framework for completing assessments that are broad-based in scope but not necessarily exhaustive. Additional details regarding the assessment of people with acquired communication impairments appear in Chapters 14–18.

QUESTIONS

6.1. Why is criterion-referenced assessment preferable to norm-referenced assessment for making AAC decisions?

6.2. What are six principles that can be used to guide an initial assessment related to seating and positioning for AAC assessment?

6.3. What are some specific questions that need to be answered in a direct selection assessment, and how can these be addressed?

6.4. Describe the issues involved in cognitive assessment of people with complex communication needs and two approaches to accomplishing this.

6.5. What are the six components of switch control, and how do they affect selection of a cursor control technique for scanning?

6.6. Describe four formats that can be used in a comprehensive symbol assessment.

6.7. Why is assessment of single-word vocabulary important, and how can this be done?

6.8. Describe three strategies that can be used to assess morphosyntactic knowledge during an AAC assessment.

6.9. Describe five components that should be examined in a literacy assessment and how to assess each of them.

6.10. Describe five considerations that should be addressed in a visual assessment and how each of them is related to AAC.

CHAPTER 7

Principles of Decision Making, Intervention, and Evaluation

Once the assessment process has been completed, the augmentative and alternative communication (AAC) team can finalize decisions about intervention and evaluate the outcomes. In Chapter 5, we discussed the importance of using a team approach to both AAC assessment and intervention planning. During implementation, the person with complex communication needs (CCN), his or her family, and the interventionists involved must continue to work together to share information about preferences and strategies. In this chapter, we discuss a number of general principles that can be used during the intervention phase and thereafter. Chapters 8–18 contain specific intervention guidelines and techniques for people with various types of disabilities who rely on AAC.

OPPORTUNITY BARRIER INTERVENTIONS

The reason for assessing the nature of opportunity barriers during the assessment (see Chapter 5) is to facilitate appropriate interventions at this stage of the process. Opportunity barriers may be related to policies, practices, facilitator knowledge and/ or skill deficits, or restrictive attitudes that limit the extent to which AAC is available or implemented.

Policy Barriers

Policy barriers in the form of "official" written laws, standards, or regulations that govern the contexts in which people with CCN find themselves will need to be resolved through advocacy efforts aimed at changing the restrictive legislation or regulations. In the United States, the Assistive Technology Act Amendments of 2004 (PL 108-364) and the Americans with Disabilities Act (ADA) of 1990 (PL 101-336) have led to the dissolution of many barriers that formerly made AAC services inaccessible to many people who needed them. For example, until 2001, the policy of

Medicare (the U.S. federal health insurance program for people over age 65 and those with disabilities) was that AAC devices were "convenience items" and were not eligible for funding. After many months of work by a coalition of dedicated AAC professionals, this policy was changed in 2001, and speech-generating devices (SGDs) are now considered to be "durable medical equipment" and are funded by Medicare. Similarly, in 2010, professionals, people with CCN, and family members worked with government officials in British Columbia (Canada) to expand SGD availability to all individuals with CCN over the age of 19. These are both good examples of the remediation of policy barriers that were achieved by advocates who collaborated to institute change.

Practice Barriers

Practice barriers are procedures or conventions that have become common in a family, school, or workplace but that contradict official policies that allow for service provision. Advocacy efforts are often needed to address practice barriers, but these efforts should almost always be combined with educational and sensitization efforts as well. A good example of an intervention aimed at remediating practice barriers is the *Communication Supports Checklist for Programs Serving Individuals with Severe Disabilities,* which was developed by the National Joint Committee for the Communication Needs of Persons with Severe Disabilities to help AAC teams "develop a shared understanding and vision" for their programs (McCarthy et al., 1998, p. 7). The book contains a Communication Bill of Rights, which is presented in Table 7.1, as well as numerous self-assessment checklists that AAC teams can use to assess their current practices and plan related interventions, as needed. In general, practice barriers are easier to eliminate than policy barriers, especially if policies are already in place to support the need for change.

Since the summer of 1998, the Quality Indicators for Assistive Technology (QIAT) Consortium has focused its efforts on developing a set of descriptors that can serve as guidelines for assistive technology service delivery in schools. The most recent version of these descriptors (QIAT Consortium, 2009) and an assessment matrix can be downloaded from the QIAT web site.

Knowledge and Skill Barriers

Knowledge barriers stem from a lack of information on the part of facilitators or other people that results in limited opportunities for communication by the person with CCN. Knowledge barriers, which can occur even when policies and practices in support of communication are in place, are best remediated through educational efforts such as in-service training, courses, workshops, directed readings, and so forth. Related to these are skill barriers, which occur when team members have difficulty with the actual implementation of an AAC technique or strategy despite even extensive knowledge. Skill barriers are what one experiences after coming back from an exciting course or workshop only to realize that actually implementing all of the new information is a formidable task! Educational efforts need to be directed toward providing guided practice, coaching or mentoring, technical assistance, and other individualized "hands-on" efforts. Working with other colleagues who have more experience in the area or asking someone to brainstorm about strategies for translating theory into practice are also good examples of appropriate skill-building strategies.

Table 7.1.   Communication Bill of Rights

All persons, regardless of the extent or severity of their disabilities, have a basic right to affect, through communication, the conditions of their own existence. Beyond this general right, a number of specific communication rights should be ensured in all daily interactions and interventions involving persons who have severe disabilities. These basic communication rights are as follows:

1. The right to request desired objects, actions, events, and persons, and to express personal preferences, or feelings.

2. The right to be offered choices and alternatives.

3. The right to reject or refuse undesired objects, events, or actions, including the right to decline or request all proffered choices.

4. The right to request, and be given, attention from and interaction with another person.

5. The right to request feedback or information about a state, an object, a person, or an event of interest.

6. The right to active treatment and intervention efforts to enable people with severe disabilities to communicate messages in whatever modes and as effectively and efficiently as their specific abilities allow.

7. The right to have communicative acts acknowledged and responded to, even when the intent of these acts cannot be fulfilled by the responder.

8. The right to have access at all times to any needed augmentative and alternative communication devices and other assistive devices, and to have those devices in good working order.

9. The right to environmental contexts, interactions, and opportunities that expect and encourage persons with disabilities to participate as full communicative partners with other people, including peers.

10. The right to be informed about people, things, and events in one's immediate environment.

11. The right to be communicated with in a manner that recognizes and acknowledges the inherent dignity of the person being addressed, including the right to be part of communication exchanges about individuals that are conducted in his or her presence.

12. The right to be communicated with in ways that are meaningful, understandable, and culturally and linguistically appropriate.

Reprinted with permission from Guidelines for Meeting the Communication Needs of Persons With Severe Disabilities. National Joint Committee for the Communication Needs of Persons With Severe Disabilities. Available from www.asha.org/ policy or www.asha.org/njc. Copyright 1992 by National Joint Committee for the Communication Needs of Persons With Severe Disabilities. All rights reserved.

Attitude Barriers

Finally, some opportunity barriers are related to attitudes that restrict or prevent communication participation. Sometimes, the beliefs held by an individual are problematic; at other times, the culture of a service delivery agency or school system acts as a barrier. Often, attitude barriers persist even when policy and practice barriers do not. For example, we know of a group home run by a very progressive agency that had clear policies related to the importance of providing supports to enable the men who lived there to make choices and control their own lives as much as possible. In fact, in this group home, the general practice was in compliance with this policy; the men were encouraged to participate in designing meal menus, decorating their home, determining their own activity schedules, and so forth. However, one particular staff member's attitude presented an opportunity barrier in that he did not believe that the men should be allowed to have words and phrases that he found to be distasteful or profane programmed into their AAC devices. Usually, attitude barriers such as this one are best approached by providing information about the issue of concern, providing time for open discussion of ideas about the issue, and modeling appropriate practices. However, despite such efforts, this staff member was not willing to listen to the men's arguments that the devices were *their* voices—not his!—and that they were entitled to program them as they wished. In the end, his employment was terminated at the insistence of the men who lived in the home because he was simply unable to incorporate a new way of thinking into his existing repertoire. In some cases, advocacy efforts are the only way to resolve an attitude barrier.

PLAN AND IMPLEMENT INTERVENTIONS FOR TODAY AND TOMORROW

Once a plan is in place to deal with the identified opportunity barriers over time, team members can compile and access assessment information and use it to make decisions about AAC interventions that best match the individual's profile of capabilities and constraints. Such decisions should be made using the principles of evidence-based practice (EBP), "the integration of best and current research evidence with clinical/educational expertise and relevant stakeholder perspectives to facilitate decisions for assessment and intervention that are deemed effective and efficient for a given stakeholder" (Schlosser & Raghavendra, 2003, p. 263). EBP does not mean that either clinical reasoning or the perspectives of people with CCN and their families are discounted when making decisions about optimal AAC techniques and strategies. It does mean that, in addition to these important components, a third component—current research evidence—is added to the mix. Thus, AAC teams who claim that they use EBP must be familiar with and consider the results of research when making clinical decisions.

"Providers must not only do the right thing, they must do the right thing right" (Parnes, 1995).

Fortunately, one of the positive outcomes of the emphasis on EBP has been the generation of a number of integrative reviews of AAC research. In such reviews, authors examine existing research related to a specific type of intervention (e.g., communication aids with voice output), using meta-analysis or other techniques. They also provide summary statements regarding (for example) the type(s) of individuals for whom the intervention has been shown to be effective, the benefits that have been shown to result from use of the technique, the optimal conditions for generating positive outcomes, and so forth. This information can be used fruitfully by AAC teams during intervention planning. For example, if research suggests that a specific technique is likely to be successful when implemented with some types of communicators but not others, the team can use this information to determine the likelihood of a positive outcome for the individual to whom they are providing support. Some examples of integrative reviews that have appeared since 2000 are provided in Table 7.2.

With regard to EBP, Schlosser noted the difference between efficacy and effectiveness, as follows: *Efficacy* pertains to the "probability of benefit [of an AAC intervention] to individuals in a defined population...under ideal conditions of use," whereas *effectiveness* pertains to the "probability of benefit [of an AAC intervention]...under average conditions of use" (2003a, pp. 16–17).

Table 7.2. Examples of integrative reviews of research evidence in augmentative and alternative communication (AAC)

Topic of review	Author(s)
AAC for people with developmental disabilities	Schlosser & Sigafoos, 2006; Sigafoos, Drasgow, & Schlosser, 2003
AAC for individuals with deaf-blindness	Sigafoos et al., 2008
Communication interventions (including AAC) for individuals with severe intellectual disabilities	Snell, Chen, & Hoover, 2006; Snell et al., 2010
Effectiveness of aided and unaided AAC strategies for promoting generalization and maintenance	Schlosser & Lee, 2000
Effectiveness of the Picture Exchange Communication System (PECS) in children with autism	Flippin, Reszka, & Watson, 2010; Lancioni et al., 2007; Preston & Carter, 2009; Tien, 2008
Effects of AAC on natural speech production in people with developmental disabilities and/or autism	Millar, 2009; Millar, Light, & Schlosser, 2006; Schlosser & Wendt, 2008
Graphic symbol techniques and manual signing for individuals with autism	Wendt, 2009
Use of speech-generating devices by individuals with autism	Schlosser, Sigafoos, & Koul, 2009
Literacy interventions for individuals with physical and developmental disabilities who use aided AAC	Machalicek et al., 2010
Presymbolic communication interventions	Olsson & Granlund, 2003
Selecting graphic symbols for requesting	Schlosser & Sigafoos, 2002
Speech and AAC interventions for children with Rett syndrome	Sigafoos et al., 2009
Use of AAC with infants and toddlers with disabilities	Branson & Demchak, 2009
Use of microswitches and speech output systems for people with severe or profound intellectual or multiple disabilities	Lancioni, O'Reilly, & Basili, 2001
Communication between nurses and people with complex communication needs who use AAC	Finke, Light, & Kitko, 2008
Efficacy of AAC interventions with persons with chronic severe aphasia	Koul & Corwin, 2003

The EBP process described by Schlosser and Raghavendra (2003) can be used to make decisions about the intervention components that are most likely to lead to positive outcomes for a given individual. The six steps or phases of this process are as follows: 1) ask a well-built question (Schlosser, Koul, & Costello, 2007); 2) select evidence sources (e.g., textbooks, research databases, and journals); 3) search the literature (Schlosser & Sigafoos, 2009; Schlosser, Wendt, Angermeier, & Shetty, 2005); 4) examine the evidence systematically (Schlosser, Wendt, & Sigafoos, 2007); 5) apply the evidence to make decisions on behalf of the specific individual who will rely on AAC; and 6) evaluate the outcome of the decisions over time. As noted previously, integrative research reviews (see Table 7.2) can be very useful to AAC teams who have limited time or resources with regard to executing steps 2–4 of this process.

An international journal entitled *Evidence-Based Communication Assessment and Intervention* offers appraisals of studies and reviews related to communication assessment, intervention (including AAC), diagnosis, and prognosis. It is published four times per year by Informa Healthcare. In addition, the National Center for Evidence-Based Practice in Communication Disorders of the American Speech-Language-Hearing Association (ASHA) compiles systematic reviews from around the world on a variety of communication topics, including AAC; they are available on the ASHA web site.

In general, two sets of AAC-related decisions should be made from the outset: those aimed at "today" and those aimed at "tomorrow" (Beukelman, Yorkston, & Dowden, 1985). The relationship between decisions for the present and decisions for the future is depicted in Figure 7.1. The "today" decisions should aim to meet the person's immediate communication needs and match the existing capabilities and constraints identified during the assessment process. The "tomorrow" decisions are based on projections of future opportunities, needs, and constraints, as well as capabilities that are likely to result from instruction and practice. Both decisions are critical to the long-term success of an intervention plan. Typically, communication interventions for people with CCN consist of three components: 1) interventions designed to increase natural abilities, 2) interventions that utilize environmental adaptations, and 3) interventions that incorporate AAC strategies and techniques.

Natural-Ability Interventions

The first decision that the team must make often involves the relative emphasis to be placed on natural-ability interventions and adaptive approaches. Of course, this consideration depends on the origin, stage, and course of an individual's communication disability. For example, an individual with end-stage amyotrophic lateral sclerosis (ALS) will not benefit from interventions designed to increase natural speech, whereas a preschool child with autism may benefit from extensive attention in this area.

A common issue for families of people with CCN is their concern that AAC interventions will inhibit the individual's natural-ability development. For example, the family of a young adult with traumatic brain injury whose limited speech cannot be

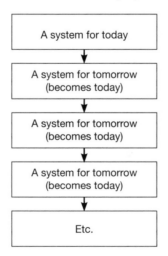

Figure 7.1. The longitudinal nature of augmentative and alternative communication (AAC) interventions for today and tomorrow.

understood by unfamiliar people may perceive a team's recommendation to provide an AAC system as an indicator that the team will no longer exert therapeutic efforts to improve the individual's speech. Or the family of a child with severe cerebral palsy may perceive the team's recommendation of a head mouse as an indication that the team will discontinue current therapeutic interventions to improve the child's upper-extremity motor function for writing.

Clearly, the first step in resolving such concerns is to provide both reassurances and concrete evidence that natural-ability interventions will not be discontinued. In reality, the evidence for one position and the accuracy of predictions concerning future improvements in natural abilities are often weak at best (see Schlosser, 2003b). Thus, compromise is a reasonable solution in most cases, considering a combination of both natural-ability and AAC approaches. Often, we approach compromise with the analogy of an investment portfolio, in which negotiable percentages of professional time are allocated to (for example) natural speech and AAC "investments," respectively. Thus, the team might decide to invest 50% of available intervention time in therapies to increase natural speech (and/or motor skills) and 50% of its time to AAC system development and use, or 10% to natural-ability areas and 90% to the area of AAC, or whatever reasonable compromise can be reached by the team. When a compromise is reached, it is critical that the team follow through with the negotiated plan and meet regularly to share progress or lack thereof so that adjustments can be made in the "investment portfolio" accordingly. In Chapters 8–18, we discuss natural-ability interventions in more detail as they pertain to specific disabilities across the life span.

Environmental Adaptation Interventions

The second intervention component in the access strand of the Participation Model (see Figure 5.1) involves resolving communication difficulties through environmental adaptations. These adaptations can be divided into two main categories: space and location adaptations and physical structure adaptations.

Space and location issues are specific to each intervention and should be readily solvable by the AAC team in most cases, assuming that consensus building has been effective, as discussed previously. Space adaptations may be necessary for removing physical barriers that interfere with use of an AAC system. For example, a woman who has experienced a brainstem stroke and lives in a residential care home may be unable to bring her communication device into the cafeteria because the tables and chairs are too close together for the device to pass between them when mounted on her power wheelchair. Or a college student with a spinal cord injury may not be able to install his speech recognition computer system in his dormitory room because there is not enough space. In the first case, the necessary adaptations are simple: move the chairs and tables farther apart; in the second case, more complex space accommodations will be necessary.

Location adaptations are more related to the location of the person with CCN than to the equipment. For example, we know of a girl who used a communication book and was seated in the back of the classroom, making it difficult for her to interact regularly with the teacher. This problem was resolved by moving her toward the front of the room so that the teacher could readily access her communication book.

Physical structure adaptations go beyond space and location adjustments and may also be necessary for accommodating the communication system or for facilitating its use. Obvious examples include adapting a bed with an adjustable swing arm in order to mount an AAC system for an individual who is partially bedridden, and widening doorways to allow passage of wheelchair-mounted equipment. Physical structure adaptations related to making public places accessible are required in the United States by the ADA.

Augmentative and Alternative Communication Interventions

The third intervention component in the access strand of the Participation Model (see Figure 5.1) involves the use of specific AAC strategies and techniques. In Chapters 8–18, we discuss this component in detail as it pertains to individuals with both developmental and acquired disabilities.

"Learning to use a communication device should not be a challenge. Leading an active interesting life, while using the device to communicate with others, should be the challenge" (Michael Williams, a man with cerebral palsy who relies on AAC, in Rackensperger, Krezman, McNaughton, Williams, & D'Silva, 2005, p. 183).

Augmentative and Alternative Communication Interventions for Today

It is important to first consider AAC technique(s) that meet the person's immediate needs within the available opportunities and that are accurate, efficient, and nonfatiguing. An accurate system is one that the individual can use to produce intended messages with a minimal number of communication breakdowns and errors. An efficient system enables an individual to produce messages in an acceptable amount of time, without the need for extensive practice or training. A nonfatiguing system enables the person to communicate for as long as necessary without becoming excessively tired or experiencing significantly reduced accuracy or efficiency. An AAC system that is accurate, efficient, and nonfatiguing must match the person's current linguistic, cognitive, sensory, and motor abilities as closely as possible. It should also be selected in consideration of existing constraints and unresolved opportunity barriers. The "system for today" should require a minimum of training and practice in order for the individual to use it effectively to communicate messages about his or her most important and immediate needs. Of course, some initial instruction or training will need to occur in most situations, but both the length and complexity of training should be minimized.

"When we first got the [AAC device], Ana had very poor head control. Getting the light to hit the right squares became a daily battle. But she carried on with a determination I found extraordinary. She must have known that this device was eventually going to liberate her, at least from the confines of speechlessness. I have never been so proud of my daughter as I was during those times" (Cy Berlowitz, describing his daughter who has severe cerebral palsy, in Berlowitz, 1991, p. 16).

Augmentative and Alternative Communication Interventions for Tomorrow

Decision making for tomorrow should be concurrent with decision making for today, under most circumstances. That is, as the AAC team implements a communication system that matches the individual's current abilities and immediate needs, it should also develop plans for broadening the individual's skill base in preparation for a system for tomorrow. These plans might involve providing instruction to improve specific motor, symbol recognition, social-pragmatic, or literacy skills. They might involve remediating identified barriers that limit the quantity or quality of communication opportunities. For individuals with degenerative conditions such as ALS, Parkinson's disease, or Rett syndrome, plans need to anticipate the future loss of motor, communication, and other skills and prepare the person accordingly. Whatever the focus of planning for tomorrow, the goal should be to institute an intervention that will enable more of the person's communication needs to be met and/or to maintain or increase the accuracy, efficiency, and ease of use of the current system.

The system for tomorrow can be an expansion or extension of the system for today, or it can involve a different device or technique. For example, the main component of the AAC system for "today" for a child with cerebral palsy was a series of eye-gaze communication displays with color photographs that were used during various activities throughout the day, to support his language and communication development. An expansion of this symbol system for tomorrow involved introducing Picture Communication Symbols for the same messages by placing them next to the photographs and then gradually enlarging them as the child became familiar with the new symbols (Figure 7.2). Simultaneously, the child was engaged in motor training activities using computer games and digital books to teach him to use a head switch for scanning. Once he learned to use his switch in this relatively easy (and motivating) context, his eye-gaze system was gradually discontinued and replaced with an SGD for communication (see Figure 7.3). Once the system for tomorrow has been instituted, it becomes the new system for today, and planning can begin immediately for yet another tomorrow. Thus, a longitudinal AAC plan should always be two-pronged by including plans for both today and tomorrow—although the time between successive "tomorrows" is likely to lengthen as the AAC system comes closer and closer to meeting all of the person's communication needs.

In some cases, it might be fairly obvious what the system for today should be, but not so clear how to plan for tomorrow. This is often the case if the individual's cognitive and/or motor impairments are very severe. In such cases, it is often advisable to institute multiple and simultaneous training programs for tomorrow, each designed to improve the person's ability to control and use a different motor site. For example, consider Karl, a young man with severe athetoid cerebral palsy and good literacy skills. It was apparent from assessment that a simple orthographic eye-gaze system combined with dependent auditory scanning (a "20 questions" approach) was the best match for his current abilities. It was also apparent that, in order for him to gain access to a more efficient and comprehensive system, he would need to achieve increased control of at least one motor movement sequence. It was not at all clear, however, which motor movement sequence could be taught best. Therefore,

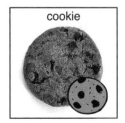 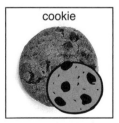 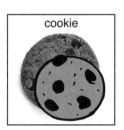 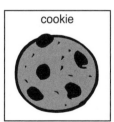

Figure 7.2.   Gradually introducing a symbol for tomorrow to replace a photograph for today.

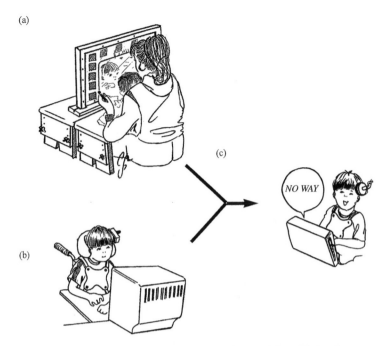

Figure 7.3.   a, b) For "today," a child communicates via eye pointing while learning to use a head switch for scanning; c) for "tomorrow," he uses scanning to a operate a speech-generating device. (From Goossens', C., Crain, S., & Elder, P. [1995]. *Engineering the preschool environment for interactive symbolic communication.* Birmingham, AL: Southeast Augmentative Communication Conference Publications; reprinted by permission.)

training programs designed to increase his ability to operate a single switch using his head, right hand, and left foot were instituted at the same time. It became apparent that his head control was improving at the fastest rate, and after 6 months of work, he was able to use a head switch to control a single-switch scanner accurately, efficiently, and without undue fatigue. When the logical direction for tomorrow is not clear, a multiple-target approach is vastly preferable to (and certainly less frustrating than) one in which single training targets are tested in succession until the best one is selected.

Provide Instruction to People with Complex Communication Needs and Their Facilitators

Both people with CCN and their facilitators are likely to require at least some instruction in the use of the AAC system for today and more extensive instruction in skill-building for tomorrow. Instruction in AAC techniques has come a long way from the days when one or two professionals did the majority of such work in isolated therapy rooms. It is now well established in the AAC literature that much, if not most, of the focus of intervention should take place in natural contexts such as classrooms, homes, community environments, and workplaces. Instructional plans that emphasize natural context interventions are more likely to result in better response generalization (to novel targets within the same response class) and better stimulus generalization (to novel people, environments, materials, and situations) than instructional plans that emphasize isolated skill training in artificial settings do (see Calculator & Black, 2009).

"I found the best way for me to learn anything is to just jump in and use the technology or whatever. This forces me to learn fast and be highly motivated. My rationale was the more I use [my AAC device] the more I will learn" (Dan, a man with cerebral palsy, in Rackensperger et al., 2005, p. 175).

Facilitators will also require various types of training, depending on the AAC system itself and the person who uses it. For example, facilitators may require training in partner-assisted scanning techniques or in how to interpret specific communicative gestures and vocalizations. Facilitators may also need to learn how to program and maintain electronic AAC devices, or how to set up a microswitch or head mouse for someone who uses these access techniques. In Parts II and III of this book, we present facilitator training programs and strategies that can be used with individuals who rely on AAC because of specific conditions or disabilities (see Kent-Walsh & McNaughton, 2005).

MEASURE AND EVALUATE INTERVENTION OUTCOMES

In the past decade, outcome evaluation has received increased attention in the AAC field. Schlosser defined outcome research in AAC as "the process of demonstrating, under average or less-than-average conditions,…the acquisition, maintenance, and generalization of behavior change (i.e., effectiveness)" (2003a, p. 22). We emphasize that outcome evaluation should measure parameters that are important both to the person with CCN and to his or her family. Thus, evaluators should be less concerned about establishing precise, cause-and-effect relationships between specific intervention components and specific changes than about answering the more general questions "Can the person participate successfully in activities and contexts that are meaningful to him or her?" and "Has the person's social network expanded in meaningful ways as a result of the AAC intervention?" (Blackstone & Hunt Berg, 2003a, 2003b; Calculator, 1999; Schlosser, 2003c). Thus, the evaluation of intervention effectiveness in the Participation Model (Figure 5.1) requires an examination of the person's ability to participate successfully in the specific activities and contexts that were identified as important during the initial needs assessment. If the desired level of participation is not achieved, the Participation Model requires reexamination and remediation of the opportunity and access factors that may be barriers (see Figure 5.1).

Several additional approaches to outcome evaluation are also available and may be useful as an adjunct to the Participation Model process. These include specific measures of functional limitations as well as general measures of consumer satisfaction and quality of life.

Functional Limitations

Functional limitations refer to "limitations in performance at the level of the whole… person" (Nagi, 1991, p. 322). Measurements of the impact of AAC interventions at this level seek to judge improvements in specific, functional skills. A number of parameters can be measured in this regard, such as how many times a person with CCN initiates interactions, responds to a partner's message, repairs communication breakdowns, makes choices, engages in social conversations, and so forth (Calculator, 1999). Parameters such as these can be measured by frequency counts and traditional language sampling procedures.

Automated systems such as the Universal Language Activity Monitor (U-LAM) can be used to record language samples for analysis from people who rely on electronic AAC devices (see Romich et al., 2004). Goal Attainment Scaling can also be used to measure an individual's progress toward specific, functional communication goals (see Granlund & Blackstone, 1999; Hanson, 2007; Schlosser, 2004). Finally, in the United States, ASHA (2003) published the National Outcomes Measurement System (NOMS), which includes 15 functional communication measures that are designed to describe changes in an adult's functional communication ability over time. The NOMS is available through the ASHA web site.

Consumer Satisfaction

Measuring consumer satisfaction with AAC services and interventions is regarded as a key means of obtaining outcome data (Cook & Polgar, 2008; Weiss-Lambrou, 2002). In this context, satisfaction refers to a person's opinion of the impact of a service, specific AAC technique, or overall AAC intervention. One measure that can be used in this regard is the Quebec User Evaluation of Satisfaction with Assistive Technology (QUEST 2.0; Demers, Weiss-Lambrou, & Ska, 2002). QUEST 2.0 was the first standardized tool designed specifically for assistive technology services and consists of questions in 12 areas; it is intended for use by adults regardless of disability and can be either self-administered or completed with assistance (Weiss-Lambrou, 2002).

QUEST 2.0 has been field tested at research centers in Canada, the United States, and the Netherlands and has been translated and validated in several languages, including French and Chinese. It assesses satisfaction with factors such as simplicity of use, effectiveness, durability, repairs and servicing, and various aspects of service delivery. QUEST 2.0 can be ordered through the Institute for Matching Person and Technology, Inc.

A related approach is the measurement of perceived "communication satisfaction" that results from an AAC intervention. This measurement can be obtained by interviewing people with CCN and their facilitators (e.g., parents and teachers) about how well the person with CCN is able to communicate as a result of intervention (e.g., Bruno & Dribbon, 1998; Culp & Ladtkow, 1992). For example, Slesaransky-Poe (1997) developed the Consumer Survey on Communicative Effectiveness, which asks adults who rely on AAC to rate their level of satisfaction regarding communication, independence, productivity, and community inclusion. Hamm and Mirenda (2006) developed the Communication Survey, which examines both the degree of importance of and a person's satisfaction with various communication contexts, partners, and functions.

Quality of Life

"Outcomes measurement should be consumer driven, flexible, and enduring. The result of AAC interventions should be an improved quality of life for people who use AAC. The results of outcomes measurement also should be used to improve cost-effectiveness and to improve the quality of equipment and services" (consensus statement developed by participants in Alliance '95, an international conference on AAC outcome evaluation, in Blackstone & Pressman, 1995).

Outcome evaluation related to quality of life (QOL) focuses on the impact of the AAC intervention on a person's ability to access and participate in preferred school, community, home, recreational, and vocational environments. The importance of outcome evaluation at this level has become increasingly recognized since the mid-1990s (Blackstone & Pressman, 1995; DeRuyter, 1995; Heaton, Beliveau, & Blois, 1995). QOL evaluations can be used to answer questions about whether an AAC intervention has resulted in (for example) increased self-determination, social inclusion, independence, participation in the community, gainful employment, academic achievement, and/or educational inclusion (Blackstone & Pressman, 1995).

The PROQOLID (Patient-Reported Outcome and Quality of Life Instruments Database) web site aims to identify and describe outcome and quality-of-life measurement instruments and facilitate access to them (Emery, Perrier, & Acquadro, 2005). It contains descriptions and reviews of more than 600 instruments and can be accessed at no charge.

Structured interviews can be used to elicit information related to QOL, as exemplified by the work of Cambridge and Forrester-Jones (2003) in the United Kingdom. Several formal QOL measures have also been used in the AAC field. For example, the Psychological Impact of Assistive Devices Scale (PIADS; Jutai & Day, 2002); and the Matching Person and Technology instruments (Galvin & Scherer, 1996) were both developed specifically to measure QOL as a result of assistive technology use. The ASHA Quality of Communication Life Scale (Paul et al., 2004) provides information about the psychosocial, vocational, and educational effects of communication impairment in adults. It can be used to assist with treatment planning, prioritization of goals, counseling, and documentation of outcomes. Hamm and Mirenda (2006) and Lund and Light (2006) used the Quality of Life for Persons with Physical and Sensory Disabilities instrument (Renwick, Brown, & Raphael, 1998) to measure outcomes for people who rely on AAC. Schlosser (2003c) reviewed a number of additional QOL instruments that were developed for various groups of people with disabilities.

The Quality of Life for People with Physical and Sensory Disabilities instrument can be obtained from the Quality of Life Research Unit at the University of Toronto. The Psychological Impact of Assistive Devices Scale is available from the Assistive Technology Research Lab at the University of Ottawa. The Matching Person and Technology instruments are available from the Institute for Matching Person and Technology, Inc. The Quality of Communication Life Scale is available from the American Speech-Language-Hearing Association and Pearson Assessments.

FOLLOW-UP

According to the principle of interventions for today and tomorrow, most AAC interventions never end! That is, once an individual has mastered a device or system for today, parallel training and practice can begin to prepare for one that is even more accurate, efficient, and nonfatiguing for tomorrow. Once these new skills are acquired, today becomes yesterday, tomorrow becomes today, and planning can begin for a new tomorrow.

If the person using AAC is a child, this cycle is likely to require repetition at each transition—from preschool to kindergarten, from elementary school to junior high, from junior high to secondary school, and from secondary school to either employment or postsecondary schooling. Adults with either congenital impairments (e.g., cerebral palsy) or acquired, nondegenerative impairments (e.g., stroke) are likely to need system alterations less frequently, unless their employment, residence, or family status changes markedly. Children or adults with degenerative disorders (e.g., Rett syndrome, ALS, multiple sclerosis), however, may require frequent system changes as their abilities deteriorate and living situations change. Finally, most individuals who rely on AAC will require additional modifications to their systems as they approach retirement age, begin to shift priorities, and experience changes in ability that occur as a result of aging (see Light, 1988).

"Whose outcome is it anyway? Is it the outcome of the people that control the money, the persons who want the quickest intervention at the lowest price? Is it the outcome of the program administrator who is always looking to put up good numbers in order to make his program look effective? Or might it be the outcome of the potential user of AAC? Will he receive and be trained in an AAC system he can use effectively so he can go forth and do battle...?? Isn't this the outcome we all could be working towards?" (Williams, 1995, p. 6).

QUESTIONS

7.1.   Why are opportunity barrier interventions important in AAC?

7.2.   What strategies can be used to address the five types of opportunity barriers?

7.3.   What is the principle of AAC intervention for today and tomorrow?

7.4.   What are the three main components that are used to make evidence-based practice decisions?

7.5.   What are the six steps of the evidence-based practice process?

7.6.   Why are strategies aimed at increasing natural motor and speech ability important as part of an AAC intervention?

7.7.   What is the difference between intervention efficacy and intervention effectiveness?

7.8.   Why is facilitator training an important component of AAC intervention?

7.9.   What types of AAC-related questions would be answered by evaluations of functional limitations, consumer satisfaction, and quality of life?

7.10.   Name two specific instruments or processes that can be used to measure functional limitations, consumer satisfaction, and quality of life of people with complex communication needs.

Augmentative and Alternative Communication Interventions for Individuals with Developmental Disabilities

Augmentative and Alternative Communication Issues for People with Developmental Disabilities

This chapter provides a context for the information presented in Part II, which addresses the communication needs of individuals who are acquiring communication and language skills for the first time. These individuals have disabilities that were either present since birth or acquired early in life and that significantly affect one or more aspects of development (e.g., communication/language, physical, sensory, social, cognitive). Augmentative and alternative communication (AAC) techniques are used routinely with people who experience developmental disabilities such as cerebral palsy, intellectual disability, autism spectrum disorders, deaf-blindness, and childhood apraxia of speech. In this chapter, each of these conditions is defined and explained briefly in terms of its description, prevalence, and major characteristics. An overview of the AAC issues most pertinent to each impairment follows.

> "A healthy mind holds no boundaries or limitations. We, as non-speaking people, are likely to be more expressive or vocal than people who can speak. If we write out who we are as individuals and keep writing about our own identities, then others will see who we really are" (Tony Diamanti, a man with cerebral palsy, in Diamanti, 2000, p. 98).

CEREBRAL PALSY

In 2007, the Executive Committee for the Definition of Cerebral Palsy, a international group of scientists and researchers, described cerebral palsy as "a group of permanent disorders of the development of movement and posture, causing activity limitation, that are attributed to nonprogressive disturbances that occurred in the developing fetal or infant brain" (Rosenbaum, Paneth, Leviton, Goldstein, & Bax, 2007, p. 9). It is estimated that the incidence of cerebral palsy is approximately 1 in 500 live births and varies little across industrialized countries; the prevalence in developing countries has not yet been established (Pakula, Van Naarden Braun, & Yeargin-Allsopp, 2009). It appears that the overall prevalence of cerebral palsy has not changed significantly since the mid-1990s, despite improved neonatal intensive care (Winter, Autry, Boyle, & Yeargin-Allsopp, 2002). Despite the multiplicity of problems associated with cerebral palsy, most individuals with this condition live to adulthood. These individuals, however, do have a significantly lower life expectancy compared with the general population (Strauss & Shavelle, 1998).

There are a number of etiologies that result in early lesions or malformations of developing brain tissue. Until the 1980s, it was thought that most cases of cerebral palsy were caused by a lack of oxygen to the brain during the birth process; however, it is now clear that this is rarely the case (Moster, Lie, Irgens, Bjerkedal, & Markestad, 2001). Rather, prematurity and problems during intrauterine development account for the majority of cases (Croen, Grether, & Selvin, 2001; Pakula et al., 2009). Among children born prematurely, the primary cause is damage to the white matter of the brain that occurs after birth as a result of cerebral hemorrhage or other problems. In children born at term, brain malformations that occur during intrauterine development account for the majority of known causes. In approximately 38% of people with cerebral palsy (whether they were born prematurely or at term), there is no identifiable cause (Pellegrino, 2002). However, cerebral palsy occurs more commonly among multiple births and in children who were conceived through the use of assisted reproductive technologies such as in vitro fertilization (Pakula et al., 2009). Existing research also provides evidence that environmental factors interact with genetic characteristics to produce risk (Pakula et al., 2009).

The Augmentative Communication Online Users Group (ACOLUG) is an Internet discussion group open to all people who communicate through AAC and to families of children who use AAC. To subscribe, go to the ACOLUG web site and click on the link labeled "Subscribe or Unsubscribe."

Characteristics

Individuals with cerebral palsy primarily experience difficulty with motor skills, which vary depending on the location of the brain lesion. The most common condition, spastic cerebral palsy, results in hypertonia (increased muscle tone). It may manifest as diplegia, in which the legs are affected more than the arms; hemiplegia, in which one side of the body is primarily affected; or quadriplegia, in which there is diffuse and severe damage affecting all four limbs as well as the trunk and oral-motor structures (Pellegrino, 2002). A second condition, dyskinetic cerebral palsy, is characterized by involuntary movements as well as changing patterns of muscle tone across the day (often, spasticity when awake and normal or even decreased tone when asleep). One subtype, dystonic cerebral palsy, involves rigid posturing of the neck and trunk, whereas another subtype, athetoid cerebral palsy, is marked by the presence of abrupt, involuntary movements of the extremities that result in difficulty regulating movement and maintaining posture. Finally, ataxic cerebral palsy, which can be associated with either increased or decreased muscle tone, causes problems with balance and positioning the trunk and limbs in space. Individuals with ataxia have a characteristic wide-based, unsteady gait when walking and have difficulty controlling the arms and hands when reaching. In addition, some individuals have mixed cerebral palsy, which includes more than one type of motor pattern (e.g., spastic-athetoid cerebral palsy). Needless to say, the wide diversity of motor problems associated with cerebral palsy presents significant challenges to AAC teams serving this population.

Communication impairments are common sequelae to cerebral palsy. Articulation disorders and impaired speech intelligibility are present in approximately 38% of children with cerebral palsy (Ashwal et al., 2004); language delays or disorders are also common, at least in part because the predominant motor impairments often restrict children's access to language-learning experiences and opportunities in the early years. The speech problems are associated with poor respiratory control as a result of muscular weakness and other factors, laryngeal and velopharyngeal dysfunction, and oral articulation difficulties that result from restricted movement in the oral-facial muscles. The incidence of dysarthria varies in relation to the type and degree of motor impairment. Other communication characteristics (e.g., overall language delay) appear to be associated with the problems of intellectual disability, hearing impairment, and learned helplessness that often co-occur with cerebral palsy (Pakula et al., 2009).

A number of associated conditions are common in people with cerebral palsy. Approximately one third to two thirds of all children with cerebral palsy also have some degree of intellectual disability (Pakula et al., 2009); individuals with hemiplegia and spastic diplegia are the least likely to be affected. In addition, it is not uncommon for individuals with cerebral palsy to have visual problems that may include eye muscle imbalances (e.g., strabismus), visual field cuts, visual-perceptual problems, and/or loss of visual acuity (especially farsightedness), any of which can significantly affect educational and communication programming. The incidence of hearing, speech, and language impairments is estimated to occur in approximately 30% of individuals with cerebral palsy, and the underlying brain injury precipitates seizure activity in roughly 40%–50% of individuals with cerebral palsy (Pellegrino, 2002). Feeding problems, growth difficulties, emotional/behavioral disorders such as attention-deficit/hyperactivity disorder, and learning disabilities are often present as well.

"I do not like when people pity me. Like those ladies in the shops or people on the streets. They stare at me as if I were a weirdo. I really hate that look. I want people to accept me as I am. Sometimes, I just want to stick my tongue out at them. But I never do. I think to myself, it's not worth it. Often, I ask myself the question, why don't people want to understand me, isn't it so simple?" (Magdalena Rackowska, a woman from Poland with cerebral palsy, in Rackowska, 2000, p. 88).

Particular Issues Regarding Augmentative and Alternative Communication

Three issues require special attention from AAC teams that plan and implement AAC interventions for people with cerebral palsy: the use of a team approach, the need for balanced interventions, and the need to plan ahead for adulthood.

Team Approach to Intervention

Communication interventions for individuals with cerebral palsy require the expertise of a team of professionals from a number of disciplines, perhaps more so than with any other developmental disability. During the assessment process, the wide variety of motor impairments in this population necessitates the involvement of professionals such as occupational and physical therapists, orthotics specialists, and rehabilitation engineers in order to determine the appropriate communication system for each individual. Professionals should be familiar with positioning and seating adaptations that must be developed on an individual basis in order to ensure optimum stability and the movement efficiency necessary to access a communication system. The team should also be familiar with the wide range of communication options available, as well as with the special considerations necessary to achieve the optimal match between the user and the system. The importance of such individualization was emphasized in a U.S. study by Lafontaine and DeRuyter (1987), in which they reported that, across 64 individuals with cerebral palsy who were assessed and provided with AAC devices, a total of 17 different types of communication devices were prescribed. These devices included several different types of nonelectronic devices such as picture or word boards and 13 different types of electronic devices. Although 47% of the individuals in Lafontaine and DeRuyter's study were able to access their devices through the use of a finger, the remainder used a number of alternative access techniques, including optical indicators, chin pointers, joysticks, and a variety of switches for scanning. Similarly diverse patterns of AAC system use have been reported more recently in countries such as Scotland (Murphy, Markova, Moodie, Scott, & Boa, 1995), Australia (Balandin & Morgan, 2001), and Israel (Hetzroni, 2002). In developing countries such as South Africa (Alant, 1999), this diversity may not be seen because the types of available AAC systems are more restricted.

In addition, because visual acuity and visual-perceptual problems also affect decisions regarding the size, spacing, and figure–ground contrast of the symbols chosen for communication, a comprehensive assessment by a pediatric ophthalmologist or another team member trained to assess these issues is often required (DeCoste, 1997). Perceptual impairments (e.g., hearing loss) can impede the process of learning to read or spell, requiring input from professionals such as speech-language pathologists or educators who specialize in remediation of these problems. Finally, but certainly of no less importance, the input of speech-language pathologists and both general and special educators will be necessary during the assessment process to train those who rely on AAC and their facilitators and to manage the intervention process.

"For an AAC user, the development of one's voice poses [a]...challenge because AAC devices can be limiting. A symbol or word might not appear on a board. A voice synthesizer might not have the right intonation. All of this can limit or change what is trying to be said....Because I rely on AAC, it has taken me many years to learn how to communicate effectively. I now use a combination of 'agencies,' including speech, written words, telecommunications, a word board, and a voice output device. All of these devices allow my 'voice' to be heard" (Nola Millin, a young woman with cerebral palsy, in Millin, 1995, p. 3).

Balanced Approach to Intervention

Beukelman (1987) emphasized the need for a "balanced approach" to communication programming for people with complex communication needs (CCN) in general. In the case of people with cerebral palsy, emphasis on AAC needs to be balanced with motor development training, speech therapy, and academic instruction, as necessary. For example, some individuals will require extensive motor training in order to use alternative access methods such as an eye tracker, head mouse, or switch for scanning. However, in the search for a technique that an individual can use immediately, a frequent mistake is to abandon such motorically demanding options. The result is that long-term efficiency is often sacrificed for short-term gains. Instead, a longitudinal program designed to meet the person's immediate communication needs with a number of readily accessible approaches, which also "invests in the future" through a systematic motor or speech therapy program to train more complex skills, is often more fruitful and, ultimately, more balanced (see Treviranus & Roberts, 2003, for additional discussion of this issue).

This principle also applies to the selection of multimodal communication systems for individuals with cerebral palsy. A number of AAC techniques may be used in different contexts and with different people to communicate a variety of messages (see Light, Collier, & Parnes, 1985a, 1985b, 1985c). In addition, although speech, gestures, and facial expressions may be severely affected as a result of motor impairment, this does not mean that people with cerebral palsy should be discouraged from using these natural modes for communication (Hustad & Shapley, 2003). Rather, a balanced approach calls for efforts to encourage and support the use of such multimodal systems, including training of both individuals and their communication partners concerning the most effective techniques to use in various situations. For example, an individual may be able to communicate with family members very effectively using natural speech and gestures that they are able to understand, whereas he or she may rely on AAC techniques with unfamiliar partners (Blackstone & Hunt Berg, 2003a, 2003b).

"I like to believe my transition to adulthood, independent living and employment started to happen on the day my parents learned of my diagnosis of cerebral palsy—they started taking me to therapies, and a preschool program, and to expand their expectations over time....The longer you put off educational and rehabilitation activities, the less likely it is that you will witness the things that you want" (Anthony Arnold, a man with cerebral palsy who relies on AAC, in Arnold, 2007, p. 94).

Plan for Adulthood

According to a U.S. Census Bureau estimate, only 30% of people with a severe disability were employed either full or part time in 2005, compared with 83.5% of people with no disability (Brault, 2008). In the Census Bureau report, the "severe disability" category included many individuals with cerebral palsy in addition to individuals with other disabilities. Nonetheless, the U.S. figures are almost identical to those reported in a 2005 Danish study of adults with cerebral palsy alone, which found that 29% were competitively employed, compared with 82% of people without a disability (Michelsen, Uldall, Mette, & Madsen, 2005). This study also found that only half of individuals with cerebral palsy who did not have an intellectual disability and who completed a regular school program had gained employment by ages 21–35.

"I think that right from the time that a young person is about 12...we need to start thinking about where they're going to be....You need to start having those discussions earlier rather than later because the actual transition is stressful enough but if it's done with some certainty and some natural expectations it's a much easier step to take" (the mother of Josh, a young man with cerebral palsy who relies on AAC, in Lund & Light, 2007, pp. 328–329).

Of course, employment may not be the primary or the only goal for all individuals with cerebral palsy. Most individuals will also consider other options such as postsecondary education, volunteering, participation in meaningful recreation and leisure activities, or some combination of these (McNaughton & Kennedy, 2010). The point is that long-term planning for adulthood is not an optional activity; although it is essential for most people who use AAC, it is especially so for individuals with cerebral palsy and limited speech. The need for long-term planning for these individuals is compounded by their need to rely on AAC devices and techniques that can accommodate a wide range of interpersonal, academic, and employment demands that are communicative in nature. For example, individuals who attend postsecondary educational institutions need to be able to interact with both instructors and classmates, request accommodations and/or alternative assignments as necessary, direct the activities of personal care attendants, complete assignments, search library resources, send and receive e-mail, and participate in a wide variety of both in-class and after-class instructional activities (Horn & May, 2010). In both paid employment and in many volunteer settings, people must be able to access both work-related and social vocabulary, multitask (i.e., take notes while communicating via voice output, or communicate while driving a power wheelchair), and produce messages both spontaneously and rapidly (McNaughton, Arnold, Sennott, & Serpentine, 2010; McNaughton, Light, & Arnold, 2002). Without advance planning and preparation, AAC systems are not likely to meet all of these demands, and even if they do, people with cerebral palsy are not likely to have the skills required to utilize them. It is essential that AAC teams (including family members) begin to plan for postschool transitions during the school years, starting as early as possible.

For extensive and detailed information about postschool transition planning, see *Transition Strategies for Adolescents and Young Adults Who Use AAC* (McNaughton & Beukelman, 2010) and the webcasts by Beth Anne Luciani and David McNaughton on the AAC-RERC (Rehabilitation Engineering Research Center on Communication Enhancement) Webcasts page.

INTELLECTUAL DISABILITY

According to the most recent definition by the American Association on Intellectual and Developmental Disabilities (AAIDD), intellectual disability is characterized by "significant limitations both in intellectual functioning and adaptive behavior as expressed in conceptual, social, and practical skills. This disability originates before the age of 18" (Schalock et al., 2010). The assumptions underlying the AAIDD definition emphasize that appropriate supports can have a significant impact on the ability of individuals with intellectual disability to live, work, recreate, and learn successfully in community environments typical of their same-age peers. A process for determining the need for and providing individualized supports has replaced the outdated classification system in previous definitions, in which people were categorized as having a mild, moderate, severe, or profound intellectual disability on the basis of an IQ score (Thompson et al., 2009).

In much of North America and parts of Europe, the Supports Intensity Scale (SIS; Thompson et al., 2004) is used to evaluate an individual's support needs across seven life domains (home living, community living, lifelong learning, employment, health and safety, social, and protection and advocacy) as well as to identify exceptional medical and behavioral support needs. The results can be used to plan and implement individualized supports in relevant areas. The SIS is available in print, on a CD-ROM, and on the American Association on Intellectual and Developmental Disabilities Supports Intensity Scale web site.

According to the World Health Organization (2001), the prevalence of intellectual disability is believed to be between 1% and 3% worldwide, with higher rates in developing countries because of the higher incidence of early childhood brain infections and of injuries and anoxia at the time of birth. A common worldwide cause is endemic iodine deficiency, which constitutes the world's greatest single cause of preventable brain damage and intellectual disability (Delange, 2000). Additional causes include genetic conditions (e.g., Down syndrome and fragile X syndrome); problems during pregnancy (e.g., the child of a mother who drinks alcohol while pregnant can be born with fetal alcohol spectrum disorder); health problems such as whooping cough, measles, or meningitis; and exposure to environmental toxins such as lead or mercury.

In a survey of speech-language pathologists in the state of Florida, 34% of school-age individuals who required AAC were reported to have an intellectual disability (Kent-Walsh, Stark, & Binger, 2008). A similar survey of speech-language pathologists in Pennsylvania indicated that 38% of preschool-age children with AAC needs had a primary diagnosis of developmental delay (i.e., intellectual disability). Demographic surveys in countries as diverse as New Zealand (Sutherland, Gillon, & Yoder, 2005) and Israel (Weiss, Seligman-Wine, Lebel, Arzi, & Yalon-Chamovitz, 2005) also suggest that children with intellectual disabilities constitute the largest proportion of school-age individuals who require AAC supports. AAC teams can and should deliver communication services of some type to these individuals regardless of the degree of impairment (National Joint Committee for the Communication Needs of Persons with Severe Disabilities, 2003a, 2003b).

Particular Issues Regarding Augmentative and Alternative Communication

Individuals with intellectual disabilities have only been recognized as appropriate candidates for AAC intervention since the mid-1980s. Indeed, some school districts, adult services agencies, and residential facilities still inappropriately maintain "candidacy" criteria to ascertain whether such individuals are likely to qualify for AAC services (National Joint Committee for the Communication Needs of Persons with Severe Disabilities, 2003a, 2003b). Nonetheless, since the mid-1980s, important positive changes have occurred in societal and professional attitudes toward these individuals. People with intellectual disabilities increasingly are being provided with the opportunities and technology needed to assist them to communicate in inclusive, dynamic environments. However, three issues remain as particular concerns for AAC teams that provide support to people with intellectual disability who rely on AAC: opportunity barriers, the relationship between communication and problem behavior, and the diversity of needs within this population.

Opportunity Barriers

When the first edition of this book was published in 1992, we identified "opportunity barriers" as one of the specific issues affecting the use of AAC by individuals with intellectual disabilities. Opportunities for the use of AAC can exist only when responsive communication partners interact in inclusive home, school, and community environments (Mirenda, 1993). Sadly, 20 years later, many people with intellectual disabilities continue to live, work, and recreate in segregated environments in which the only people available to them as communication partners are other individuals with CCN or paid staff members. In addition, the notion persists in many places that AAC instruction with this population should be conducted in highly structured settings until some arbitrary criterion is reached; only then is the individual exposed to natural situations in which communication skills are actually required. Unfortunately, given the generalization difficulties common in people with intellectual disabilities, this approach is usually futile. In an extensive discussion of this issue, Calculator and Bedrosian noted that "there is little justification for conducting communication intervention as an isolated activity because communication is neither any more nor less than a tool that facilitates individuals' abilities to function in the various activities of daily living" (1988, p. 104). The presence of inclusive, natural communication opportunities will directly affect the vocabulary selected as well as the instructional techniques used and must be considered an integral part of any AAC intervention. The availability of such opportunities will also affect the extent to which AAC is used to support truly functional communication that is both motivating and life enhancing for the individual using it.

"Do not try to control me. I have a right to my power as a person. What you call non-compliance or manipulation may actually be the only way I can exert some control over my life" (from "A Credo for Support," by Kunc & Van der Klift, 1995).

Problem Behavior

Most people with intellectual disabilities do not engage in socially inappropriate behaviors. Behavior problems, however, do occur in these individuals more often than in people without disabilities (Batshaw & Shapiro, 2002), for reasons that should be quite obvious—a lack of preferred and functional places to go, people to be with, things to do, and ways to communicate. For decades, the primary strategies that were used to "manage" the behavior of people with intellectual disabilities included incarceration (i.e., institutionalization), medication, and the use of aversive (i.e., punitive) behavior modification techniques. In the mid-1980s, the emphasis shifted to the use of proactive, ecological strategies to prevent problem behaviors, as well as numerous strategies for teaching functional communication skills as alternatives (Sigafoos, Arthur, & O'Reilly, 2003; Sigafoos, Arthur-Kelly, & Butterfield, 2006). This shift has great relevance for the AAC field because many individuals with intellectual disabilities do not use speech as their primary mode of communication. It is critically important that facilitators working with individuals who engage in problem behavior familiarize themselves with the literature on communication approaches for behavioral support so that they can act as both interventionists and advocates in this regard. Many of the strategies that are used most often to support individuals with problem behaviors involve either AAC input strategies such as visual schedules, contingency maps, and rule scripts (Bopp, Brown, & Mirenda, 2004; Mirenda & Brown, 2007, 2009) or AAC output strategies such as those used to teach choice making and functional communication training (Bopp et al., 2004; Tiger, Hanley & Bruzek, 2008).

Different Strokes for Different Folks

As noted previously, the term *intellectual disability* is really an "umbrella" term that encompasses a large range of syndromes and conditions that result in, among other things, cognitive impairment. Individuals with some of the conditions that fall under this umbrella (e.g., Angelman syndrome, Down syndrome) commonly experience significant problems with spoken communication in addition to cognitive impairments, whereas individuals with other conditions (e.g., Williams syndrome and Prader-Willi syndrome) do not (Dykens, Hodapp, & Finucane, 2000). Furthermore, even those individuals who do have difficulty with communication are not necessarily alike with regard to the nature of their impairments. For example, individuals with Down syndrome usually develop adequate speech for functional communication (Dykens et al., 2000), but those with Angelman syndrome often do not (Didden, Korzilius, Duker, & Curfs, 2004).

Given this diversity, the nature of remedial interventions directed at both natural speech development and AAC will vary considerably among people with intellectual disabilities, depending on the specific disability involved (Wilkinson & Hennig, 2007). Thus, AAC team members should be alert to the importance of understanding the language, communication, and social-relational characteristics; learning strengths; and overall developmental patterns that are typical for individuals with specific intellectual disabilities so that intervention can be staged and implemented with these characteristics in mind (Ogletree, Bruce, Finch, Fahey, & McLean, 2011). It is also important to remember that many individuals with intellectual disabilities may have multiple diagnoses (e.g., Down syndrome and autism; see Rasmussen, Bšrjesson, Wentz, & Gillberg, 2001), which can further complicate both their developmental profiles and the nature of their intervention needs. On the other hand, it is also important to remember that most AAC strategies and techniques can be applied to individuals across the range of specific syndromes and conditions; we will discuss these generic approaches in Chapters 9–13.

"I think in pictures. Words are like a second language to me. I translate spoken and written words into full-color movies, complete with sound, which run like a VCR tape in my head. When somebody speaks to me, his words are instantly translated into pictures" (Temple Grandin, a professor with autism, in Grandin, 1995, p. 19).

AUTISM SPECTRUM DISORDERS

It is increasingly accepted that the term *autism spectrum disorder* (ASD) encompasses a wide range of social-communication impairments (Wing, 1996). Although the etiology of autism is not known, a large body of research is available to demonstrate that it is not caused by family or emotional factors (Wing, 1996). Considerable research is being focused on identifying a number of genetic, neurological, and environmental factors that may cause the syndrome. The prevalence of ASD is estimated at 1 in 88 individuals and occurs in all racial, ethnic, and socioeconomic groups (Centers for Disease Control and Prevention, 2012). It is well established that focused educational and related interventions from an early age can make a real difference with regard to outcomes (National Research Council, 2001).

For information about current North American research on the causes of ASD, visit the web sites of the International Society for Autism Research, the Studies to Advance Autism Research and Treatment network, and Autism Speaks. For information about assessment and diagnosis, visit the First Signs web site.

Characteristics

On one end of the autism spectrum are individuals who may also have intellectual disabilities and require extensive educational, behavioral, and community supports. On the other end are socially eccentric or socially "shy" individuals who may live independently, hold down jobs, get married, and/or raise children (see Aston 2001, 2003; Stanford, 2002). Between these two extremes are most people with ASD, who require a variety of supports, especially in the core area of social communication.

Social, Communication, and Language Impairments

Individuals with ASD experience a wide range of complex issues related to both the means and the forms of language and communication (see Mirenda & Iacono, 2009). Estimates are that about 40% of children with an ASD do not develop speech, and another 25%–30% of children will have some words at 12 to 18 months of age and then lose them (Johnson, 2004; Schneider, 2004). If speech does develop, certain impairments are common, including echolalia, repetitiveness, literalness of meaning, monotonous intonation, and idiosyncratic use of words or phrases.

Most striking in individuals with ASD are a number of verbal and nonverbal impairments of social interaction that are apparent early in life. Researchers have documented several core symptoms that are diagnostic "red flags." These include no big smiles or other warm, joyful expressions by 6 months or thereafter; no back-and-forth sharing of sounds, smiles, or other facial expressions by 9 months or thereafter; no babbling by 12 months; no back-and-forth gestures, such as pointing, showing, reaching, or waving by 12 months; no words by 16 months; no two-word meaningful phrases (without imitating or repeating) by 24 months; and any loss of speech or babbling or social skills at any age (Wiseman, 2006).

"As she grew, the problem of her speech took precedence over all the others. It was through speech that she must join the human race" (Clara Claiborne Park, referring to her daughter with autism, in Park, 1982, p. 198).

Most people with ASD have receptive and/or expressive language impairments as well. Comprehension problems are often masked by unusual skills in other areas that make it seem that people with ASD understand everything that is said to them. Indeed, many people with ASD have visuospatial and visual-memory skills that far surpass their apparent abilities in the language area, which may account for reports of unusual reading and spelling abilities (hyperlexia; Newman et al., 2007). Individuals with ASD may also use visuospatial splinter skills to compensate for a lack of linguistic understanding by memorizing routines and attending to the subtle situational cues that accompany spoken language (Mirenda & Erickson, 2000).

"As a child, the 'people world' was often too stimulating to my senses. Ordinary days with a change in schedule or unexpected events threw me into a frenzy, but Thanksgiving or Christmas was even worse. At those times our home bulged with relatives. The clamor of many voices, the different smells—perfume, cigars, damp wool caps or gloves—people moving around at different speeds, going in different directions, the constant noise and confusion, the constant touching, were overwhelming....This is not unusual for autistic children because they are over-responsive to some stimuli and under-sensitive to other stimuli" (Temple Grandin describing her experience as a child with autism, in Grandin & Scariano, 1986, pp. 24–25).

Cognitive and Processing Impairments

Underlying the speech, language, and communication impairments of ASD are a number of developmental and cognitive processing issues that directly affect social and communication interventions. Research suggests that, on average, 41% of individuals with ASD also have an intellectual disability; this co-occurrence is less common than previously thought (e.g., Bölte & Poutska, 2002). This difference may be due to changes that have occurred over time in the diagnostic criteria for ASD, the positive impact of early intervention, and/or other factors. In addition, researchers in the United Kingdom have provided evidence that people with ASD have impaired "theory of mind"—the ability to attribute independent mental states to oneself and others in order to explain behavior. This impairment could account for the inability of even the most capable individuals to take the perspective of others into account in social situations. Further, Prizant (1983) described people with ASD as "gestalt processors," referring to their tendency to process the gestalt, or "whole," of a situation or utterance rather than its component parts; this tendency could account for much of the echolalic language frequently observed in these individuals, at least during the early stages of language development.

Particular Issues Regarding Augmentative and Alternative Communication

Overall, it is clear that ASD is an extremely complex and varied disorder, both within and across individuals. This complexity presents numerous challenges with regard to both speech-based and AAC interventions. Three issues deserve specific mention: the importance of early intervention, the need for AAC interventions to be situated in social contexts, and the use of speech-generating devices (SGDs).

Early Intervention

There are several elements that research has shown to be critical in intervention programs for individuals with ASD. The most important of these are

1. Start early.
2. Start early.
3. Start early.
4. Start early.
5. Start early!

In their comprehensive report issued in 2001, the National Research Council's Committee on Educational Interventions for Children with Autism strongly recommended that entry into intervention programs should begin as soon as a diagnosis is seriously considered (not necessarily confirmed). The committee also concurred that "active engagement in intensive instructional programming" (p. 219) should be provided to children at least up to age 8 for a minimum of 25 hours per week on a year-round basis and should consist of "repeated, planned teaching opportunities" (p. 219) conducted in both one-to-one and very small group sessions. They also recommended that emphasis be placed on the use of evidence-based instructional techniques in six main areas: 1) functional, spontaneous communication using verbal and/or AAC modalities; 2) developmentally appropriate social skills with parents and peers; 3) play skills with peers; 4) various goals for cognitive development, with emphasis on generalization; 5) positive behavioral supports for behavior problems; and 6) functional academic skills, as appropriate.

The committee acknowledged that a wide range of instructional approaches may be used to accomplish these goals. These include discrete trial teaching (Smith, 2001); incidental teaching (McGee, Morrier, & Daly, 1999); other structured teaching approaches based on applied behavior analysis (e.g., Leaf & McEachin, 1999; Sundberg & Partington, 1998); the Developmental, Individual-Difference, Relationship-Based Model (DIR; Greenspan & Weider, 1999); the SCERTS® Model (Social Communication, Emotional Regulation, and Transactional Support; Prizant, Wetherby, Rubin, Laurent, & Rydell, 2006a, 2006b; Rubin, Laurent, Prizant, & Wetherby, 2009); the Early Start Denver Model (Rogers & Dawson, 2010); and many others. Although the committee did not recommend a specific curriculum or approach, they stressed the importance of goal-directed, evidence-based, individualized programs that meet the needs of both children with ASD and their families. It is beyond the scope of this chapter to either summarize or critique the various ASD intervention approaches; however, we emphasize that families are continuously faced with the task of deciding what to do for their child with ASD and how best to do it. Some of the decisions may affect the extent to which AAC techniques of various types will be accepted and used by the family (e.g., in some applied behavior analytic programs, manual signing may be accepted but graphic symbols may not be; see Mirenda, 2003b, and Sundberg, 1993). Thus, AAC interventionists may need to work with other professionals whose views are quite divergent from (and perhaps even incompatible with) their own; this will require considerable skill at negotiation and collaboration.

Howard Shane and his colleagues at Children's Hospital Boston are developing a Visual Immersion Program (VIP) that provides a wide variety of visual supports designed to support the communication needs of individuals with ASD in practical everyday exchanges (Shane, O'Brien, & Sorce, 2009; Shane & Weiss-Kapp, 2008). A webcast by Howard Shane and colleague Meghan O'Brien describing the VIP is available on the AAC-RERC web site.

Communication in a Social and Developmental Context

Because ASD profoundly affects the very nature of communication as a social mediator, it is critically important that AAC interventions emphasize the pragmatic aspects of communication rather than merely aspects related to form (Duchan, 1987). To quote Rees (1982, p. 310), "morphology plus syntax plus semantics does not equal communication" for individuals with ASD. Especially for beginning communicators, the development of spontaneous communication as a dynamic, interpersonal process is critical. Related to this fact is the need to teach the individual to use communication skills in the context of naturally occurring routines related to functional activities in daily life.

It is also important that interventions start at the individual's level of social, communicative, and cognitive development and build skills in a natural developmental progression. A number of researchers have demonstrated that the developmental profiles of children with ASD, unlike those typically found in children with intellectual disabilities, are characterized by an uneven distribution of skills; this is often referred to as "developmental discontinuity" (Fay & Schuler, 1980). On a sensorimotor assessment battery, for example, children with ASD tend to perform markedly better in the areas of object permanence and tool use (causality) than in areas requiring interpersonal interaction, such as gestural or vocal imitation, use of adult-as-agent (means-ends), symbolic understanding, or language comprehension (Curcio, 1978; Wetherby

& Prutting, 1984). This information has direct implications for AAC interventions because it is important to gear such interventions to the person's *social and linguistic* abilities rather than to the child's *object* abilities. For example, manual sign or other formalized communication systems (e.g., pictorial systems) are often recommended for individuals with ASD who do not speak. This recommendation presumes that the problem is simply lack of an output mode and that communicative intent or language is intact. In fact, many individuals with ASD have neither the language nor the social base on which communication must be built, even though they demonstrate substantial abilities in nonlanguage areas such as fine and gross motor skills or areas that involve object manipulation (e.g., puzzle assembly). Formal language or communication approaches with individuals who show evidence of significant developmental discontinuity should be preceded by interventions designed to build imitation, joint attention, and natural gestural communication skills (see Prizant et al., 2006a, 2006b; Rogers & Dawson, 2010). Premature initiation of formal language-based AAC (or speech) approaches will often result in nonfunctional, stereotypical behavior, with resulting frustration on the part of both the child and his or her facilitators.

Visit the AAC-RERC web site for webcasts on the use of speech output technology to support literacy instruction and language development. Visit the Pennsylvania State University Literacy Instruction for Individuals with Autism, Cerebral Palsy, Down Syndrome and Other Disabilities web site for additional webcasts related to literacy development for students with ASD and other developmental disabilities.

Speech Output

A number of studies have demonstrated that SGDs and other speech-output technologies can be used effectively with individuals with ASD to teach both communication (Schlosser, 2003d; Schlosser, Sigafoos, & Koul, 2009) and literacy skills (Koppenhaver & Erickson, 2009; Light & McNaughton, 2009a). This growing research base is encouraging and should alleviate previous concerns about the appropriateness of speech-output technology with this population. Potential advantages of SGDs for individuals with ASD include 1) the fact that speech output combines attention getting with the communicative act itself; 2) the availability of high-quality speech output that can act as a readily understandable "social bridge" to both familiar and unfamiliar communicative partners (Trottier, Kamp, & Mirenda, 2011); and 3) the ability to program SGDs with whole messages (e.g., DO YOU WANT TO COME OUTSIDE AND PLAY WITH ME?) in addition to single words and phrases, thus increasing communicative efficiency and reducing potential communication breakdowns. Powerful speech output devices have become increasingly available via devices such as the Apple iPad and iPod Touch, which can be used as dynamic display SGDs with the addition of relatively inexpensive applications such as Proloquo2Go (Kagohara et al., 2010; Sennott & Bowker, 2009).

DEAF-BLINDNESS

People with deaf-blindness (also referred to as dual sensory impairment) have varying degrees of both vision and hearing loss that significantly impairs their ability to acquire information via the auditory and visual channels (Rönnberg & Borg, 2001). The usual legal definition of deaf-blindness is a visual acuity of 20/200 or less with a moderate to profound hearing loss (i.e., a loss of 60–90 dB or greater; Ladd, 2003).

People who are deaf-blind can be classified into two groups: those who are congenitally deaf-blind and experienced the onset of both hearing and visual impairments between birth and age 2 (Munroe, 2001); and those with acquired deaf-blindness, for whom the onset of visual and hearing impairments occurs later in life. The most common causes of congenital deaf-blindness include intrauterine infections (e.g., congenital rubella), congenital brain damage, and chromosomal abnormalities (e.g., CHARGE syndrome). Acquired deaf-blindness can also be caused by genetically inherited disorders (e.g., Usher syndrome), as well as aging, postnatal or early childhood infections, and acquired brain injury (Munroe, 2001). Recent estimates indicate that more than 10,000 children and youth (from birth to age 21) and approximately 35,000–40,000 adults in the United States are deaf-blind (Miles, 2008). Canadian data suggest that approximately 55% to 70% of people who are deaf-blind become so after age 2 (Munroe, 2001; Watters, Owen, & Munroe, 2005).

Information about communication for individuals with acquired and congenital deaf-blindness can be found at A-Z to Deafblindness, the American Association of the Deaf-Blind, the National Consortium on Deaf-Blindness, and DeafblindResources.org.

Cognitive and Communication Abilities

As noted previously, deaf-blindness can occur as either a congenital or an acquired condition; most individuals in the latter group are those with Usher syndrome, which involves mild to severe congenital deafness and progressive blindness as result of retinitis pigmentosa (Rönnberg & Borg, 2001). Of course, any combination of deafness and blindness can also co-occur (e.g., congenital blindness and acquired deafness, progressive decline in both hearing and vision simultaneously). In a Canadian study of 182 individuals with congenital and acquired deaf-blindness, Dalby et al. (2009) found that the former group was three to five times more likely to have moderate to severe impairments in cognition, activities of daily living, and social interactions. In the absence of effective alternatives to speech, most congenitally deaf-blind individuals are likely to remain at a prelinguistic stage of communication development (Bruce, 2005). In the study by Dalby et al. (2009), 21.6% of those with congenital impairments were always or usually understood by others, compared with 81% of those with acquired impairments. In terms of language comprehension, a similar pattern was seen, with 5.7% of those in the congenital group but 39.4% of those in the acquired group able to understand others clearly.

"When I did become blind, I was extremely frustrated. Communication was hard, to say the least, with my family. I suffered through it, and I stuck in there. We made our way through. I had friends and family coming over that helped me. I learned signs and they learned signs as well. That's now how we communicate" (an adult with acquired deaf-blindness, in Watters et al., 2005, p. 20).

Particular Issues Regarding Augmentative and Alternative Communication

Because of the challenges presented by the dual auditory and visual processing limitations, AAC teams need to consider a wide range of AAC options, many of which are unique to this population. In particular, it is important to recognize issues related to the timing of the dual sensory impairments (i.e., congenital versus acquired later in life), the important role played by intervenors, and the need for systematic instruction.

Congenital and Acquired Impairments

Clearly, the timing and severity of both hearing and vision losses in people who are deaf-blind greatly affect the development of communication abilities as well as other areas of functioning. Dalby et al. (2009) found that 62.4% of individuals with acquired deaf-blindness communicated via speech or speech reading. Other commonly used communication techniques for these individuals include tactile fingerspelling, one- or two-handed tactile sign language, adapted national sign language (e.g., American, Swedish), and electronic aids such as the Screen Braille Communicator and the DeafBlind Communicator.

"I wish I had known about nonverbal ways to communicate with my daughter Sara when she was much younger. When Sara was 10, we were introduced to a wonderful educator who specialized in nonverbal communication. [She] came to Sara's class to talk to the school team about object communication and calendar boxes. It changed our lives for the better. Sara learned that objects represented activities and she loved the power that this knowledge gave her in school and at home" (Janette Peracchio, Sara's mother, in National Consortium on Deaf-Blindness, 2011).

In contrast, Dalby et al. (2009) found that only 23.9% of those with congenital deaf-blindness were able to speak; this group communicated primarily via adapted or manually coded sign language (68.1%) or idiosyncratic signs, gestures, or behaviors (78.4%). In a review of AAC research for people with congenital deaf-blindness, Sigafoos et al. (2008) found that tangible symbols (e.g., a cup to request a drink) was used with the largest number of participants. This was followed by communication boards or books with line-drawing symbols that were often enlarged and/or presented on dual displays so that both the person with deaf-blindness and his or her communication partner had access to a display. Textured symbols, whereby various arbitrarily selected textures were used to request desired items, were employed in three studies; sometimes the textures were used as symbols on microswitches or SGDs. Conventional, unaided AAC techniques including gestures, manual signs, and fingerspelling were taught to a few participants across five different studies. Surprisingly, only 2 of 17 studies focused on multimodal communication (e.g., gestures plus manual signs plus tangible symbols). Sigafoos et al. (2008) noted the need for more research to examine the use of multimodal AAC, to determine how preintervention assessments can be used to select AAC techniques systematically, and to compare different instructional procedures and AAC options for this population.

"We realized that Andy lived in a bubble. He could only access information as far as he could hear and see. Because he is profoundly deaf and has vision in only one eye, his bubble is quite small. We didn't want Andy to grow up isolated from people and the world. We wanted him to be independent. If he was to be independent, then he needed to learn, and if he was to learn, he needed access to information and communication. It was overwhelming for us to provide all that Andy needed on our own. The only way was with the help of a trained person who could compensate for his hearing and vision losses. An INTERVENER!" (Andy's parents, in Prouty & Prouty, 2009, p. 2).

Role of the Intervener

An increasing number of children and adults who are deaf-blind are supported in school and community settings by trained interveners. Interveners receive specialized, in-depth training in deaf-blindness and related educational strategies so that they can provide continual access to both information and communication for the individual they support (Alsop, 2004). The intervener's role is to 1) facilitate access to environmental information usually gained through vision and hearing; 2) facilitate the development and/or use of receptive and expressive communication skills by the individual who is deaf-blind; and 3) develop and maintain a trusting, interactive relationship that can promote social and emotional well-being (Alsop, Blaha, & Kloos, 2000). In this role, the intervener is an integral member of a student's educational team and/or an adult's support system in the community. In fact, in many cases, a longtime intervener may know more about an individual's communication strengths and needs than any other professional, including the AAC specialist! Thus, it is important to include the intervener in all AAC assessment and intervention decisions and to seek his or her advice and expertise as needed.

Information about interveners and intervener training is available from the National Consortium on Deaf-Blindness, DeafblindResources.org, and the Canadian Deafblind Association. Information about assessment and instructional techniques for children who are congenitally deaf-blind can be found at the SPARKLE web site.

Need for Systematic Instruction

Perhaps more so than people with any other type of developmental disability, individuals with congenital deaf-blindness require careful, systematic instruction in order to use any communication system, even for basic functions such as requesting. Innovative training procedures must be employed to overcome the limitations imposed by their dual sensory impairments while simultaneously promoting functional use of multiple modes of communication. Sigafoos et al. (2008) found that the most commonly reported instructional procedures included 1) presenting a discriminative stimulus, 2) prompting communicative behavior, 3) fading prompts, and 4) providing differential reinforcement for correct responses. Behavioral techniques such as behavior chain interruption, the system of least prompts, mand-model and error correction, and match-to-sample techniques were also employed in some studies (see Chapter 10 for details about these procedures). The most frequent target skills taught across the 17 studies reviewed were choice making and requesting (a preferred object, help, a break from a task, etc.), followed by recruiting attention from a caregiver. Only 4 of the 17 studies targeted social conversational skills such as greeting others, responding to greetings from others, asking questions, and answering questions.

CHILDHOOD APRAXIA OF SPEECH

Childhood apraxia of speech (CAS) is a congenital, neurological speech sound disorder "in which the precision and consistency of movements underlying speech are impaired in the absence of neuromuscular deficits (e.g., abnormal reflexes, abnormal tone)" (American Speech-Language-Hearing Association [ASHA], 2007, pp. 3–4). Because there is no clear consensus about the criteria for diagnosis, ASHA (2007) recommended that the term *suspected CAS* be used to describe these children.

CAS can occur as result of either a known or an unidentified neurological impairment. The prevalence is estimated at 1–2 children per 1,000 (Shriberg, Aram, & Kwiatowksi, 1997), although no sound epidemiological data are available (ASHA, 2007). Individuals with suspected CAS often come from families with a history of speech and/or language problems (Lewis, Freebairn, Hansen, Iyengar, & Taylor, 2004), and there appears to be a genetic basis for the disorder, at least in some cases (Shriberg, 2006).

Characteristics

The behavioral features of CAS are difficult to identify on the basis of existing research, and deficits may occur in any or all of the following: nonspeech motor behaviors, motor speech behaviors, speech sounds and structures (i.e., word and syllable shapes), prosody, language, metalinguistic/phonemic awareness, and literacy. With regard to motor speech behaviors, there is some consensus on the validity of three features: 1) inconsistent errors on consonants and vowels in repeated productions of syllables or words, 2) lengthened and disrupted coarticulatory transitions between sounds and syllables, and 3) inappropriate prosody, especially in the realization of lexical or phrasal stress (ASHA, 2007).

A series of brief "letters to parents" of children with suspected CAS was published in the April 2000 issue of *Language, Speech, and Hearing Services in Schools.* In plain language, the letters explain the speech characteristics, nature, and causes of CAS, as well as associated problems and treatment approaches (Hall, 2000a, 2000b, 2000c, 2000d).

Particular Issues Regarding Augmentative and Alternative Communication

Two issues related to AAC intervention for children with CAS deserve special mention: the use of AAC as a secondary strategy and the need for a multitier approach to intervention.

Augmentative and Alternative Communication as a Secondary Strategy

Because CAS is primarily a motor speech disorder, AAC is typically used as a secondary intervention while treatment primarily focuses on improving natural speech production (ASHA, 2007). As Blackstone noted, "Every intelligible word/phrase is worth it" (1989, p. 4). ASHA (2007) recommended that intensive speech therapy be provided in frequent (e.g., two to four times per week), relatively short (e.g., 30–45 minute) sessions that employ strategies based on the principles of motor learning theory. Such strategies include distributed practice across a variety of activities, settings, and situations, and the use of multiple exemplars of target speech sounds (Strand & Skinder, 1999). DeThorne, Johnson, Walder, and Mahurin-Smith (2009) suggested a number of alternative strategies aimed at facilitating early speech development as well, including AAC.

One of the major concerns voiced by parents of children with suspected CAS is whether the provision of AAC techniques will inhibit speech development and/ or production. A number of case studies of children with suspected CAS who use

AAC have offered evidence that should alleviate this concern. Although speech may not improve as a result of AAC use (Bornman, Alant, & Meiring, 2001; Culp, 1989), it does not appear to decrease and may improve over time (Blischak, 1999; Cumley, 1997; Cumley & Swanson, 1999; Waller et al., 2001). Furthermore, children with suspected CAS often show evidence of significant language delays that can be traced to their inability to "practice" language in their early years (Stromswold, 1994). Delayed language development is a high price to pay for either waiting for speech to develop naturally or devoting 99% of available therapy time to speech intervention. Rather, it is critically important to provide children with suspected CAS with one or more appropriate AAC modalities from an early age so that they have ample opportunities to use and "play" with language (Binger, 2008a). For example, Cumley and Swanson (1999) provided a case study example of a preschool child with suspected CAS who was provided with an SGD with Picture Communication Symbols organized by activity. Her mean length of utterance increased from 2.6 words per utterance without AAC to 4.6 words per utterance with AAC supports. Similar improvements in language development following the introduction of AAC have been noted in other reports as well (e.g., Harris, Doyle, & Haaf, 1996; Waller et al., 2001).

Additional information about speech interventions for CAS is available through the Apraxia-Kids and Prompt Institute.

A Multitier Model for Use of Augmentative and Alternative Communication

Ball and Stading (2006) proposed a multitier model for providing AAC to children with suspected CAS, based on their functional natural speech and their communication needs. The model includes five tiers: traditional AAC, AAC for speech supplementation, AAC for communication breakdowns, AAC for literacy and academics, and AAC for practice.

"I am eternally grateful that M could get the [SGD] one year before entering grade one, although I wish it was one year earlier. I would like to recommend that children start with the [SGD] from at least the age of three years. The earlier they experience themselves as speakers, the better" (the mother of M., a 6.5-year-old Afrikaans-speaking boy with suspected CAS, in Bornman et al., 2001, p. 631).

Traditional Augmentative and Alternative Communication   Individuals with suspected CAS whose speech is largely unintelligible, who use primarily one-word utterances, and who are unable to communicate effectively with family members, peers, and teachers are likely to benefit from multimodal AAC interventions. These interventions include aided techniques such as communication books or wallets and SGDs (Blackstone, 1989; Bornman et al., 2001) and unaided techniques such as gestures and manual signs. The advantage of aided AAC techniques is that they are more intelligible to unfamiliar communication partners than are gestures and manual signs. The main disadvantages are the vocabulary and portability constraints that they can impose on the person with CAS. Kravitz and Littman (1990) emphasized the importance of providing an adequate number of vocabulary items, noting that for many individuals with suspected CAS, communication books and SGDs may be nonfunctional unless they have 400–500 vocabulary items. It is also important to make aided AAC techniques readily available and portable because most individuals with suspected CAS are ambulatory. SGDs and communication displays can be transported using shoulder straps, carrying cases, or briefcases. In addition, communication miniboards can be made available on walls, mealtime place mats, car dashboards, refrigerators, bathtub tiles—in short, in any and all of the places the individual may go—so that opportunities and vocabulary for communication are abundantly available (Blackstone, 1989).

It is important to design aided AAC displays in ways that are most likely to facilitate both language development and social competence. Activity-specific symbol displays (either low-tech or on an SGD) can be arranged using a Fitzgerald key (e.g., subjects, verbs, adjectives, and objects from left to right, respectively) so that the individual learns to create longer and more complex messages that are grammatically accurate (Binger & Light, 2007; Cumley & Swanson, 1999). At the same time, preprogrammed messages can be provided on an SGD to facilitate small talk (see Chapter 3), predictable social interactions (e.g., ordering a meal at a fast-food restaurant, telling a knock-knock joke), storytelling, and other types of exchanges involving messages that can be anticipated in advance.

"I cannot stress enough how important it is to be doing the right type of therapy with an apraxic child. We had almost no progress for a year with language stimulation therapy. Now, with visual, tactile, and auditory cues and lots of repetition, we are on our way to sentences! We are so very proud of [Kennedy]!" (Traci, Kennedy's mother, in the *Apraxia-Kids Monthly* newsletter ["Traci," 2003, p. 7]).

Augmentative and Alternative Communication for Supplementation   Many individuals with suspected CAS can produce single-word speech that is reasonably intelligible but struggle with multiword utterances, and may restrict the number of words they are willing to attempt as a result. Such individuals will often benefit from one or more versions of speech supplementation via AAC. Individuals who are literate may benefit from the use of alphabet supplementation, whereby they simply point to the first letter of each word on an alphabet display as they speak. This process slows down their rate of speech and at the same time provides their communication partner with information that may make partially intelligible words more "guessable."

Alternatively, symbol displays similar to those used in more traditional AAC applications can be used, with the individual pointing to key symbols in conjunction with speech. Such displays can be especially useful for topic setting, which is often challenging for a person with suspected CAS. When the person attempts to introduce a new topic of conversation with one or more poorly articulated words, his or her communication partner is required to guess what the word is from a virtual universe of possibilities. If the person can narrow the range of possibilities by referring to one or more symbols on a display, the communication partner may find it easier to guess the spoken words that are difficult to understand.

Augmentative and Alternative Communication for Communication Breakdowns   People with suspected CAS who are able to rely on speech as their primary mode of communication and who are able to produce multiword utterances may still encounter difficulty when communication breakdowns occur due to unintelligible words or phrases. For example, Blockberger and Kamp (1990) reported on the use of natural speech in addition to gestures, manual signs, and SGDs with school-age children with suspected CAS. The children and their families generally preferred to use natural speech and unaided approaches, and resorted to aided AAC techniques only when communication breakdowns occurred. Clarification and repair strategies may include the use of alphabet or symbol supplementation displays, gestures, body language or pantomimes, and/or pointing to environmental cues (Blackstone, 1989). A preprogrammed message (either written or on an SGD) that assists the communication partner to resolve the breakdown may also be useful (e.g., TRY ASKING ME THE QUESTION SO I CAN ANSWER YES OR NO).

"I just wanted to let everyone know that my son Samuel, 10 years old, just gave his first ever oral report in school. It was on the planet Mercury, and he had a wonderful model and used cards for guidance, but didn't read word-for-word off the cards. I wish I had been there! I can tell he was very proud of himself and was waiting for people to come by at the planet fair and ask him questions….By contrast, last year in third grade his oral biography project was taped sentence-by-sentence at home, and then he played the tape to the class, and gave the oral report just to the speech therapist. What a difference in a year!…With more time and confidence, I now feel that he may not automatically present as someone with a speech disorder the rest of his life" (Trina, Samuel's mother, in the *Apraxia-Kids Monthly* newsletter ["Trina," 2004, p. 5]).

Augmentative and Alternative Communication for Academics and Literacy
As noted previously, many individuals with suspected CAS struggle with literacy in addition to speech production, especially with regard to the phonological skills that form the foundation of literacy learning (Light & McNaughton, 2009a). This difficulty with literacy can result in difficulty with academics in general because most of what children learn in school requires the ability to read, write, and spell. In addition, many children with suspected CAS also exhibit fine motor planning problems that affect handwriting abilities. AAC teams should consider providing augmented writing supports such as computers even before the child enters school to ensure that the motor planning problems do not stand in the way of academic progress.

AAC symbol displays can be used to provide symbols with text for reading, to highlight words when reading out loud, and to provide voice output that may assist with correct speech production (Ball, 2008). For example, Binger, Kent-Walsh, Berens, del Campo, and Rivera (2008) taught the mother of a Latino preschooler with suspected CAS to model two-symbol responses to *wh-* questions during a storybook reading activity. The girl began to produce two-symbol responses to her mother's questions after eight story reading sessions and continued to do so with new books 8 weeks later. Ball (2008) suggested that SGDs can also be used to facilitate phonemic awareness by enabling a child to activate digitized phonemes and then combine them to produce words via synthetic speech (see Figure 8.1). Similarly, Blischak (1999) provided instruction in rhyming—one component of phonologic awareness—to three children with suspected CAS, using an SGD with synthetic speech. Although the use of SGDs to promote literacy development in children with suspected CAS requires empirical examination, such strategies appear to have potential.

Augmentative and Alternative Communication for Practice   As noted previously, ASHA (2007) recommended that intensive speech therapy for children with CAS be provided two to four times per week in 30- to 45-minute sessions. In addition, parents are often asked to provide structured speech practice at home between therapy sessions by providing appropriate stimuli, asking the child to produce the targets, and providing feedback based on their judgment of accuracy. However, several barriers may negatively impact the effectiveness of parent-led practice. These

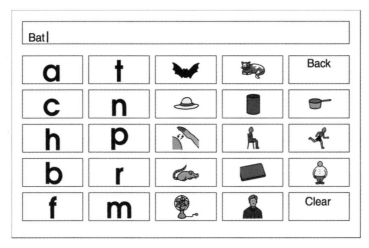

Figure 8.1.   Speech-generating device display with phonemes needed to make -*at* and -*an* words (e.g., *bat, mat, can, fan*). (From Ball, L. [2008]. Childhood apraxia of speech: Augmentative & alternative communication strategies. In J. Wambaugh, N. Alarcon, L. Shuster, & L. Ball [Eds.], *Traditional and AAC approaches for apraxia of speech in adults and children.* Miniseminar presented at the American Speech-Language-Hearing Association annual conference, Chicago. The Picture Communication Symbols ©1981–2012 by DynaVox Mayer-Johnson LLC. All Rights Reserved Worldwide. Used with permission.)

barriers include limited parental time available to devote to such practice (Pappas, McLeod, McAllister, & McKinnon, 2008) and parental provision of speech models that are less than optimal (Gardner, 2006). The use of SGDs or digital devices with speech output to enable individuals with CAS to practice natural speech without direct parent involvement has been suggested as an alternative (Ball, 2008).

In the few research studies that have examined this option, digital images (e.g., computerized pictures, photographs) are displayed on a computer screen, and a digitized speech model is provided to label or otherwise describe the image (e.g., Choe, Azuma, Mathy, Liss, & Edgar, 2007; Nordness & Beukelman, 2010). For example, Nordness and Beukelman (2010) used Microsoft PowerPoint (2004) for Macintosh with audio and video clips of participants' speech-language pathologists modeling each of 10 target words. The children were provided with five practice trials of each target word for a total of 50 trials, randomly ordered, and were asked to practice for 10 minutes daily. Results were compared with parent-led and no practice conditions and suggested that computer-led practice offered an increase in overall practice time above and beyond that achieved with parent-led practice only. Although this study used a computer rather than an SGD to provide images and speech models, there is no reason that an SGD with appropriate symbols could not be used to provide a similar type of practice experience. Other types of digital devices (e.g., iPad, iPod Touch) with applications that provide good speech models and allow voice recording of a child's imitative responses (e.g., ArtikPix) can also be used to provide motivating opportunities for independent practice.

QUESTIONS

8.1.   Differentiate between spastic, dyskinetic, ataxic, and mixed cerebral palsy and discuss the AAC-related implications of each.

8.2.   Describe three particular considerations in delivering AAC services to people with cerebral palsy.

8.3.   How is intellectual disability currently defined and evaluated?

8.4.   Describe three particular considerations in delivering AAC services to people with intellectual disabilities.

8.5.   How do the characteristics of autism spectrum disorders affect the provision of AAC services and supports?

8.6.   What does current research say about the use of SGDs with people with autism and CCN?

8.7.   What are the two main types of deaf-blindness, and what are the communication and AAC implications of each?

8.8.   Describe the role of the intervener as a member of the AAC team of an individual who is deaf-blind.

8.9.   How is suspected childhood apraxia of speech defined?

8.10.   Describe the five tiers of Ball and Stading's (2006) model for AAC intervention for children with CAS.

CHAPTER 9

Supporting Participation and Communication for Beginning Communicators

In this and subsequent chapters, we use the term *beginning communicator* to refer to any individual (regardless of age) who has one or more of the following characteristics:

- He or she relies primarily on nonsymbolic modes of communication such as gestures, vocalizations, facial expressions, and body language. These behaviors may be nonintentional (i.e., they function as communication only when they are interpreted by others) or intentional (i.e., they are used with indices of communicative intent, such as persistence, joint attention, and use of alternative modes when communication breakdowns occur; see Ogletree, Bruce, Finch, Fahey, & McLean, 2011).
- He or she is learning to use aided or unaided symbols to represent basic messages related to communicative functions such as requesting, rejecting, sharing information, and engaging in social interaction.
- He or she uses nonelectronic communication displays and/or simple switches or speech-generating devices for both participation and early communication.

Beginning communicators may be young children with various types of disabilities whose communication is developing in accordance with their chronological age. They may be children, adolescents, or adults with developmental disabilities who are at an early stage of language development. They may be individuals who are in the early stages of recovery following a severe acquired brain injury or some other significant neurological trauma. Regardless of their age or the etiology of their communication impairment, they require support to learn (or relearn) basic communication skills that enable them to have a positive impact on their environment and the people around them. In this chapter, we discuss interventions for beginning communicators that are related to opportunity and participation, nonsymbolic communication, and beginning symbol use. In Chapter 10, we discuss strategies to support language development and broad-based symbolic communication.

Many terms have been used in the child language literature to refer to what we mean by the term *nonsymbolic communication*. These include *partner-perceived communication* (Wilcox, Bacon, & Shannon, 1995), *prelinguistic communication* or *potential communicative acts* (Sigafoos, Arthur-Kelly, & Butterfield, 2006), and *early augmentative and alternative communication (AAC) behaviors* (Siegel & Cress, 2002). What these terms have in common is that they refer to both intentional (i.e., illocutionary) and unintentional (i.e., perlocutionary) behaviors (McLean & Snyder McLean, 1988; Ogletree et al., 2011) that may be either conventional or unconventional in form and that do not involve the use of symbolic modes such as pictures, manual signs, or printed words.

Relationship Between Communication and Problem Behavior

It is not unusual for beginning communicators to exhibit nonsymbolic behaviors that create challenges for those with whom they live, learn, play, and/or work. These might include behaviors such as tantrums, hitting, screaming, pushing, various forms of self-injurious behavior, and many others. Numerous authors have suggested that many problem behaviors can be interpreted as communicative in nature and treated as such (Carr et al., 1994; Donnellan, Mirenda, Mesaros, & Fassbender, 1984; Durand, 1990; Reichle & Wacker, 1993). Throughout this chapter, communication interventions related to individuals who exhibit problem behaviors are discussed in the context of other communication interventions.

Three important principles are common to both nonsymbolic and symbolic communication interventions for problem behaviors. First is the principle of functional equivalence: Often, the most appropriate intervention involves teaching the individual an alternative behavior that serves the same function as the problem behavior. This principle means that interventionists must undertake a comprehensive functional behavioral assessment (FBA) to identify the function(s) of the behavior(s) of concern so that they can design and teach appropriate alternatives (see Bambara & Kern, 2005; Crone & Horner, 2003; Dunlap et al., 2010; Hieneman, Childs, & Sergay, 2006; and Sigafoos et al., 2006, for examples of FBA procedures). For example, if the function of the behavior is to get attention, the new behavior must result in attention; or if the behavior allows the individual to avoid nonpreferred events, the new behavior must also allow the individual to accomplish this.

 A number of Internet resources on FBA are available through the Center for Effective Collaboration and Practice and the Office of Special Education Programs (OSEP) Technical Assistance Center on Positive Behavioral Interventions and Supports.

The second principle, the principle of efficiency and response effectiveness, states that people communicate in the most efficient and effective manner available to them at any given point in time. This principle means that an alternative behavior must be at least as easy for the individual to produce as the problem behavior is and must also be as effective in obtaining the desired outcome. If the new behavior is more difficult or less effective, the old behavior will persist. Finally, the third principle is the principle of goodness-of-fit, which says that sometimes the most appropriate response to problem behaviors is to create a better fit between the person and his or her environment. This principle usually requires altering relevant aspects of the environment based on the results of the FBA. The following case study report provides an example of the third principle.

A Greek man named Christos had autism, a seizure disorder, and rapid-cycling bipolar disorder in addition to complex communication needs (CCN; Magito-McLaughlin, Mullen-James, Anderson-Ryan, & Carr, 2002). He engaged in frequent, highly disruptive behavior problems including self-injury, aggression toward others, property destruction, and running away. An FBA revealed that virtually all of Christos's behaviors were aimed at enabling him to escape or avoid nonpreferred environmental or social events (e.g., crowding; overheating; interactions with large, male staff members; lack of access to community activities). When Christos's environment was altered to achieve a better fit with his needs and preferences, the rate and intensity of his problem behaviors decreased dramatically. Some of the interventions used in this regard included moving him to his own apartment with support, hiring Greek-speaking staff members who shared his interests, teaching him self-control and communication skills, providing him with a visual schedule so he could predict upcoming events, and getting him more involved in preferred activities with his family and community.

Unfortunately, like Christos, many nonsymbolic communicators live in isolated, noninteractive environments; engage primarily in boring, nonpreferred tasks; and are forced to adhere to rigidly structured schedules over which they have no control or choice on a daily basis (see Brown, 1991). As Carr, Robinson, and Palumbo (1990) noted in their now-classic discussion of this issue, the appropriate response in such situations is to focus on changing the environment or the sequence of events, not the person. As we learn more and more about the relationship between problem behavior and communication, it becomes increasingly important to remember that it is critical to provide opportunities for communication and control in the context of meaningful, interactive activities and environments.

THE PARTICIPATION MODEL
AND BEGINNING COMMUNICATORS

The communication opportunity component of the Participation Model (Figure 5.1) refers to the contexts in which communication occurs. Within the Participation Model, planning and implementation of augmentative and alternative communication (AAC) interventions require assessment of the individual's participation and communication needs in natural contexts such as community, home, and school environments. As discussed in Chapter 5, the Participation Model requires that the participation patterns of typically developing peers in relevant environments first be assessed for comparison. The participation patterns of a person with CCN are then assessed in the same contexts and compared with those of the peers. Finally, interventions are designed to increase the participation of the beginning communicator to match peer levels more closely. For infants and toddlers, this step requires analyzing the interaction patterns of peers in home and community settings. For preschoolers and school-age children, teams also need to conduct this kind of examination in the classroom. When supporting adults who are beginning communicators, teams should perform participation analyses in home, community, and work environments. In the sections that follow, we provide specific strategies for minimizing or eliminating communication opportunity barriers and for arranging optimal environments to support beginning communicators across the age range.

RESOLVING OPPORTUNITY BARRIERS
AND ENHANCING PARTICIPATION FOR YOUNG
CHILDREN WITH COMPLEX COMMUNICATION NEEDS

Throughout this book, we use the generic term *young children* to refer to all individuals involved in early intervention, including infants, toddlers, and preschoolers. A number of principles guide AAC interventions for young children. First, AAC teams should be aware that norm-referenced assessment tools cannot accurately and meaningfully measure the abilities of most individuals with CCN, especially when they are very young; thus, it is important not to ascribe undue credence to the results of such assessments. Second, it is critical to build on young children's strengths rather than focus on their impairments. Finally, AAC interventions with young children should operate under the assumption that all children have the potential to make significant skill gains.

In addition to following these basic principles, AAC teams should conduct communication interventions with the view that long-term outcome predictions are inappropriate when addressing the needs of young children. Thus, without exception, strategies for supporting the development of natural speech should always be included in communication interventions for this age group. Similarly, teams should include strategies for supporting the development of literacy skills (e.g., reading, writing) in all intervention plans, even for children who may seem unlikely to acquire such skills (Light & Kent-Walsh, 2003). In addition, AAC professionals should base their intervention strategies on the assumption that general-education kindergarten placement is the goal for all young children, although some may need substantial supports in order to participate optimally in this setting. This aggressive approach can result only in positive outcomes for children with CCN and will guard against the all-too-frequent later realization that a child might have developed a number of important skills if he or she had received adequate communication and literacy instruction in the early years. Interventions designed to increase communication opportunities as well as those designed to teach specific communication and social interaction skills are usually necessary for positive outcomes.

Early Intervention Services

During the first few years of a child's life, his or her primary caregivers usually deliver early intervention services in the home. Family members generally learn to provide appropriate inputs and supports, including those related to communication, from teachers and therapists who visit the home regularly. Starting at approximately 3 years of age, a child may attend a preschool program for at least part of the day, in which he or she receives direct services from professional staff. There is no doubt that preschool environments that include at least some typically developing children are preferable to classrooms in which all children have CCN, simply because of the rich opportunities for social interaction and communication that are available in inclusive settings (Romski, Sevcik, & Forrest, 2001). In this chapter and subsequent chapters, we assume that some amount of regular, systematic inclusion with peers without disabilities exists in the preschool setting; if it does not, this should be recognized as an opportunity barrier and targeted for remediation.

For young children with disabilities, "peer-related social competence is clearly aligned with issues of personal independence and...personal choice. The ability to achieve successfully and appropriately interpersonal goals involving one's peers is empowering in perhaps the most meaningful sense of the term" (Guralnick, 2001, p. 496).

Communication Opportunities

Table 9.1 displays an example of a participation analysis and intervention plan for a preschool-age child's daytime activities at school. In this example, the AAC team identified participation discrepancies between the teachers' expectations of a child with CCN and the child's peers. The team then designed a variety of environmental, instructional, and assistive device adaptations to reduce those discrepancies during routines that occurred throughout the child's day. In all cases, the basic opportunity principle of the Participation Model was reflected: the first step to increasing communication is to increase meaningful participation in natural contexts that are conducive to communication. From the perspective of the child with CCN, such contexts include a number of common characteristics: they should be highly motivating, familiar, and valued by the child and his or her family, and they should provide numerous opportunities for

Table 9.1. Sample participation analysis and intervention plan for a preschooler with complex communication needs (CCN)

Activity	How do peers participate? (What is expected?)	How does the child with CCN participate?	Intervention plan
Music (group)	Choose songs, sing repetitive parts of songs, perform hand or body movements to songs	Does not choose or sing, does not put on record, makes hand and body movements with aide's assistance, mostly sits and watches/listens	Provide songs that child can turn on with a switch to sing along, provide picture symbols representing songs so child can choose, continue to imitate hand/body movements with aide
Snack time (group)	Wash hands with help, ask for snack item and drink, ask for help as needed, eat/drink appropriately, take dirty plate/cup to sink, wash hands/face with help	Washes hands with help; does not ask for snack, drink, or help; needs help to eat and drink; does not take plate/cup to sink; needs help to wash hands and face	Provide real object choices of snack and drink options, look for eye gaze or reach to indicate choice, talk to physical therapist about using prone stander at sink so that child can participate in cleanup routine
Pretend-play time (solo or small group)	Engage in doll play in kitchen or grooming area, block and car play, dress-up play; children are expected to play with peers while teacher encourages verbal language use	Tues. and Thurs.: sits in wheelchair and watches peers play in an area; Mon., Wed., and Fri.: practices switch use with battery-operated toys and paraprofessional	Encourage peers to use child's lap tray as a play surface, adapt toys with Velcro so child can pick up toys with adapted Velcro glove, use Fisher-Price stove and sink on lap tray instead of large play kitchen furniture, adapt battery-operated blender and mixer for switch activation, use activity frame to display small items within reach

meaningful, sustained social and communicative interactions (Light et al., 2005). Some strategies for increasing opportunities for communication participation in preschool settings are summarized in the sections that follow.

Creating Predictable Routines at Home and in the Preschool Classroom

Daily living routines can provide many opportunities for communication if care-givers structure them with this purpose in mind. In most homes and classrooms, routines such as dressing, bathing, eating, toileting, and (for children with mobility impairments) position changing occur at regular times and intervals throughout the day. If this is not the case, these routines should be regularized as much as possible so that the child can begin to anticipate their occurrence. In addition, caregivers should perform the steps of these routines in roughly the same sequence each time so that the child can begin to anticipate what happens next. Whenever possible, caregivers should allow sufficient time to carry out each routine so that communication instruction can occur concurrently with the activity. Specific strategies for using regular, predictable routines to teach communication skills are discussed later in this chapter.

Adaptive Play

Play is an activity that is "done for its own sake, rather than as a means to achieving any specific end....[It is also] spontaneous and voluntary, undertaken by choice rather than by compulsion....Play includes an element of enjoyment, something that is done for fun" (Musselwhite, 1986, pp. 3–4).

Because the primary "business" of young children is play, their communication occurs primarily in play contexts. Thus, increasing participation in play activities automatically increases the quality and quantity of communication opportunities (Brodin, 1991). Unfortunately, in some preschool classrooms, the "fun" component of play is often ignored and play becomes, quite literally, the child's "work." This observation is not to imply that educators cannot use play as a vehicle to promote the development of gross motor, fine motor, social, cognitive, self-help, and (of course) communication skills. In fact, whenever possible, it is desirable to "telescope" goals and activities by working on one primary and one or more secondary goals simultaneously in a play context. For example, a "dress the doll" activity can provide a context within which a child can practice fine motor skills related to dressing, as well as social and communication skills with peers. What is critical is that the activity *remain playful* and not become one in which toys are used as vehicles for work. This requires careful selection of play materials and the ways they are used.

In order for play activities to foster the development of communication skills, parents and educators must select toys and play materials with interaction goals in mind. For example, some types of toys (e.g., blocks, balls, toy vehicles, puppets) have been found to be more facilitative of peer interactions than others that are primarily used in solitary play (e.g., books, paper and crayons, playdough, puzzles; Beckman & Kohl, 1984). Other important considerations in selecting a toy include safety, durability, motivational value for children with various types of disabilities, attractiveness, and reactivity (Light, Drager, & Nemser, 2004). Reactivity refers to the extent to which the toy "does something" (e.g., produces sound, sustains movement, creates a visual display). Research has demonstrated that young children with disabilities engage in longer periods of manipulative play with reactive toys than with nonreactive toys (Bambara, Spiegel-McGill, Shores, & Fox, 1984). Finally, parents and teachers should select toys for both realistic and imaginative play so that children have opportunities both to acquire and practice new skills and to pretend.

Another way to increase the probability that children will play with toys is to make the toys easy to hold, carry, and manipulate. This is particularly important for children with motor impairments because the quality of early communication is related to a child's ability to manipulate objects (Granlund & Olsson, 1987). Numerous play adaptations can be implemented at home or at school, including activity frames, adjustable easels, learning boxes, play boxes, and other means of stabilizing and presenting manipulable toys so that they are accessible to children with limited hand and arm control. Toys can also be attached to lap trays with Velcro or elastic cords so that they are within reach. Books can be adapted with small foam or carpet tape squares pasted on the corners to separate the pages for easier turning (these are often called "page fluffers"). Small magnets or squares of Velcro can be attached to toys so that the child can pick them up with a headstick or mitten with the same material affixed to it. Toys with movable parts (e.g., levers, knobs) can be adapted with plastic or Velcro extenders for children with sensory or motor impairments. Figure 9.1 illustrates some of the many possible toy adaptations.

A number of excellent online resources focus on selecting and adapting toys to increase meaningful communication participation in preschool settings for young children with disabilities. These include the Let's Play! Projects, Do2Learn, and Simplified Technology web sites.

If a child with CCN has access to battery-operated toys and appliances (e.g., blenders, slide projectors), these items may also require modifications to accommodate motor and/or sensory impairments. Parents and school staff can either purchase the switches through commercial distributors or manufacturers or construct them inexpensively at home or at school using readily available components (e.g., see the handouts page at the Simplified Technology web site for directions). It is important to emphasize that playing with battery-operated toys should serve as the means to an end (i.e., participation in play routines and activities), not as an end in itself. All too often, children with motor or other impairments can be found sitting in the corner of a classroom with a paraprofessional, playing with a battery-operated toy and a microswitch while the other preschoolers are having fun playing house, garage, or dress-up! Unfortunately, this poor practice is often compounded when teachers provide a child with only one or two battery-operated toys for switch activation, apparently under the assumption that a monkey (or a bear, or a dog) hitting a drum (or crashing a pair of cymbals, or riding in a car) is so fascinating that it will sustain the child's attention for an extended period of time, day after day! None of these practices reflect an understanding of the principles of child development in general, the Participation Model, or the appropriate use of microswitch technology, and they are almost certain to result in the widespread lament, "We spent all that money to buy a switch and a toy and the child is bored with it after 2 minutes!" Table 9.2 summarizes some suggestions for using microswitches to enhance inclusive participation in home and preschool activities for children.

Communication opportunities can also arise or be created in the context of music, movement, puppetry, acting, and other fine arts activities for young children. Like other play activities, these may require adaptations in order to be accessible to children

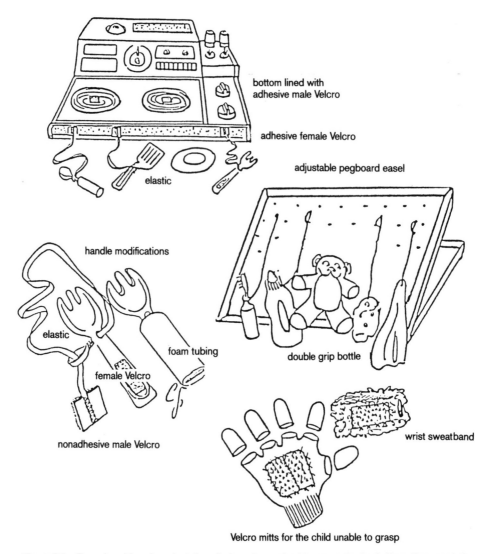

bottom lined with
adhesive male Velcro

adhesive female Velcro

elastic

adjustable pegboard easel

handle modifications

elastic

foam tubing

double grip bottle

female Velcro

nonadhesive male Velcro

wrist sweatband

Velcro mitts for the child unable to grasp

Figure 9.1.   Examples of toy play adaptations that can be made at home or at school. (From Goossens', C. [1989]. Aided augmentative communication intervention before assessment: A case study of a child with cerebral palsy. *Augmentative and Alternative Communication, 5,* 17; reprinted by permission of Informa Healthcare.)

with disabilities. For example, many songs can be adapted so that they are easily represented through manual signs or pictorial symbols and incorporated throughout the preschool day. Music-and-movement activities (e.g., fingerplay songs such as "Where Is Thumbkin?") and gross motor games (e.g., Red Light, Green Light) are also excellent vehicles for teaching basic cognitive and communication skills such as following directions, imitation, sequencing, and concept development. However, many standard movement activities and songs require one or more of the following modifications to be used for communication purposes: 1) simplifying target movements so that the child can participate meaningfully (this is also a good place to incorporate movement goals identified by motor therapists); 2) slowing the speed of the song or activity; 3) making directions shorter, simpler, and more repetitive; 4) simplifying the vocabulary; 5) pairing words with manual signs; 6) accompanying movements with sounds or words to encourage speech; and 7) including visual aids or concrete materials for children who

Table 9.2.   Suggestions for using microswitch technology to enhance participation of preschoolers with complex communication needs

Environment	Activity	Participation via microswitch technology
School	Activity transitions	Child activates switch attached to an iPod, with a recording of the teacher singing the cleanup song or saying, "Time to get ready for _____," or whatever the transition routine involves.
	Snack time	Child uses a switch to operate a toy car or truck that "delivers" the snack of the day to each of his or her friends at the snack table.
	Free play time	Child uses a switch to operate a simple computer game with a peer; child controls battery-operated toys in various centers (e.g., blender, car, spinner).
Home/school	Playtime	Child in a crib activates a switch placed near a mobile body part to turn on a toy that provides stimulating and enjoyable feedback (e.g., a light display, a music tape, a mobile).
	Pretend play time	Child uses a switch to activate a battery-operated car, truck, robot, toy blender, or toy mixer, depending on the theme of the pretend play.
	Art time	Child uses a switch to operate a Paint 'N' Swirl device (AbleNet, Inc.) to make a swirly design pattern; child provides power for electric scissors used by a peer or adult to cut paper.
	Story time	Child uses a switch to operate a recording of an adult reading the repeated story line in the "story of the day" as an adult reads the rest of the story out loud.
	Cooking	Child activates a switch to operate a blender to make a milkshake, a mixer to make cake batter, or a food processor to make salad.
	Music time	Child activates a switch to turn on a CD player or an iPod recording of a same-gender child singing his or her part in a song.

do not yet engage in pretend play (Musselwhite, 1985). Activities such as acting (Stuart, 1988) and puppetry (Musselwhite, 1985) can also serve to create communication opportunities. For example, the teacher can attach a puppet to the child's foot or wrist rather than to his or her hand, or the child's wheelchair can be decorated so that it can be used as a prop or stage in a play or puppet show.

Sherazad is a 4-year-old Indo-Canadian girl who lives with her mother, father, and brother. She uses a ventilator as a result of a high spinal cord injury from a fall when she was 2 years old. She cannot speak, and others must provide all of her personal care needs. She is learning to use a sip-and-puff switch in the context of daily activities at home and in her preschool. For example, with her switch, she can turn the lights on and off in the classroom; turn music on and off during music time; help to make blender drinks daily during snack time; and play adapted versions of Candy Land, Chutes and Ladders, and other children's games using a battery-operated spinner attached to her switch. Paper templates with colored or numbered sections are fitted under the spinner dial. When she sips on her switch, the spinner spins around, and when she puffs, it stops. Her game partner then moves her token to the color or the number of spaces selected (Canfield & Locke, 1997). She can also play computer games with her friends; operate a battery-operated toy mixer, blender, and microwave during "house play" time; tell the teacher to turn the pages of a book during storytime by activating a small communication device with a single recorded message; and operate electric scissors and a hot glue gun to make art projects with a helper during art time. Once Sherazad enters kindergarten, she will use the switch to type letters and words with an AAC device at the same time that her classmates learn to write letters with pencil and paper.

RESOLVING OPPORTUNITY BARRIERS AND ENHANCING PARTICIPATION FOR SCHOOL-AGE INDIVIDUALS WITH COMPLEX COMMUNICATION NEEDS

Where do typically developing children and adolescents find communication opportunities, meet communication partners, and learn to communicate in a variety of ways? As most parents know, these opportunities all occur primarily at school, when children interact with classmates and other peers. However, a number of studies have shown that communication opportunities for beginning communicators may be severely limited even in schools, especially when these students are placed in self-contained classrooms with similar students (e.g., Sigafoos, Roberts, Kerr, Couzens, & Baglioni, 1994). Since the mid-1980s, the school reform movement in North America and elsewhere has emphasized the importance of including students with disabilities in general education classrooms along with their typically developing peers. Research indicates that inclusive education with appropriate supports greatly increases the likelihood that students with CCN will have numerous, daily opportunities for natural communication with a variety of partners (Calculator, 2009; Jorgensen, McSheehan, & Sonnenmeier, 2010; Katz & Mirenda, 2002).

Of course, there is no guarantee that just because students with CCN are enrolled in general education classrooms, they will be included in the educational and social milieu of the school in ways that promote communication. Several factors may limit communication opportunities: 1) potential communication partners may fail to recognize or make use of naturally occurring events related to communication; 2) partners may preempt communication by anticipating students' wants and needs; and 3) students with CCN may have limited repertoires of communicative behaviors, making it less likely that others will offer them opportunities to communicate (Sigafoos et al., 1994). As a result of these factors, it may be necessary to engineer school environments and support teachers and paraprofessionals to create explicit opportunities for communication. Some simple strategies that can be used in this regard include withholding an item needed to complete or engage in an activity so that the student has an opportunity to request it; inserting regular, frequent opportunities for symbol use into classroom activities (e.g., by asking questions that are relevant to a specific lesson or context, such as *What do we need to do next?*, *Whose turn is it now?*, and *Where is the boy in the story going?*); interrupting an ongoing activity to create an opportunity for requesting or protesting; providing a wrong or incomplete item in response to a request (e.g., providing part of a toy so that a child has to ask for the rest); and delaying assistance in order to create the need to ask for help (Sigafoos, 1999; Sigafoos & Mirenda, 2002; Sigafoos, O'Reilly, Drasgow, & Reichle, 2002). If such strategies are used, it is important that they be incorporated throughout the day in general education activities and contexts.

"If she needs something, if she needs help opening the paint, she'll tap one of the other kids and hand them the jar like, 'You know, I can't get this cover off.' And they have gotten so they've been as excited as I have. 'Hey, Holly wants me to open it! Holly asked me to do it! She's communicating!'" (a mother whose daughter was enrolled in a general education classroom, in Giangreco, 1996, p. 252)

It is also important to acknowledge that inclusive education presents considerable challenges to those who provide classroom support, in that students with CCN in general education classrooms usually have a broader range of communication needs than do students in special education classrooms. In general education class-rooms, students need to be able to ask and answer questions on a number of topics, give reports, participate in instructional groups, and participate in a wide variety of social exchanges (Kent-Walsh & Light, 2003). In inclusive social environments, students encounter communication opportunities that go far beyond simple request-ing, rejecting, and identifying wants and needs as they interact with classmates and friends. For example, if an adolescent is sitting in the cafeteria and eating lunch with his high school classmates, he probably does not have to communicate many wants and needs because his needs (at least for food and drink!) have already been met. However, he may be asked by his friends to share information about what he did last weekend, about an upcoming school musical or football game, or about a favorite TV show or video game. In order for students to be fully included in social as well as educational activities, it is critically important that they have strategies for com-munication in areas such as information sharing, social closeness, and social etiquette (Light, 1988). In Chapters 10 and 13, we present extended discussions of strategies for supporting social communication and for including students who rely on AAC in general education classrooms. In addition, a number of person-centered planning models have been developed in this regard.

Person-Centered Planning

Who is there to talk to? For most individuals with CCN, the answer is family members, adults who are paid to be communication partners or facilitators, and perhaps other people with disabilities. These are all perfectly acceptable communication partners—but they should not be the *only* communication partners. Imagine what it would be like, day after day, to communicate only with your parents, your teachers, and other people who have at least as much difficulty as you do in getting messages across!

Most of the time, a systematic approach is required in order to develop and im-plement plans that enable people with CCN to transition from restrictive settings in which few communication partners are available to those that are more inclusive. Person-centered planning (O'Brien & Lyle O'Brien, 2002) is a process that can has been used in this regard and that enables people with disabilities and their facilitators to "focus on opportunities…to develop personal relationships, have positive roles in community life, increase their control of their own lives, and develop the skills and abilities to achieve these goals" (Mount & Zwernik, 1988, p. 6). Person-centered planning is as much a process for organizational change as for individual planning, and it consists of several basic steps. First, a "vision plan" is developed from a group interview of the person with CCN and the people who are involved in his or her life, to gather information about past events, relationships, places, preferences, choices, ideas about the future, obstacles, and opportunities. The goal of this first step is to develop a collective vision of the future that emphasizes the person's capacities and gifts rather than his or her impairments and problems (O'Brien & Pearpoint, 2007). Next, the person with CCN and other members of the group develop both short- and long-term goals based on the vision plan. Finally, facilitators make commitments of various types and levels to help the individual carry out the plan over time.

PATH and Social Networks

Two person-centered planning processes have been used extensively with people with CCN. The first, PATH (Planning Alternative Tomorrows with Hope), is an eight-step planning process that can be used to bring together a person with CCN and the individuals in his or her social network for the purpose of short- and long-term planning (O'Brien & Pearpoint, 2007; Pearpoint, O'Brien, & Forest, 2008). The second, Social Networks (Blackstone & Hunt Berg, 2003a, 2003b), was designed specifically for use with individuals with CCN, to help teams collect and interpret information in order to plan AAC interventions in inclusive settings. A central component of this model involves identifying communication partners across five "circles of communication partners" that constitute the social network of the person using AAC (see Figure 9.2): 1) life partners (e.g., close family members); 2) relatives and close friends (i.e., people with whom the person enjoys spending time and has a close relationships); 3) neighbors and acquaintances (e.g., classmates, co-workers); 4) people who are paid to interact with the student with CCN (e.g., teachers, classroom assistants); and 5) unfamiliar partners with whom the individual interacts occasionally (e.g., shopkeepers, community helpers). The Social Networks Inventory and planning approach can be used to assist AAC team members to both recognize areas of strength and identify areas that require attention across the five circles.

Written materials and training videotapes on person-centered planning and PATH are available from Inclusion Press in Toronto. Social Networks inventories and DVDs are available through Augmentative Communication, Inc. The Social Networks assessment and implementation materials are available in Catalan, Chinese, Danish, French, German, Hebrew, Italian, Norwegian, Russian, Spanish, and Swedish in addition to English.

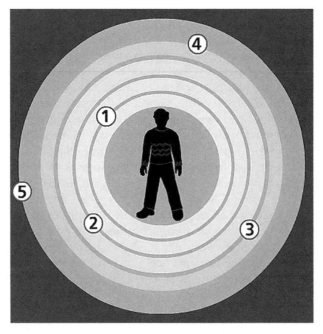

Figure 9.2.   Circles of communication partners: 1) life partners; 2) close friends and relatives; 3) acquaintances; 4) paid workers; 5) unfamiliar communication partners. (From Blackstone, S., & Hunt Berg, M. [2003a]. *Social networks: A communication inventory for individuals with complex communication needs and their communication partners–Inventory booklet* [p. 30]. Monterey, CA: Augmentative Communication, Inc.; reprinted by permission.)

RESOLVING OPPORTUNITY BARRIERS AND ENHANCING PARTICIPATION FOR ADOLESCENTS AND ADULTS WITH COMPLEX COMMUNICATION NEEDS

Since the mid-1970s, a number of authors have argued that adolescents and adults who are beginning communicators should be fully included in the community and should participate in the same types of vocational, recreational and leisure, and other activities as typical adults (McNaughton & Bryen, 2007; Meyer, Peck, & Brown, 1991). In this regard, older individuals with CCN must have access to a community-referenced support model, within which they can learn the skills needed to participate in activities that are age appropriate, functional (i.e., directly useful in their daily activities), taught in the actual community or vocational environments in which they are needed, and taught with reference to the cues and corrections that are naturally available (Falvey, 1989; Ford & Mirenda, 1984). Such activities may occur in home, recreational and leisure, community, vocational, or school environments. Person-centered planning models, such as the PATH and Social Networks approaches described previously, can be used to develop individualized plans and strategies for accomplishing this goal.

Adoption of a community-referenced approach to instruction has a direct, positive impact on the quantity and quality of the participation and communication opportunities that are available to adults who rely on AAC. Because of increased involvement in the community, an individual may, for example, need to order food in a restaurant, cheer for the local basketball team, ask for help at a college library, or chat with co-workers at break time—the list of natural opportunities for things to say and people to say them to becomes endless! Careful analysis of the settings in which adolescents and adults with CCN participate helps to identify the opportunities available for communication and to ensure that necessary adaptive and AAC techniques are included in an intervention.

An "ecological inventory" process has been used successfully for this purpose for many years. In brief, the ecological inventory process is similar to the first few steps in the Participation Model and involves the following (Reichle, York, & Sigafoos, 1991):

- Observe a peer without disabilities engaging in the activity of interest.
- Write a step-by-step list of the skills required.
- Assess the skills of the adult with CCN against the skill inventory to identify discrepancies.
- Design communication supports and instructional programs to teach needed skills.

Figure 9.3 provides excerpts from an ecological inventory completed for an adult in a community environment, along with suggested participation and communication adaptations in discrepancy areas. AAC teams can apply this basic format to activities at home, in the workplace, or in the community. If the individual is not supported to participate in functional, age-appropriate activities in a wide variety of settings, this restriction should be considered an opportunity barrier and targeted for remediation.

InterAACtion: Strategies for Intentional and Unintentional Communicators (Bloomberg, West, Johnson, & Caithness, 2004) is a manual and DVD aimed at facilitators who support adults with developmental or multiple disabilities who rely on AAC. It is available through the Scope Communication Resource Centre in Australia.

THE BOTTOM LINE

Over and over again, friends, parents, professionals, and community members have documented the positive impact of inclusive social opportunities on the communication abilities of people who are beginning communicators. There is simply no doubt about it: The availability of genuine and motivating communication opportunities in inclusive settings is at least as important to the success of a communication

Environment: Prendle's Drug Store
Target Individual: Sarah, age 20
Activity: Purchasing personal care items
Set-up: In the store with a friend who also needs to do some shopping, friend is wheeling Sarah in wheelchair

Skill (as performed by a peer without a disability)	Participation (person with a disability)	Possible participation or communication adaptations
1. Enter store.	–	Pause before entering, wait for signal indicating anticipation/acceptance.
2. Greet salesperson at jewelry counter, if present.	+ (vocalized)	In addition, consider single message loop tape with greeting that can be activated with microswitch by left hand.

	Items to Purchase			
Repeat for each item:	**1**	**2**	**3**	
3a. Walk/wheel along front of store, looking down each aisle until desired aisle is identified.	–	–	–	Encourage Sarah to look down aisle, pause and look for accept signal, proceed down aisle after signal.
3b. Walk/wheel down aisle.	–	–	–	Friend can wheel her slowly down aisle.
3c. Locate correct section.	–	–	–	As she wheels past the sections, look for an accept signal and stop.
3d. Examine options.	P	P	P	Friend can hold up two options at a time to make this easier.
3e. Choose desired item.	P	P	P	Look for eye gaze or arm movement toward one of the two options presented. If none, try another two options.
3f. Converse with friend as desired/needed.	P	–	P	Consider a multiple message loop tape with topic-setter statements that can be activated with micro-switch by left hand: "Have you seen any good movies lately?"
3g. Check to see if next item is in the aisle. If yes, go to Step 3a. If no, go to Step 2.	–	–	–	Friend can push her down aisle again slowly, looking for signal to stop.

4. Locate checkout stand.	–	Wheel to front of store and pause within view of stand, pause and wait for a signal to proceed.
5. Greet cashier.	P (smiled slightly)	Consider single message loop tape as in Step 2.

Figure 9.3. Excerpts from an ecological inventory with suggestions for participation and communication adaptations (*Key:* + = performed independently; – = not attempted; P = prompted).

intervention as is the availability of an appropriate access system. This is perhaps more true for people who are just learning the basics of communication than for anyone else because these individuals may have the fewest personal resources and the most need for assistance from others. If the communication partners of these individuals do not include a substantial number of people who are not paid to interact with them, who are not likely to leave for a new job next year, and who do not believe that their primary task is to make the individual more like everyone else, the communication interventions are almost certainly going to have a limited impact!

Once the AAC team has created communication opportunities and contexts and has identified communication partners, it can begin to plan a multimodal and multielement approach for building communication skills. For many beginning communicators, initial interventions may be aimed at strengthening their existing repertoires of nonsymbolic communication behaviors.

Support Helps Others Use Technology (SHOUT) is a nonprofit society in the United States that was organized primarily to help adults who rely on AAC to overcome barriers related to employment. SHOUT sponsors the annual Pittsburgh Employment Conference for Augmented Communicators. In Canada, Speaking Differently is a society aimed at improving the quality of life of adults with CCN.

SENSITIZING AND TRAINING FACILITATORS TO RESPOND TO NONSYMBOLIC COMMUNICATION

As mentioned in previous chapters, we use the term *facilitator* to refer to an individual who assumes or is assigned responsibility for supporting the communication of individuals with CCN. Teaching facilitators to identify and respond to the nonsymbolic communication signals of beginning communicators is important for at least two reasons. First, and most obviously, contingent responding teaches an individual that his or her behavior has an impact on the behavior of others in meaningful and predictable ways. When a parent consistently responds to a child's vocalizations by approaching, or when a support worker routinely responds to an adult's arm wave by moving away, the child and the adult learn that their behaviors have "communicative power" over the behaviors of others.

Second, and perhaps less obviously, contingent responding by facilitators can prevent the development of problem behaviors that serve a communicative purpose. Green, O'Reilly, Itchon, and Sigafoos (2005) described the mechanism that explains how this works.

Sami communicates exclusively through undifferentiated vocalizations, arm reaches, and uncoordinated arm movements. Sometimes, caregivers and others notice and respond appropriately to Sami's behaviors; sometimes, they notice but do not respond appropriately because they interpret her behaviors inaccurately; and sometimes, they fail to notice Sami's behaviors entirely. In response to the inconsistent (or absent) responses of her caregivers, Sami intensifies the quality of her behaviors over time so that "the vocalization now becomes a scream, the reach becomes an aggressive grab, and initially uncoordinated arm movements might even become self-injurious face slapping" (Green et al., 2005, p. 54). Sami's caregivers definitely respond to the intensified behaviors, and they probably exert extra effort to figure out what they mean as well—and as a result, Sami learns that screaming, grabbing, and self-injurious behaviors are more efficient at obtaining a desired result than the subtle, nonsymbolic behaviors she displayed initially were. Had her caregivers responded more consistently in the first place, Sami's challenging behaviors probably would not have emerged and persisted.

Distinguishing and Responding to Signals for Communication

Individuals who communicate primarily through gestures and vocalizations initially do so when the need arises rather than in response to queries or directives from their communication partners. Initially, an individual's spontaneous signaling behavior is not intended to be communicative but simply occurs at random. When facilitators consistently interpret and respond to such behaviors as if they are intentional, the individual gradually learns to initiate them intentionally. Unfortunately, although most adults are attuned to conventional gestures and vocalizations of typical children and adults, they often either ignore or misinterpret many of the idiosyncratic behaviors exhibited by children and especially adults with CCN (Rowland, 1990). In particular, facilitators may find it difficult to distinguish intentional from unintentional behaviors (Carter & Iacono, 2002; Iacono, Carter, & Hook, 1998) because these distinctions are often quite subtle. However, these distinctions are important so that facilitators can respond differentially to intentional rather than unintentional behaviors in order to strengthen the former, a process often referred to as shaping. Siegel and Cress (2002) and Carter and Iacono (2002) summarized some of the indicators of intentionality that have been noted by a number of investigators; these are displayed in Table 9.3.

"Parents rely heavily on their own intuition and ability to interpret their child....[This] involves a great degree of guesswork....Parents are often regarded with suspicion about the validity of their interpretations. They often hear from other people that they over-interpret the child and that their comprehension is only an expression of wishful thinking....[However], parents have a unique competence in knowing their children and understanding their children's communication" (Brodin, 1991, p. 237).

Parent and Facilitator Training

A number of evidence-based facilitator training programs are available to teach adults who support beginning communicators across the age range to use the prin-

Table 9.3.   Indicators of intentional communicative behaviors

1. Is there an alternating gaze between an object (i.e., goal) and a facilitator (i.e., joint attention)?
2. Is there body orientation to indicate that a signal is being directed toward a facilitator?
3. When a signal is produced, is there a pause before it is repeated that might indicate that the communicator is awaiting a response from a facilitator?
4. When a signal is produced and the facilitator responds, does the signal terminate?
5. When a signal is produced and the facilitator responds, does the communicator show either satisfaction or dissatisfaction with the response?
6. When a signal is produced and the facilitator does not respond, does the communicator persist by repeating or changing the signal?
7. Is the signal ritualized (i.e., the same every time) or does it have a conventional form (e.g., pointing, shaking head)?

Sources: Siegel and Cress (2002); Carter and Iacono (2002).

ciples reviewed in the previous sections to support both nonsymbolic and symbolic communication. These include *Communicating Partners* (MacDonald, 2004), *It Takes Two to Talk* (Pepper & Weitzman, 2004), *More than Words* (Sussman, 1999), the van Dijk approach (Nelson, van Dijk, Oster, & McDonnell, 2009), the SCERTS® Model (Social Communication, Emotional Regulation, and Transactional Support; Prizant, Wetherby, Rubin, & Laurent, 2003; Prizant, Wetherby, Rubin, Laurent, & Rydell, 2006a, 2006b), and *InterAACtion: Strategies for Intentional and Unintentional Communicators* (Bloomberg et al., 2004). In addition, a number of general strategies can be used for facilitator instruction regardless of the skills being taught. Kent-Walsh and McNaughton (2005) described eight general steps required for facilitator training, which are summarized in Table 9.4. In the sections that follow and in subsequent chapters, we describe numerous strategies that can be taught to facilitators using this basic framework.

In 2007–2008, Augmentative Communication Community Partnerships Canada (ACCPC) developed, piloted, and evaluated a project to train "communication assistants" to act as facilitators for people who rely on AAC. Results indicated that the provision of trained communication assistants significantly increased participants' ability to communicate and participate in their communities and their feelings of dignity, empowerment, autonomy, and privacy (Collier, McGhie-Richmond, & Self, 2010). Information about the training program is available through the ACCPC web site.

STRATEGIES FOR RESPONDING TO AND EXPANDING NONSYMBOLIC COMMUNICATION

Three of the essential building blocks of communication are spontaneous signals for getting attention, accepting, and rejecting. Even individuals who have a limited repertoire of gestural or vocal behaviors can usually be taught to communicate us-

Table 9.4.   Eight steps for communication facilitator instruction

Step	Description
1. Introduce the target strategy and measure the facilitator's current use and commitment to learning it	Observe the facilitator with the person with complex communication needs (CCN) and assess the frequency and accuracy of target strategy use; review results with facilitator and secure commitment to learn the strategy.
2. Describe the strategy	Describe the target strategy and its component steps, and explain its potential positive impact on the person with CCN.
3. Demonstrate the strategy	Model use of the target strategy with the person with CCN while "talking through" the steps involved.
4. Verbal practice	Ask the facilitator to describe the strategy and all of the steps required to implement it.
5. Controlled practice and feedback	Provide prompting and verbal feedback to the facilitator as he or she attempts to implement the strategy with the person with CCN.
6. Advanced practice and feedback	Gradually fade instructor prompts and feedback as the facilitator practices use of the strategy in multiple situations within the natural environment.
7. Reassess facilitator skill and commitment for long-term strategy use	Observe the facilitator's independent use of the strategy and compare to the results from Step 1; assist the facilitator to develop a long-term action plan for continued strategy use.
8. Generalization	Facilitator implements the strategy with the person with CCN across a wide range of settings and situations.

Source: Kent-Walsh and McNaughton (2005).

ing nonsymbolic signals for these purposes. Attention-getting signals are those the individual uses primarily to initiate social interactions with others, such as laughing, crying, or making eye contact. Questions such as *How does (name) let you know that she wants you to pay attention to her?* or *What does (name) do to let you know he wants you to talk to him?* will often encourage parents or other familiar caregivers to provide examples of behaviors that serve this function. Acceptance signals are those used to communicate that whatever is currently happening is tolerable, okay, or enjoyable. Familiar communication partners are usually able to describe these behaviors if asked questions such as *How do you know when (name) likes something?* or *How do you know when (name) is happy?* Rejection signals are used to communicate that the individual finds his or her current status unacceptable, not enjoyable, or intolerable for some reason. Partners will often describe these behaviors when asked questions such as *How do you know when (name) doesn't like something?* or *How do you know when (name) is unhappy or in pain?* Note that the ability to signal acceptance and rejection is not the same as the ability to respond to yes/no questions—the latter involves a much more sophisticated set of skills. Acceptance and rejection signals may be overt and obvious, such as smiling, laughing, frowning, or crying, or may be very subtle, such as averted eye gaze, increased body tension, increased rate of respiration, or sudden passivity.

Most individuals are able to signal acceptance and rejection in some way, although this may be quite idiosyncratic. If clear, intentional, and socially appropriate attention-seeking, acceptance, and rejection signals are not part of an individual's communication repertoire, initial interventions should include strategies for developing these behaviors.

Teaching Attention-Seeking Signals and Gestures

It is particularly important that facilitators be attuned to attention-seeking behaviors initiated by the individual. Initially, facilitators should respond to any intentional behaviors that are socially and culturally acceptable and that appear to function to get attention so that the person can repeatedly experience the communicative results of his or her efforts (Smebye, 1990). For example, a facilitator might respond to a behavior such as pounding on a lap tray or vocalizing loudly as an indicator of a desire for attention. After a repertoire of acceptable attention-seeking behaviors has been established and is used intentionally, facilitators can then begin to limit their responses to the most desirable and frequent behaviors only.

Simple technology can serve to enhance the salience of attention-getting behaviors, especially for individuals whose behaviors are quite subtle and easily missed. For example, researchers have used switch-activated attention-getting devices (e.g., call buzzers) and single-message audio recordings that say COME HERE PLEASE for this purpose.

> In one study, an *interrupted behavior chain* strategy was used to teach use of attention-getting devices to three children with CCN and significant intellectual, sensory, physical, and medical disabilities who were extremely limited in their ability to participate in daily school routines (Gee, Graham, Goetz, Oshima, & Yoshioka, 1991). Teachers identified three or four routines that could be interrupted to provide opportunities during the school day for the students to use their attention-getting devices. For example, one such opportunity occurred during a transfer activity when a student, Erik, was told it was time to get out of his wheelchair and had his straps loosened and tray removed, but was not then moved. Erik's teacher waited for him

to initiate a gestural or vocal behavior to call attention (e.g., extending his arms, making agitated noises, whimpering) and then prompted him to activate a switch mounted in an appropriate location and connected to one of the attention-getting devices described previously. When the device was activated after the teacher's prompting, the routine continued as planned (i.e., Erik was moved from the wheel-chair). Over time, the teacher faded the instructional prompts for switch activation by pausing for a few seconds to give Erik a chance to initiate switch activation with-out prompting. All three students learned to activate their attention-getting switches independently across several such routines within no more than 60 instructional opportunities. This study demonstrated clearly that well-planned instruction using appropriate contexts and technology can result in the acquisition of at least simple attention-seeking behaviors, even by individuals with very severe disabilities.

Relationship to Problem Behavior

Unfortunately, attention-getting signals for many nonsymbolic communicators take the form of socially unacceptable behaviors, such as screaming, grabbing, hitting, throwing tantrums, engaging in self-injurious behaviors, and others. Since the 1980s, a technique known as functional communication training (FCT) has been used widely in response to such behaviors. FCT involves a set of procedures designed to reduce problem be-haviors by teaching functionally equivalent communication skills. As noted previously, FCT requires a thorough assessment to identify the function (i.e., communicative mes-sage) of the behavior of concern, as well as systematic instruction to teach new com-municative behaviors (Sigafoos, Arthur, & O'Reilly, 2003). Mirenda (1997) and Bopp, Brown, and Mirenda (2004) reported that a large number of FCT interventions involv-ing people who rely on AAC have focused on teaching alternative attention-getting behaviors. This has been accomplished by teaching use of nonsymbolic communica-tive behaviors such as tapping or waving a hand or arm (Kennedy, Meyer, Knowles, & Shukla, 2000; Lalli, Browder, Mace, & Brown, 1993; Sigafoos & Meikle, 1996), activating a microswitch with the recorded message PLEASE COME HERE (Northup et al., 1994; Peck et al., 1996), and activating an electronic communication device with attention-getting messages such as I WANT TO BE WITH THE GROUP (Durand, 1993) or WOULD YOU HELP ME WITH THIS? (Durand, 1999). Systematic teaching strategies such as prompting and fad-ing can be used to teach the new attention-getting behaviors in natural contexts, with brief attention provided in all cases as a response. Several authors have provided useful descriptions of the key steps required to plan and implement FCT/AAC interventions for individuals with developmental disabilities (see Bopp et al., 2004; Sigafoos, Arthur, & O'Reilly, 2003; Tiger, Hanley, & Bruzek, 2008).

 First Things First: Early Communication for the Pre-Symbolic Child with Severe Disabil-ities (Rowland & Schweigert, 2004) is a manual designed for parents and profession-als. It includes strategies for assessment as well as for teaching basic communication messages such as asking for more, gaining attention, and making choices. It is avail-able from Design to Learn.

Teaching Use of Accept/Reject Signals and Gestures

The basic principles of contingent interpretation and responsiveness are also the cor-nerstones for building communicative signals that serve the functions of acceptance or rejection (Sigafoos & Mirenda, 2002; Sigafoos et al., 2002). Often, these signals are quite subtle; for example, an individual might not display behavior changes when he or she is content but might whimper slightly when distressed or uncomfortable. In other cases, a person might exhibit more overt indicators such as limb movements, smiling, or crying. Initially, it is necessary for facilitators to respond to and comply with any communicative behaviors that can be socially and culturally tolerated, in order to strengthen the behaviors over time and teach the power of communication. Occasionally, facilitators express concern about the implications of this strategy, worrying that people will become "spoiled" if they always "give them what they want." This need not be a concern if facilitators are attuned to the amount and level of responsiveness the individual needs so that they can decide when to begin to respond intermittently to these signals and/or shape them into less subtle forms.

Relationship to Problem Behavior

Some individuals utilize socially unacceptable gestural behaviors to signal acceptance or rejection or to engage in social interactions with others. For example, both stereotypic behaviors (e.g., spinning objects, rocking back and forth) and aggressive behaviors (e.g., tantrums, self-injurious behaviors) often serve as rejection messages that serve an escape function (Durand & Carr, 1987, 1991; Kennedy et al., 2000). Other individuals may flap their hands, squeal repetitively, or become aggressive when they are happy or excited, which are two clear occasions for sending acceptance messages. Individuals may also initiate and maintain social interactions with a variety of socially inappropriate behaviors. As is the case with inappropriate forms of attention getting, FCT can be used to teach alternatives to inappropriate acceptance, rejection, and social interaction signals.

> Monica used to bang loudly on her wheelchair lap tray when she did not want to eat the food her mother offered to her. Her mother began to watch to see whether Monica produced more subtle rejection cues before she started banging. She noticed that occasionally Monica would purse her lips and turn her head away first, so Monica's mother started to respond to this behavior whenever it occurred by removing the rejected food. At the same time, when Monica banged on the lap tray, her mother prompted her to turn her head instead. Over a 2-month period, Monica's lip pursing and head turning increased and she stopped banging on the tray almost completely because she now had another way to tell her mother no thanks! By utilizing the principles of FBA and FCT, Monica's mother both taught a new communicative alternative and prevented a problem behavior from persisting.

> "When it is time to go out to recess, the paraprofessionals in Mrs. Hennessey's grade 3 classroom make sure everyone is dressed properly in coats, gloves, and hats. Sarah, a paraprofessional, directs Ken (a student with trisomy 13) toward the coat rack. She holds his hand and they swing their arms back and forth slightly as they walk. While smiling at Ken, Sarah's voice is warm as she says to him, It's almost time for recess now, what do you need to do? Ken returns the smile and looks delighted as he reaches for his coat. He obviously enjoys the attention Sarah pays him and uses his nonsymbolic behaviors (e.g., reaching, smiling) to communicate with her" (Siegel-Causey & Guess, 1989, p. 28).

Scripted Routines

Scripted routines can be used to provide structured opportunities for beginning communicators to practice using attention-getting, acceptance, and rejection signals in the context of naturally occurring activities (e.g., Keen, Sigafoos, & Woodyatt, 2001; Siegel & Wetherby, 2000). Table 9.5 displays part of a scripted routine created for Adam, a young man with deaf-blindness and severe physical disabilities, to use during a dressing routine at the swimming pool. As can be seen from this example, scripted routines usually consist of five elements, depending on the type of routine and the person's disability. These five elements—touch cue, verbal cue, pause, verbal feedback, and action—are described with reference to Table 9.5.

1. *Touch cue.* Touch cues provide information in addition to spoken words and occur before each step in a routine. The touch cue for a step should be the same each time, and all facilitators should use the same cues. Touch cues are critical for individuals with one or more sensory impairments (e.g., vision, hearing, or both) and are often useful for other nonsymbolic communicators as well. For example, in Step 2 of Table 9.5, the touch cue associated with putting on Adam's swimsuit is the suit brushing against his wrist.

Table 9.5.   Example of a scripted routine for Adam

Touch cue (how facilitator gives nonverbal information)	Verbal cue (what facilitator says)	Pause for at least 10 seconds, look for a response	Verbal feedback (what facilitator says while performing the action)	Action (what facilitator does after the person accepts or a second pause is over)
1. Rub seat belt under Adam's elbow. Release buckle so that a sound is made.	*Time to get ready for a swim.*	Pause, observe	*Okay, I hear you making a noise; let's put on your swimsuit.*	Continue to Step 2.
2. Rub swimsuit against his wrist.	*It's time to put on your swimsuit.*	Pause, observe	*Oh, you moved your foot; okay, let's get undressed.*	Continue to Step 3.
3. Unzip coat.	*It's time to take off your coat.*	Pause, observe	*I see you moved your arm; here, I'll help you take off your coat.*	Continue to Step 4.
4. Rub Adam's back.	*Let's lean forward now.*	Pause, observe	*I hear you making a noise; good, you can lean forward now.*	Lean him forward.
5. Pat his right arm where the sleeve ends.	*Time to pull out your arm.*	Pause, observe	*I see you trying to move your arm; I'll help you get it out.*	Remove right arm from sleeve.
6. Move loose coat across his back and pat his left arm where the sleeve ends.	*Let's take out the other arm now.*	Pause, observe	*Good for you, you're trying to move the other arm. Let's take it out.*	Remove left arm from sleeve.
7. Tap his right shoe, hard.	*Time to take off your shoe.*	Pause, observe	*I hear you making a noise to tell me to take off your shoe.*	Untie and remove right shoe.
8. Tap left shoe, hard.	*Time to take off your other shoe.*	Pause, observe	*You moved this foot; I guess you want the other shoe off.*	Untie and remove left shoe.

2. *Verbal cue.* The verbal cue is what the facilitator says while providing the touch cue. For example, while rubbing Adam's swimsuit against his wrist before putting it on, the facilitator says, "It's time to put on your swimsuit" (Step 2, Table 9.5). Facilitators should not be rigid about the precise structure of verbal cues and should provide essential information as naturally as possible, using short, simple phrases or sentences. Facilitators should always use verbal cues, even with individuals who have hearing impairments, because most of these individuals have at least some residual hearing.

3. *Pause.* After each pair of touch and verbal cues, the facilitator pauses for 10–30 seconds and observes the person for a response. For Adam, a response is likely to be a motor movement or vocalization that appears to be intentional or can be interpreted as intentional. If the person responds with a signal that can be interpreted as acceptance after the pause, the facilitator continues the routine. If the individual gives a rejection signal, the facilitator stops the routine briefly and then tries again, explores an alternative way of proceeding, or terminates the routine altogether. If neither type of signal is produced, the facilitator repeats the paired touch and verbal cues and waits 10–30 seconds again for a signal. If the individual still gives no signal, the facilitator acknowledges this verbally and continues the routine. The length of the pause depends largely on the individual's level of responsiveness and the extent of motor involvement. Individuals with severe motor impairments require much longer pauses in order to have time to formulate and produce signals.

4. *Verbal feedback.* After the individual's acceptance signal, verbal feedback in the form of a comment about what the person did and what action the facilitator will do in response is provided in conjunction with the appropriate action. For example, after pausing (Step 2, Table 9.5), Adam's facilitator says, "Oh, you moved your foot; okay, let's get undressed."

5. *Action.* For each step in the scripted routine, the facilitator performs an action after providing verbal feedback. The action is the actual step in the routine that was identified through a task analysis. The facilitator may have to assist an individual who is unable to perform the action independently; the amount of assistance provided should be adjusted to the individual's needs. It is important to remember that the point of a scripted routine is not to teach the person to perform the action; rather, it is to facilitate the development of communicative signaling within the context of a familiar activity.

Scripted routines have also been referred to as *joint action routines* (McLean, McLean, Brady, & Etter, 1991; Snyder-McLean, Solomonson, McLean, & Sack, 1984) and *planned dialogues* (Siegel & Wetherby, 2000; Siegel-Causey & Guess, 1989). Additional examples for creating scripts and adapting activities for communication can be found in these publications.

To teach scripted routines for play to young children, facilitators can utilize a simplified format similar to the one described in Table 9.5, but without the touch and verbal cues. For example, the facilitator can create an interactive routine for singing "Row, Row, Row Your Boat" by sitting on the floor facing the child while holding his or her hands. As the facilitator sings the song, he or she rocks to and fro in a boatlike motion with the child. Once the routine has been established and the child is seen to enjoy it, the facilitator pauses after every 1–2 lines in the song and watches for any indication that the child wants to continue the game. The facilitator can apply this basic format—action, pause to elicit a communicative signal, action—to other interactive games and songs as well. Individuals older than 5 years of age can engage in scripted routines in the context of age-appropriate social or recreational activities such as swimming, playing video or pinball games, going to school dances, participating in relay races, and so forth.

> Over a 6-month period, Adam gradually began to participate in the dressing and undressing routine for swimming by moving his left arm or leg or by vocalizing during the pauses in the routine (see Table 9.5). At first, these movements occurred infrequently, but they gradually became more common as his support staff responded to them. Additional scripted routines were introduced during mealtimes, position changes, and bath time. Now, Adam has changed from a 27-year-old man who spent 99% of his day either sleeping or passively allowing people to care for him to a 45-year-old man who spends most of his day actively involved in home and community activities. He operates a large switch positioned by his head to activate an attention-getting buzzer and uses numerous tangible symbols on a speech-generating device to make choices, express his preferences, and participate in social routines. His communication skills continue to develop as his social network expands and as he is increasingly included in his community.

Gesture Dictionaries

After facilitators have instituted a range of interventions to teach signals for attention getting, acceptance, and rejection, most beginning communicators gradually develop a repertoire of vocalizations and gestures for communication. Many of these signals may be idiosyncratic, such that only a few familiar facilitators (e.g., parents, support workers) are able to understand and respond to them consistently. People who are less familiar with the person may have difficulty understanding and interpreting these messages accurately, resulting in communication breakdowns. For example, a child's baby sitter may not know that the child's way of asking someone to change the channel on the television is to walk over to the television and tap on it repeatedly. If the sitter tries to dissuade the child from engaging in this seemingly destructive act, the child's efforts may intensify until both individuals are frustrated and dissatisfied.

Communication breakdowns may be avoided by using a "gesture dictionary," in which descriptions of the person's gestures, along with their meanings and suggestions for appropriate responses, are compiled. The dictionary can take the form of a wall poster in a classroom or home, or it can be an alphabetized notebook with cross-referenced entries. For example, in the previous situation, the baby sitter might look in the child's gesture dictionary under *T* for *tap* or *television*. Under either (or both) words, the sitter might find a description of the tapping behavior, its meaning, and how to respond (e.g., "Tapping means he wants you to change the channel on the television. Prompt him to sign HELP, and then change the channel for him"). Table 9.6 displays a portion of a gesture dictionary created for Shawn, an adolescent with visual and cognitive impairments. The gesture dictionary can also be used for individuals well beyond preschool age; in fact, this technique is often used to orient new staff to the communication patterns of students with CCN in new classrooms or of adults in group homes and other residential environments that have a high staff turnover.

Table 9.6. Example of a gesture dictionary for Shawn

What Shawn does	What it means	What facilitator should do
Makes the T sign by his chin	Wants to go to the bathroom	Acknowledge and provide assistance
Makes "ssssh" sound	"Yes"	Respond according to situation
Shakes head back and forth	"No"	Respond according to situation
Reaches his hand out to another person	"I want to shake your hand" (greeting)	Shake his hand
Claps another's hand when offered	"I'm feeling sociable or affectionate"	Give him a high five, fist bump, etc.
Wraps both arms around his abdomen, arms crossed at chest and hands tapping both shoulders	"I want a hug"	Encourage him to shake your hand or give a high five, or give him a hug if appropriate
Hands flat across mouth	Wants food	If mealtime or near mealtime, ask him to wait and set the timer; if between meals, offer choices using food samples
Hand sideways to mouth	Wants a drink	Acknowledge and offer choices using drink samples
Hand to mouth with teeth grinding	"I'm really hungry!"	Provide a small amount of bland food (he has an ulcer)

The gesture dictionary has also been called a *communication diary* (Bloomberg, 1996), *communication dictionary* (Siegel & Wetherby, 2000), and *communication signal inventory* (Siegel & Cress, 2002). Regardless of what it is called, this type of support consists of three components: descriptions of what the person does (communicative behavior), what it means (function or message), and how facilitators should react (consequence).

INTRODUCING SYMBOLIC COMMUNICATION: VISUAL SCHEDULES AND "TALKING SWITCH" TECHNIQUES

A number of strategies for communication participation are applicable to individuals who have developed the basic skills of attention getting, accepting, and rejecting and are being introduced to symbolic communication. It is important to expand the repertoires of these individuals to include basic skills such as following a symbol schedule and engaging in simple social routines. Because the use of symbolic techniques such as manual signing and the use of object or graphic symbols require joint attention, we begin with a brief discussion of this important skill. We then summarize a few of the most common introductory symbol techniques.

Establishing Joint Attention

For typically developing children, joint attention (JA) is the ability to shift one's attention between a communication partner and an object or another person. In most children, JA emerges gradually and sequentially over a 6-month period—children first begin to check a partner's attentional focus at 9–12 months, then begin to respond to a partner's pointing at 11–14 months (e.g., partner points and says *Look there!*), and finally begin to direct a partner's attention themselves at 13–15 months (e.g., by showing an item and alternating eye gaze between it and the partner; Carpenter, Nagell, & Tomasello, 1998). When AAC is used, JA interactions are unique in that they are "quadratic…in nature, because they involve the [person with CCN], the communication partner, the AAC system, and the target object, such as toy or book" (Smith, McCarthy, & Benigno, 2009). Thus, it is important to introduce communication symbols in ways that facilitate rather than interfere with JA.

One strategy for reducing the JA demands of aided AAC with beginning communicators involves manipulating the position of AAC symbols during an interaction. Smith, McCarthy, and Benigno (2009) explored this issue experimentally and found that typically developing infants made more frequent and longer bids for JA when a communication device was held directly in front of them (i.e., aligned with the direction of their eye gaze) than when it was positioned off to the side. Similarly, Clibbens, Powell, and Atkinson (2002) found that mothers of infants and toddlers with Down syndrome who were learning manual signs typically signed within the child's existing focus of attention rather than off to the side or in another position. In addition to alignment, the extent to which facilitators respond to a beginning communicator's focus of attention is also associated with the frequency and duration of coordinated JA (Benigno, Bennett, McCarthy, & Smith, 2011). Thus, it appears that beginning communicators are most likely to be engaged when AAC symbols are presented in their line of visual regard and when facilitators provide comments that are contingent on the focus of attention (see also Light et al., 2005).

Visual Schedules

A *visual schedule* (also known as a calendar system, schedule system, or activity schedule) represents the main activities in a person's day with symbols and may serve several purposes: 1) to introduce an individual to the idea that one thing (i.e., a symbol) can represent another (i.e., a referent); 2) to provide an overview of the sequence of activities across a day and provide specific information about what will happen next; and 3) to facilitate smooth transitions from one activity to the next, especially for individuals who have a high need for predictability (Flannery & Horner, 1994). The visual schedule strategy originally came from the work of Stillman and Battle (1984) and other practitioners supporting individuals with deaf-blindness. It is also widely used with people who have visual, intellectual, or multiple disabilities (see Bopp, Brown, & Mirenda, 2004; Hodgdon, 1996; McClannahan & Krantz, 1999; Mesibov, Browder, & Kirkland, 2002; Rowland & Schweigert, 1989, 1990, 1996; Vicker, 1996). Schedule systems can be effective in home, school, and community settings for beginning communicators across the range of age and ability (see Bopp et al., 2004). Table 9.7 describes how to create and use a visual schedule.

Visual schedules can incorporate real objects, tangible symbols, photographs, line-drawing symbols, or written words in age-appropriate daily appointment books, wall displays, or other formats (see Hodgdon, 1996, and McClannahan & Krantz, 1999, for examples). Schedules can also be created using computer technologies such as Microsoft PowerPoint and various software programs for digital videotape editing (Rehfeldt, Kinney, Root, & Stromer, 2004). Numerous schedule applications are also available for tablet computers such as the Apple iPad, Samsung Galaxy, and so forth. Instruction in the use of a visual schedule is generally conducted in loosely structured naturalistic formats, with a hierarchy of prompts that are gradually faded.

Table 9.7.   Creating and using a visual schedule

Prepare the visual schedule

1. *List, in chronological order, the individual's daily schedule* across relevant home, school, and community environments. The list should include all of the activities he or she does every day or during a relevant portion of the day.

2. *Identify symbols that can be used to represent each of the activities.* For most beginning communicators, these symbols are likely to be real object, partial object, or photographic symbols; for example, a brush might represent morning grooming activities, a milk container might represent eating breakfast, and socks might represent getting dressed. Collect the symbols in one place (such as a cardboard box) so that they are readily available. The same objects should be used to represent an activity every time.

3. *Construct a way to display the symbols.* Real or partial object symbols can be placed in a series of shallow containers arranged in a left-to-right order (e.g., a series of empty shoe boxes or cardboard magazine holders taped together, a series of transparent plastic bags hung on cup hooks, or a long cardboard box with cardboard dividers taped into it at intervals). If photographs or other graphic symbols are used, they can be placed on the pages of a photo album or in some other portable carrier.

4. *Devise a method for identifying finished activities.* For real object symbols, this can be a "finished box" into which the person with complex communication needs (CCN) can deposit each object after finishing the activity. If photographs or other graphic symbols are used, the individual can simply turn them over or move them to a "finished" area at the end of each activity.

5. *Construct the schedule.* Using the display, arrange the symbols in chronological order to represent at least four or five activities in the person's day.

Use the visual schedule

1. Before each activity, prompt the person with CCN to go to the schedule display and select the next symbol in the sequence. Prompt the person to take the symbol to the related activity.

2. When the activity is completed, prompt the person with CCN to discard the symbol in the manner determined previously. Note that the discarded symbols should be readily accessible to the individual at all times so that he or she has the option of using them to ask to do that activity again. If this happens, facilitators should make *every attempt* to respond to the request and allow the individual to engage in the activity the symbol represents.

3. Look for signs that indicate that the person with CCN is making the connection between a symbol and the activity it represents. Such signs might include 1) taking a symbol and then wheeling or walking to the place where the activity typically occurs (e.g., to the bathroom for grooming, to the table for eating) and 2) smiling or laughing when selecting a symbol for a preferred activity.

Figure 9.4 provides an example of a schedule used at home and in the community by a preschooler who has Down syndrome, and Figure 9.5 provides an example of one used by an adolescent with autism.

A videotape/DVD entitled *PrAACtically Speaking* is designed for staff who support adults with developmental disabilities and CCN in community settings. It features examples of gesture dictionaries and visual schedule systems in addition to other strategies for interaction. An information booklet accompanies the video, which is available from the Australian organization Yooralla.

"Talking Switch" Techniques

A number of simple "talking switch" devices can also be used to introduce the use of symbols and provide limited-context communication using voice output. Talking switch devices are small, battery-powered aids that can be programmed to speak one or more messages when activated. A facilitator simply records a human voice message, music, or another sound (e.g., a dog barking), and the person using the device plays the recording with a simple switch activation. Ideally, the person who records a voice message should be the same age and gender as the person who uses

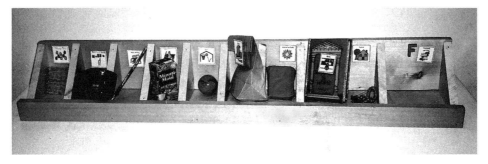

Figure 9.4. Object schedule used at home and in the community by a preschooler. (The Picture Communication Symbols ©1981–2012 by DynaVox Mayer-Johnson LLC. All Rights Reserved Worldwide. Used with permission.)

it. Activation may be either direct (i.e., an individual with sufficient fine motor skills simply activates the device with his or her hand) or remote. In the latter case, some type of switch (e.g., one that is operated by the head) is connected to the device in some way. Such simple voice-output techniques may be especially appropriate for beginning communicators who are learning to employ microswitches to participate in predictable communicative exchanges (see Rowland & Schweigert, 1991).

The most obvious context for using a single-message talking switch is one in which an individual participates in a preferred activity. In this case, a single symbol

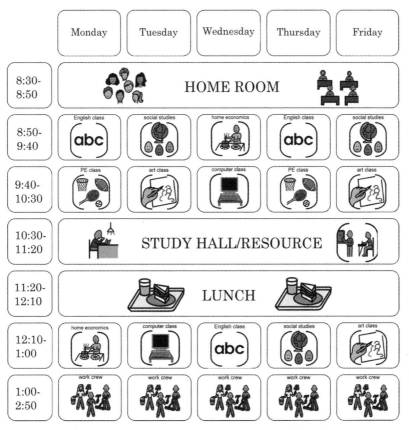

Figure 9.5. Visual schedule for school used by an adolescent with autism. (The Picture Communication Symbols ©1981–2012 by DynaVox Mayer-Johnson LLC. All Rights Reserved Worldwide. Used with permission.)

representing a relevant message should be fastened to the switch prior to use. The type of symbol (e.g., real object, tangible symbol) can vary, depending on the needs and abilities of the individual (see Chapter 6 for assessment information). The talking switch is then programmed to speak a related message; for example, it might be used in a preschool or elementary school classroom in the following situations:

- During opening "circle time" (e.g., the child activates a message to sing his or her part in the greeting song)
- At transition times (e.g., the child activates a recording of someone singing the cleanup song or of a voice saying TIME TO CLEAN UP!)
- Whenever a request for continuation or turn taking is appropriate (e.g., the child plays a recording that says MORE, PLEASE or MY TURN)
- Any time the schedule dictates that a specific activity take place (e.g., in the morning the child plays a recording that says TAKE OFF MY COAT, PLEASE)
- Any time an interjection during an activity is appropriate (e.g., WOWEE! COOL!)

Book reading activities provide an especially rich context for introducing talking switches and communication symbols to beginning communicators. For example, Trudeau, Cleave, and Woelk (2003) described a group reading activity with two pre-schoolers with cerebral palsy and CCN. The group facilitator used adapted books and related props (King-DeBaun, 1993, 1999), Picture Communication Symbols, and a talking switch device with a repeated story line (e.g., "THEN I'LL HUFF, AND I'LL PUFF, AND I'LL BLOW YOUR HOUSE IN" from Joseph Jacobs's *The Story of the Three Little Pigs*; in the public domain), along with scaffolding and a variety of prompting strategies, to include the children in book reading interactions with their mothers. Similarly, talking switches have been used to increase communicative interactions and participation during book reading with children with autism (Bedrosian, 1999), Rett syndrome (Koppenhaver, Erickson, & Skotko, 2001; Skotko, Koppenhaver, & Erickson, 2004), and moderate to severe intellectual disabilities and visual impairment (Bellon-Harn & Harn, 2008).

Older individuals with CCN can employ talking switch techniques for similar purposes in age-appropriate contexts during activities such as

- Participating in events that require specific contextual messages (e.g., singing "For He's a Jolly Good Fellow" to a co-worker, singing "Happy Birthday" at a party)
- Cheering (or booing) a favorite sports team on television or in person (e.g., GO CANUCKS!)
- Conversing on the telephone by activating a single message—a nice way for beginning communicators to keep in touch with friends and relatives (e.g., HI, GRANDMA, IT'S CHARLIE. GUESS WHAT? I WENT TO THE ZOO LAST WEEK)
- Greeting (e.g., HI, HOW ARE YOU TODAY?) or saying farewell (e.g., GOOD-BYE, GOOD TO SEE YOU, LET'S GET TOGETHER SOON)
- Making single requests in predictable situations (e.g., I'D LIKE A CHEESEBURGER AND SMALL FRIES, PLEASE)
- Initiating conversations or introducing topics (e.g., SO, HOW WAS YOUR WEEKEND?)
- Making introductions (e.g., HI, MY NAME IS GEORGE. WHAT'S YOURS?)

In some cases, beginning communicators might be able to understand all of the words in such messages, although in other cases, they may participate beyond their level of receptive language understanding.

Jeremiah is a young man with multiple disabilities who communicates primarily with facial expressions and body language. When he uses his talking switch to say the blessing before dinner with his family, he does not understand all of the words, nor did he recognize the PRAY symbol on his switch when he first began to participate in this activity. However, Jeremiah smiles broadly when it is time for him to hit his switch, and he appears to enjoy participating in this routine. As he led his family in the blessing every evening, he learned basic concepts such as cause and effect (hit the switch and your whole family talks!); and, over time and with repeated use, he also came to recognize the PRAY symbol as representing this activity.

A more advanced type of talking switch device is capable of multiple recorded messages in a fixed sequence. The messages are played one at a time by successive switch activations. This type of device might enable a person to (for example)

- Tell his or her half of a knock-knock joke, waiting between each switch hit for the partner to take a turn
- Recite a series of scripted lines in a class play
- Dictate a series of words in a spelling test to the rest of the class, one at a time
- Engage in simple, predictable conversations that involve turn taking
- Participate in singing predictable songs with repeated lines (e.g., "Old MacDonald had a horse…a pig…a cow…")

Like single-message talking switches, multiple-message switch devices are only as limited as the opportunities provided to the person communicating with them and the imagination of his or her facilitators!

Many types of talking switches (with both single- and multiple-message capacity) are available from companies such as AbleNet, Inc.; Adaptivation, Inc.; and Enabling Devices.

QUESTIONS

9.1. What is meant by the term *beginning communicator?* To whom does this description refer?

9.2. What three principles are important to nonsymbolic and symbolic interventions for problem behavior?

9.3. What are predictable routines, and why are they important for young children who rely on AAC? Give five examples of how predictable routines can be used to encourage communication at home and at preschool.

9.4. What is person-centered planning, and why is it important? Describe two person-centered planning processes that can be used with people who rely on AAC.

9.5. Why is facilitator training an important part of an AAC intervention? Describe the eight-step facilitator training process proposed by Kent-Walsh and McNaughton (2005).

9.6. How can attention getting and use of accept/reject signals be taught to a beginning communicator, and why are they important targets for instruction?

9.7. What are the components of a scripted routine, and when can this technique be used?

9.8. What are the three components of a gesture dictionary, and what are some of the purposes of this technique?

9.9. What are visual schedules, and how can they be used?

9.10. What are talking switch techniques, and how can they be used?

CHAPTER 10

Language Development and Intervention

Challenges, Supports, and Instructional Approaches

> Dig in, get the support of both the school and the social services agencies, get the devices funded, and [then] make us work our little tails off until we master enough language to become competent communicators. (advice to augmentative and alternative communication [AAC] teams from Gus Estrella, a man with complex communication needs [CCN], in Estrella, 2000)

Gus Estrella reminds us that successful use of AAC requires more than symbol displays, selection techniques, and voice output. These are some of the tools of AAC, to be sure—but they are not at the heart of the matter, any more than a piano is at the heart of Ludwig van Beethoven's reputation as a master pianist! Once AAC tools are in place, it is a person's ability to use language interactively that ultimately leads to communicative competence. In this chapter, we summarize what we know about language development in people with CCN and how to support language learning and development in general. In Chapter 11, we continue this discussion with descriptions of specific strategies for supporting communicative competence across language domains.

LANGUAGE DEVELOPMENT IN PEOPLE WHO RELY ON AUGMENTATIVE AND ALTERNATIVE COMMUNICATION

Language is what allows us to talk, read, write, understand what others say, and learn about the world. When we have language, we can combine words in unique ways to describe our perceptions, thoughts, and experiences using spoken, pictorial, or written phrases and sentences. Regardless of the cultural, cognitive, social, and other factors that influence language development, all languages are composed of five domains: phonology, semantics, syntax, morphology, and pragmatics. Because

255

phonology relates primarily to the ability to read, spell, and write, we discuss this important domain in the context of literacy intervention for people who rely on AAC in Chapter 12. Brief summaries of current knowledge about the challenges faced by people with CCN in each of the other four language domains are provided in the sections that follow.

Semantics

Semantics refers to understanding words and how they relate to one another. For example, a school-age child with intact semantic knowledge knows that the words *pin*, *pan*, and *pen* refer to three different objects and can discriminate among them. People with CCN face a unique set of challenges in acquiring semantic knowledge because their input language (i.e., the language they hear from others) is usually speech but their output language (i.e., the language they use to communicate to others) is some type of symbol. Thus, they need to learn not only the meanings of the spoken words they hear but also the meanings of the related symbols they use. This asymmetry between input and output creates a number of instructional and learning challenges (see Smith & Grove, 2003), as follows:

- The landmark work of Hart and Risley (1995, 1999) clearly indicates that children who are talked to more by adults, especially in the context of mutual or parallel activities that are social or playful rather than goal directed, develop larger vocabularies. However, adults tend to talk less to young children with CCN than to young, typically developing children, in part because children with CCN are less able to respond (Blockberger & Sutton, 2003).

- Often, individuals with CCN do not select the lexicon (i.e., the corpus of words from which a specific word can be selected) for their AAC displays; rather, they rely on facilitators to do so for them. Hence, an individual's external lexicon (i.e., the words on his or her communication display) may not reflect his or her internal lexicon (i.e., the words in his or her head; Blockberger & Sutton, 2003; Nelson, 1992; Smith & Grove, 1999, 2003; Sutton, 1999).

- As they communicate with symbols on their communication displays, people with CCN rarely receive symbol feedback from their partners, particularly if they overextend words. For example, if a child with CCN uses the symbol cow to refer to a dog, a facilitator might tell her the correct word verbally *(No, that's not a cow, that's a dog)* but not show her the correct symbol on her communication display, even if it is there (Smith & Grove, 2003; von Tetzchner & Martinsen, 1992).

- There may be less "convergence" between semantic and conceptual organization in some graphic symbol sets and systems (e.g., Blissymbolics) than in others (e.g., Picture Communication Symbols; Schlosser, 1999a, 1999b).

Underlying these concerns is the question of how individuals with CCN learn new symbol–referent relationships. Until 12 months of age, most typically developing children learn to comprehend new words at a fairly slow rate as the adults around them label and repeat words during interactions in familiar routines (Nelson, 1988). Then, between 12 and 15 months of age, most children begin to acquire new vocabulary words much more rapidly (i.e., after one or two exposures), a phenomenon referred to as "fast mapping" (Carey & Bartlett, 1978; Dollaghan, 1987). The ability to fast map accounts, at least in part, for the rapid growth in the vocabulary size of young children; by one estimate, they learn an average of nine new words each day and know at least 14,000 words by the time they are 6 years old (Carey, 1978)!

Can children with CCN fast map? Several experimental and intervention studies suggest that the answer is yes (Drager et al., 2006; Romski et al., 2010; Romski, Sevcik, Robinson, Mervis, & Bertrand, 1996; Wilkinson & Albert, 2001; Wilkinson & Green, 1998). For example, a study by Romski et al. (1996) involved 13 youth with little or no functional speech and moderate-to-severe intellectual disabilities. Each participant received four exposure trials to each of four novel objects labeled with both nonsense words and abstract symbols (i.e., lexigrams) on a speech-generating device (SGD). After four exposures, researchers tested participants' ability to both comprehend and produce the lexigrams immediately as well as 1 day and 15 days later. Seven of the participants fast mapped the symbol meanings and retained their comprehension of some of the words for up to 15 days, and generalized this knowledge from comprehension to production. The finding that at least some individuals with CCN are able to fast map has implications for how AAC teams teach new vocabulary symbols and build semantic knowledge. Specific instructional techniques in this regard will be discussed in Chapter 11.

Syntax

Syntax refers to the rules for putting words into sentences; for example, if a person understands English syntax, then he or she would know that *I like this cake* is preferable to *Like I this cake,* even though listeners might comprehend both. We know quite a bit about the syntactic difficulties of individuals who communicate with graphic symbols from two reviews (Binger & Light, 2008; Blockberger & Sutton, 2003). The most commonly reported syntactic characteristics of people with CCN include

- A predominance of one- or two-word messages, both in spontaneous and elicited conditions (e.g., Nakamura, Newell, Alm, & Waller, 1998; Soto, 1999; Sutton & Morford, 1998; Udwin & Yule, 1990)
- A prevalence of simple clauses (e.g., *I like cake*), with limited use of complex structures such as questions, commands, negatives, and auxiliary verbs (Soto & Toro-Zambrana, 1995; van Balkom & Welle Donker-Gimbrère, 1996)
- Use of constituent word orders that differ from the individual's spoken language background, regardless of the AAC modality used (e.g., Smith & Grove, 1999, 2003; Trudeau, Morford, & Sutton, 2010). For example, for the sentence *The dog eats the bone,* a person with CCN who uses symbols might produce a sentence in subject-object-verb order (e.g., DOG BONE EAT), verb-subject-object order (EAT DOG BONE), or even object-verb-subject order (BONE EAT DOG). Even individuals with more advanced language skills often have difficulty with word order in compound sentences (e.g., producing GIRL BLUE BOX HELP BOY IN SHOPPING CART for *The girl helps the boy putting the blue box in the shopping cart;* Smith & Grove, 2003)
- Omission of words that appear frequently in the individual's language, such as verbs and articles, even when these words are available on the communication display (Soto & Toro-Zambrana, 1995; van Balkom & Welle Donker-Gimbrère, 1996)
- Extensive use of multimodal combinations (e.g., gesture + symbol, vocalization + symbol), word overextensions (e.g., DOG instead of COW), and other metalinguistic strategies that compensate for a lack of needed symbols (Light, Collier, & Parnes, 1985c; Mirenda & Bopp, 2003; Sutton, Soto, & Blockberger, 2002)

Why do these unusual syntactic patterns frequently occur in the messages of people who rely on AAC? The earliest explanation, known as the deficit hypothesis, suggested that most individuals with CCN have underlying language deficits, a notion that has since been disproved (see Kraat, 1985, for the most notable review of evidence against this assumption). In its place, language researchers have proposed the modality-specific hypothesis, which suggests that the unusual graphic symbol utterances produced by people with CCN reflect the asymmetry between what they hear (i.e., spoken language) and how they communicate, and are a function of the differences between the two (Sutton et al., 2002; Smith & Grove, 2003). For example, the graphic symbol message ME SISTER GO ORANGE BOY FISH MOVIE FUNNY might be produced to mean "My sister and I went to see the movie *Finding Nemo* [a movie about an orange male fish] and we thought it was funny" even by someone who has intact language ability. This might occur because the symbols needed to construct a grammatically correct message (e.g., MY, AND, I, WENT, THOUGHT, WAS) are not included on the communication display, and the specific movie title, *Finding Nemo*, is also unavailable. If this is the case, constructing a telegraphic message using the symbols that *are* on the display and describing the movie hero as ORANGE BOY FISH, with the expectation that the communication partner will either know the required background information or ask clarifying questions to assist with co-construction, is a good compensatory strategy. It is probable that both display-related and language practice–related factors contribute to the differences seen in the language patterns of people with CCN, although additional research is needed to develop a comprehensive theoretical model of language development that can be tested systematically.

Morphology

The rules for building and changing words are referred to as morphology. For example, knowing that *pin* refers to one object and *pins* refers to more than one object or that *walk* describes a current action whereas *walked* describes a past action indicates an individual's morphological awareness. Most studies have demonstrated that individuals with CCN experience marked difficulties with both receptive and expressive morphology (e.g., Bruno & Trembath, 2006; Kelford Smith, Thurston, Light, Parnes, & O'Keefe, 1989; Redmond & Johnston, 2001; Sutton & Gallagher, 1993). A 2003 study by Blockberger and Johnston illustrates this difficulty. The researchers assessed mastery of three grammatical morphemes (possessive -'s, third-person singular -s, and past tense -ed) in children with CCN (5–17 years of age) and in children who were typically developing. The children were matched by Peabody Picture Vocabulary Test–Revised (Dunn & Dunn, 1981) scores and had comparable chronological ages. The researchers found that participants with CCN of all ages scored significantly lower on three tasks that probed acquisition of morphological understanding and use: a comprehension task involving picture selection, a grammaticality judgment task, and a structured written word (fill-in-the-blank) task. It is not clear why people with CCN regularly experience problems with morphology, but at least four explanations are possible:

- The symbols needed to indicate (for example) plural, possessive, or past tense may not be available on a communication display, so the person using that display is unable to practice using them (Blockberger & Johnston, 2003).
- Individuals with CCN omit morphemes because they choose efficiency over accuracy as a strategy for enhancing the speed of communication (Blockberger & Sutton, 2003; Light, 1989a; Mirenda & Bopp, 2003).

- Individuals with CCN are not taught the morphological rules that apply to various situations (Blockberger & Johnston, 2003; Sutton & Gallagher, 1993).

- The AAC modality itself influences output and precludes the need for conventional English morphemes (Smith, 1996; Smith & Grove, 1999, 2003). Smith (1996) provided an example by referring to the Picture Communication Symbol (PCS) symbol for SIT, which is a line drawing of a person sitting on a chair. When asked to symbolize the sentence *The girl is sitting on the chair,* one of Smith's research participants simply pointed to the symbol for SIT, rather than combining the symbols FOR GIRL, SIT, ON, and CHAIR. In fact, this participant was correct— the form of the symbol for SIT itself precludes the need for constructing the utterance word by word! It is likely that similar occurrences contribute to other difficulties with grammatical morphology, but research to examine this issue is still in its infancy.

"An American movie titled *Field of Dreams* was about a man building a baseball field in his cornfield. A voice told him, 'If you build it, they will come.' The same voice is speaking for people using augmentative and alternative communication. It says, 'If you build language, effective and independent communication will come'" (Van Tatenhove, 1996).

Pragmatics

Difficulties with semantics, syntax, and morphology notwithstanding, there is no doubt that, in the end, the most important aspect of language development for people who rely on AAC is related to pragmatics. Pragmatics refers to the communicative functions of language and the rules for using language contextually for social purposes (Iacono, 2003). Communicative functions include, for example, the ability to request, comment, repair/clarify, reject/protest, and solicit information by asking questions.

Numerous studies from around the world have indicated that the range and general patterns of communicative functions produced by individuals with CCN tend to be restricted primarily to responses and requests, regardless of the context (e.g., Basil, 1992; Carter, 2003a, 2003b; Iacono, 2003; Light, Collier, & Parnes, 1985b; Sutton, 1999; Udwin & Yule, 1991; von Tetzchner & Martinsen, 1992). During interactions with speaking partners, many people who rely on AAC tend to occupy a respondent role; they seldom initiate conversations, respond primarily when obligated to do so, and produce utterances that are only as long as they need to be to get a message across (Calculator & Dollaghan, 1982; Collins, 1996; Light, Collier, & Parnes, 1985b; von Tetzchner & Martinsen, 1992). Naturally speaking partners, on the other hand, tend to control conversational topics, ask many questions (especially those requiring yes/no and single-word responses), and spend a significant amount of time repairing and/or averting breakdowns during conversations with people with CCN (Basil, 1992; Iacono, 2003; Light et al., 1985b). However, Müller and Soto (2002) found that when two people who rely on AAC interact with one another, their conversations appear to be much more "equal" than when they interact with natural speakers. Thus, it may be that the phenomenon of conversational asymmetry is at least in part a function of an imbalance in conversational "power" rather than a function of pragmatic difficulties per se in people who rely on AAC.

Summary

Many individuals who rely on AAC are able to use symbols and/or writing to communicate eloquently about their life experiences; for example, in 2000, people with CCN from around the world shared their poems, stories, and narratives in a book entitled *Beneath the Surface* (Williams & Krezman, 2000). Clearly, these individuals have mastered the intricacies of language and are able to pass their knowledge on to others. However, many individuals with CCN face both receptive and expressive language difficulties that, at least in part, stem from the fact that their language-learning experiences are very different from those of individuals who can speak. As Nelson so eloquently noted,

> How can [we] assess what words and structures a young child knows if the only words and structures available [to] the child…have been provided by someone else? How can [we] know whether a preliterate child might actually have a variety of words in mind to express a concept or communicate a feeling, but cannot because the words are inaccessible for expression?…How can [we] know if a child can generate multiword utterances if the child's computer is preprogrammed with frequently used phrases? (1992, p. 4)

How, indeed? Strategies specifically aimed at language development need to be an integral part of every AAC intervention. In the section that follows, we describe some of the most commonly used and/or promising methods for supporting language development.

"Over the years,…[Adam] has added some of the structure, rules, and intricacies of language. He added these in the same way he adds to his vocabulary: when he wants and needs them to communicate, when he's given the words with which to do them, and when it isn't too much trouble to use them! Come to think of it, that's just about the way my daughter developed her language, and she doesn't use AAC. The only difference between the kids was that my daughter didn't have to wait for someone to give her a way to express those words" (the mother of Adam, a 9-year-old boy who relies on a variety of AAC techniques, in Gregory & McNaughton, 1993, p. 22).

SUPPORTING LANGUAGE LEARNING AND DEVELOPMENT

In Chapter 9, we emphasized the importance of providing meaningful, motivating opportunities throughout the day for beginning communicators to practice using gestures, body language, vocalizations, visual schedules, and talking switches as they begin to communicate. The need for such opportunities is no less important as AAC teams continue to support the development of a range of communicative functions that require symbol use. In this section, we review the most important considerations related to language development and symbolic communication.

Symbols and Language

One of the challenges in representing language for people with CCN who do not (yet) know how to read involves how to "translate" spoken language into a visual form without losing specificity and flexibility. There is wide variability in the extent to which existing AAC symbol sets (see Chapter 3) enable individuals to communicate precisely, using closely related but linguistically distinct words and concepts such as *eat, ate,* and *eating; mouse* and *mice; small* and *smaller;* and *boy, boys, boy's,* and *boys'.*

Do certain symbol approaches facilitate language development (or certain aspects thereof) more than others?

The answer depends on whom you ask! For example, proponents of Blissymbolics have stated for many years that this symbol system allows people who use it to learn about the rules of morphology, syntax, and message construction:

> Blissymbolics is a language with a wide vocabulary, a grammar which allows for sentences in past, future and present tenses, and markers for possession, plurality, questions and commands....It is a totally generative system with each new symbol interpretable by the receiver through analysing the component parts. (Blissymbolics Communication International, 2012)

Similarly, manually coded language systems such as Signing Exact English use modified and supplemented American Sign Language signs to give a clear and complete visual presentation of spoken English. Many other symbol sets, such as Picture Communication Symbols (DynaVox Mayer-Johnson), incorporate specific symbols that can be used to indicate, for example, past and future tense (e.g., *ran, will run*) or relative size (e.g., *big, bigger, biggest*) but not plural (e.g., *cat, cats*) or possessive forms (e.g., *cat, cat's*).

In the end, it is clear that some individuals who rely on AAC symbols—regardless of the type—develop complex, generative language whereas others do not (see Goldstein, 2002; Mirenda, 2003b; Soto & Toro-Zambrana, 1995; Williams & Krezman, 2000). However, little empirical evidence is available to suggest that any one type of symbol is more facilitative of language development than any other. What we *do* know is that many commercially available AAC symbols are not immediately transparent to young children (Mirenda & Locke, 1989; Light, Worah, et al., 2007) and appear to represent early language concepts in ways that are quite different from how children themselves represent them (Lund, Millar, Herman, Hinds, & Light, 1998; Light, Worah, et al., 2007). Thus, perhaps the best advice for now is to find ways to integrate manual signs, photographs, pictures, digital images, and formal symbol sets into AAC systems that are highly motivating, interactive, individualized, and designed to support both language and literacy development over time (Pierce, Steelman, Koppenhaver, & Yoder, 1993).

Organizational Strategies

When an individual uses graphic symbols on an AAC display, those symbols must be organized to promote maximally efficient and effective communication. This is particularly crucial when an individual has a large number of symbols in his or her system. Organizational strategies that fall into two main categories—grid displays and visual scene displays—are commonly used. On a grid display, individual symbols, words, and/or phrases are arranged in a grid pattern according to one of several organizational schemes. In a visual scene display (VSD), events, people, objects, and related actions are inherent components of a contextual scene (Blackstone, 2004). Specific types of grid and scene displays are discussed in the sections that follow, along with what we know about their role in promoting language learning and development.

Semantic-Syntactic Grid Displays

The first type of grid display organizes vocabulary items according to the parts of speech and their relationships within a syntactic framework (Brandenberg &

Vanderheiden, 1988). By mapping the symbols according to spoken word order and/ or usage, this strategy is intended to facilitate language learning, although there is no direct empirical evidence that this actually occurs. A commonly used semantic-syntactic display strategy is the Fitzgerald key or some modification thereof (McDonald & Schultz, 1973). The original form of the Fitzgerald key organized symbols from left to right into categories such as *who* (i.e., nouns), *doing* (i.e., verbs), *modifiers, what, where, when,* and so forth, with frequently used phrases and letters clustered along the top or bottom of the display. Regardless of the categorization strategy used, symbols on semantic-syntactic displays are often color coded by category to allow easier visual access. Figure 10.1 provides an example of a generic semantic-syntactic grid display.

Taxonomic Grid Displays

A second grid display strategy involves grouping symbols according to superordinate categories such as *people, places, feelings, foods, drinks,* and *action words.* Research with typically developing children suggests that they do not find this type of organizational structure useful until sometime between ages 6 and 7 (Fallon, Light, & Achenbach, 2003). Thus, this strategy may not be appropriate for individuals with CCN who are developmentally younger than age 6. The impact of taxonomic grid displays on language learning and development has not been investigated to date.

Activity Grid Displays

Perhaps the most popular grid display strategy involves organizing vocabulary according to event schemes, routines, or activities; some researchers refer to these as *schematic grid layouts* (e.g., Drager, Light, Speltz, Fallon, & Jeffries, 2003; Fallon et al., 2003). Each display contains vocabulary items that are specific to an activity (e.g., birthday party) or to certain subroutines within an activity (e.g., getting ready for the party, singing the birthday song and eating cake, opening presents, and playing

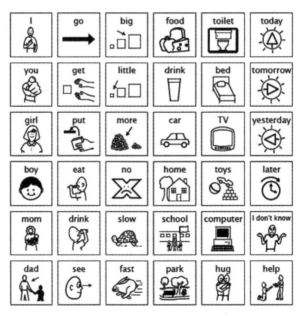

Figure 10.1. Generic semantic-syntactic grid display using a Fitzgerald key. (The Picture Communication Symbols ©1981–2012 by DynaVox Mayer-Johnson LLC. All Rights Reserved Worldwide. Used with permission.)

games; Drager et al., 2003). Each display contains symbols for people, places, objects, feelings, actions, descriptors, prepositions, and other vocabulary items that are relevant to the specific activity or subroutine. Typically, vocabulary items are organized on activity displays in syntactic categories—for example, nouns might be grouped together in one area, verbs might be grouped together in another, and so forth. Thus, activity displays provide a vehicle for participation while promoting language development and complex expressive output (e.g., multiword combinations). Figures 10.2 and 10.3 provide examples of activity displays that a child might use at school to engage in a plant lesson during science class and to play space explorers with friends at recess.

The advantage of this organizational strategy is that facilitators can construct new displays relatively quickly using vocabulary items that are appropriate to a specific activity or event. This enhances the probability that vocabulary words for specific contexts will be available when they are needed, to construct both single- and multiword utterances. Unfortunately, many individuals with CCN do not have access to vocabulary items that they can combine flexibly. Rather, they only have access to single communication boards containing a limited number of symbols that represent nouns for wants and needs (e.g., preferred objects, toys, and food/drink items), plus a few verbs such as EAT, DRINK, and the inevitable TOILET or BATHROOM. Thus, it is not surprising that their language development often lags behind that of their speaking peers. In contrast, multiple activity displays, each of which contain a focused set of symbols, enable facilitators to provide relevant vocabulary items from a variety of semantic categories for specific activities across the day. Activity-specific displays can be used in combination with a generic communication board or supplemental border display containing core vocabulary words that are likely to apply across activities (e.g., LET ME, MORE, GET, NO/DON'T, FINISHED, UH-OH, GOOD). Nonelectronic activity displays can be mounted in specific locations, such as on the wall (e.g., in each room of a home, at the child's height), on an aquatic flotation device at the swimming pool (e.g., a kickboard or an inner tube), or on the dashboard of a car.

Pragmatic Organization Dynamic Display

The Pragmatic Organization Dynamic Display (PODD; Porter, 2007) is a grid display system that combines a number of vocabulary organization strategies to support communication for different functions. For example, activity displays are used for predictable activities, whereas taxonomic category displays are used for less predictable, generative messages. Efficient communication is the overriding factor determining the selection, organization, and placement of vocabulary in PODD communication books. For example, the first pages of a PODD book generally include words and phrases that can be used to express messages that are contingent on an ongoing activity, need to be interpreted in relation to the partner's previous utterance, or need to be said quickly. In addition, PODDs incorporate a number of navigational strategies (e.g., symbols that direct a communication partner to take an action, such as TURN THE PAGE or GO TO [CATEGORY]), pragmatic starters (e.g., I WANT SOMETHING or I'M ASKING A QUESTION), and symbols for conversational repair (e.g., THAT'S NOT WHAT I'M SAYING or I DON'T UNDERSTAND). PODD page sets include predictably associated vocabulary in all sections or categories of a communication book to increase the efficiency of communication with word combinations. Thus, vocabulary words may be repeated in multiple locations throughout a PODD book in order to reduce the number of page turns required to produce a sentence. Although research on the extent to which the PODD system promotes language development is still

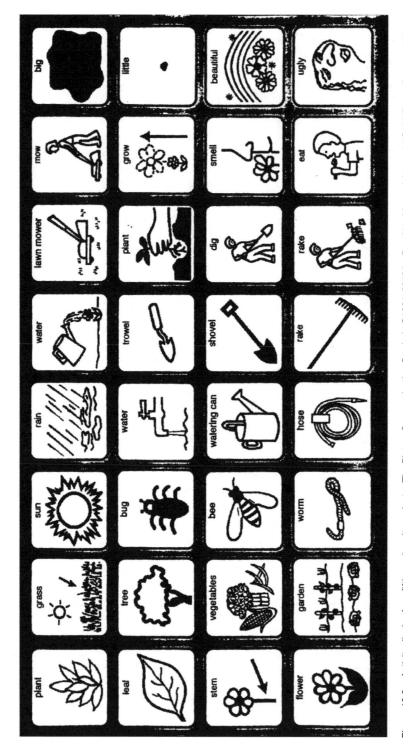

Figure 10.2. Activity display for a fifth-grade unit on plants. (The Picture Communication Symbols ©1981–2012 by DynaVox Mayer-Johnson LLC. All Rights Reserved Worldwide. Used with permission. As previously published in Downing, J. [2005]. *Teaching communication skills to students with severe disabilities* [2nd ed., p. 103]. Baltimore: Paul H. Brookes Publishing Co.)

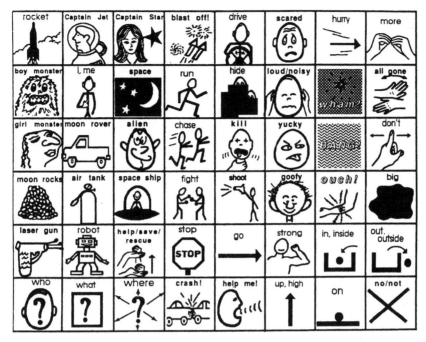

Figure 10.3. An activity display for playing space explorers. (The Picture Communication Symbols ©1981–2012 by DynaVox Mayer-Johnson LLC. All Rights Reserved Worldwide. Used with permission.)

required, its increasing popularity—especially in Australia, New Zealand, and parts of North America—suggest that AAC teams find it to be a powerful organizational strategy for both communication and learning. Figure 10.4 illustrates the taxonomic organization scheme and some of the navigational features of a PODD book.

A complete description of the PODD system and templates for constructing PODD communication displays are available on a CD-ROM entitled *Pragmatic Organization Dynamic Display Communication Books: Direct Access Templates* (Porter, 2007) distributed by DynaVox Mayer-Johnson.

Visual Scene Displays

Visual scene displays (VSDs; Blackstone, 2004; Shane & Weiss-Kapp, 2008) are similar to activity displays in that they contain symbols that are associated with specific activities or routines. However, the vocabulary on a VSD is organized schematically rather than in a grid format. Ideally, a VSD image depicts both the environmental and interactional context of an event that is personally relevant to the person with CCN (Dietz, McKelvey, & Beukelman, 2006). For example, a VSD for the activity of going to the playground might be a photograph of a playground with swings, a slide, a teeter-totter, and a jungle gym (i.e., the environmental context). A number of children might be playing on the equipment (i.e., the interactional context), including the child with CCN him- or herself (providing personal relevance). If the VSD is on an SGD, an associated message is spoken when hidden "hot spots" on the photograph are activated; for example, in Figure 10.5, touching the woman might produce the message THIS IS MY GRANDMA, OPENING HER GIFTS ON MOTHER'S DAY.

Research suggests that VSDs are easier for young, typically developing children (as young as age 2.5 years) to learn and use than either activity grid displays

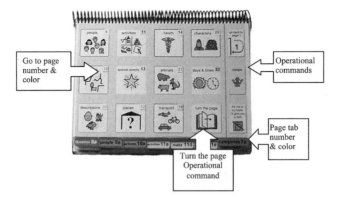

Figure 10.4. Taxonomic organization and navigation strategies in a Pragmatic Organization Dynamic Display (PODD) communication book. (Reprinted with permission from Pragmatic Organization Dynamic Display [PODD] communication books: A promising practice for individuals with autism spectrum disorders, by G. Porter & J. M Cafiero. *Perspectives on Augmentative and Alternative Communication, 18,* 121–129. Copyright 2009 by American Speech-Language-Hearing Association. All rights reserved. The Picture Communication Symbols ©1981–2012 by DynaVox Mayer-Johnson LLC. All Rights Reserved Worldwide. Used with permission.)

or taxonomic grid displays (Drager, Light, et al., 2004; Drager et al., 2003; Fallon et al., 2003). There is also some evidence that young children with developmental disabilities (e.g., autism spectrum disorders) can learn to use VSDs quite rapidly and take more social turns during interactions when they use VSDs compared with grid displays (Drager, Light, & Finke, 2009). VSDs have also been shown to support fluent, appropriate communication between adults with moderate-to-severe aphasia and their communication partners (McKelvey, Dietz, Hux, Weissling, & Beukelman, 2007; Seale, Garrett, & Figley, 2007). Research on the long-term impact of VSDs on language development is still needed.

Hybrid Displays

Finally, symbols can be organized on hybrid displays that incorporate elements of both VSD and grid layouts. For example, the VSD might consist of a photograph of

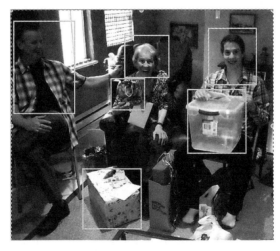

Figure 10.5. Visual scene display on a speech-generating device of a family gathering for Mother's Day. Hot spots (rectangles) around some parts of the photo show areas that speak a related message when activated; hot spots are invisible on the actual display. Photo courtesy of Pat Mirenda.

a child carving a pumpkin with her grandfather on Halloween, with conventional AAC symbols placed around the outside of the display to depict associated messages (see Figure 10.6). As is the case with regular VSDs, research examining the impact of hybrid displays on language development is still required.

VSDs can be incorporated into some SGDs with dynamic screen displays, including those available from DynaVox Mayer-Johnson and Prentke Romich Company. VSD applications are also available for the iPad and iPod touch, including Scene Speak (Good Karma Applications, Inc.) and Scene and Heard (TBox Apps).

Message Units: From Sentences to Morphemes

The size of the message units that are made available to individuals with CCN is another factor that undoubtedly affects language development. Message units can range in length from one symbol that equals one paragraph (e.g., a HAMBURGER symbol, accompanied by the printed message *Hello. I would like a hamburger with tomato and lettuce, no mustard, no ketchup, and extra onions. Thank you*) to one symbol that equals one morpheme marker (e.g., an arrow pointing to the left that indicates past tense, or an arrow pointing to the right that indicates future tense). In between these two extremes are symbols that represent sentences (e.g., a single symbol that means LEAVE ME ALONE), phrases (e.g., a single symbol that means I WANT or I DON'T WANT), and individual words (e.g., HAPPY, SLEEP). The related question that confronts AAC teams is, How does use of different message unit lengths affect both long- and short-term language development?

The short answer is this: We really don't know, because almost no research has examined this issue to date. Thus, decisions regarding the appropriate length

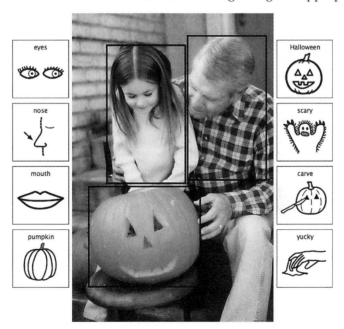

Figure 10.6. Hybrid display on a speech-generating device of a child carving a pumpkin with her grandfather on Halloween. Hot spots (rectangles) around some parts of the photo show areas that speak a related message when activated; hot spots are invisible on the actual display. (The Picture Communication Symbols ©1981–2012 by DynaVox Mayer-Johnson LLC. All Rights Reserved Worldwide. Used with permission.)

of message units are typically made on an individual basis, using a combination of clinical experience and theoretical knowledge derived from typical language development. The fact is that good rationales exist for the selection of both longer (e.g., paragraph- and sentence-length) message units and shorter ones (e.g., phrase-, word-, and morpheme-length units). Longer message units speed up the communication process, which is often both slow and cumbersome, especially for individuals who access their AAC systems through scanning (Blockberger & Sutton, 2003; Paul, 1997). In addition to functionality, longer message units require fewer cognitive/ linguistic resources and thus may be advantageous for individuals who fatigue easily, are minimally motivated to communicate, and/or are just learning AAC techniques (i.e., beginning communicators). Finally, longer message units permit individuals with CCN to produce messages that actually exceed their productive language ability (Light, 1997). For example, Jason, a beginning communicator with Down syndrome, might select a photograph of himself to activate a spoken message on his SGD, MY NAME IS JASON; WHAT'S YOUR NAME?—a message that he would not be able to construct himself using individual symbols.

On the other hand, longer message units may impede communication accuracy and flexibility, as illustrated in the following anecdote:

> Tim vocalized to get his mother's attention, then looked at his mom, looked at his dinner, looked back at his mom, frowned, then selected the line drawing of the *DOG* from his computer-based AAC system (thus retrieving the preprogrammed message *"My dog's name is Skippy"*). After numerous attempts, Tim's mother eventually determined that Tim intended to communicate the intrinsic message "dog," not the extrinsic message produced by the speech synthesizer, and that he was trying to tell her to give his dinner to his dog because he didn't like it. (Light, 1997, p. 65)

For Tim, having only a sentence-level message associated with the symbol DOG actually slowed down his communication and forced his mother to play "20 questions" in order to understand what he really meant. Clearly, the ability to communicate more flexibly is one of the advantages of shorter message units such as words and morpheme markers. Having opportunities to manipulate word- and morpheme-length units is also likely to enhance language development because the ability to break down and analyze message components is directly under the control of the individual who relies on AAC (Blockberger & Sutton, 2003). Hence, correct language structures can be reinforced and expanded (e.g., Child: WANT BALL; Father: *Oh, you want the RED BALL* [points to symbols while saying *red ball*]; *here you are!*), and incorrect structures can be corrected through modeling (e.g., Child: HAT ME [shows hat]; Teacher: *What a nice hat you have! Try saying it this way:* MY HAT [points to symbols while saying *my hat*]). Finally, the provision of shorter message units reduces the need for the individual to have to "translate" the language he or she hears (input modality) into the language he or she is able to use (output modality; Smith & Grove, 1999, 2003).

Given the clear advantages and disadvantages of these contrasting approaches to message unit size, perhaps the best solution at the present time is the compromise suggested by Blockberger and Sutton:

> The possible benefits of more grammatically complete and correct output must be carefully weighed against the cost in terms of the longer time it will take to produce that utterance....The answer may lie in continuing to provide...phrases or sentences for certain functional situations [while] ensuring that the individual has the opportunity and AAC tools to segment and construct the linguistic forms in other situations. (2003, p. 97)

Research is needed to clarify the long-term impact of message length on language development. In the meantime, AAC teams must consider the pros and cons of providing symbols to represent both short and long message units for each individual and context, and then rely on clinical judgment to make decisions that seem optimal.

INSTRUCTIONAL APPROACHES

In order to use symbols effectively, individuals with CCN must learn both their meanings, alone and in combination (receptive language), and how to produce them in communicative contexts (expressive language). Some instructional approaches treat receptive and expressive language as separate entities, whereas others take a more holistic perspective. In the sections that follow, we describe a number of instructional approaches that can be used to support receptive and/or expressive language development in general. In Chapter 11, we provide more focused discussion of how these strategies can be employed with beginning and advanced communicators to teach specific communicative functions and language structures.

Explicit Instruction and Incidental Teaching

Explicit instruction (Reichle & Drager, 2010) is grounded in the traditions of both experimental (e.g., Remington & Clarke, 1993a, 1993b) and applied behavior analysis (e.g., Johnston, Reichle, Feeley, & Jones, 2012). Teaching is conducted in small teaching units (often referred to as "trials") that consist of a stimulus (e.g., the facilitator holds up a cookie and asks *What's this?*), a prompt (e.g., from an array of two photographs, one of a cookie and one of a shoe, the facilitator gestures toward the COOKIE symbol), a correct response by the learner (e.g., he or she points to the COOKIE photo), and a reinforcer (e.g., the facilitator says *Yes, that's a cookie; good for you!* and gives the learner a piece of cookie). Trials are repeated and prompts are faded gradually until the learner can produce the correct response independently.

A number of strategies can be used by facilitators for prompting and error correction in the context of explicit instruction. Prompts are often provided in the form of facilitator modeling (e.g., a facilitator signs FINISHED to prompt a learner to do so, or touches the symbols DOG EAT BONE to prompt production of this multiword utterance). Prompts can also be provided in the form of an expectant facial expression, gesture or point, verbal cue (e.g., *Say "thank you" to the man for helping us*), and/or a physical prompt (e.g., a parent shows a child how to activate his SGD by moving his finger to the symbols HOT DOG YUCKY when he clearly does not like the taste). Similarly, a number of strategies can be used to provide instructional feedback contingent on message construction. A facilitator may use a recast by attending to a learner's message and responding with a more complete or correct form of it. For example, if a child uses an SGD to create the two-symbol utterance BIG CAR, a parent might provide an expansion recast by saying *Yes, that's a big red car* while modeling BIG RED CAR on the SGD. Alternatively, if there is more than one car in sight, the parent might provide a corrective recast by saying *I see two big cars* while modeling BIG CAR + s on the SGD.

Explicit instruction is often combined with incidental teaching (Cowan & Allen, 2007; Hart & Risley, 1982) to teach communication and language skills in the context of everyday activities and routines. Incidental teaching procedures have several elements in common. First, a facilitator arranges the environment to create communication opportunities that will be motivating to the learner. Next, the facilitator provides instruction by using gestures, modeling, verbal cues (often referred to as *mands*), and/or physical prompts to elicit the target communication behavior. For example, during a cooking activity, a facilitator might use a mand-model procedure (Rogers-Warren & Warren, 1980) by asking *What are you doing?* while a learner is making toast. If the learner fails to respond, the facilitator might say *Show me what you are doing* (a mand). If this still fails to elicit a correct response, the facilitator might then shape the learner's hands to produce the signs MAKE TOAST while saying *Make toast.* Regardless of the procedure that is used, the facilitator responds to the desired communicative behavior in a manner that is functionally related to it. For example, if the learner asks for a desired item or activity (e.g., WANT HAT), the facilitator provides it (e.g., *Okay, here's your hat*); but if the learner labels an item or activity (e.g., MAKE TOAST), the facilitator confirms or expands on the utterance (e.g., *Yes, that's right; I bet that toast will taste good*). Table 10.1 summarizes seven incidental teaching procedures that can be employed to teach both aided and unaided AAC symbol use across a range of pragmatic functions (Harris, Doyle, & Haaf, 1996; Iacono, Mirenda, & Beukelman, 1993; Nigam, Schlosser, & Lloyd, 2006; Remington, Watson, & Light, 1990; Romski & Ruder, 1984). Specific applications of explicit instruction and incidental teaching will be provided in detail in Chapter 11.

Explicit instruction may be the most efficient approach for individuals who require a large number of practice trials to learn a basic core of signs or symbols (e.g., Hodges & Schwethelm, 1984; Iacono & Parsons, 1986; Romski, Sevcik, & Pate, 1988). Similarly, if an individual requires corrective feedback on a regular basis during communication interactions, he or she may come to view communication as a negative

Table 10.1. Incidental teaching procedures

Procedure	Description
Mand-model	When a person with complex communication needs (CCN) approaches or is engaged with a preferred item or activity, the facilitator asks a question (e.g., *What do you want?*, *What's that?*). If no response is forthcoming or if an expanded response is preferred, the facilitator models the desired response (Rogers-Warren & Warren, 1980). For example, after a parent points to a doll while a child is playing with it and asks *What's that?*, the parent models the sign DOLL if child does not respond or responds incorrectly.
Expectant time delay	A facilitator asks a question, models a symbol, or places a desired item in view and then provides an extended wait (i.e., pause), accompanied by an expectant facial expression and eye contact (Halle, Baer, & Spradlin, 1981; Kozleski, 1991a). For example, a parent points to a picture in a storybook, asks *Who's that?*, and then waits expectantly to provide an opportunity for the child with CCN to sign or point to a symbol.
Missing/out-of-reach item	An item needed for an activity is missing. For example, during dinner preparation, a parent lays out salad ingredients but "forgets" to provide a bowl, so the child with CCN needs to ask for it (Cipani, 1988).
Incomplete presentation	An initial request is followed by incomplete presentation of the requested item. For example, after asking for toast with jam, an adult with CCN is provided with bread but no jam or butter, and needs to request these items separately (Duker, Kraaykamp, & Visser, 1994).
Interrupted behavior chain	An ongoing activity is interrupted to create a need for requesting. For example, an adult with CCN who is proceeding through a cafeteria line must ask the attendant for certain items before proceeding to the next station (Carter & Grunsell, 2001; Goetz, Gee, & Sailor, 1983).
Wrong-item format	The individual is provided with a wrong item following a request. For example, after asking for a cup of tea, an adult with CCN is provided with a cup of coffee instead, creating the need to use a repair strategy to clarify the original request (Sigafoos & Roberts-Pennell, 1999).

Source: Sigafoos and Mirenda (2002).

experience. In such situations, a facilitator may use explicit instruction to build a repertoire of accurate sign or symbol productions while avoiding repeated errors (Remington, 1994). In most situations, a complementary blend of explicit and incidental teaching techniques is preferred (e.g., Nigam et al., 2006; Reichle & Brown, 1986; Reichle, Rogers, & Barrett, 1984; Reichle, Sigafoos, & Piché, 1989; Sigafoos & Couzens, 1995; Sigafoos & Reichle, 1992; Sigafoos & Roberts-Pennell, 1999).

Conversational Coaching

Hunt, Alwell, and Goetz (1988, 1990, 1991a, 1991b) introduced a strategy that holds promise for teaching individuals to use graphic or SGD-based AAC displays in conversational interactions. This strategy requires a facilitator to provide unobtrusive conversational coaching to the person with CCN and his or her communication partners (e.g., friends, parents, co-workers). In order to do so, a facilitator provides gestural, physical, indirect verbal, and direct verbal prompts (typically, in a least-to-most-directive hierarchy) to teach the basic conversational skills of commenting, asking partner-focused questions, answering questions, and taking nonobligatory turns (e.g., using head nods, smiles, and vocalizations to indicate interest). First, the person with CCN is prompted to initiate a conversation by pointing to a picture, remnant, or symbol, either to ask a question (e.g., DO YOU WATCH DANCING WITH THE STARS?) or make a comment (e.g., I LOVE AMERICAN IDOL). Next, the conversational partner responds to the question or comment, makes one or more additional comments about the topic, and ends his or her turn by asking a question. The facilitator then prompts the person with CCN to answer the question, comment as desired, and ask another question; prompts are faded as quickly as possible over time. A loose form of this cycle (depicted in Figure 10.7) is repeated until the conversation reaches its natural end point. Several studies regarding this strategy have indicated that school-age children and adolescents with developmental disabilities can learn to initiate and maintain augmented conversations independently after several weeks of instruction (Hunt, Alwell, & Goetz, 1988, 1991a, 1991b; Storey & Provost, 1996). Similar strategies have also been used to teach adults with developmental disabilities and CCN to participate in conversational exchanges (Dattilo & Camarata, 1991; O'Keefe & Dattilo, 1992; Spiegel, Benjamin, & Spiegel, 1993).

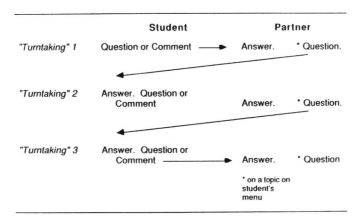

Figure 10.7. Turn-taking cycle for conversational coaching. (From Hunt, P., Alwell, M., & Goetz, L. [1991b]. Interacting with peers through conversation turn taking with a communication book adaptation. *Augmentative and Alternative Communication, 7,* 120; reprinted by permission of Informa Healthcare.)

Coaching strategies can also be taught to family members or peers, with the goal of teaching them to provide AAC instruction during natural social routines. For example, Trottier, Kamp, and Mirenda (2011) taught six typically developing classmates of Ian and Max, two 11-year-old boys with autism, to provide instruction on SGD use during social game routines at school. The classmates required approximately 2 hours of coaching to learn how to provide modeling, gestural, and verbal coaching to Ian and Max, whose spontaneous social communication increased substantially as a result (e.g., *Oh, no!, I'm winning!, You're cheating!, How many do you have?*). Similar results were also reported for three preschoolers with autism who were coached by their peers to use SGDs during play routines (Trembath, Balandin, Togher, & Stancliffe, 2009), and for a 30-year-old woman with moderate intellectual disability who was coached by her mother to use an SGD during social exchanges (Cheslock, Barton-Hulsey, Romksi, & Sevcik, 2008). From studies such as these, it appears that both children and adults can be taught to provide coaching aimed at increasing social communication by people who rely on AAC.

Strategy Instruction

A considerable body of research has demonstrated the effectiveness of instructional strategies developed in conjunction with the strategy instruction model (SIM; Ellis, Deshler, Lenz, Schumaker, & Clark, 1991) for teaching a wide range of skills. Light and Binger (1998) used adapted SIM instruction to teach a variety of social interaction skills to individuals with CCN. AAC strategy instruction consists of eight basic steps:

1. Define the specific goal (i.e., target skill) to be taught.
2. Explain the skill to the person with CCN and why it is important.
3. Demonstrate how to use the skill or have the person observe someone else applying the skill while saying "think-aloud" statements that explain when to use it.
4. Ask the person with CCN or significant others (as appropriate) to think of a situation in which he or she might use the skill.
5. Set up situations for the person with CCN to use the skill, either during natural interactions or during a combination of role playing and actual interactions. Use several different settings, partners, and sets of materials during instruction. Start instruction in situations that are less demanding, and as the individual develops competence, introduce more demanding situations.
6. Provide guided practice for the person to use the target skill in naturally occurring situations or role playing. Always give the person an opportunity to use the skill spontaneously, and prompt only as required using a least-to-most cueing hierarchy (natural cue, expectant pause, general point and pause, and model). Provide feedback on both appropriate use of the skill and problem areas after each instructional session.
7. Evaluate progress regularly to measure the effects of instruction. Practice until the person with CCN uses the skill spontaneously in 80% of opportunities during instructional sessions on at least two consecutive occasions.
8. Conduct probes in novel settings with novel partners to evaluate the generalized effects of instruction, and offer "booster sessions" of role playing and practice, as needed, to facilitate generalization.

Strategy instruction has been used to teach a variety of conversation initiation, maintenance, repair, and termination skills to children and adults who rely on AAC (e.g., Light & Binger, 1998). Elements of this approach have also been used to teach grammar skills (Binger, Maguire-Marshall, & Kent-Walsh, 2011; Lund & Light, 2003) and to train AAC facilitators to support communication (Kent-Walsh & McNaughton, 2005). We discuss specific uses of strategy instruction in Chapter 11.

Language Modeling Techniques

A number of language modeling techniques have been developed for AAC instruction over the years. These include aided language stimulation (ALgS; Elder & Goossens', 1994; Goossens', 1989; Goossens' & Crain, 1986a; Goossens', Crain, & Elder, 1992), the System for Augmenting Language (SAL; Romski & Sevcik, 1992, 1993, 1996), and aided language modeling (ALM; Drager et al., 2006). All three of these techniques are based on the premise that, by observing symbols as they are used by facilitators during motivating activities, an individual "can begin to establish a mental template of how symbols can be combined and recombined generatively to mediate communication during the activity" (Goossens' et al., 1992, p. 101). Because these techniques mimic the way natural speakers learn to comprehend language, they are intended to teach language in a very natural way that reduces the need for more explicit instruction.

Aided Language Stimulation

In aided language stimulation (ALgS), a facilitator "highlights symbols on the user's communication display as he or she interacts and communicates verbally with the user" (Goossens' et al., 1992, p. 101). For example, a facilitator might say, *Let's build a big house*, while pointing to the symbols BUILD, BIG, and HOUSE on an eye-gaze vest or board, SGD, or activity display. Obviously, in order for this type of communication to occur, symbol displays must be readily accessible to the facilitator and must contain the key vocabulary items for activities that occur across the day. Table 10.2 details the steps for selecting vocabulary for ALgS displays, and Figures 10.8 and 10.9 depict examples of ALgS displays that could be used in a preschool setting and a community setting, respectively.

  Specific to ALgS are a variety of instructional techniques that facilitators use to indicate symbols while they are talking; these include 1) index finger pointing, 2) index finger pointing with a small squeaker concealed in the palm of the hand to draw attention to the display, 3) pointing to each symbol with a small flashlight or squeeze light (referred to as shadow light cuing), and 4) using a "helping doll" with an elongated pointer (e.g., a small dowel) taped to one hand of the doll (Goossens', 2010; Goossens' et al., 1992). Regardless of the technique used, the aim is to provide both speech and symbol input during activities throughout the day, in much the same way as total communication is used to combine speech and manual signs.

Because ALgS requires that, as much as possible, communication displays be available for each activity in a person's school and/or home setting, this technique can be very labor intensive. To meet this need, DynaVox Mayer-Johnson offers CD-ROMs of Picture Communication Symbols for more than 100 activities, called *Communication Displays for Engineered Preschool Environments* and *Communication Displays for Engineered Adolescent Environments*. These CD-ROMs replace the previous ALgS books by Goossens', Crain, and Elder (1994) and Elder and Goossens' (1996).

Table 10.2.   Aided language stimulation vocabulary selection

Example: Doll play
1. *Choose* an augmentative and alternative communication (AAC) modality that incorporates pictorial symbols (e.g., eye gaze, a communication board, a speech-generating device).
2. *Delineate* a variety of doll play activity themes (e.g., cooking, doctor, kitchen, baby care).
3. *Delineate* subthemes associated with the activities (e.g., baby care: changing diapers, mealtime, dressing/undressing, grooming, bedtime).
4. *Select* vocabulary to reflect the interactions that can occur within each subtheme (e.g., baby care—changing diapers: *stinky, wet, dry, change, pin, cry, no way, yucky, put on, take off, baby, Mommy, wipe, bottom, powder, diaper, finished*).
5. *Add* vocabulary commonly used across subthemes (e.g., *more, yes, no, help*).
6. *Develop* symbol displays for each subtheme that incorporates vocabulary from Steps 4 and 5, and post in the relevant activity area for easy access (e.g., in the doll play area of the classroom).
7. *Point to* the symbols during verbal interactions with the child with complex communication needs during the activity, and support the child if he or she attempts to use the symbols as one component of a multimodal communication system.

Sources: Goossens' (1989); Goossens' and Crain (1986a, 1986b).

A number of case studies and anecdotal reports have documented the effectiveness of interventions incorporating ALgS (e.g., Basil & Soro-Camats, 1996; Goossens', 1989; Heine, Wilkerson, & Kennedy, 1996) or a version thereof called Natural Aided Language (Cafiero, 1998, 2001). In addition, several research studies have examined the impact of ALgS with preschoolers and school-age children with a range of complex communication needs (Bruno & Trembath, 2006; Dada & Alant, 2009; Harris & Reichle, 2004) and with adults with developmental disabilities (Beck, Stoner, & Dennis, 2009). Results provide evidence that participants can learn to recognize and use new symbols (Harris & Reichle, 2004; Dada & Alant, 2009), compose more syntactically complex aided messages (Bruno & Trembath, 2006), and take more communicative turns during group activities (Beck, Stoner, & Dennis, 2009) as a result of

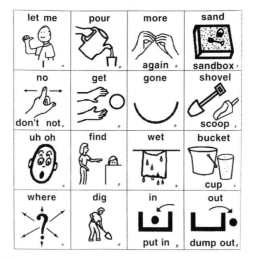

Figure 10.8.   Aided language stimulation display for a young child during a sand play activity. (From Goossens', C., Crain, S., & Elder, P. [1994]. *Communication displays for engineered preschool environments: Books 1 and 2* [p. 128]. Solana Beach, CA: Mayer-Johnson. The Picture Communication Symbols ©1981–2012 by DynaVox Mayer-Johnson LLC. All Rights Reserved Worldwide. Used with permission.)

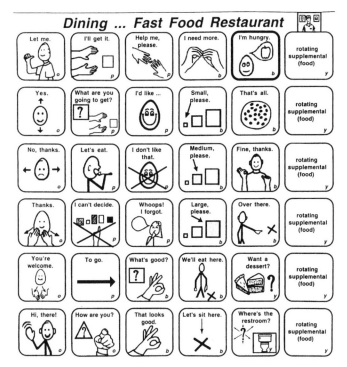

Figure 10.9. Aided language stimulation display for an adolescent or adult in a fast food restaurant. (From Elder, P., & Goossens', C. [1996]. *Communication overlays for engineering training environments: Overlays for adolescents and adults who are moderately/severely developmentally delayed* [p. 195]. Solana Beach, CA: Mayer-Johnson. The Picture Communication Symbols ©1981–2012 by DynaVox Mayer-Johnson LLC. All Rights Reserved Worldwide. Used with permission.)

ALgS instruction. In addition, results of an observational study suggest that parents are able to learn to use basic ALgS techniques with their young children at home during (for example) mealtime, dressing, toileting, and bedtime routines (Jonsson, Kristoffersson, Ferm, & Thunberg, 2011).

System for Augmenting Language

The System for Augmenting Language (SAL) approach (also known as augmented communication input; Romski & Sevcik, 2003) is similar to ALgS, with two notable exceptions: the use of an SGD is a critical component of the intervention (Romski & Sevcik, 1992, 1993, 1996), and SAL instructional techniques are much simpler than the elaborate procedures for elicitation used in ALgS. In SAL, communication displays using graphic symbols with a printed word gloss are constructed for a learner's SGD, and communication partners learn to activate symbols on the device to augment their speech input in naturally occurring communication interactions. For example, a teacher might say, *Johnny, let's go outside and play,* while pointing to the symbols OUT-SIDE and PLAY on the SGD. Thus, Johnny sees the teacher model the use of the symbols at the same time that he hears both the teacher and the SGD say the words. Aside from this, "loosely structured naturalistic communicative experiences [are] provided to encourage, but not require, the children to use symbols when natural communicative opportunities [arise]" (Romski & Sevcik, 1992, p. 119). Because SAL, like ALgS, relies heavily on facilitators' use of the technique on an ongoing basis, a variety of strategies are also included to ensure that partners' perceptions and experiences with the technique remain positive.

In 1996, Romski and Sevcik described the outcomes of a 2-year longitudinal investigation of the use of SAL with 13 ambulatory students with CCN (i.e., 10 or fewer spoken words). All of the students had moderate-to-severe intellectual disabilities, were in primary or secondary school classrooms., and were provided with portable SGDs in inclusive home and school settings. Vocabulary words were represented on the SGDs using arbitrary symbols called lexigrams that were accompanied by their printed English equivalents. Communication partners learned to operate the devices and to use them in accordance with the basic principles of SAL, as described previously.

Over the course of the study, all of the SAL students learned to use the lexigrams, in combination with gestures and vocalizations, to request items, assistance, and information; to make comments; and to answer questions, among other functions. In addition, meaningful and functional symbol combinations spontaneously emerged in the repertoires of 10 of the 13 students (e.g., WANT + JUICE, HOT DOG + GOOD, JUICE + PLEASE; Wilkinson, Romski, & Sevcik, 1994). In addition, some students learned to recognize the printed words displayed on their SGDs, and some also showed increases in intelligible spoken word productions (Romski & Sevcik, 1996). In a 5-year follow-up study, Romski, Sevcik, and Adamson (1999) found that the students continued to convey more conversationally appropriate, clearer (i.e., less ambiguous), and more specific information to an unfamiliar adult partner with their SGDs than without them. Romski, Sevcik, Adamson, and Bakeman (2005) also compared the 13 participants with comparable youth who were able to talk and with youth without either speech or SAL experience. In general, the SAL participants fell in the middle of the range, communicating better than the participants without speech or SAL experience yet not quite as well as the natural speakers. These follow-up studies serve to support the distinct contributions the SAL experience made to the participants' communicative interactions over the long term.

Most recently, a version of SAL was used in a study of 62 toddlers (ages 21–40 months) with a range of developmental disabilities who had fewer than 10 intelligible spoken words (Romski et al., 2010). The children were assigned at random to one of three interventions: augmented communication input (AC-I, similar to SAL), augmented communication output (AC-O), and spoken communication (SC). The children's parents were taught to implement the intervention with their children during play, book reading, and snack routines. Children in the SC group were not provided with SGDs but were encouraged to produce the target spoken words using speech. Children in the AC-O group were provided with SGDs and prompted to use them to communicate, whereas children in the AC-I group were provided with facilitator modeling on SGDs but were not prompted to use the SGDs themselves. Results indicated that children in both the AC-I and AC-O groups made significant gains in the use of target symbols on the SGDs after just 18 sessions of parent-coached intervention, and more children produced the target spoken words in both of the augmented groups than in the SC group. These results provide evidence that language modeling can be used to promote symbol learning in very young children with CCN and that augmented communication does not hinder—and may in fact support—their speech production.

Aided Language Modeling

Aided language modeling (ALM) is the most recent addition to the AAC modeling literature. Similar to other modeling techniques, an ALM facilitator provides models that combine symbols and speech, typically during highly motivating interactive play or story reading activities. In order to do so, the facilitator typically points to a referent in the environment (e.g., a doll), then points to a symbol of the referent (e.g., a picture of a doll or the written word *doll*) while simultaneously saying the related word (e.g., *doll*). Variations of this technique have also been used, depending on the context and the skill being taught. ALM requires fewer facilitator skills than ALgS and, unlike SAL and subsequent versions of it, does not require an SGD (although one can be used).

In the first ALM study, Drager et al. (2006) taught new vocabulary symbols to two preschoolers with autism. Both children demonstrated increased symbol comprehension and production within a short period of time and maintained the gains up to 3 months later. Binger and Light (2007) used a version of ALM to teach two-symbol combinations to five preschoolers with developmental disabilities, some of whom also had suspected childhood apraxia of speech. In this study, a facilitator pointed to two symbols (e.g., FEED + DOLL) while labeling them with speech or SGD output (e.g., *feed doll* or FEED DOLL), and then followed this with a complete spoken sentence (e.g., *It's time to feed the doll!*). Four of the five participants learned to produce a wide range of two-symbol messages following less than 4 hours of instruction and maintained this ability over a 2-month period. Most recently, educational assistants (Binger, Kent-Walsh, Ewing, & Taylor, 2010) and parents (Binger, Kent-Walsh, Berens, Del Campo, & Rivera, 2008; Kent-Walsh, Binger, & Hasham, 2010; Rosa-Lugo & Kent-Walsh, 2008) have been taught to use ALM or a version thereof with preschoolers and school-age children during story reading activities. Target skills in these studies included turn taking, production of novel semantic concepts, and production of multisymbol messages. Results indicate that parents and educational assistants can learn ALM strategies in a short period of time with appropriate instruction (see Kent-Walsh & McNaughton, 2005) and that child participants can acquire new communication and language skills as a result. The use of ALM to teach specific language structures will be described in detail in Chapter 11.

QUESTIONS

10.1. What are three issues or practices that affect semantic knowledge in people with CCN?

10.2. What are four common characteristics related to the use of syntax by people with CCN, and what might account for them?

10.3. What are four explanations for the morphological difficulties that are commonly experienced by people with CCN?

10.4. What are four common vocabulary organizational strategies, and how does each of them appear to affect language learning and ability in people with CCN?

10.5. What are the advantages and disadvantages of short (i.e., word-level) versus long (i.e., phrase- or sentence-level) message units for people with CCN?

10.6. What are explicit instruction and incidental teaching, and how are they related?

10.7. Describe four incidental teaching procedures, and give an example of each.

10.8. What are the main components of the conversational coaching cycle?

10.9. What are the eight steps involved in strategy instruction?

10.10. Describe the three main language modeling techniques, and discuss their similarities and differences.

CHAPTER 11

Instruction to Support Linguistic and Social Competence

No longer can we select communicative target behaviors for both the [augmentative and alternative communication (AAC)] user and partner from a magician's hat without considering the effects of these behaviors on perceptions of the AAC user's communicative competence. (Bedrosian, Hoag, Calculator, & Molineux, 1992, p. 1110)

In 1989, Light proposed a definition of communicative competence for people who rely on AAC. She argued that the development of communicative competence is a complex process that relies on knowledge, judgment, and skills in four domains: operational, linguistic, social, and strategic (Light, 1989b). Operationally, individuals who rely on AAC must learn to apply the necessary motor (Treviranus & Roberts, 2003), cognitive (Rowland & Schweigert, 2003), and visual/auditory skills (Kovach & Kenyon, 2003) needed for operation of their AAC systems, whether the systems involve the use of manual signs, graphic symbols, or speech-generating devices (SGDs). Linguistically, people who rely on AAC need to learn the linguistic code(s) of their AAC systems (e.g., Blissymbols, manual signs) as well as the semantic, morphosyntactic, pragmatic, and other skills required by the language(s) spoken in their homes and social communities (Blockberger & Sutton, 2003; Mineo Mollica, 2003; Romski & Sevcik, 2003; Smith & Grove, 2003). Social competence skills include those needed for functional choice making, requesting, and rejecting as well as those related to pragmatic discourse strategies such as initiating, maintaining, repairing, and terminating conversations (Brady & Halle, 2002; Iacono, 2003; Light, Parsons, & Drager, 2002; Sigafoos & Mirenda, 2002; Sigafoos, O'Reilly, Drasgow, & Reichle, 2002). Social domain skills also include those that relate to interpersonal dynamics, such as knowing how to put partners at ease, actively participate in conversations, and so forth (Light, Arnold, & Clark, 2003). Finally, strategic skills are those that allow people who rely on AAC to "make the best of what they do know and can do" (Light, 1996, p. 9; see also Mirenda & Bopp, 2003). Light's description of these four domains and their importance for people who communicate with AAC led the field in a new direction that resulted, ultimately, in a 2003 book entitled *Communicative Competence for Individuals Who Use AAC: From Research to Practice* (Light, Beukelman, & Reichle, 2003). In this book, AAC researchers and clinicians from around the world described the four components of communicative competence in detail, along with implications for practice.

In this chapter, we build on Light et al.'s (2003) book and on research that has appeared since it was published to discuss specific strategies that have been shown to be effective for teaching many of the skills required for communicative competence. In particular, we focus on skills in the linguistic and social domains, as these comprise the fundamental building blocks of most communicative interactions. We begin with a discussion of strategies aimed at building semantic knowledge that, for people who rely on AAC, requires an understanding of symbol–referent relationships (e.g., that the sign for *happy* or the graphic symbol for *jump* refers to the respective emotion or action). We then proceed to discuss strategies for teaching multiword combinations, grammatical concepts, and the use of morphemes (e.g., *-s, -ing*). Finally, we focus on pragmatics with a discussion of instructional strategies aimed at teaching functional communication skills to beginning communicators (e.g., choice making, requesting, rejecting) as well as skills for conversation and discourse. It is important to note that instruction across these domains and skill areas can (and should) be provided simultaneously, just as occurs with individuals who use speech to communicate. Parents do not teach their young children one language or communication skill at a time—rather, they provide models and supports across a range of skills simultaneously, as should teachers and other facilitators in a person's life. AAC teams need to remember that language and communication skills are intimately interrelated and that it is important to support development across domains in addition to focusing on building specific skills.

SUPPORTING SEMANTIC DEVELOPMENT

As we discuss in Chapter 10, individuals who rely on symbols to communicate face a rather formidable learning challenge. Like their peers who can speak, they must first learn the meanings of the spoken words they hear (i.e., comprehension)—but then, unlike their peers, they must "translate" those words into either unaided or aided symbols in order to use them to communicate (i.e., expression). Two primary approaches—explicit instruction and language modeling (see Chapter 10)—have been used to teach language comprehension and symbol–referent relationships.

Explicit Instruction

An explicit instructional approach to semantic development is based on the principles of stimulus control and the premise that symbol–referent learning is fundamentally a match-to-sample task (Wilkinson & McIlvane, 2002). Thus, to teach symbol comprehension, a facilitator arranges structured teaching trials that require a learner to match symbols to their referents (typically, during initial instruction, the referents are objects). For example, a facilitator might place photographs of a cup and an apple on a table, give the learner a cup that is identical to the one in the photo, and prompt the learner to place the cup with the photo of the cup (Franklin, Mirenda, & Phillips, 1996). Over subsequent trials, prompts are gradually faded and new objects and symbols are introduced systematically, until the learner is able to match identical objects and their symbols without instruction. Once this goal has been achieved with identical objects and symbols, nonidentical matching instruction begins, wherein the learner is taught to match objects with symbols that differ in one or more ways (e.g., a red apple to a green apple symbol; the sign DOG to the spoken word *dog*). Additional explicit instructional techniques (e.g., stimulus fading and stimulus shaping; Reichle & Drager, 2010) can be combined with this basic approach to teach symbol comprehension and production in a structured format (see Wilkinson, 2005; Wilkinson & Albert, 2001; Wilkinson & Green, 1998).

Naturally occurring communicative interactions such as choice-making routines and picture book reading activities can also be used to provide explicit symbol–referent instruction (Rowland & Schweigert, 2000b; Soto & Dukhovny, 2008; Stephenson, 2009b). For example, during a choice-making routine (e.g., snack time), a facilitator might offer a choice of one preferred and one nonpreferred item (e.g., a puzzle and a sock) and ask, *What do you want?* After the learner chooses one of the items (in this case, the puzzle), the facilitator then offers two symbols, one of which corresponds to the item selected (i.e., a picture of the puzzle) and one of which does not (i.e., a picture of a sock) and asks, *Which one?* If the person selects the symbol that represents the previously chosen item (i.e., the picture of the puzzle), he or she receives the item; but if the person selects the incorrect symbol (i.e., the picture of the sock), the person receives neither item. An unsuccessful comprehension check is followed by a second trial in which the facilitator provides an appropriate prompt to elicit a correct response or uses an error correction procedure of some type (Kozleski, 1991b; Sigafoos & Couzens, 1995). Regardless, the person always receives the chosen item following a successful comprehension check. Alternatively, facilitators may implement the reverse version of this procedure, in which the person first selects a symbol representing a desired item, and the facilitator then provides him or her with a corresponding item and a distractor item. Again, a correct response occurs only if the person selects the item represented by the selected symbol.

Language Modeling

The language modeling approach to semantic development is based on research describing how typically developing, speaking children acquire new vocabulary words as they grow and develop. As described in Chapter 10, several variations of language modeling have been described in the AAC literature—all of which involve, at a minimum, a facilitator who 1) points to key graphic symbols while speaking, in the context of a motivating, interactive activity; and 2) provides opportunities for the learner to use the symbols during the activity. For example, consider an interaction between Martha, the facilitator, and George, an adolescent with autism who uses a Picture Communication Symbol (PCS) display. They are baking cookies together. Martha points to symbols (shown here in capital letters) on George's display while talking (spoken words are in italics):

Martha: *Let's get the cookie mix* COOKIE MIX *and the bowl* BOWL. *I'll put the cookie mix* COOKIE MIX *in the bowl* BOWL. [puts the box in the bowl without opening it, thus providing a contextual cue to elicit George's use of the symbol OPEN]

George: [laughs but does not point to OPEN]

Martha: *Uh-oh! I guess I did something wrong here! I wonder what the problem is?* [pauses for 5 seconds to give George time to point to OPEN]

George: [vocalizes agreement that something is wrong but does not point to the symbol]

Martha: [gestures toward the symbols on George's display, and pauses for another 5 seconds]

George: [watches but does not respond]

Martha: *I forgot to do something with the cookie mix* COOKIE MIX *box.* [5-second pause]

George: [still does not point to OPEN]

Martha: [points to OPEN on George's display]

George: OPEN

Martha: *Oh! Right! I need to open* OPEN *the cookie mix* COOKIE MIX *before I put it in the bowl* BOWL*! Thank you, George!* [opens box]

The utility of language modeling to teach symbol–referent relationships was first documented empirically by Romski and Sevcik (1996). Since that time, AAC specialists and/or researchers have provided additional evidence in support of this approach to teach new symbol vocabulary to both preschoolers (Drager et al., 2006; Harris & Reichle, 2004) and school-age children (Dada & Alant, 2009). Others have taught parents and educational assistants to support the acquisition and/or production of semantic concepts via language modeling, with positive results (Kent-Walsh, Binger, & Hasham, 2010; Romski et al., 2010; Rosa-Lugo & Kent-Walsh, 2008). It is important to note that, to date, no studies have compared the relative efficiency and effectiveness of explicit instruction and language modeling approaches for semantic development. As noted in Chapter 10, some authors have suggested that the ability to "fast map" (i.e., acquire new vocabulary words or symbol–referent associations after only a few exposures) is necessary in order for language modeling to be effective, but only a few studies (e.g., Drager et al., 2006; Harris & Reichle, 2004) have evaluated fast mapping skills in the participants. Thus, at this juncture, it seems that explicit instructional and language modeling strategies should be combined in a judicious mixture to support semantic development.

SUPPORTING SYNTACTIC DEVELOPMENT

In 2008, Fey provided a useful description of interventions designed to support syntactic development in children who are able to speak, as follows:

> Put very simply, in languages like English, syntax is the key to determining who did what to whom….In interventions for young speaking children with language impairments, syntax is a consideration from the very outset of intervention (Bloom & Lahey, 1978). For example, even in the single-word stage, before word combinations are targeted, clinicians select potential pivot words (e.g., *more, gimme, all gone, done, not, away, bye bye*) and true relational words (e.g., *push, eat, throw, hot, yucky*) along with commonly used nouns, in anticipation of their later use as building blocks in multi-word constructions. Once 40–60 words are productive in the child's lexicon, the focus switches to multi-word constructions. (p. 44)

In the same article, Fey proceeded to lament the fact that early syntax is often neglected as a focus of intervention for many individuals who rely on AAC. An examination of the AAC literature confirms this observation; with the exception of a few single-subject or case studies (e.g., Harris, Doyle, & Haaf, 1996; Liboiron & Soto, 2006; Remington, Watson, & Light, 1990; Soto, Yu, & Kelso, 2008; Spiegel, Benjamin, & Spiegel, 1993), almost no intervention research has addressed this domain to date. Thus, it is not surprising that many authors have noted differences in syntax use by people who rely on AAC and have offered various explanations to account for these differences (see Chapter 10 and Binger & Light, 2008). Regardless, it is clear that focused instruction related to syntactic development is usually required. Fey provided "five principles underlying grammar interventions for speaking children that could be useful for developing such a program for AAC users" (2008, p. 45). Fey's five principles and the implications thereof are summarized in Table 11.1.

Since 2000, AAC researchers have documented the utility of a number of instructional strategies for teaching syntax/grammar, many of which incorporate Fey's principles. These studies have used both strategy instruction and language modeling, combined with elements of incidental teaching (see Chapter 10), to teach a range of syntactic structures.

Strategy Instruction

Lund and Light (2003) provided evidence that strategy instruction (Light & Binger, 1998; see Chapter 10) can be used to teach both comprehension and production of grammatical constructs. The participants were two adults with cerebral palsy who

Table 11.1. Five principles for syntax/grammar interventions with people who rely on augmentative and alternative communication (AAC)

Principle	Example/implication
1) The basic goal of all grammar interventions should be to help people with complex communication needs (CCN) improve in the use of grammar so they become better communicators in conversation, narration, exposition, and other textual genres in written and oral modalities.	The functionality of grammatical targets is paramount. Consider questions such as "What kinds of meanings does the person produce with single graphic symbols?" and "What kinds of symbol combinations would make the person's messages more complete and more readily interpretable?"
2) The specific goals of grammatical intervention should be based on the person's functional readiness and need for the targeted forms.	Observe the person's performance in communicative contexts and select target goals to teach syntactic constructs that are sometimes used correctly or for which the person demonstrates a need but consistently does not use or use correctly.
3) The social, physical, and linguistic contexts of intervention should be manipulated to provide frequent opportunities for both facilitator models of specific grammatical targets and use (or misuse) of these grammatical targets by the person with CCN.	Arrange the environment (objects, activities) and the linguistic context (i.e., partners' communicative behaviors) to create a real need for the target grammatical constructs. Provide numerous language models of the target construct (via speech + symbols) and wait for the person to respond.
4) Immature AAC utterances should be systematically contrasted with more grammatically complete forms, using sentence recasts.	Recasts are responses to the productions by a person with CCN that maintain the meaning of the person's attempts but add grammatical detail and/or information to complete the meaning (Camarata & Nelson, 2006). Incorrect productions by the person with CCN should be followed with recasts that model the target grammatical construct.
5) Telegraphic models should be avoided and replaced by grammatical models in well-formed phrases and sentences.	Spoken models and recasts should be grammatically correct and complete (e.g., *The doll is crying* rather than *Doll cry*), even when simultaneous symbol models cannot correspond one-to-one with the target grammar (e.g., in this example, because symbols for *the, is,* and/or *-ing* are not available on the communication display).

used SGDs to communicate. The target constructs included the use of adjective phrases (e.g., *blue sweater*), auxiliary inversions (e.g., *Who did Susie see?*), possessive pronouns (e.g., *theirs, his*), and infinitive constructs using *to* (e.g., *I need to buy a new shirt*). The grammatical constructs were selected because the participants' incorrect understanding and use of these forms resulted in frequent communication breakdowns and negative perceptions by others of their communicative competence, which limited their employment options.

For each construct, instruction consisted of three main components: 1) an explanation of the target grammatical rule; 2) practice identifying correct and incorrect forms of the construct in both spoken and written forms (e.g., *He wore his new shoes* versus *He wore his shoes new*); and 3) practice correcting incorrect forms on an SGD, with think-aloud statements provided by the facilitator to model the thought processes required to correct errors (e.g., for the incorrect sentence *He wore his shoes new*, a facilitator might say, "Remember the rule that the adjective always comes before the noun. *New* is the adjective and *shoe* is the noun. Let's fix it."). Both participants acquired the target grammatical constructs and, with one exception, showed evidence of maintenance up to 8 weeks later. The strategy instructional framework is likely to be useful to teach syntactic forms that were not targeted in this study, although additional research is needed to explore this.

Language Modeling

Various language modeling techniques (see Chapter 10) can also be used to support the use of multisymbol utterances by people with complex communication needs (CCN). In their extensive description of the System for Augmenting Language (SAL), Romski and Sevcik (1996) noted that meaningful and functional symbol combinations emerged in the repertoires of 10 of their 13 participants (e.g., WANT +JUICE, HOT DOG + GOOD, JUICE + PLEASE; see also Wilkinson, Romski, & Sevcik, 1994). Similarly, Bruno and Trembath (2006) used aided language stimulation (ALgS; Goossens', Crain, & Elder, 1992) to teach the use of multisymbol combinations to nine children at a summer camp for people with CCN. ALgS was used to model two- and three-symbol messages that included subjects, verbs, prepositions, objects, or places during theater and story writing activities. Syntactic complexity improved for seven of the nine participants after only 5 days of intervention.

Binger and Light (2007) used aided language modeling to teach production of agent + action (e.g., DOG BITE), action + object (e.g., BITE COOKIE), and agent + object (e.g., DOG COOKIE) symbol combinations to five preschoolers with developmental disabilities. In this study, facilitators first provided a two-symbol speech + symbol model during a pretend play activity (e.g., DOG SPILL while saying *dog spill*) and then provided a complete spoken model (e.g., *The dog spilled the tea*). Expectant delays (5-second pauses with an expectant look) were inserted into the activity after each pretend play action, to provide opportunities for the children to produce symbol utterances. Four of the five children learned to produce a variety of multi-symbol utterances after less than 4 hours of instruction. Language modeling can also be combined with incidental teaching techniques such as the mand-model (Iacono, Mirenda, & Beukelman, 1993; Nigam, Schlosser, & Lloyd, 2006) and time delay procedures (Binger, Kent-Walsh, Berens, del Campo, & Rivera, 2008; Binger, Kent-Walsh, Ewing, & Taylor, 2010) to teach multisymbol utterances. In the latter two studies, parents or educational assistants were taught to implement the language modeling intervention.

SUPPORTING THE USE OF GRAMMATICAL MORPHEMES

Morphology refers to the comprehension and use of grammatical markers that alter word meanings in important ways. For example, adding *-ed* to a word changes it from present to past tense (e.g., *work, worked*); adding *-s* changes it from singular to plural (e.g., *boy, boys*); and adding *-'s* changes it from a simple noun to a possessive (e.g., *dog, dog's*). As described in Chapter 10, people who communicate through AAC often omit morphemes from their utterances (e.g., BOY JUMP may used to mean *The boys jump* or even *The boys jumped*), for a variety of reasons.

A few studies have examined the use of language modeling techniques to teach the use of morphemes to people with CCN (see Binger & Light, 2008). Bruno and Trembath (2006), in the AAC camp study described previously, used ALgS to teach the use of the morphemic structure auxiliary verb + main verb + *ing* (e.g., *is fly + -ing*), with some success. More recently, Binger, Maguire-Marshall, and Kent-Walsh (2011) taught morpheme production to three school-age children with cerebral palsy or suspected childhood apraxia of speech who used SGDs. The target morphemes, which were taught during a book reading activity, included *-ing, -'s, -ed, -s* for both plural and third-person singular (e.g., *pig + -s, her + -s*), and auxiliary verb + main verb + *ing* (e.g., *is fly + -ing*). During the intervention, a facilitator read a participant-selected book out loud while providing aided language models that consisted of grammatically complete spoken utterances plus messages produced on an SGD that contained a target morpheme. For example, for a book about a monster, the facilitator read *The monster is eating monster snacks* and then modeled HE IS EAT + -ING. During book reading sessions, if a participant created a message with incomplete or incorrect morphemes, the facilitator provided a recast by modeling a correct utterance on the SGD followed by a complete spoken sentence. Structured probe trials were conducted at the beginning of each session to assess participants' ability to use the target morphemes accurately. Interestingly, results suggested that teaching the morphemes one at a time was not the optimal strategy; all three participants learned to use the target constructs quickly in isolation but none maintained their use when they were probed simultaneously. The results suggest that, although aided language modeling appears to be a viable approach for teaching morpheme use, explicit instructional procedures related to discrimination learning may also be required to teach learners to recognize when each of the markers is required (see Binger, 2008b, for additional discussion of this issue).

SUPPORTING PRAGMATIC LANGUAGE DEVELOPMENT

In the remainder of this chapter, we focus on instructional techniques that can be used to teach pragmatic language use in the forms of functions such as requesting, commenting, rejecting, and engaging in conversations. These and other functions enable people with CCN to get what they want, avoid or escape from what they don't want, and engage in conversations in order to both share information with others and participate in social interactions for their own sake, among other things. At the end of the day, it is for the sake of fulfilling these pragmatic functions of language that the semantic, syntactic, and morphemic skills discussed in this chapter are required. We begin the discussion of pragmatics with strategies to teach basic, functional skills (e.g., choice making and requesting), and we then examine strategies for supporting conversational and other types of interactions. This is the longest section of the chapter because pragmatic language use is the domain in which the majority of AAC intervention research has been focused.

Teaching Choice Making and Requesting

Do you remember the discussion about teaching people to accept and reject in Chapter 9? The development of nonsymbolic behaviors to signal acceptance and rejection shows an implicit awareness of preference. Preference is evident when an individual indicates acceptance and rejection after he or she is offered options *one at a time.* For example, when Maxwell's dad tries to help him put on his red shirt, he squirms around and begins to whine. When his dad gets the message and offers his Vancouver Canucks shirt instead, Maxwell smiles and cooperates with dressing.

In the above example, Maxwell showed that he preferred the Canucks shirt and could communicate his preference with gestures. The development of preferences and a way to communicate them through nonsymbolic means is a necessary first step to choice making. People who don't have preferences find it difficult to make choices—think of the last time you went shopping and couldn't find anything you really liked! You might have bought something anyway, but it was more difficult to make the choice because nothing really caught your eye. The same thing applies to people who are learning to make choices, at least in the beginning of instruction—if they don't have preferences, they will find it hard to make choices. In particular, this applies to older individuals who have spent years in institutional settings in which they were provided with few opportunities to express their preferences or make choices. As these individuals move into the community, they may need to be exposed to many, many new activities, environments, foods, drinks, and people before they begin to develop preferences and communicate them through acceptance and rejection signals. (See Chapter 9 for a discussion of opportunity strategies related to this concern.) Once they have developed such preferences, they can learn to make choices among them or requests for them.

Types of Choice Making and Requesting

You may be wondering how choice making and requesting are related. Choice making occurs when an individual selects a preferred item or activity from two or more options, either independently or when someone else offers them. Thus, choice making is not always self-initiated and does not always occur in the context of a communicative interaction. For example, when Donna goes to the store to buy new shoes, she may use one of two basic strategies to make her choice:

- She can wait until a clerk approaches her to offer help and then tell the clerk what type of shoe she has in mind. She can then wait until the clerk shows her some options *(Which of these do you like?),* try them on, and make her selection from the offered options (an elicited choice with visual supports).

- She can look around the store, try on a few pairs of shoes, and then decide to purchase a specific pair without consulting anyone (a self-initiated, independent choice).

In both of these scenarios, Donna makes a choice by the time she leaves the store with her new shoes. She never, however, makes a *request,* because one of the two essential components of a request interaction does not occur. The first of these is that another person must be inclined to provide mediation or assistance if asked to do so; in Donna's case, the shoe store clerk might have fulfilled this role but is never asked to do so. The second component of requesting is that the individual who attempts to gain access to a specific activity or item (e.g., new shoes) must be unable to do so without the assistance or mediation of another person (Sigafoos & Mirenda, 2002). Because it is possible for Donna to purchase new shoes without asking for help or advice from the clerk, this component is not fulfilled. Requesting always involves a communication interaction between two people, whereas choice making may or may not.

If you recall, one of the principles of intervention within the Participation Model (Figure 5.1) is to match the requirements of the communication system for "today" to the skills that are currently in a learner's repertoire. In this case, this means that the format(s) used for choice making and requesting should be selected on the basis of skills that are currently in a person's repertoire. If this is not done, the result is likely to be incorrect choices or requests and frustration for everyone involved! Table 11.2 summarizes a variety of choice making and requesting formats that are defined by the symbolic, memory, and initiation requirements of the task. The table can be used to select one or more formats that are likely to lead to success for an individual, as well as to emphasize that an individual's ability to make a choice or request in a specific context does not guarantee his or her ability to make a choice or request in other.

Teaching Elicited Choice Making

Elicited choices are initiated by someone *other than* the person who relies on AAC. In this section, we will examine some of the issues involved in teaching elicited choice making.

Providing Choice-Making Opportunities

People who are learning to make elicited choices need frequent, meaningful opportunities to control their environments in this way. Thus, the AAC team's first step in teaching choice making is to identify when, where, and by whom choices can be offered to an individual throughout the day. Some occasions for choice making are obvious: deciding what food to eat or drink, what music to listen to, which television show to watch, and which clothes to wear. Other instances may be less obvious, such as choosing who to sit next to during an activity, how to complete an activity, and the order in which to complete a multicomponent task (e.g., a personal care routine in the morning).

Many choice-making opportunities can be embedded in high-interest, fun activities. For example, Dante is a boy with Down syndrome who loves animals. His mother sets out an array of plastic animals, plastic food, and doll clothes, and then manipulates the animals for Dante while asking him to make choices. She starts by asking, "Which animal wants to eat breakfast?" while holding up a bear and a lion. After Dante gestures toward the bear, she sits it on a toy chair in front of a toy table and asks, "What does he want to eat?" while presenting photographs of cereal and eggs. Dante looks at the EGGS symbol, and his mother says, "He wants eggs? Does he want green eggs or blue eggs?" and holds up symbols representing these two colors. Dante and his mother continue with this pretend play activity until several animals have "eaten" breakfast and "selected" clothes to wear to school—amidst much laughter and silliness! This example serves as a reminder that motivation is one of the key components of successful choice making. In fact, without a motivating context, no one is likely to exert the effort required to make choices that are meaningful!

Age Appropriateness   The options available during choice-making opportunities for beginning communicators should be appropriate for people of the same age who do not have disabilities. With sufficient exposure and encouragement from friends and others, most adolescents and adults with disabilities will acquire sensi-

Table 11.2. Choice making and requesting formats

Format	Example	Choice gesture	Yes/no response	Visual scan of an array	Verbal language comprehension	Symbol knowledge
		Motor, visual, verbal language, and symbol requirement(s)				
Simple choice with visual support	Mary first holds up an empty cup and asks, "Do you want coffee?" Eva either accepts or rejects using a gesture. If yes, she gets coffee; if no, Mary then holds up an empty juice box and asks, "Do you want juice?" Eva either accepts or rejects. Mary continues to hold up one object or symbol at a time until Eva accepts.	X	X			
Simple choice without visual support	Mary first asks, "Do you want coffee?" Eva either accepts or rejects using a gesture. If yes, she gets coffee; if no, Mary then asks, "Do you want juice?" Eva either accepts or rejects. Mary continues to offer one option at a time until Eva accepts.	X	X		X	
Elicited ("offered") choice with visual support	Alfred's teacher puts *both* a red crayon and a blue crayon on the table and asks, "Which one do you want?" Alfred points to or looks at the one he wants.	X		X		
Elicited choice without visual support	Alfred's teacher says, "Do you want a red crayon or a blue crayon?" Alfred points to the symbol BLUE CRAYON on his communication display.	X		X	X	X
Self-initiated choice	Julia looks at the sandwiches available in the cafeteria at her workplace and places the one she wants on her tray.	X		X		
Elicited request	On the playground, Fred's classmate asks, "What do you want to do next?" Fred makes the manual sign SWING.				X	X
Self-initiated request	Josie sees an item that she wants on a high shelf in the store. She approaches a clerk and initiates a request by pointing first to a HELP symbol and then to the item.	X		X		X

tivity to age-appropriate cultural norms. Unfortunately, these individuals may have had limited exposure to age-appropriate experiences, and when presented with such unfamiliar options, they may express no interest or may continue to choose options that are age inappropriate. This presents communication facilitators with a dilemma: Do we offer age-inappropriate options when teaching choice making because these are more motivating for the individual, or do we offer only age-appropriate options, although the person shows little interest in them?

The principle of developing systems for today and tomorrow discussed in Chapter 7 offers a solution to this dilemma. According to this principle, decisions for today should meet immediate communication needs and match current capabilities and constraints identified during assessment. Decisions for tomorrow should be based on projections of future opportunities, needs, constraints, and capabilities as a result of instruction. In terms of the choice-making dilemma, the principle of today and tomorrow suggests that for today, choice-making options should be those that are valued by the individual, regardless of their age appropriateness. Nevertheless, the principle also demands that the facilitator take concurrent steps to expose the individual to a variety of age-appropriate options so that they can be incorporated into the individual's choice-making repertoire for tomorrow. Although the "today" decision may be necessary to provide motivation, it is certainly not an acceptable long-term solution.

For more than a decade, an international team of researchers has investigated the use of microswitches for choice making by individuals with complex, multiple disabilities requiring pervasive supports. For example, in one study, an adolescent who had never before participated in choice making learned to choose first between food and drink options and then between two specific foods or drinks, using a series of microswitches (Singh et al., 2003). In two other studies, nonsymbolic communicators with significant disabilities learned to associate spoken words with specific microswitches to activate preferred leisure media (e.g., music, tape-recorded stories; Lancioni, Singh, O'Reilly, & Oliva, 2003; Lancioni, Singh, O'Reilly, Oliva, Dardanelli, & Pirani, 2003). Results suggested that the ability to make choices and control environmental stimulation is related to increases in various indices of happiness (Lancioni, Singh, et al., 2007). Summaries of this important and innovative work have been provided by Lancioni, Singh, O'Reilly, and Oliva (2005) and Lancioni et al. (2008).

Choice-Making Arrays   When arranging for multiple choice-making opportunities throughout the day, facilitators should select the types of choices that will be available and how many choices to offer at one time. Usually, initial choice arrays utilize two options, progressing gradually to three, four, and so forth, as the individual learns to visually scan and select from more options. Large choice arrays for individuals with physical impairments may require aids such as an eye-gaze board, scanning device, or another system that displays the options so that they are motorically accessible.

With regard to the nature of the choices available, the facilitator has several options for teaching initial choice making. He or she may 1) provide two preferred options (Rowland & Schweigert, 2000a), 2) provide one preferred and one nonpreferred option (DePaepe, Reichle, & O'Neill, 1993; Frost & Bondy, 2002), or 3) use one preferred option and one "nothing" or "distractor" option (Rowland & Schweigert, 2000b). (Note that a fourth option promoted by some in the past, which involves using one preferred and one aversive item, does not appear in our list of acceptable strategies.) No empirical data are available to guide decisions in this area, and reasonable arguments can be made in support of each option (Sigafoos & Mirenda, 2002). Our preference, particularly during initial instruction, is to start out with two preferred or acceptable options because this is the most natural choice format (Rowland & Schweigert, 2000a). If there are indications that the person is having difficulty making choices—for example, if he or she frequently chooses an option and then rejects it, or if he or she always chooses the item on one side of the array—one of the other array formats might help to clarify the task. Other strategies to consider for individuals who seem to find initial choice making difficult include spacing options closer together or farther apart, aligning them vertically rather than horizontally, and holding them out of reach from individuals who are impulsive (Mirenda, 1985).

Choice-Making Items or Symbols   During choice-making opportunities for individuals who are just learning the concept of choice, facilitators may employ real, meaningful items (e.g., drinks, foods, toys) rather than symbols of those items. For example, a facilitator might offer a woman who is learning to make choices both a toothbrush and a washcloth and ask, What should we do first? during a personal care routine. The facilitator can then help her to use whichever object she chooses. There is no correct or incorrect answer during such early choice-making interactions because the person is learning the concept "what you point to/reach for/look at, you get." Even this basic concept may be novel for many individuals, especially those who have not been provided with opportunities to make choices in the past. Facilitators may need to offer such individuals motivating choices many times each day before they begin to understand what choice making is all about.

Symbols can also be used from the outset of instruction to teach elicited choice making within a "no wrong answer" format. For example, Sean's teacher embeds choices while she reads the book *Brown Bear, Brown Bear, What Do You See?* by asking, "What do you think he sees next?" and providing the symbols RED BIRD, YELLOW DUCK, BLUE HORSE, and so forth. It really does not matter whether Sean guesses correctly or not because his teacher can provide supportive feedback in either case (*Look, you were right!* or *No, he didn't see a yellow duck; he saw a blue horse*). The point here is to give Sean choice-making opportunities in the context of a motivating activity, not to assess accuracy.

Darcy is a 23-year-old with cerebral palsy who lived and attended school in a hospital setting for 15 years. She now lives in a group home with four other women. When she moved into the community, she had no formal communication system, although she could communicate her preferences quite well through facial expressions, vocalizations, and body language. Darcy's family wanted her to be able to make choices and communicate her wants and needs with greater clarity. To accomplish this, Darcy's support staff first made decisions about her daily schedule based on her observed preferences, and provided her with real objects in a visual schedule system to represent each of the activities in her day. Through repeated exposure and practice during a 3-month period, she learned to recognize the objects as representing specific activities. Then her support staff began using the object symbols to offer Darcy elicited choices among activities and constructed her daily schedule based on those choices. At the same time, her support staff constructed multiple symbol activity displays and used them to provide Darcy with aided language models (see Chapter 10) at home and in the community. For example, when she went to the community library, her facilitator pointed to key symbols on a library display as they checked out books together (e.g., WAIT, PUT BOOK ON DESK, GIVE CARD, PUT BOOK IN BAG). Within a few months, Darcy was able to make elicited choices using PCS symbols in addition to object symbols.

Instructional Techniques for Choice Making

AAC specialists have a variety of options with regard to choice-making instruction that involves the use of symbols. One approach utilizes facilitator prompts such as verbal cues, gestures, models, and/or physical assistance within an errorless learning paradigm to teach the person to select a symbol from an array; the related item is then provided. Because this approach does not presume that there are "right" and "wrong" choices, it can be used across a wide range of choice-making activities (e.g., Locke & Mirenda, 1988; Sigafoos, Couzens, Roberts, Phillips, & Goodison, 1996). Another approach employs the comprehension check procedure (Rowland & Schweigert, 2000b) that was described previously in this chapter (see "Supporting Semantic Development"). As of the time of publication, there were no empirically validated guidelines regarding the selection of one instructional approach over another. Thus, facilitators should employ whichever approach seems to best fit the skills of the person involved and switch to another approach if the first one is not fruitful within a reasonable amount of time. Regardless of the instructional technique selected to teach elicited choice making, it is always critical for the facilitator to provide natural consequences following a selection.

Natural Consequences As noted previously, beginning communicators need to experience natural consequences in order to learn, even if this means that sometimes they do not get what they want because they were not paying sufficient attention or did not weigh the choice options adequately. A common mistake that facilitators make is to offer the individual two choice options and then to provide corrective input if the individual selects the option that the facilitator presumes or knows to be less preferred. The following scene in a kitchen illustrates this mistake:

Tom: *Do you want milk* [shows milk carton] *or juice* [shows juice container]?

Nan: [looks at and points to milk carton]

Tom: [suspects that Nan does not really want milk] *Really, do you want milk?*

Nan: [looks at and points to juice container]

Tom: *Yes, okay, you want the juice.* [gives juice]

Providing corrective feedback in this way almost certainly ensures that problems will occur later in instruction. Nan will learn that it is not necessary to pay attention or think about her response because Tom will always "make it better" in the end. Instead, it would be preferable for Tom to let the natural consequence of an incorrect choice occur and then offer an opportunity for Nan to try again, as illustrated in the following scene:

Tom: [gives Nan the milk that she chose]

Nan: [pushes the milk away and begins to whine, cry, and scream]

Tom: *Oh, you don't want milk? Okay, we'll try again in a minute.* [removes the milk, pauses for a minute, and presents a new opportunity to choose between milk and juice]

Another common feedback error occurs when a facilitator checks an individual's response for correctness by providing a second or even a third opportunity to make the same choice. The following scene between two friends who enjoy playing Wii games together illustrates this mistake:

Mark: *Do you want to play Super Mario* [shows Super Mario box] *or Zelda* [shows Zelda box]?

Zack: [gestures toward Super Mario box]

Mark: *Okay, let's try it again. Do you want to play Zelda* [shows Zelda box] *or Super Mario* [shows Super Mario box]?

Zack: [assumes he must have misunderstood the first time and gestures toward The Zelda box]

Mark: *You need to start paying attention. Do you want to play Super Mario* [shows Super Mario box] *or Zelda* [shows Zelda box]?

Zack: [does not respond because there seems to be no way to win this game!]

This "massed trial" approach to assessing the accuracy of choice making is inappropriate and almost certainly will confuse the learner because the consequence of a choice is unclear. Instead, a natural consequence should follow each choice-making opportunity so that the individual can gradually learn the effects of his or her actions.

Communication devices such as the SuperTalker and iTalk2 (AbleNet, Inc.), VoicePal (Adaptivation, Inc.), Cheap Talk 4 and Cheap Talk 8 (Enabling Devices), and ChatBox Deluxe (Saltillo Corp.) can be used by people with significant motor impairments for choice making via external switches.

It should be clear from this lengthy discussion that teaching choice making to beginning communicators involves careful planning and decision making. Because the ability to make choices lays the foundation for the ability to make requests, it is important to take the time to teach this skill systematically. Once the skills for choice making are in place, instruction for requesting can commence.

"People say I can't do something and I say, 'Watch me,'—and show them I can do it" (Larry, an adult with CCN, talking about his experience skydiving, in Angell, Stoner, & Fulk, 2010, p. 64).

Teaching Requesting

Requesting is clearly one of the most basic and essential communication skills, and is often taught early in the instructional process. The sections that follow summarize some of the most common techniques that facilitators may use to teach people to make requests. These methods include the generalized requesting approach (Reichle, York, & Sigafoos, 1991) and the Picture Exchange Communication System (PECS; Bondy & Frost, 2001; Frost & Bondy, 2002), as well as a general case approach that can be combined with both of these. Regardless of the instructional approach used, it is important to remember that the issues related to opportunity, age-appropriateness, and other factors discussed in the section on choice making are equally relevant here.

Relationship to Problem Behavior

The ability to make self-initiated requests is a skill that is related both to communication and to the reduction of problem behavior. It is not uncommon for beginning communicators to use socially unacceptable behaviors to initiate requests for desired items or activities (Durand, 1990). Mirenda (1997) and Bopp, Brown, and

Mirenda (2004) found that between one third and one half of published interventions in which AAC techniques were used to reduce problem behaviors were related to inappropriate requesting behaviors. Interventionists taught participants in these interventions to make generic (e.g., WANT, MORE, PLEASE) and/or specific requests for desired items or activities using gestures (Wacker et al., 1990), manual signs (e.g., Day, Horner, & O'Neill, 1994; Drasgow, Halle, & Ostrosky, 1998; Kennedy, Meyer, Knowles, & Shukla, 2000), tangible symbols (e.g., Durand & Kishi, 1987; Gerra, Dorfman, Plaue, Schlackman, & Workman, 1995), photographs or pictographic symbols (e.g., Frea, Arnold, & Vittemberga, 2001; Lalli, Browder, Mace, & Brown, 1993; Peck Peterson, Derby, Harding, Weddle, & Barretto, 2002), an SGD (Durand, 1993), and/or a microswitch and taped message (Steege et al., 1990; Wacker et al., 1990). Clearly, learning some form of self-initiated requesting was important to these beginning communicators.

Teaching Generalized and Explicit Requesting and Use of an Attention-Getting Signal

One of the most well-established instructional approaches for teaching generalized requesting employs a combination of explicit instruction and incidental teaching, as discussed in Chapter 10 (Reichle et al., 1991; Sigafoos & Reichle, 1992). Generalized requesting is accomplished when the individual uses a single symbol (e.g., WANT or PLEASE) to initiate requesting and then makes choices among two or more offered options. Use of a generalized request symbol requires no symbol discrimination skills because only one symbol is used to initiate the request. In order to make a self-initiated generalized request, the individual must also be able to gain the attention of his or her communication partner. Table 11.3 summarizes the instructional steps for teaching generalized requesting and the use of an attention-getting signal. This approach has been demonstrated to be effective with many individuals with developmental disabilities, including those with whom AAC interventions are often unsuccessful (e.g., individuals with Rett syndrome; Sigafoos, Laurie, & Pennell, 1995, 1996).

Picture Exchange Communication System

Some individuals have difficulty learning to make requests in the absence of verbal questions or directives to do so (e.g., *Show me the sign for what you want*). For example, Carter (2003a, 2003b) observed 23 students with severe and multiple disabilities and found that more than two thirds of their communicative interactions were requests, and more than half (57.9%) of the requests were preceded by a teacher question, directive, or physical/gestural prompt. Thus, the rate of students' self-initiated communication was quite low, suggesting the need for instructional strategies designed to encourage spontaneity. The Picture Exchange Communication System (PECS; Frost & Bondy, 2002) was designed with this goal in mind.

Requesting via PECS is taught as the first skill in a person's communicative repertoire because skills such as eye contact, imitation, facial orientation, matching-to-sample, or labeling are not required as prerequisites (Frost & Bondy, 2002). In PECS, learners are taught to *exchange* symbols for desired items rather than point to them on a communication display; the communication partner then provides the requested item or activity. PECS instructional techniques are similar to (and partially derived from) both the verbal prompt-free (Locke & Mirenda, 1988; Mirenda & Datillo, 1987; Mirenda & Santogrossi, 1985; Mirenda & Schuler, 1988) and expectant delay strategies (Kozleski, 1991a).

Table 11.3.   Teaching generalized requesting and use of an attention-getting signal

Phase 1: Assess preferences and teach elicited choice making

1. *Provide* an assortment of potentially reinforcing items (e.g., toys, food, drinks) on a tray of some sort.
2. *Hold the tray* within the individual's reach for 10–20 seconds, and encourage him or her to select an item.
3. *Accept* the individual's reach or point as an indicator of a selection.
4. *Remove* the tray, *provide* the item, and *record* the selected item as data.
5. If no response occurs within 10–20 seconds, remove the tray, wait, and try again.
6. Repeat Steps 1–6 until Steps 3–4 occur three times in a row.
7. Repeat over 3–4 days to determine the individual's preferences and how long each practice session should last.

Phase 2: Teach use of a generic WANT symbol

1. *Place* a WANT symbol (e.g., the Picture Communication Symbol WANT) in front of the individual within reach.
2. *Offer* a tray with various items on it (as in Step 1 above) and ask, "What do you want?"
3. When the individual attempts to reach for a desired item:
    a.   *Note* the item for which he or she was reaching.
    b.   *Move* the tray and its items well out of reach.
    c.   Physically (not verbally) *prompt* the individual to touch the WANT symbol.
4. After the WANT symbol has been touched, *provide* the desired item.
5. Over subsequent trials, gradually *fade* the physical prompt until the individual is consistently and independently touching the WANT symbol in response to the question "What do you want?"
6. Practice Steps 1–5 in a variety of natural contexts with a variety of items (e.g., at breakfast with food items, at the library with books, during a grooming session with self-care items). *Do not* practice in one context only, or the individual will not learn that the WANT symbol can be used anytime and anyplace.

Phase 3: Teach use of an attention-getting signal to initiate requests

1. Be sure the WANT symbol is readily available to the individual.
2. Identify a gestural or aided attention-getting signal that will be taught. Some possibilities include tapping a listener's arm or shoulder (gesture), raising a hand until attended to (gesture), ringing a bell (aided), and activating a call buzzer (aided). If an aided attention-getting signal is selected, be sure it is readily accessible to the individual.
3. Use a physical prompt to teach the individual to use the signal to get a partner's attention.
4. The partner then approaches the individual and repeats Steps 2–6 in Phase 2.
5. Over subsequent trials, fade the prompt used to teach the attention-getting signal until the person can initiate use of it independently.
6. Insure that the attention-getting signal is available to the individual during as much of the day as possible to encourage spontaneous requests.

Sources: Keogh and Reichle (1985); Reichle, York, and Sigafoos (1991).

Instruction in PECS begins after an assessment of potential reinforcers for the person who is learning to communicate. In Phase 1 of PECS instruction, the person learns to pick up a single symbol (e.g., photograph, line drawing) and hand it to a facilitator, who gives the person the associated item (e.g., food, drink, toy). Initially, an assistant to the facilitator provides only physical and gestural cues (i.e., no verbal cues such as *What do you want?* or *Give me the picture*) to prompt the learner to initiate this exchange. Over time, the assistant gradually fades the prompts until the symbol–item exchange is made unassisted. In Phase 2, the assistant gradually moves away so that the person learns to find the symbol, take it to the facilitator from a distance, and exchange it for the desired item with assistance. In Phase 3, the number of symbols available is increased and procedures for teaching symbol discrimination are implemented, using one of the comprehension check procedures described previously. Once the individual has mastered basic requesting, the facilitator then extends the program in Phases 4–6 to construct simple sentences (e.g., I WANT, I SEE, and/or I

HEAR...), respond to the question *What do you want?*, and employ descriptive symbols related to color, size, number, and so forth (see Frost & Bondy, 2002, and Bondy & Frost, 2009, for additional information).

PECS has been shown to be highly successful with regard to the development of functional communication skills in beginning communicators across the age range (including adults). These individuals include those with autism spectrum disorders (Bondy & Frost, 2009), global developmental disabilities (Bock, Stoner, Beck, Hanley, & Prochnow, 2005; Chambers & Rehfeldt, 2003; Rehfeldt & Root, 2005; Stoner et al., 2006), cerebral palsy (Almeida, Piza, & LaMonica, 2005), blindness (Lund & Troha, 2008), and deafness (Okalidou, & Malandraki, 2007). In a summary of research regarding PECS and SGDs, Lancioni, O'Reilly, et al. (2007) noted that, of 173 individuals involved in PECS-related publications, there was substantial progress in all but three cases. In a later review, Preston and Carter noted that, although additional research is needed, "PECS stands as a promising intervention with some empirical support" (2009, p. 1483) for children and adults with developmental disabilities who have little or no speech.

General Case Instruction

Facilitators have relied on general case instruction since the early 1980s to teach functional living skills (Horner, McDonnell, & Bellamy, 1986) and communication skills (Chadsey-Rusch, Drasgow, Reinoehl, Halle, & Collet-Klingenberg, 1993; Chadsey-Rusch & Halle, 1992; Halle & Drasgow, 1995; Reichle & Johnston, 1999) to people with CCN. General case instruction involves analyzing the relevant stimulus and response classes associated with particular tasks or situations and teaching individuals both when to respond and when not to respond under a variety of conditions (Chadsey-Rusch et al., 1993). General case instruction can be used in conjunction with either of the instructional techniques discussed previously for teaching what some authors have referred to as "conditional requesting" (see Reichle & Johnston, 1999; Sigafoos, 1998; Sigafoos & Mirenda, 2002).

> As an example of general case instruction, consider Cay, a young woman with cerebral palsy who uses a wheelchair for mobility and has difficulty with fine motor skills. In order to teach Cay to request assistance by pointing to a generic HELP, PLEASE symbol on her lap tray, her facilitator first identified a number of diverse situations across relevant environments in which she would be likely to require assistance (i.e., positive exemplars). Such situations included, among others, a food preparation activity during which Cay would need assistance to open tightly closed containers, a shopping outing when she would encounter doors that she could not open herself, and a dressing activity in which she would require someone to fasten buttons and snaps on her clothes. Cay's facilitator also identified specific situations in which Cay would not require assistance (i.e., negative exemplars); some of these included opening loosely closed containers during food preparation, entering stores with electronic doors that opened automatically, and putting on clothes with Velcro fasteners. Next, her facilitator conducted a task analysis to identify the steps involved in the task (e.g., recognizing the need for help, gaining a listener's attention, asking for help, and saying thank you) as well as some of the task variations that Cay might encounter at each step. For example, "recognizing the need for help" would require Cay to recognize various types of containers, doors, and clothing items for which she both would and would not require assistance.

Once Cay's facilitator completed these preparatory steps, instruction was conducted across a number of facilitators in order to enhance generalization. All facilitators provided verbal and modeling prompts that they faded quickly to teach Cay to use her HELP, PLEASE symbol in the situations that were identified as positive exemplars and to refrain from doing so when she encountered negative exemplars. Both positive and negative exemplars were included from the outset of instruction. Once Cay acquired the basic skill of asking for help in the contexts identified as positive exemplars, her facilitators arranged opportunities for her to practice this skill in novel (i.e., untrained) settings and situations.

Although the general case technique requires more time and instructional planning than teaching in only one or two restricted contexts, research suggests that it is also more likely to result in spontaneous use and generalization of newly acquired communication skills (see DePaepe et al., 1993, for additional examples of the use of this approach).

Teaching Basic Rejecting

Communicative rejecting is defined as "the use of behavior that works through the mediation of a listener and enables the person to escape from or avoid objects, activities, or social interactions" (Sigafoos, Drasgow, Reichle, O'Reilly, & Tait, 2004, p. 33). Communicative rejecting functions as an escape (i.e., leave-taking) response when it is used to terminate an ongoing event. For example, Olivia screams when the evening news comes on the television and she wants her mother to change the channel. Communicative rejecting functions as an avoidance (i.e., refusal) response when it allows an individual to evade an event that has not yet occurred. For example, when told that it is time to go to school, Yasmeen sits down on the floor in her living room and refuses to get up. As can be seen in both of these examples, rejecting—like requesting—is often expressed through problem behavior.

Relationship to Problem Behavior

Many individuals are highly motivated to escape or avoid undesired items or activities and often use problem behaviors such as aggression, tantrums, and self-injury to do so. Mirenda (1997) and Bopp et al. (2004) found that between one third and one half of studies in which communicative alternatives to problem behaviors were taught involved the escape function. Interventions that have incorporated numerous AAC techniques to teach communicative rejecting, including gestures (Lalli, Casey, & Kates, 1995), a tangible symbol for BREAK (Bird, Dores, Moniz, & Robinson, 1989), manual signs (e.g., Drasgow, Halle, Ostroksy, & Harbers, 1996; Kennedy et al., 2000; Peck et al., 1996), picture symbols (Wacker, Berg, & Harding, 2002; Choi, O'Reilly, Sigafoos, & Lancioni, 2010), a card with the word *break* or *done* printed on it (e.g., Brown et al., 2000; Peck et al., 1996; Peck Peterson et al., 2002), a microswitch with a taped message such as STOP! (Hanley, Iwata, & Thompson, 2001; Steege et al., 1990), and an SGD (Durand, 1993, 1999). There is no doubt that functional communication training to teach communicative rejecting is critically important in almost all situations when a problem behavior is used for the purpose of escape, avoidance, or both.

Teaching Generalized and Explicit Rejecting

Communicative rejecting can be taught in both generic and specific forms using AAC techniques. The generic form involves teaching the individual to indicate NO by gesturing, producing a manual sign, pointing to or giving a picture symbol, activating an SGD, or using other modalities. The advantage of teaching a generalized rejecting behavior is that it can be used in a variety of situations to indicate both escape (i.e., "I don't want to do this anymore") and avoidance (i.e., "I don't want to do this at all!"). The disadvantage is that it might not be easy to interpret exactly what the person is trying to reject or why (Sigafoos et al., 2002). For example, Trina and her classmates are following an obstacle course during physical education class in the school gymnasium. When Trina signs NO while navigating the course, her teacher does not know whether Trina wants to 1) take a short break from the course (escape), 2) refrain from engaging in an upcoming obstacle (avoid), 3) leave the gymnasium altogether for the rest of the class (escape), or 4) escape or avoid in some other way. On the positive side, Trina's signing NO is vastly preferable to her previous rejecting behaviors, which involved loud screaming and having a tantrum.

There are six main steps involved in teaching generalized rejecting (Sigafoos et al., 2004). First, the AAC team identifies nonpreferred items or events and the existing behaviors that are used by the person to escape or avoid those items or events. Second, the team determines the appropriateness of the current rejecting behaviors in the contexts in which they occur. If a behavior is deemed effective and appropriate (e.g., use of a head shake to indicate NO), it can be accepted; but if it is socially unacceptable, inefficient, or difficult to interpret, instruction should be instituted. Third, an acceptable form of communicative rejecting (e.g., a gesture, manual sign, graphic symbol) is selected to suit the individual who requires instruction and the context in which the intervention will occur. The new behavior should be at least as efficient and effective as the current, inappropriate rejecting behavior(s). Fourth, opportunities for rejecting are created across a range of contexts by, for example, providing a nonpreferred item or activity (Duker & Jutten, 1997; Reichle, Rogers, & Barrett, 1984) or providing a wrong item (e.g., Sigafoos & Roberts-Pennell, 1999; Yamamoto & Mochizuki, 1988). Fifth, prompts are provided to elicit the new rejecting response when an opportunity occurs, with the prompts faded gradually over time. Finally, the communicative behavior is reinforced consistently by removing the rejected object or stopping the rejected activity immediately, each time the new rejecting behavior is produced. Once an individual learns a rejecting behavior, it is important for facilitators to honor it even in situations that may not be clear cut, such as when the individual rejects a preferred item because he or she does not wish to have more (e.g., rejecting a third cup of coffee although the first two were accepted; Sigafoos et al., 2002, 2004).

After a new rejecting behavior is well established, systematic modifications and extensions can be made as needed. For example, signals for increasingly longer delays (e.g., *Jeff, do just one more problem and then you can take a break* or *Two more peas and you're done!*) can be inserted between the communicative rejecting behavior and removal of a nonpreferred item or activity (see Tiger, Hanley, & Bruzek, 2008). Similarly, instruction for teaching rejecting may be combined with instruction in other communicative domains, especially when escape or avoidance of specific activities are not in the person's long-term best interests (Sigafoos et al., 2002). For example, even when an individual uses an appropriate communicative form (e.g., a picture symbol) to refuse to take a needed medication or to refuse to go to school, it may be impossible for facilitators to comply. In such cases, use of a visual schedule (Chapter 9) to ensure predictability, clarify the non-negotiability of specific activities, and remind the person about upcoming preferred activities may be helpful. In this regard, Mirenda (2003c) described the successful use of a visual schedule with Alec, a 17-year-old with autism, in which symbols representing required, non-negotiable activities (e.g., taking his medication, attending a scheduled class at school) were marked with a large red dot in the upper left corner to signify "no choice," whereas symbols representing activities over which Alec had some control were marked with a green dot.

Teaching *Yes* and *No*

It should be obvious from the preceding discussions that teaching individuals to respond to yes/no questions—which some authors have referred to as "discriminated rejecting" (Sigafoos et al., 2004, p. 35)—is another skill set that is relevant to most beginning communicators. It is important to note that this seemingly simple task is actually quite complex; for example, consider the following yes/no questions:

- *Do you want to go to the park?* (yes/no requesting/rejecting)
- *Do you like to go to the park?* (yes/no communication of preference)
- *Is this the park?* (yes/no labeling)
- *Did you go to the park yesterday?* (yes/no information sharing)

It should be evident from these examples that the apparently simple act of "teaching yes/no" actually involves teaching an individual how to use both of these words to respond to a wide range of linguistically diverse questions. Sometimes, the result is that the person will receive a preferred item or will engage in a preferred activity—but this is not always the case! In fact, there is no reason to anticipate that individuals who learn to use yes/no appropriately for requesting or rejecting will automatically generalize this usage to answer other types of questions (Sigafoos et al., 2004).

Unfortunately, yes/no instruction has received very little research attention, especially with beginning communicators who rely on AAC. In the few studies that do exist, yes/no has been taught solely in the context of requests for preferred and nonpreferred items or activities. For example, Reichle et al. (1984) used explicit instruction to teach an adolescent to respond to two questions: 1) *What do you want?* when presented with a tray of preferred items and 2) *Want one?* when presented with a tray of nonpreferred items. The adolescent was taught to produce a manual sign for WANT in response to the first question and a manual sign for NO in response to the second. Similarly, Duker and Jutten (1997) used explicit instruction (prompting, fading, and reinforcement) to teach three men with significant disabilities to produce YES or NO gestures. The men were asked, *Do you want this one?* and presented with either highly preferred or nonpreferred items. Although the three men all learned to use YES and NO gestures to answer the question, accurate responding did not generalize to a novel setting without additional instruction. As these two studies indicate, there is a real need for focused research examining exemplary practices for teaching both yes/no for requesting/rejecting and yes/no for other question forms to beginning communicators who rely on AAC.

Clinicians in the United Kingdom have developed a wide range of Talking Mats and related symbols that are designed to support people with CCN to make choices, express their views and opinions about the supports they receive and want, and make decisions about their own care and treatment. Talking Mats is a "dynamic low-tech communication framework that uses…three sets of picture symbols that are presented to the person with [CCN]—Topics being explored, Options relating to each topic, and a Visual Scale to allow participants to indicate their general feeling about each option" (Murphy & Cameron, 2008, p. 233). Talking Mats resources are available to support self-determination by people with CCN and intellectual disabilities, aphasia, and dementia, and to support goal setting and other areas related to personal planning. Information about resource materials, DVDs, and training can be accessed through the Talking Mats web site.

Supporting Communication for Social Interaction

The abilities to make choices, request, reject, answer yes/no questions, and make decisions are all important communicative functions without which daily life would be difficult, if not impossible. But imagine what it would be like if *all* you could communicate about involved these few functions. There would be no joking or teasing, no back-and-forth conversations, no answering or asking questions, no playing games or hanging out with friends—in other words, no ability to participate in the types of social interactions that constitute the majority of what most people communicate about, day in and day out! Individuals with CCN—no matter how basic or how sophisticated their communication abilities may be—also need access to AAC techniques that support social interaction, as well as instruction in how to participate in these interactions successfully. In Chapter 10, we introduced general approaches that can be used to teach social interaction skills, including strategy instruction, conversational coaching, and language modeling. In this chapter, we review techniques for teaching specific skills in this domain.

"I am alone in my thoughts. I am alone among other people. My identity is locked in my mind....The inability to speak, or the inability to communicate one's own words fluently, is the greatest disability a person can have in the social circle of life" (Tony Diamanti, a man with cerebral palsy who uses AAC, in Diamanti, 2000, p. 98).

Introduction Strategies

Most of us introduce ourselves briefly when we meet someone new. Similarly, individuals who communicate through AAC need to have a way to introduce themselves and the skills required to do so. Such introductions usually include three components: 1) basic information about the person, perhaps including some mention of his or her disability; 2) information about the person's means of communication; and 3) information about what the communication partner can do to facilitate the interaction. Light and Binger (1998, p. 104) provided an example of an introduction strategy produced by Maureen, a 44-year-old woman with cerebral palsy, using an SGD:

HI. MY NAME IS MAUREEN KRAMER. I UNDERSTAND WHAT IS SAID TO ME. I USE THIS COMPUTER TO COMMUNICATE; I JUST TYPE IN MY MESSAGE AND THE COMPUTER SPEAKS IT OUT. YOU CAN READ THE SCREEN IF YOU DO NOT UNDERSTAND. PLEASE WAIT PATIENTLY WHILE I AM TYPING ON THE COMPUTER. WHEN I SEND YOU A MESSAGE, TRY TO GUESS WHAT I AM COMMUNICATING. CHECK WITH ME TO SEE IF YOU ARE CORRECT. I NOD MY HEAD TO SAY "YES" AND SHAKE MY HEAD TO SAY "NO." IF YOU DO NOT UNDERSTAND, PLEASE LET ME KNOW. THANKS!

Light, Binger, Dilg, and Livelsberger (1996) reported that use of an introduction strategy positively influenced perceptions of the communicative competence of people with CCN, as rated by 30 adults and 30 adolescents without prior AAC experience and by 30 AAC professionals. In a related study, experimenters successfully used strategy instruction (Chapter 10) to teach the use of introductory strategies to individuals who relied on AAC (ages 12–44 years) with cerebral palsy, autism, acquired brain injury, or developmental disabilities (Light & Binger, 1998). The participants in this study communicated using a variety of AAC techniques that included eye gazing, gestures, some speech, and various SGDs.

Several studies have demonstrated the importance of a brief introductory message, called a *floorholder*, in both face-to face and telephone interactions by people who rely on SGDs. For example, Bedrosian, Hoag, and McCoy (2003) examined sales clerks' reactions to the floorholder PLEASE WAIT WHILE I PREPARE MY MESSAGE that was delivered by a person using an SGD. They found that sales clerks assigned higher ratings of social competence to the person with CCN when a floorholder was used than when it was not. Similarly, Hanson and Sundheimer (2009) examined business owners' reactions to telephone calls made by people who relied on SGDs with and without the floorholder PLEASE WAIT, I'M USING A COMPUTER TO TALK. Overall, they found that 30% of calls that started with a floorholder were completed successfully, compared with 18% that did not; and calls with a floorholder that started as soon as a person answered were almost three times more successful than those in which the floorholder occurred after a 3-second delay. These results emphasize the importance of providing even a brief warning that message construction may take longer than usual when AAC techniques are employed.

Initiation and Topic-Setting Strategies

Initiation and topic-setting strategies allow people who rely on AAC to start and establish topics of conversation. In this section, we discuss initiation and topic-setting approaches that include visual supports, collections, remnants, conversation books, joke cards, and dual communication boards.

Visual Supports   Simple visual supports of various types can be used to help children in particular initiate interactions with peers. For example, two 10- to 12-year-old boys with cerebral palsy and severe intellectual disabilities were provided with communication "badges" that they used to initiate play activities (Jolly, Test, & Spooner, 1993). During free-play time at school, four badges that featured photographs of preferred activities were attached to the boys' lap trays with Velcro. They were taught to pull off a badge and hand it to a classmate in order to initiate a play activity. Similarly, three preschoolers with autism and their peers were each given a colored PCS symbol representing the message CAN I PLAY?, which was glued to a large key-shaped form and laminated (Johnston, Nelson, Evans, & Palazolo, 2003). The symbol could be worn as a necklace or attached to each child's belt loop or pocket. Through explicit instruction (Chapter 10), the children with autism learned to show the symbol to their peers to gain entry to play groups, and they also showed evidence of reduced off-task behavior. Simple visual supports such as badges and initiation cards can also be used to initiate interactions and topics (see Figure 11.1).

Collections   Many individuals of all ages enjoy collecting various types of favorite objects. Even preschoolers may begin to accumulate collections of items such as Pokémon cards, bracelets, toy cars, squirt guns, or stuffed animals. Older individuals may collect stamps, hockey cards, political buttons, or baseball caps—the possibilities are endless! If facilitators display them appropriately, such collections can be used to stimulate interactions between individuals who rely on AAC and their peers across the ability range. For example, a teenager might wear a different message button from his or her collection to school every day, or a teacher might display a child's toy robot collection on a bulletin board at school. Facilitators can also remind

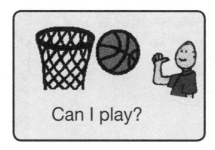

Can I play?

Figure 11.1.   Scott's card for asking to join his friends in play. (The Picture Communication Symbols ©1981–2012 by DynaVox Mayer-Johnson LLC. All Rights Reserved Worldwide. Used with permission. As previously published in Downing, J. [2005]. *Teaching communication skills to students with severe disabilities* [2nd ed., p. 163]. Baltimore: Paul H. Brookes Publishing Co.)

both adults and children to comment on a new addition to the collection and could encourage the child's peers to look at the collection items and talk with the child about them. Items in some collections may also be shared as play or personal materials (e.g., toy cars, jewelry).

Remnants   Remnants or scraps saved from recent activities can provide another way for individuals who are able to use basic symbols to tell people about past events, such as those that occurred during the school day or over the weekend. Remnants can be placed in a small photo album for portability, and can allow a person with CCN to both initiate topics and answer questions such as *What did you do at school/work/home today?* or *What did you do over the weekend?* Typically, each remnant is accompanied by a caption (usually written by a facilitator) that describes each event and asks a related question (e.g., ME AND MY DAD WENT TO FUN LAND FOR MY BIRTHDAY. HAVE YOU EVER BEEN THERE?). Cue cards can also be included in the book to prompt the communication partner to ask additional questions, such as ASK ME WHO I WENT WITH or ASK ME WHAT FUNNY THING HAPPENED THERE.

Remnants have been used successfully to support conversational interactions between preschoolers and their parents (Marvin & Privratsky, 1999) and between individuals with severe and/or global aphasia and their family members (Garrett & Huth, 2002; Ho, Weiss, Garrett, & Lloyd, 2005). In addition, remnants can be very useful for individuals who are able to speak but who have poor articulation that makes their speech difficult to understand, such as those with suspected childhood apraxia of speech (Binger, 2007; Cumley & Swanson, 1999). Once such an individual has narrowed down the topic of conversation by referring to a remnant, his or her communication partner may find it easier to guess the parts of the individual's speech that are difficult to understand.

Conversation Books   Conversation books are collections of remnants, photographs, or drawings that can be used to initiate and maintain conversational topics (Hunt, Alwell, & Goetz, 1990). For example, one page in a communication book might display a picture of the characters in a television program and a written message stating, I LIKE WATCHING THE SIMPSONS ON TV. WHAT DO YOU LIKE TO WATCH? (see Figure 11.2). Several similar pages that introduce different topics can be included in the book, which can be either a simple photo album or one that allows a 10-second voice message to be recorded on each page (i.e., a Talking Photo Album). In the latter case, the person relying on AAC simply pushes a button on each page to speak the message that has been recorded to describe each photo or remnant.

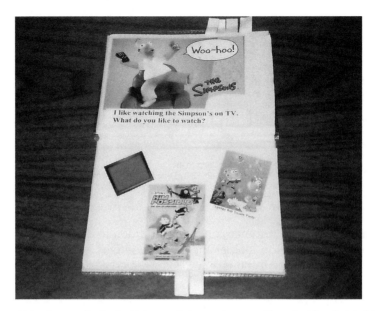

Figure 11.2. Conversation book with images that support conversations about favorite television programs. Photo by Lavada Minor. (From Downing, J. [2005]. *Teaching communication skills to students with severe disabilities* [2nd ed., p. 167]. Baltimore: Paul H. Brookes Publishing Co.; reprinted by permission.)

The Talking Photo Album is available from Augmentative Communication, Inc., in the United States and from Bridges and Special Needs Computers in Canada.

Joke Cards Individuals who have a keen sense of humor may enjoy initiating interactions with simple joke cards. We use small file cards with a riddle written on one side and the answer on the other. For example, one side might have a picture or symbol of a chicken on a road with the caption WHY DID THE CHICKEN CROSS THE ROAD? and on the bottom the direction PLEASE TURN OVER FOR THE ANSWER. The other side would bear a picture of the chicken on the opposite side of the road and the punch line, TO GET TO THE OTHER SIDE. The facilitator can teach the person to approach an appropriate partner and hand him or her card, riddle side up (color coding the correct side might be helpful). Some individuals may use joke cards without really understanding the language of the joke themselves—but who understands that chicken joke anyway? The person is learning how to initiate an interaction and (most important) how to make a friend laugh and share a positive exchange—both valuable communication skills for beginning communicators.

Facilitators can make a slightly more advanced form of the joke card by using either paper-and-pencil or electronic knock-knock jokes. The format of this joke (with which most people in North America are familiar) lends itself readily to simple conversational turn taking. In the paper-and-pencil version, a series of pictures representing the parts of the joke facilitates its telling. For example, Tomas first touches a picture of someone knocking on a door accompanied by a written label such as WANNA HEAR A COOL JOKE??? KNOCK, KNOCK…After his partner Rajinder responds *Who's there?*, Tomas touches the next picture (e.g., a picture of plates and bowls labeled DISHES). Rajinder responds, *Dishes who?*, and Tomas touches the final picture, a photo of himself with the caption DISHES ME. WHO IS YOU? and everyone groans together!

As noted in our discussion of talking switch techniques in Chapter 9, simple communication devices such as the Step-by-Step Communicator (AbleNet, Inc.) or the Chipper (Adaptivation, Inc.) can also be used to tell knock-knock jokes and riddles.

Dual Communication Boards   Another technique for conversational initiation and interaction involves the use of dual communication boards (e.g., Heller, Allgood, Ware, Arnold, & Castelle, 1996; Heller, Ware, Allgood, & Castelle, 1994). The individual using AAC and his or her conversational partner receive identical boards with symbols on them that both people can understand and use appropriately. A facilitator then uses both explicit instructional procedures (e.g., graduated prompting) and conversational coaching to teach the person using AAC to initiate, take turns, ask and answer questions, and so forth. The dual display format has been shown to decrease communication breakdowns by promoting natural turn taking and allowing both partners to interact at natural distances. Some evidence also suggests that communication partners who are not familiar with AAC prefer dual displays to the more typical single-display format (Heller et al., 1994). AAC teams have implemented this technique successfully with individuals who have severe to profound hearing impairments and reduced vision in community-based vocational sites.

"When I was in high school, I was called names and made fun of. And all I had was a letter board to communicate with. So you think you don't have any friends at school? Do you ask other students questions about themselves, about the homework assignments, and school activities? Sometimes you need to focus on them first before they will focus on you" (Randy Kitch, a disability rights activist who relies on AAC, in Light, Arnold, & Clark, 2003, p. 376).

Partner-Focused Questions

It might seem obvious that the ability to ask people to talk about themselves is fundamental to successful social interactions. Unfortunately, AAC instruction often focuses primarily on teaching people to make requests, answer questions, and make comments, but not on teaching them to ask questions about their conversational partners' thoughts, feelings, and experiences (Blackstone & Wilkins, 2009; Light, Arnold, & Clark, 2003). Many individuals require specific instruction to teach the use of partner-focused questions such *How was your weekend?*, *What do you think?*, *What's up?*, and *How do you feel about that?* Light, Corbett, Gullapalli, and Lepowski (1995) found that the use of such questions was positively related to perceptions of the communicative competence of people with CCN by observers both with and without prior AAC experience. In a related study, Light, Binger, Agate, and Ramsay (1999) used strategy instruction to teach the generalized use of partner-focused questions to individuals who relied on AAC and who ranged in age from 10 to 44 years. The study included individuals with cerebral palsy, intellectual disability, or acquired brain injury who used various combinations of eye gazing, speech, gestures, line drawings, and SGDs.

A specific form of a partner-focused question is the response-recode (R-R) strategy (Farrier, Yorkston, Marriner, & Beukelman, 1985). When a person responds to a question and then asks a related question in return (e.g., *My favorite coffee drink is cappuccino; what's yours?*), he or she has used the R-R form. O'Keefe and Dattilo (1992) taught the R-R strategy to three adults with developmental disabilities who used AAC techniques in conversations about preferred leisure activities. Two participants used communication boards, and one used an SGD; in addition, all three used gestures, facial expressions, and a few spoken words. During instruction, a facilitator initiated a topic by asking a question and then provided the participant with explicit instruction to elicit the R-R form. All three individuals learned to produce generalized R-R forms that were maintained over time. Family members and caregivers reported lasting changes in the participants' conversational repertoires and agreed that the R-R skill was "fundamental to true conversational involvement" (O'Keefe & Dattilo, 1992, p. 231).

Nonobligatory Turns and Comments

Nonobligatory turns follow a partner's comment or statement and include interjections such as *Cool, No way, Yeah,* and *Uh-huh,* as well as more substantive comments on the conversational topic. These social interjections place few linguistic demands on the person who relies on AAC but still provide important social feedback to let a communication partner know that the person with CCN is attending to and interested in the interaction. Light, Binger, Bailey, and Millar (1997) found that the ability to take nonobligatory turns was related to positive perceptions of the communicative competence of people with CCN. They taught this skill to individuals (4–21 years of age) with developmental disabilities, intellectual disabilities, cerebral palsy, or autism. The participants' communication systems consisted of speech, gestures, communication boards with line drawings and/or printed words, manual signs, and assorted SGDs. Following strategy instruction, five of six individuals in this study were able to take nonobligatory turns in conversations with new people in new settings.

In a related study, Buzolich, King, and Baroody (1991) reported the successful use of explicit instruction that utilized graduated prompting plus time delay (see Chapter 10) to teach commenting to three students who relied on SGDs. The comments consisted of phrases such as THIS IS FUN, SOUNDS GOOD, YUCK!, and I DIDN'T LIKE IT. The students were provided with instruction during a regular communication group that occurred daily in their classroom. All three students learned to produce the comments appropriately using a range of SGDs, and two students generalized this ability to novel contexts. Commenting can also be supported by providing appropriate symbols and instruction to individuals who use low-tech communication displays and books (see Figure 11.3).

Regulatory Phrases

Regulatory phrases allow individuals who rely on AAC to manage and control aspects of interactions that are related to the operation of their AAC systems. Such phrases might provide directions to the communication partner with regard to positioning (e.g., CAN YOU COME OVER HERE WHERE I CAN SEE YOU?), effective use of the AAC system (e.g., SAY EACH LETTER AS I POINT TO IT), obtaining and securing conversational turns (e.g., I HAVE SOMETHING TO SAY), and signaling the need to repair a communication breakdown (e.g., WAIT, LET ME SAY IT DIFFERENTLY).

Buzolich and Lunger (1995) provided a case study in which a clinician taught Vivian, an adolescent who relied on AAC, to interact with her classmates by using a variety of regulatory phrases that were programmed into her SGD. Instruction was provided through both role playing and conversational coaching with peers. Although Vivian did not use more regulatory phrases during postintervention probes, she did initiate more topics, repair more conversational breakdowns, and use a wider variety of conversational strategies after instruction.

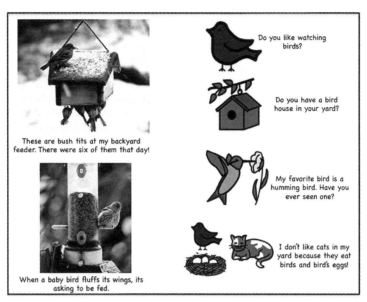

These are bush tits at my backyard feeder. There were six of them that day!

When a baby bird fluffs its wings, its asking to be fed.

Do you like watching birds?

Do you have a bird house in your yard?

My favorite bird is a humming bird. Have you ever seen one?

I don't like cats in my yard because they eat birds and bird's eggs!

Figure 11.3. AAC display used by an adult with Down syndrome to comment about the birds in her backyard. (The Picture Communication Symbols ©1981–2012 by DynaVox Mayer-Johnson LLC. All Rights Reserved Worldwide. Used with permission.)

Partner reauditorization occurs when a speaking partner repeats and expands an aided message without rising intonation. For example, imagine that an individual with CCN points to a symbol for TV during a conversation with a friend. Reauditorization occurs when the partner then says, *Oh, you watched TV last night.* This strategy can be useful to increase the rate of a communication interaction because it allows the communication partner to guess the meaning of a telegraphic message produced by the person with CCN (Mirenda & Bopp, 2003). Four studies have provided evidence that reauditorization does not affect perceptions of the communicative competence of people who rely on AAC, either positively or negatively (Bedrosian et al., 1992; Bedrosian, Hoag, Johnson, & Calculator, 1998; Hoag & Bedrosian, 1992; Hoag, Bedrosian, Johnson, & Molineux, 1994).

Conversational Repairs

Conversational repair strategies are sometimes needed to resolve communication breakdowns that occur during interactions. Such breakdowns may occur during conversations with individuals who rely on AAC because of difficulties related to message intelligibility or comprehensibility, conversational timing, partner unfamiliarity with AAC, and numerous other factors (Brady & Halle, 2002). The need for a repair strategy by a person with CCN may be signaled when the communicative partner requests clarification (e.g., *What?*, *Pardon me?*), responds to a communicative attempt inappropriately (e.g., by changing the topic or providing erroneous information), or does not respond to a communicative attempt at all (Bedrosian, Hoag, & McCoy, 2003; Brady & Halle, 2002).

Halle, Brady, and Drasgow (2004) described two basic types of repair strategies, repetitions and modifications; the latter type can be further subdivided into additions, reductions, and substitutions. Repetition (i.e., saying, signing, or pointing to the same message again) may be the least effective strategy, especially when the source of the breakdown is poor intelligibility. Additions involve adding a new element to the original message (e.g., signing JUICE again while also pointing to a glass), whereas reductions involve deleting an element (e.g., pointing emphatically to a single symbol for HELP rather than to the symbols I + WANT + HELP). Substitutions involve using a completely different message than the original utterance (e.g., activating LEAVE ME ALONE on an SGD rather than the more polite CAN I HAVE SOME TIME TO MYSELF?).

Halle et al. (2004) emphasized that beginning communicators in particular often use problem behavior to repair communication breakdowns. For example, consider an interaction between Mrs. Sherman, a teacher, and Henry, a student who uses vocalizations, gestures, body language, and pictures to communicate. Mrs. Sherman is sitting at her desk in the morning, talking to Jelissa, one of Henry's classmates, when Henry enters the room:

Henry:	[stands by Mrs. Sherman's desk and hums quietly]
Mrs. Sherman:	[does not notice Henry and continues talking to Jelissa]
Henry:	[taps his hand softly on the side of the desk]
Mrs. Sherman:	[does not notice Henry and continues talking to Jelissa]
Henry:	[grabs a handful of Mrs. Sherman's hair and pulls]
Mrs. Sherman:	*Henry, NO!!!! That hurts! You must not pull my hair! You need to go to the principal's office so he can call your mother and tell her what you did!*

Of course, readers have the advantage of having "insider information" that was not available to Mrs. Sherman about the subtle communicative messages underlying Henry's humming and tapping. It seems clear to us that Henry's humming was an attempt to initiate a "Good morning!" conversation with Mrs. Sherman, and that tapping was a repair strategy that he used when she did not hear his humming. However, Mrs. Sherman would surely be surprised with this analysis because both behaviors were so subtle that she did not recognize them at all. She only "heard" Henry when he finally resorted to the more blatant (but less socially acceptable) behavior of hair pulling that, unfortunately, did not have a positive communicative outcome. This is a typical example of a situation in which instruction in the use of one or more appropriate repair strategies is urgently needed. Fortunately, Henry received explicit instruction to teach him to tap Mrs. Sherman gently on the shoulder if she did not notice his humming. This served two purposes: it resolved the hair pulling problem and it resulted in Henry learning a generic substitution strategy for failed communicative initiations.

Unfortunately, aside from common sense and a few case studies (see Brady & Halle, 2002, and Halle et al., 2004), little research is available to provide guidance about how to teach repair strategies to beginning communicators who rely on AAC. However, Halle et al. (2004) offered a number of suggestions that are based on research outcomes related to functional communication training in general, including the following:

1. Identify current and future situations in which use of a repair strategy might be relevant because of communication breakdowns.

2. Select two or more forms to teach as repairs. Teaching at least two forms is important so that (as was the case with Henry) if the first is unsuccessful, the person has another alternative. All of the repair strategies taught should be both socially appropriate and sufficiently transparent to communicative partners to communicate the intended message.

3. Teach the repair strategies using graduated prompting procedures in naturally occurring routines and contexts. As much as possible, ignore problem behaviors that occur in response to communication breakdowns.

4. Encourage communication partners to respond to appropriate repairs as soon as they occur with the behavior indicated by the repair.

5. Monitor use of the new repair strategies and teach additional ones as needed.

QUESTIONS

11.1. What are the four components of communicative competence proposed by Light (1989b), and why are they important for AAC intervention?

11.2. How can explicit instruction and language modeling be used to support semantic development in people who rely on AAC?

11.3. What are the five principles underlying grammar interventions for people who rely on AAC that were proposed by Fey (2008)?

11.4. How can strategy instruction and language modeling be used to support semantic development in people who rely on AAC?

11.5. How can language modeling be used to support the development of grammatical morpheme use in people who rely on AAC?

11.6. What are elicited and self-initiated choices, and how can they be taught?

11.7. Describe two strategies that can be used to teach basic requesting.

11.8. Describe the six main steps involved in teaching basic rejecting.

11.9. Describe two strategies that can be used to teach the use of *yes* and *no.*

11.10. What are five strategies that can be used to enable people to initiate and establish conversational topics?

11.11. What are nonobligatory turns and regulatory phrases, and how can both of them be taught?

11.12. What are the two basic types of repair strategies, and how can conversational repairs be taught?

CHAPTER 12

Literacy Intervention for Individuals with Complex Communication Needs

Janice C. Light and David B. McNaughton

> Teaching literacy skills is the single most empowering thing that we can do for individuals who require [augmentative and alternative communication (AAC)].
> (Lindsay, 1989)

It is difficult to overestimate the importance of literacy skills in today's society. The acquisition of reading and writing skills fosters cognitive development and enhances learning; allows fuller participation in education; increases access to employment opportunities; facilitates the use of a wide range of technologies; supports the development of social relationships (e.g., through texting and social networking web sites); fosters personal expression; and allows access to enjoyable leisure pursuits. With rapid technological developments and increased reliance on the Internet, literacy skills continue to assume even greater importance in daily life, leading Moore, Bean, Birdyshaw, and Rycik to conclude that all individuals

> will need advanced levels of literacy to perform their jobs, run their households, act as citizens, and conduct their personal lives. They will need literacy to cope with the flood of information they will find everywhere they turn. They will need literacy to feed their imagination so they can create the world of the future. (1999, p. 99)

Although literacy skills are essential in the lives of all citizens, they carry even greater importance in the lives of individuals with complex communication needs

---

Note: Letters and words shown in italics in this chapter were actually presented to the student in regular type.

(CCN) who rely on AAC. Access to literacy skills significantly expands the communication options available to individuals with CCN. Without access to literacy skills, these individuals must rely on others to provide graphic or other symbols to represent the language concepts that they wish to express. With access to literacy skills, these individuals are able to use text-based AAC systems and independently generate any message that they desire. According to Light and Kelford Smith, literacy skills provide individuals who rely on AAC with "the opportunity to initiate topics, to develop ideas, to provide clarification, to communicate independently, to interact with a diverse audience, and to express ideas, thoughts, and feelings" (1993, p. 10). In addition, because literacy skills are highly valued in today's society, the acquisition of these skills also serves to significantly enhance others' perceptions of the competence of individuals with CCN as well as to increase their own self-esteem. Acquisition of literacy skills can reduce the opportunity barriers imposed by others and facilitate the inclusion of individuals with CCN in school, at work, and in the community.

"Brent (a 5-year-old with cerebral palsy) learned to read and type as a preschooler. At his transition meeting for kindergarten, the occupational therapist on his school team remarked, 'If Brent does not go on to college, it will be our fault. He has already proved that he can learn. Now it is up to us to make sure that he has the opportunity to learn'" (Light & McNaughton, 2005).

Given the importance of literacy skills, it is encouraging to find clear evidence that individuals with CCN can indeed learn to read and write despite their limited access to speech (e.g., Koppenhaver, Evans, & Yoder, 1991; Light & McNaughton, 2009b, 2011). This evidence of positive literacy outcomes extends across individuals with a wide range of disabilities (e.g., autism, cerebral palsy, childhood apraxia of speech, Down syndrome, multiple disabilities), across a wide range of ages (e.g., preschoolers, school-age children, adolescents, adults), and among those who rely on a wide range of AAC systems (e.g., manual signs, low-tech communication boards, and speech-generating devices [SGDs]) (e.g., Koppenhaver et al., 1991; Light & McNaughton, 2009a, 2011; Light, McNaughton, Weyer, & Karg, 2008). Unfortunately, despite this evidence of the potential for positive literacy outcomes, the typical outcomes for individuals with CCN are far from encouraging. The research suggests that many of these individuals are nonliterate and many others demonstrate significant difficulties with reading and writing skills compared with their typically developing peers (Berninger & Gans, 1986; Kelford Smith, Thurston, Light, Parnes, & O'Keefe, 1989; Koppenhaver & Yoder, 1992; Lund & Light, 2006). In fact, it has been estimated that up to 90% of individuals who rely on AAC enter adulthood without acquiring functional literacy skills, severely restricting their communication, their educational and vocational outcomes, and their overall quality of life (Foley & Wolter, 2010). What accounts for these poor literacy outcomes?

FACTORS THAT AFFECT LITERACY LEARNING

Learning to read and write requires the integration of knowledge and skills across a variety of domains, including 1) orthographic processing (i.e., processing and identification of letters and letter patterns); 2) phonological processing (i.e., detection and manipulation of the sound structures of speech and mapping of letters to sounds and sounds to letters); 3) context processing (i.e., use of vocabulary knowledge, syntactic/ grammatical knowledge, and world knowledge to derive meaning from text or encode meaning into text); and 4) meaning processing (i.e., integration of orthographic, phonological, and contextual processing to build a coherent understanding of the meaning of the text or to encode meaning into coherent text; see Adams, 1990). "Good" readers are able to recognize letters and letter sequences automatically; they are able to recognize sound patterns, manipulate sounds easily, and map sounds to letters (and vice versa) rapidly; they are able to access word meanings quickly and use context and world knowledge to help with unfamiliar words; and they are able to integrate these skills with ease to derive meaning from the text or to encode meaning into text (Adams, 1990; National Reading Panel [NRP], 2000). In contrast, "poor" readers may have weak knowledge of letter patterns and may struggle to recognize letters and letter sequences; they may have difficulty with auditory discrimination and phonological awareness activities; they are more likely to have limited vocabulary knowledge; and they must devote more attention and resources to basic word recognition and decoding/encoding activities, leaving fewer resources to construct the meaning of the text and monitor their comprehension. There are a wide range of factors that may contribute to literacy outcomes (both positive and negative), including both intrinsic and extrinsic factors.

Intrinsic Factors that Affect Literacy Learning

Intrinsic factors are factors directly related to the needs and skills of the learner. Literacy learning is more challenging for individuals with CCN because of intrinsic factors that may include one or more of the following:

- Visual impairments that limit their perception of printed text and their ability to recognize and discriminate between letters

- Hearing impairments that limit their perception of the sounds of spoken language and thereby affect the translation of spoken language into written code (and vice versa)

- Motor impairments that limit or complicate physical access to reading materials and writing implements (e.g., pencils, pens, computer keyboards, or other technologies)

- Cognitive impairments that impact working memory and other processing skills that are required to learn to read and write

- Language impairments that limit the semantic, syntactic, and morphological knowledge (i.e., knowledge of vocabulary, grammar and sentence structure) required to understand and produce written texts

- Speech impairments that impact the accurate and consistent translation of spoken language into written language (and vice versa)

- Lack of experiences and world knowledge that restrict understanding of texts as well as limit the production of cohesive written texts on a range of topics

- A history of limited participation and lack of success in literacy activities that result in a lack of motivation

The challenges in literacy learning are further compounded when individuals with CCN face significant health problems that may jeopardize their well being, the consistency of their performance, and the time and attention given to literacy instruction. It is essential to realize that these intrinsic challenges are *not* reasons to neglect literacy instruction; rather, they are reasons to ensure that individuals with CCN are provided with systematic, effective, evidence-based instruction to support literacy learning. Comprehensive assessment of an individual's needs and skills by a knowledgeable multidisciplinary team is required prior to literacy intervention to determine strengths and areas of difficulty (see Chapter 6 for discussion of assessment processes). Although some intrinsic factors may not be amenable to change, the multidisciplinary AAC team should focus on maximizing sensory/perceptual, motor, cognitive, language, world knowledge, and speech function to as great an extent as possible in order to support literacy learning.

Krista was 8 years old when we first met her. She faced numerous challenges including significant speech, motor, vision, and hearing impairments. However, these challenges were not an excuse to deny her the opportunity to participate in literacy instruction; rather, the challenges were the impetus for us to ensure that we provided Krista with consistent, systematic, evidence-based literacy instruction, adapted to meet her needs and skills. This literacy instruction resulted in her successful acquisition of basic reading and writing skills, which in turn resulted in increased educational and social opportunities for her (Light, McNaughton, et al., 2008).

Extrinsic Factors that Affect Literacy Learning

In addition to intrinsic factors, literacy learning is also affected by a wide range of extrinsic factors related to the environment. Literacy learning does not occur in isolation; rather, it is deeply embedded within a series of interrelated contexts including the physical context (i.e., the amount and the nature of literacy materials in the individual's environment), the functional context (i.e., the time and organization of literacy activities within the day), the social context (i.e., the quality of interaction with literate partners during literacy experiences), the language context (i.e., the language available/used during literacy activities), and the cultural context (i.e., the value, expectations, and priority accorded to literacy learning by the family, school, and broader community; Light & Kelford Smith, 1993).

The Physical and Functional Contexts for Literacy Learning

Research suggests that the homes of children who rely on AAC have an array of reading and writing materials and models of others reading and writing, similar to the homes of children without disabilities (Light & Kelford Smith, 1993). What differs, however, is the children's access to these literacy materials: Children with CCN are reported to have less frequent access to reading materials and significantly less access to writing materials than their peers without disabilities (Koppenhaver & Yoder, 1993; Light & Kelford Smith, 1993). Parents of children with CCN report that they spend significantly more time completing activities of daily living with their children (e.g., feeding, toileting, dressing) than parents of children without disabilities do, leaving much less time for literacy-related activities at home. These differences extend beyond the home to the classroom as well. Koppenhaver (1991, cited in Koppenhaver & Yoder, 1993) reported that teachers typically allocated less than 60 minutes per day for literacy instruction and that students spent approximately 40% of that time waiting for instruction, out of the room, or otherwise off task. This resulted in approximately 35 minutes of reading and writing instruction per day for students with CCN—significantly less than their peers without disabilities. Furthermore, many students with CCN are assigned to self-contained special education classrooms, resulting in decreased academic expectations and even fewer opportunities for literacy learning at school (Machalicek et al., 2010).

The Social Context for Literacy Learning

Not only do children who rely on AAC have fewer literacy experiences than their peers without disabilities, but the quality of these experiences also differs. Typically developing children usually participate actively in literacy experiences with their parents and teachers by commenting, asking questions, and answering questions. In contrast, research suggests that individuals who rely on AAC have few opportunities to participate in meaningful ways in literacy activities; the interactions tend to be dominated by parents or teachers (e.g., Kent-Walsh, Binger, & Hasham, 2010; Light, Binger, & Kelford Smith, 1994). Individuals with CCN often have limited or no access to AAC during literacy activities; as a result, given their limited access to speech, they have few, if any, means to communicate during literacy activities (e.g., to ask questions about the text, comment on the text, relate it to their own experiences). The social context is influenced by the language context, including the language available to the individual who relies on AAC and the language used by partners during literacy activities.

The Language Context for Literacy Learning

By definition, written language is an encoding of speech. The printed letters or graphemes on a page have no meaning in and of themselves; rather, their meaning is derived from their representation of the sounds (phonemes) of speech and the blending of these sounds to represent words. In typical development, acquisition of literacy skills is thus founded on the oral/spoken language skills that develop early in life. In contrast, individuals with CCN have limited or no access to speech themselves and typically rely on multiple modes to communicate, including both unaided and aided AAC symbols (e.g., gestures, manual signs, and graphic symbols displayed on communication boards and/or SGDs). Unlike traditional orthography (written language) that maps spoken language at a phonemic level (i.e., the level of speech sounds), most unaided and aided AAC symbols map spoken language at the semantic level (i.e., the level of word meaning). Furthermore, most AAC symbols are not true language systems (Light, 1997). To date, we do not have a full understanding of the impact of graphic (or other) AAC symbols on literacy acquisition (Bishop, Rankin, & Miranda, 1994). It is critical to ensure that individuals with CCN have access to AAC systems that support communication, language development, and the transition to traditional orthography.

The Cultural Context for Literacy Learning

One potential explanation for the reduced emphasis on literacy experiences and instruction for individuals with CCN may be found in parental and teacher expectations. In several studies, parents of children who rely on AAC rated their children's acquisition of reading and writing skills as less important than a range of other skills such as communication and making friends (Light & Kelford Smith, 1993; Marvin & Miranda, 1993; Trenholm & Miranda, 2006). Furthermore, Light and McNaughton (1993) found that parents and teachers of individuals with CCN had few expectations that their children would acquire literacy skills. Low expectations instigate a vicious cycle of literacy failure: Parents and teachers have low expectations and therefore devote limited time and effort to literacy activities; in turn, individuals with CCN have few opportunities to learn literacy skills; and as a result, parents and teachers observe limited progress, which confirms their low expectations for successful literacy outcomes. Concerted intervention is required to break the cycle of low expectations and poor literacy outcomes for individuals who rely on AAC.

Sandra has severe cerebral palsy. She was 13 years old when we first met her. She did not know how to read or write and had never had the opportunity to participate in literacy instruction. After 8 weeks of appropriate instruction, Sandra had learned to decode regular words and was able to apply these decoding skills during shared book reading activities. With appropriate support and instruction, she was well on her way to becoming a competent reader and writer. She told us about the low expectations that she had experienced: "They said I'd never read." Clearly, Sandra proved those expectations wrong. Visit the Student Success Stories section of the Pennsylvania State University web site for Literacy Instruction for Individuals with Autism, Cerebral Palsy, Down Syndrome and Other Disabilities for more information about Sandra.

Instructional Factors that Affect Literacy Learning

Literacy skills are not innate. Most individuals require concerted, appropriate, and effective instruction to learn to read and write. In fact, the first 3 to 4 years of formal schooling are largely devoted to learning to read and write. One of the main factors contributing to poor literacy outcomes for individuals with CCN has been the lack of effective evidence-based literacy interventions adapted to meet the needs of individuals who have limited or no speech (Berninger & Gans, 1986). Most literacy curricula are designed for typically developing children or for children who are at risk in the area of literacy development but who can use speech to participate.

Fortunately, over the past decade there has been increased attention to the development of literacy interventions for individuals with CCN (e.g., Browder, Ahlgrim-Delzell, Courtade, Gibbs, & Flowers, 2008; Erickson, Clendon, Abraham, Roy, & Van de Carr, 2005; Light & McNaughton, 2009a). Learning to read and write is a complex process that 1) begins well before formal schooling with the development of *emergent literacy skills;* 2) transitions to the acquisition of *basic conventional reading and writing skills,* typically through the first 3 to 4 years of formal schooling (i.e., learning to read and write); and 3) culminates in the realization of *advanced literacy skills* and the application of those skills to facilitate learning and participation in society (i.e., reading and writing to learn). The remaining sections of this chapter discuss each of these stages of literacy intervention in turn, providing a summary of the state of the art in research-based practice.

FOSTERING EMERGENT LITERACY SKILLS

The process of developing literacy skills begins very early in life, typically within the first year as children begin to learn language and are first exposed to print materials (e.g., simple books). These early years of literacy development, prior to the learning of conventional literacy skills, are referred to as the *stage of emergent literacy.* During this stage, children acquire the knowledge and skills that form the underpinnings for the development of later reading and writing skills. Specifically, they build language skills (i.e., they learn the semantic, syntactic, morphological, and narrative skills that they will require later to understand and produce written texts); they begin to make connections between spoken and written language (i.e., they learn that print carries meaning and that it represents spoken language); and they learn the basic conventions of print (e.g., how to hold a book, where to start reading, how to move from left to right in the text).

Storybook reading is a particularly important aspect of emergent literacy. During storybook reading activities, a literate partner (e.g., parent, teacher, older child) reads text to a child and talks about the story, relating it to the child's experiences while the child listens to the story, comments on events, asks questions, and/or retells parts of the story. These early story reading experiences play an important role in a child's development of language skills. During storybook reading, children are exposed to a wide variety of vocabulary and sentence structures as well as to story grammar. Furthermore, storybook reading introduces young children to the type of "displaced talk" that forms the foundation of formal education. Unlike daily life, in which the young child communicates about events that are actually occurring, displaced talk requires the child to talk about people, things, and events outside of the here and now. Storybook reading provides a supportive milieu for first introducing displaced talk because the illustrations in the book provide visual and contextual support to enhance children's understanding, and parents and teachers typically provide further scaffolding support by helping children talk about the story and relate it to their own experiences. Research on children who are typically developing and those who may be at risk in the area of literacy development suggests that storybook reading is highly correlated to later literacy outcomes (e.g., Bus, van IJzendoorn, & Pellegrini, 1995).

Challenges in Emergent Literacy Development for Individuals Who Rely on AAC

Like their typically developing peers, children who rely on AAC are regularly read to by their parents and teachers (Dahlgren Sandberg, 1998; Light & Kelford Smith, 1993). For many, storybook reading is a regular part of their daily or weekly routine. However, the nature of the storybook reading interactions of children with CCN differs significantly from that of the interactions experienced by their typically developing peers. For example, Light and Kelford Smith (1993) found that, whereas typically developing children usually choose books themselves and often choose the same book repeatedly, the parents of children who rely on AAC are the ones who usually choose the books to be read and tend to choose different books each time. As a result, storybook reading sessions may not be as responsive to the needs and interests of these children. Furthermore, without repeated readings of the same storybook, children with CCN have limited opportunities to participate in story reading activities and build their competence. Repeated readings seem to play a critical role in helping young children to develop their comprehension skills, learn inference skills, practice retelling or narrating stories, anticipate events or story lines, and participate in "pretend reading."

The research also suggests that, when parents, teachers, or paraprofessionals read to children who rely on AAC, they overwhelmingly dominate the interaction, providing few opportunities for the children to participate (e.g., Kent-Walsh et al., 2010; Light et al., 1994). Partners tend to focus only on reading the story; they provide few pauses to allow the children to initiate communication, and they seldom ask questions. When they do encourage children to participate, they tend to focus on the mechanics of the book (e.g., encouraging children to turn pages or point to pictures) rather than discussing the story to promote comprehension and develop language and communication skills. Very often, children with CCN do not have access to AAC during story reading interactions, severely limiting their communication options (Light et al., 1994) and their ability to learn emergent literacy skills.

Intervention to Promote the Development of Emergent Literacy Skills

There is a growing body of research that demonstrates the effectiveness of interventions to enhance the emergent literacy skills of individuals with CCN. At this point, most of these interventions have focused on increasing the frequency of turn taking (i.e., participation), receptive and/or expressive vocabulary knowledge, and/or the length of messages expressed by individuals with CCN during story reading interactions. In order to achieve these goals, interventions have focused on two areas: 1) providing the individual with access to AAC that includes appropriate vocabulary concepts during story reading; and 2) teaching partners (e.g., parents, paraprofessionals) to use interaction strategies that promote effective communication by individuals who rely on AAC.

Providing Access to Appropriate Augmentative and Alternative Communication for Emergent Literacy Activities

A crucial first step in fostering the emergent literacy skills of individuals with CCN is ensuring that they have access to appropriate and effective AAC to support their communication. Access to AAC can be provided in various ways, including 1) incorporating manual signs and gestures into story reading activities; 2) using objects to communicate choices during story reading (Browder, Mims, Spooner, Ahlgrim-Delzell, & Lee, 2008); 3) providing simple switches programmed with repeated story lines (e.g., Koppenhaver, Erickson, Harris, McLellan, Stotko, & Newton, 2001; Koppenhaver,

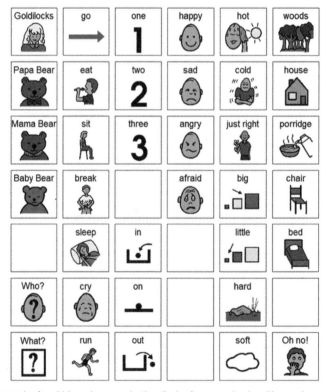

Figure 12.1.   An example of a grid-based communication display for a preschooler with complex communication needs for emergent literacy activities using the story of Goldilocks and the Three Bears. Symbols on the actual display should be in color. (The Picture Communication Symbols ©1981–2012 by DynaVox Mayer-Johnson LLC. All Rights Reserved Worldwide. Used with permission.)

Erickson, & Stotko, 2001); 4) providing low-tech communication boards with appropriate vocabulary from the story to ask questions and comment (e.g., Trudeau, Cleave, & Woelk, 2003); and 5) providing SGDs programmed with appropriate vocabulary (e.g., Bellon-Harn & Harn, 2008; Binger, Kent-Walsh, Berens, del Campo, & Rivera, 2008; Rosa-Lugo & Kent-Walsh, 2008). Several investigators have explored different ways to organize and display vocabulary in aided AAC systems to facilitate participation during story reading interactions, including traditional grid displays of AAC graphic symbols that are presented separately from the actual storybook (Binger et al., 2008; Rosa-Lugo & Kent-Walsh, 2008; see Figure 12.1); relevant AAC symbols in a circular layout around the perimeter of the actual pages of the storybook, scanned into the SGD (Wilkinson, Foderaro, Maurer, Weinreb, & O'Neill, 2011); and visual scene displays (VSDs) of scanned pages from the actual storybook with relevant vocabulary programmed directly as hotspots within these scenes (Wood Jackson, Wahlquist, & Marquis, 2011; Light & Drager, 2011; see Figure 12.2). What is clear from these studies is that provision of AAC can result in increased turn taking and improved participation during story reading interactions by individuals with CCN (e.g., Browder, Mims, et al., 2008; Mims, Browder, Baker, Lee, & Spooner, 2009) as well as expansion of the range of concepts expressed (e.g., Rosa-Lugo & Kent-Walsh, 2008) and the length of messages communicated (e.g., Binger et al., 2008).

Genevieve, a girl with Down syndrome, was introduced to manual signs and an SGD with VSDs to enhance her language and communication development when she was 8 months old. Genevieve quickly learned to use the VSDs to participate actively within shared story reading activities with her parents and older sisters. Visit the Success Stories section of the Pennsylvania State University Early Intervention for Young Children with Autism, Cerebral Palsy, Down Syndrome, and Other Disabilities web site to view a video of Genevieve participating in shared reading with her parents and older sisters with the book *Brown Bear, Brown Bear, What Do You See?* by Bill Martin Jr. On the video, she uses her SGD and manual signs to participate actively in the interaction and to express her "first word" at 9 months of age, by selecting the duck from the VSD to retrieve the speech output "duck" along with a quacking sound, and by producing a sign approximation for DUCK. Even at this young age, Genevieve is already establishing important emergent literacy skills through this shared storybook reading activity that lays the foundation for later literacy learning.

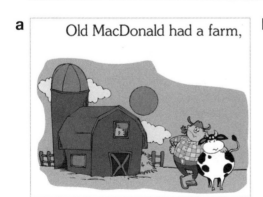 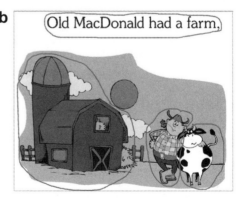

Figure 12.2. An example of a visual scene display (VSD) for a toddler with complex communication needs for emergent literacy activities with the book *Old MacDonald Had a Farm*. a) Screenshot illustrating the visual scene display of the page of the book as the child would see it on the screen of the speech-generating device; b) screenshot illustrating the hotspots embedded in the VSD. Touching each hotspot produces speech output and/or sound effects (e.g., touching the farmer produces the speech output "Old MacDonald"; touching the barn produces "farm" or a reading of the text; and touching the cow produces "cow" and then "moo"). The child does not see the hotspots highlighted in this way. Hotspots are highlighted only when they are selected. Pictures on the actual VSD should be in color.

Teaching Interaction Strategies to Literate Partners

Simply providing access to AAC is necessary but not sufficient to ensure that individuals with CCN are able to participate successfully within emergent literacy activities. Emergent literacy activities must be scaffolded by a literate partner to ensure that the learner has the opportunity to participate and receives the supports required to do so effectively. Table 12.1 summarizes a range of partner interaction strategies that positively impact the communication of individuals with CCN during story reading activities. Research suggests that a wide variety of partners (e.g., parents and educational staff from various cultural/ethnic backgrounds, including European American, African American, and Hispanic) can successfully learn to use a combination of these strategies in a short amount of time, and that such use results in increases in turn taking, use of novel semantic concepts, and production of multisymbol messages by children who rely on AAC during storybook reading interactions (e.g., Bellon-Harn & Harn, 2008; Binger et al., 2008; Binger, Kent-Walsh, Ewing, & Taylor, 2010; Kent-Walsh et al., 2010; Rosa-Lugo & Kent-Walsh, 2008; Soto & Dukhovny, 2008).

Although we most often think of storybook reading in the context of young children, older individuals who are not yet literate will also benefit from emergent liter-

Table 12.1. Partner interaction strategies that support the participation of individuals with complex communication needs in story reading activities

Strategy	Description
Select appropriate books	Allow the learner to choose books of interest
	Ensure books are at an appropriate language level to support the learner's comprehension
Introduce the topic of the book	Encourage the learner to think about the topic of the book
	Discuss related experiences
	Discuss the purpose of reading (e.g., enjoying the story, learning new information, answering questions)
Introduce new vocabulary as required	Explain new concepts to the learner (e.g., illustrate with examples, relate to prior experience)
	Teach appropriate augmentative and alternative communication (AAC) symbols to represent new concepts
Read the text of the book	Read each page of the book out loud, tracking word by word with a finger under the text as it is read aloud
	Regularly pause and provide the opportunity for the learner to ask a question or make a comment
Use time delay (wait expectantly)	Focus attention on the learner with an expectant look
	Wait at least 5–10 seconds
Ask appropriate questions	Ask questions to encourage the learner to think about the story
	Encourage the learner to make predictions
	Relate the text to the learner's prior experiences
Model use of AAC and speech	While reading or talking about the story, sign or select the appropriate aided AAC symbols from the learner's speech-generating device or low-tech communication board
Respond to communicative attempts	If the learner asks a question or makes a comment, respond by answering the question or expanding on the learner's comment by adding more information
Encourage the learner to tell the story	With repeated readings of the book, pause and encourage the learner to retell parts of the story

Source: Light and McNaughton (2009a).

acy experiences to build their language skills, make connections between spoken and written language, and introduce the conventions of print. In these situations, sports, fashion, and cooking magazines or books might replace more traditional children's storybooks. And, although storybook reading is most often discussed in the context of emergent literacy activities, it is essential for partners to continue to read and discuss texts with learners well beyond the emergent literacy stage as they develop conventional literacy skills themselves (Foley & Wolter, 2010). Reading to students and discussing texts serves a number of purposes: 1) it builds world knowledge as learners read about events that they may not experience firsthand; 2) it scaffolds cognitive development as learners access more advanced texts than they can read independently; 3) it introduces more advanced language concepts, sentence structures, and written genres (e.g., narrative, persuasive argument, expository essay), thus fostering language development; 4) it promotes more advanced comprehension and inference skills; and 5) it illustrates the pleasure of reading, thereby increasing motivation for reading instruction.

Providing Independent Access to Reading Materials

In addition to scaffolded reading activities with literate partners, it is also important to ensure that individuals with CCN have independent access to motivating and interesting reading materials as well numerous opportunities to engage with print. Access to appropriate reading materials might be facilitated by a variety of strategies: placing books in easily accessible locations, offering book choices during free time, providing the means to request favorite books, adapting books to allow easy page turning, incorporating text into daily routines at home or school (e.g., labels on activity centers, recipes, instructions), introducing books on tape or CD, providing access to books on the computer, and/or scanning books into aided AAC systems (e.g., Erickson, Koppenhaver, Yoder, & Nance, 1997; Goossens', 1989; Light & Kelford Smith, 1993; Light et al., 1994; Light & Drager, 2011; Musselwhite & King-DeBaun, 1997).

Building Narrative Skills

Story reading provides a rich context to introduce new vocabulary and sentence structures. Often, AAC intervention tends to focus on basic communication, and AAC systems tend to include only functional vocabulary. The vocabulary and sentence structures required for literacy activities differ from those used for basic face-to-face communication and may best be acquired through book reading activities. In addition to the development of semantic and syntactic knowledge to support literacy development, book reading interactions also serve to foster narrative skills (and skills in other genres). Unlike their typically developing peers, individuals who rely on AAC often have minimal opportunities for the extended types of communicative interactions required to build narrative skills. Given these limited experiences, individuals with CCN may require concerted intervention to build narrative skills. For example, Soto and colleagues described the positive effects of intervention targeting understanding and use of story structures on the linguistic and narrative complexity of stories told by children who relied on AAC (e.g., Soto, Solomon-Rice, & Caputo, 2009; Soto, Yu, & Henneberry, 2007; Soto, Yu, & Kelso, 2008). Such intervention serves to prepare students who rely on AAC with the narrative- and discourse-level language skills required to read and write extended texts successfully.

Building Emergent Writing Skills

During the stage of emergent literacy development, individuals with CCN need opportunities not only to engage in story reading and other emergent reading activities but also to engage in early "writing" activities. These emergent writing activities help children learn that they can use text to encode or express meaning. Unfortunately, many children who rely on AAC do not have regular access to early writing activities (Light & Kelford Smith, 1993). The lack of participation in early writing activities seems to reflect a lack of access, rather than a lack of interest in these writing activities. Many individuals with CCN experience motor impairments, ranging from mild to severe, that may complicate or prohibit use of conventional writing implements (e.g., crayons, markers, pencils, paintbrushes). Occupational and/or physical therapists may be able to recommend appropriate seating and positioning as well as adaptations to writing and drawing tools to facilitate reliable access and control by individuals with CCN. Computer technologies (with alternative access as required) may also facilitate access to early writing activities for individuals with CCN through drawing programs and through keyboard access.

Individuals with CCN are often denied access to computer technologies until they can demonstrate that they can use them. Such denial deprives these individuals of the *opportunity* to learn, placing them at risk to fall further and further behind their peers. Pencils are not withheld from children without disabilities until they prove that they can write; rather, they have access to pencils, crayons, markers, and other writing implements early on, before they know how to write, in order to support their learning of writing skills. Similarly, early in their development, individuals with CCN require access to technologies and/or software to serve as "electronic pencils" along with other supports for writing and drawing.

With writing tools (both electronic and conventional) in place, individuals with CCN require numerous opportunities to engage in emergent writing experiences, scaffolded by parents, teachers, or other literate adults or children. These activities might include "writing" secret messages, drawing pictures and writing stories, making signs for a pretend store, creating birthday cards, writing letters or e-mail messages, labeling photo albums of school or family experiences, and so forth. The goal here is not that the learner produce written text that is free of spelling, vocabulary, and grammatical errors, but rather that the learner develop the understanding that he or she can encode meaning through "writing." Initially, the learner may simply produce scribbles or strings of unrelated letters, and the literate partner may help by modeling written text. Later, as the learner develops some phonological awareness skills and some knowledge of letter sounds, he or she may begin to use sound spellings to encode meaning.

Tim, a 4-year-old with cerebral palsy, was provided with access to an adapted keyboard on his SGD early in life, before he had learned conventional writing skills. He liked to play with the letters on the keyboard to create written messages. He was especially delighted one day when he produced the written message "P U," using sound spelling to tease his older sister (Light & McNaughton, 2005).

Introducing Phonological Awareness and Letter–Sound Correspondences

Beyond the emergent literacy activities discussed, young children are also typically introduced to phonological awareness skills and letter–sound correspondences during this early phase of literacy development (Erickson & Clendon, 2009). For example, through preschool and child care programs, educational software, and television shows, many young children are introduced to letters and their sounds as well as to activities such as rhyming and sound blending well before they start elementary school. Introducing these skills early, during meaningful and fun activities, may be especially beneficial for children with CCN, giving them a head start on the learning of conventional literacy skills (see the section "Interventions to Teach Basic Reading Skills" for further information on these skills).

Lili, a toddler with Down syndrome who relies on speech approximations, manual signs, and an SGD to communicate, was introduced to letter–sound correspondences and phonological awareness activities at an early age during play activities with her parents and therapists. By the age of 23 months, she had already learned many letters and sounds and associated these letters and sounds with familiar words. Visit the Success Stories section of the Pennsylvania State University Early Intervention for Young Children with Autism, Cerebral Palsy, Down Syndrome, and Other Disabilities web site to see a video of Lili demonstrating her knowledge of the "daddy letter," *d.*

KEY COMPONENTS OF INTERVENTION TO TEACH CONVENTIONAL LITERACY SKILLS

Through emergent literacy activities, individuals with CCN build language skills, begin to make connections between spoken and written language, and learn the basic conventions of print. Although these skills are essential, they are not sufficient to support acquisition of functional reading and writing skills. Organized, regular instruction is also required to teach conventional literacy skills to individuals with CCN. In order to maximize effectiveness, intervention must 1) allocate sufficient time for instruction; 2) use appropriate and effective instructional techniques to teach skills that are known to support the successful acquisition of conventional reading and writing; 3) provide appropriate adaptations to ensure the active participation of individuals with speech, motor, and/or sensory/perceptual impairments; and 4) build positive rapport and ensure student motivation (Light & McNaughton, 2010). Furthermore, the AAC team must monitor the student's progress and make any adjustments required to maximize outcomes.

Allocating Sufficient Time for Literacy Instruction

Recommended practices suggest that all students in Grades 1–3 should receive at least 90 minutes of literacy instruction per day and that students who are at risk for literacy development problems should receive a total of 130–150 minutes of literacy instruction per day (Vaughn, Wanzek, Woodruff, & Linan-Thompson, 2007). Students who rely on AAC may require even more instructional time because they often have slow rates of communication and may require more time to participate in instructional activities. In a nutshell, the more time devoted to literacy instruction, the greater the gains that will be observed in a given time period. Unfortunately, in many cases, even the recommended minimum standards for instructional time are not met for individuals with CCN; rather, research suggests that many of these individuals receive only a small amount of literacy instruction per day, typically 30 minutes or less (e.g., Koppenhaver, 1991; Koppenhaver & Yoder, 1993; Mike, 1995). As noted previously, this lack of literacy instructional time may reflect, at least in part, low expectations on the part of parents and educators (Light & McNaughton, 1993; Mirenda, 2003a), a lack of knowledge and skill in adapted literacy instruction for individuals who rely on AAC (Light & McNaughton, 2009b), and/or competing demands in the home and school environments (e.g., scheduling of numerous therapies, additional time required for activities of daily living such as dressing and feeding; Light & Kelford Smith, 1993).

Every effort should be made to maximize the time allocated for literacy instruction. In order to do so, collaboration may be required among families and educational personnel, including general and special education teachers, speech-language pathologists, paraprofessionals, and/or classroom volunteers. One way to provide additional time for literacy learning is to start instruction as early as possible with children with CCN. Research has demonstrated that preschoolers (ages 3–5 years) with CCN (including those with autism, cerebral palsy, and Down syndrome) can learn to read and write when they are provided with appropriate instructional supports (Light & McNaughton, 2009a, 2011). On the other hand, although numerous benefits may result from early literacy instruction, research also demonstrates that it is never too late to learn conventional literacy skills. Light and McNaughton (2011) described the successful acquisition of literacy skills by adolescents with CCN (including those with autism, cerebral palsy, and multiple disabilities) who did not start instruction until later in their lives.

Implementing Effective Instructional Techniques to Teach Key Skills

The NRP (2000) concluded that the most effective literacy intervention combines both direct instruction in key skills and numerous opportunities to apply these skills in the context of meaningful and motivating literacy experiences. Table 12.2 provides definitions of these key literacy skills. Ultimately, these skills must be applied fluently in order for an individual to read, understand, and write meaningful texts in a variety of genres.

Typically, direct instruction aimed at teaching key literacy skills involves a most-to-least prompting hierarchy to ensure learner success. First, the instructor models a target skill for the learner; next, the instructor provides guided practice in the form of scaffolding support or prompts to help the learner perform the skill successfully; and, finally, the instructor gradually fades support until the learner is able to perform the skill successfully and independently (Archer & Hughes, 2010; Light & McNaughton, 2009a). Throughout the process, the instructor provides corrective feedback as required. Table 12.3 provides an example of these instructional procedures.

In addition to direct instruction, learners also require numerous opportunities to apply key skills within authentic reading and writing experiences. For example, if a student is learning to decode single words, the instructor might encourage him or her to apply decoding skills during shared reading activities in which the instructor reads part of a sentence and the student is responsible for decoding specific target words within the text. Providing opportunities for learners to apply newly acquired

Table 12.2.   Knowledge and skills required to support the acquisition of basic reading and writing skills

Knowledge or skill	Definition
Language skills	Knowledge and skills in vocabulary, syntax, morphology, narratives, and other genres (e.g., expository, persuasive)
Phonological awareness skills	Ability to notice, think about, and manipulate the phonemes (sounds) of words, including sound blending (e.g., blending sounds to form words) and phoneme segmentation (e.g., breaking words into component sounds)
Letter–sound correspondences	Knowledge of the sounds represented by each of the letters and of the letters used to represent different speech sounds
Single-word decoding skills	Ability to apply knowledge of letter–sound correspondences and sound blending to "sound out" words with regular spellings (e.g., *cat, pig, dad*)
Sight word recognition skills	Ability to read/recognize words without sounding them out, especially irregular words (e.g., *light, their, are*)
Application of decoding and sight word recognition skills in shared book reading	Using knowledge of letter–sound correspondences, sound-blending skills, and sight word recognition skills as required to read target words during shared book reading with a literate partner
Reading and understanding of text (reading comprehension skills)	Ability to decode or recognize by sight each word in the text, access the meanings of the words, process the words together to derive the full meaning of the text, and relate this meaning to prior knowledge and experience
Single-word encoding skills	Ability to apply phoneme segmentation skills and knowledge of letter–sound correspondences to break down regular words and spell them (e.g., *mom, run*)
Sight word spelling skills	Ability to recall and select the correct letters in sequence to spell words with irregular spellings (e.g., *said, know*)
Handwriting skills and/or keyboard knowledge	Knowledge of the correct shapes for letters and the fine motor skills to produce these shapes legibly and/or knowledge of the location of the letters on the keyboard and operational skills to select them efficiently as required using appropriate access techniques
Application of encoding and language skills in simple writing activities	Using knowledge of letter–sound correspondences, phoneme segmentation skills, and sight word spelling skills to encode appropriate words in simple sentences to communicate meaning to others
Writing meaningful texts in a range of genres	Ability to generate coherent narrative (or other genres) using appropriate vocabulary, syntax, morphology, and narrative structure; skills to spell each word in each sentence correctly in sequence (applying either encoding or sight word spelling skills); handwriting or keyboard knowledge to produce or select each letter required

Source: Light and McNaughton (2009a).

key skills during authentic literacy experiences has several benefits: 1) it provides additional opportunities to practice new skills, thus promoting acquisition and increasing fluency; 2) it promotes generalization of skills to new materials and contexts; and 3) it increases motivation by demonstrating that reading and writing are meaningful and fun.

Providing Adaptations for Individuals with Complex Communication Needs

Individuals with CCN may have motor and/or sensory/perceptual impairments in addition to significant speech impairments. Therefore, literacy instruction must be adapted to accommodate specific needs.

Table 12.3.   Direct instruction procedures for teaching basic literacy skills

Step	Participant involvement	Instructional procedures
Model	The instructor does the skill; the learner observes.	Instructor demonstrates the skill for the learner.
Guided practice	The instructor and the learner do the skill together.	Instructor provides scaffolding support/prompting to help the learner perform the skill successfully. Instructor gradually fades support as the learner develops competence.
Independent practice	The learner does the skill independently while the instructor observes and provides feedback.	Learner performs the skill independently. Instructor monitors performance and provides feedback.
Feedback	The instructor provides feedback to the learner.	If the learner performs the skill accurately, the instructor provides appropriate positive feedback. If the learner is incorrect, the instructor directs the learner's attention to the error, models the correct response, provides guided practice for the learner to complete the skill successfully, and then provides additional opportunities for independent practice.

From Light, J., & McNaughton, D. (2009a). *Accessible Literacy Learning (ALL): Evidence-based reading instruction for learners with autism, cerebral palsy, Down syndrome, and other disabilities.* Pittsburgh: Mayer-Johnson.

Adaptations to Accommodate Speech Impairments

As noted previously, most literacy curricula require students to use spoken responses to participate in instruction (e.g., saying letter sounds, blending or segmenting words orally, decoding words orally, or reading out loud). Instructors use students' oral responses to gauge their learning and to determine any areas of difficulty that require remediation. Clearly, curricular adaptations are required for individuals with significant speech impairments to 1) provide alternative response modes, 2) provide insight into areas of strength and difficulty and thus support instructional decision making, and 3) compensate for a lack of speech production and oral rehearsal.

Literacy activities can easily be adapted to support alternative response modes (e.g., manual signs, speech approximations, aided AAC symbols, letters, words) rather than spoken responses. For example, Light, McNaughton, and Fallon (2009a) described adapted instruction in decoding in which students are presented with a written word to decode; however, instead of reading a word orally, they can either sign the word, choose an AAC symbol that represents the word from their SGD or aided communication display, or choose an appropriate AAC symbol from a group of symbols provided specifically for the instructional activity. If the incorrect choices that are provided as options are selected carefully, systematic data collection and error analyses can be used to provide the instructor with insight into the learner's areas of strength and difficulty. For example, Figure 12.3 presents adapted materials that might be used for instruction in decoding. The target word is *cat*, and the student is expected to decode the word and then select the correct AAC symbol from the field of four options provided. Each of the AAC symbols provided as a response option is carefully selected to assist in the analysis of student performance, with one option representing the target word (i.e., *cat*) and the other three options each representing a change to one of the letter sounds in the target word (i.e., change to the initial letter sound, *bat*; the final letter sound, *can*; or the medial vowel, *cut*). Careful data collection and analysis of a learner's responses over numerous trials with different response plates can allow the instructor to determine areas of strength (e.g., the student performs well on initial and final letter sounds) as well as areas of difficulty (e.g., the learner demonstrates some difficulty with medial vowels). Areas of difficulty can then be targeted specifically for additional instruction.

In addition to adapted response modes to support participation and instructional decision making, adaptations may also be required to instructional procedures to support the learner in establishing the links between oral and written language. As typically developing children learn to read and write, they regularly utilize oral rehearsal to support them in translating written language into oral language or oral language into written language. For example, they may slowly sound out the letters in a word orally and then blend them out loud to decode a new word. Or they may say a word slowly to try to segment out the individual sounds to support early writing. Learners with CCN do not have easy access to the speech production skills required to perform these tasks themselves orally and thus face increased working memory demands in learning early conventional literacy skills. They may benefit from external scaffolding support, especially during the early stages of instruction, to compensate for their lack of access to oral rehearsal and to help them build subvocal rehearsal (i.e., inner voice). For example, Light and McNaughton (2009a) proposed that instructors provide guided practice during the early stages of instruction by demonstrating oral rehearsal for learners and encouraging them to develop subvocal rehearsal skills (i.e., "say it in your head"). This external scaffolding support can be gradually faded as the learner acquires the skills.

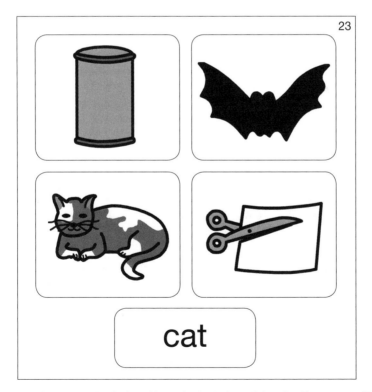

Figure 12.3.   An example of adapted instruction in single word decoding. The target word is *cat;* the response options are CAN, BAT, CAT, and CUT. (From Light, J., & McNaughton, D. [2009a]. *Accessible Literacy Learning [ALL]: Evidence-based reading instruction for learners with autism cerebral palsy, Down syndrome, and other disabilities.* Pittsburgh: Mayer-Johnson; adapted by permission. The Picture Communication Symbols ©1981–2012 by DynaVox Mayer-Johnson LLC. All Rights Reserved Worldwide. Used with permission.)

Adaptations to Accommodate Motor Impairments

Some individuals with CCN may have motor impairments that range from mild to severe. Often, these impairments limit their access to literacy materials and thus restrict their participation in literacy instruction. Input from occupational and/or physical therapists is critical to determine appropriate seating and positioning to maximize motor performance (see Chapter 6). Some individuals who have more severe motor impairments may also require alternative access to support their full participation in instructional activities as well (e.g., eye pointing, scanning, partner-assisted scanning). It is important for the AAC team (which should include a knowledgeable occupational and/or physical therapist) to determine the most effective and efficient access techniques for the individual (see Chapters 4 and 6). Moreover, because literacy instruction itself is cognitively demanding for learners with CCN, it is important that the access technique selected does not impose additional cognitive demands. For example, if a student is just learning to use eye pointing to control his or her SGD and is not yet fluent with this technique, but is able to use partner-assisted scanning easily and reliably, then initial literacy instruction should utilize partner-assisted scanning as a means of access. Eye pointing with an SGD can be introduced later on, once the learner has developed greater competence with this method. This is in accordance with the principle of designing systems for today and tomorrow discussed in Chapter 7.

Adaptations to Accommodate Sensory/Perceptual Impairments

Many individuals with CCN have visual and/or hearing impairments. Learning to read and write places an increased burden on an individual's visual and auditory skills compared with functional communication and activities of daily living. For example, learners are required to make fine discriminations between letters and sounds that may be similar in appearance and sound. As described in Chapter 6, it is important to ensure that comprehensive visual and auditory assessments by qualified professionals are completed and that accommodations are in place. Instructional accommodations for speech, motor, hearing, and/or visual impairments ensure that individuals with CCN have both the opportunity and the necessary supports to learn to read and write.

Krista was 8 years old when we first started literacy instruction with her. She had motor, vision, and hearing impairments as well as a tracheostomy, and she required numerous adaptations to support her participation in literacy instruction. To accommodate her visual impairment, we provided the following accommodations: 1) use of corrective eyeglasses; 2) use of large, clear print (i.e., 80 point Arial font); 3) use of black text on a yellow background to maximize contrast and visual attention; 4) addition of key caps (large lowercase black letters on a yellow background) on her computer keyboard; 5) positioning of reading and writing materials within 12–18 inches of her eyes; 6) adjustment of fluorescent lighting and use of materials with a matte finish to reduce glare; and 7) use of technologies with text highlighting to assist her to visually track connected text from left to right with wraparound to the next line. In order to accommodate her hearing impairment, we provided the following accommodations: 1) use of appropriate assistive hearing devices (FM system and bilateral hearing aids); 2) adjustment of initial instruction to focus on letter sounds and words that she could easily perceive and discriminate; 3) use of augmented input and other visual supports (i.e., manual sign plus speech, writing plus speech) to support learning; and 4) appropriate positioning of the instructor to maximize visual cues. In order to accommodate her motor impairment, we ensured that books had firm pages so that Krista could turn them independently and provided a keyguard to assist her in the accurate selection of letters on the computer. Finally, literacy instruction was adapted to bypass the need for spoken responses and to allow Krista to respond by using manual signs, pointing to AAC symbols from an array, or selecting AAC symbols from her SGD. These adaptations allowed Krista to participate in instruction and to successfully learn to read and write. To learn more about Krista's success, see the work of Light, McNaughton, et al. (2008) and visit the Student Success Stories section of the Pennsylvania State University web site for Literacy Instruction for Individuals with Autism, Cerebral Palsy, Down Syndrome and Other Disabilities.

Building Positive Rapport and Ensuring Student Motivation

In addition to the use of appropriate instructional content, methods, and adaptations, it is also critical to build positive rapport with the student and ensure student motivation for learning. According to retrospective reports of literate adults with CCN, the support and encouragement of adults who believed in their ability to learn was fundamental to their successful acquisition of reading and writing skills (Koppenhaver et al., 1991). Successful interventionists provide instruction in ways that reflect the belief that all students can learn, regardless of their disability; use materials and activities that incorporate students' interests; and communicate a personal interest in the student (Moje, 1996; Sturtevant & Linek, 2003). By doing so, they build a positive relationship with the student, a relationship that encourages student participation and provides increased motivation to succeed (Hamre & Pianta, 2001; Moje, 1996). Because of a lack of appropriate instruction, many individuals with disabilities, especially those who are older, come to literacy instruction with a history of failure and low expectations for success (Brophy, 2010). For these students, it is especially important for professionals to communicate their belief that the student will be successful (Gallagher & Mayer, 2008), provide instructional activities that support success from the very beginning (Light & McNaughton, 2009a; Moje, 1996), and incorporate student interests into instructional activities (Moes, 1998; Sturtevant & Linek, 2003). This approach ensures that students will believe that it is worthwhile to learn literacy skills and that these skills are attainable, thus building intrinsic motivation for learning to read.

Because of her multiple disabilities, many people assumed that Krista, described in the previous case study, had limited potential for learning. She was in a self-contained special education class at school and had not had the opportunity to participate in literacy instruction. Krista's parents advocated for her to have the opportunity to learn to read and type in order to develop to her full potential. We started with the fundamental belief that Krista could learn, regardless of the challenges she faced. We provided appropriate accommodations to address her speech, motor, visual, and hearing impairments and to ensure her access to literacy instruction and materials. We incorporated materials and activities into instruction that were meaningful to Krista and that reflected her interests, and we provided instructional supports (modeling, guided practice, and independent practice) to ensure her success from the onset of instruction (Light, McNaughton, et al., 2008). With these instructional supports, Krista successfully learned to read and type. Visit the Student Success Stories section of the Pennsylvania State University web site for Literacy Instruction for Individuals with Autism, Cerebral Palsy, Down Syndrome and Other Disabilities to read more about Krista's success and to see videos of her literacy instruction.

Monitoring the Effectiveness of Intervention

Once accommodations are in place and motivating, evidence-based literacy instruction is ongoing, instructors should provide regular assessment and evaluation of the learner's response to intervention to ensure that the instruction is as effective and efficient as possible. Although there may be some daily fluctuations in performance, students should demonstrate progress in learning skills over time. As students acquire new skills, instructors need to celebrate these accomplishments and move on to target new, more challenging skills. If students do not demonstrate progress as expected over time, it is critical for the AAC team to examine ongoing instructional data and brainstorm to determine the potential difficulty in order to adjust instruction to address the problem area. Table 12.4 summarizes factors that might contribute to a lack of progress and provides potential solutions.

TEACHING BASIC CONVENTIONAL LITERACY SKILLS: LEARNING TO READ AND WRITE

Reading and writing are synergistic processes; thus, literacy instruction for individuals with CCN should focus on both reading and writing instruction. The following sections discuss interventions to teach basic reading and writing skills.

Table 12.4. Potential causes of and solutions for instructional difficulties during literacy instruction

Possible causes of instructional difficulties	Potential solutions
Insufficient time spent on instruction	Schedule additional instructional time.
	Train others to provide instruction or skill review.
	Identify additional practice activities and opportunities.
	Set instructional priorities; focus on 1–2 skills at a time.
Instructional procedures implemented incorrectly	Use scripts to guide instruction.
	Monitor implementation to ensure consistency if multiple instructors are involved.
Learner confusion with respect to task expectations	Adapt instruction to use familiar response formats (e.g., if learner uses the Picture Exchange Communication System [PECS], adapt the task so that the learner hands the instructor the correct symbol rather than pointing to it).
	Provide additional models, demonstrating for the learner how to complete the task.
	Provide guided practice to support the learner to complete the task successfully.
Vision or hearing difficulties	Ensure reliable and valid assessments of hearing and vision.
	Ensure access to necessary aids and assistive technologies (e.g., hearing aids, eyeglasses, vision aids).
	Adapt instructional materials and procedures to optimize performance.
Lack of learner motivation	Incorporate materials and activities that reflect the learner's interests and preferences.
	Establish positive rapport with the learner.
	Celebrate achievements with the learner and others.
Too many distractions during instruction	Initially, implement instruction of new skills in a distraction-free setting.
	Gradually provide instruction in a more typical environment as the learner develops competence with target skills.
Lack of generalization of new skills	Provide additional instruction with a wider range of materials and tasks.
	Develop a variety of practice activities.

Source: Light and McNaughton (2009a).

Intervention to Teach Basic Reading Skills

According to the NRP (2000), reading and writing requires the integration of knowledge and skills across a variety of domains. Typically, literacy instruction to teach basic reading skills targets the following skills: first, phonological awareness skills (e.g., sound blending, phoneme segmentation skills) and letter–sound correspondences; then decoding skills and sight word recognition skills, as well as the application of these skills in the context of shared reading activities; and, finally, independent reading of simple texts and reading comprehension skills (see Table 12.2). The following sections discuss each of these skills, with emphasis on evidence-based interventions for individuals with CCN. Although these sections present the skills in a linear manner, discussing them one at a time, it is important to remember that learners are typically involved in instruction in several skills at any one point in time (see Table 12.5 for a sample instructional session).

Phonological Awareness Skills

Phonological awareness refers to an individual's understanding and awareness of the sound structure of language. Specifically, phonological awareness is the ability to notice, think about, and manipulate the phonemes or sounds in words (Torgesen, Wagner, & Rashotte, 1994). There are numerous phonological awareness tasks that include rhyming; segmenting words into component sounds; blending sounds to form words; determining beginning, middle, or final sounds in words; and so forth. Sound-blending (or phoneme-blending) skills are a key component required to decode new words: In order to decode, the learner must look at the letters in the target word, determine the sounds of these letters in sequence, and then blend these sounds together to determine the target word. Conversely, phoneme segmentation (or sound segmentation) skills are a key component of encoding or spelling: In order to spell a word, the learner must listen to the target word, break it into its component sounds in sequence, determine the letters that represent each of these component sounds, and then select or produce the target letters in sequence. Phonological awareness skills, especially sound blending and phoneme segmentation, are strongly correlated with later literacy outcomes such as decoding and spelling (Ehri et al., 2001).

What do we know about the phonological awareness skills of individuals with CCN? Research results support the following conclusions: 1) individuals with CCN *can* acquire phonological awareness skills, despite their severe speech impairments; however, 2) most individuals with severe speech impairments demonstrate deficits in phonological awareness compared with their peers without disabilities

Table 12.5. Sample literacy instruction session for a student with complex communication needs who has acquired phonological awareness skills and some letter–sound correspondences and is learning additional letter–sound correspondences and decoding skills

Skill targeted for instruction	Time allocated for instruction
Reading to student and talking about books	10–15 minutes
Learning new letter–sound correspondences and reviewing those previously acquired	10–15 minutes
Learning decoding skills	10–15 minutes
Applying decoding skills during shared reading	10–15 minutes
Reviewing phonological awareness skills	5–10 minutes

(Card & Dodd, 2006; Dahlgren Sandberg, 2006; Foley, 1993; Foley & Pollatsek, 1999; Vandervelden & Siegel, 1999). These findings suggest the need for concerted interventions to teach phonological awareness skills to individuals with CCN as a foundation for later literacy development.

Typically, phonological awareness interventions require beginning readers and writers to produce oral responses. Thus, adaptations are required to bypass the need for oral responses and support the participation of individuals with CCN. In the case of sound blending, adapted instruction might follow the procedures employed by Light, McNaughton, and Fallon (2009b). First, the instructor says a word slowly, extending each phoneme for 1–2 seconds (e.g., "mmmmoooommmm"). Next, the learner blends the sounds in his or her head (i.e., via subvocal rehearsal); determines the target word (e.g., *mom*); and responds by signing the target word, by making a speech approximation of the target word (if it can be understood by the instructor in context), or by selecting an AAC symbol for the target word from an array of symbols. A growing body of research has demonstrated the effectiveness of direct instruction using these types of adaptations to teach sound-blending skills to individuals with CCN, including students ranging in age from 3 to 14 years with a range of disabilities (e.g., autism, cerebral palsy, Down syndrome, childhood apraxia of speech; Browder, Ahlgrim-Delzell, et al., 2008; Fallon, Light, McNaughton, Drager, & Hammer, 2004; Light & McNaughton, 2009a, 2011).

Like sound blending, instruction in phoneme segmentation typically requires a learner to produce oral responses (e.g., to segment the first sound in a word and say it aloud). It is somewhat more challenging to design adapted instruction in phoneme segmentation to bypass the need for oral responses. If a learner has already acquired letter–sound correspondences, the instructor can say the word out loud as the learner listens to it. The learner can then segment out the target sound (e.g., the initial sound) and then select a letter that represents that sound from a keyboard or an array of letters presented by the instructor (e.g., Blischak, Shah, Lombardino, & Chiarella, 2004; Browder, Ahlgrim-Delzell, et al., 2008; Millar, Light, & McNaughton, 2004). It should be noted, however, that this form of adapted instruction requires both phoneme segmentation skills and letter–sound correspondences, thus placing added demands on the learner. Many individuals with CCN have not yet acquired letter–sound correspondences when they are introduced to instruction in phonological awareness skills, so alternative instructional approaches that focus solely on phoneme segmentation skills may be required. Such instruction might follow these procedures: 1) the instructor presents an array of AAC symbols, all starting with different sounds, and then says the initial sound of one of the symbols; 2) the learner segments the initial sound of each of the symbols subvocally, or "in his or her head"; and 3) the learner then selects the symbol whose initial sound matches the target sound presented by the instructor (or says or signs the word; Fallon et al., 2004; Light, McNaughton, Fallon, & Millar, 2009). Truxler and O'Keefe (2007) used a similar approach, but rather than presenting the response options through an array of graphic AAC symbols, they presented the options orally (e.g., "Which word has /t/ at the end: *fat, mean, horse?*"). Usually, instruction first targets segmentation of initial phonemes in single-syllable words because these tend to be stressed and are therefore easier to segment; later instruction may target segmentation of final phonemes and medial vowels (Millar et al., 2004; Vandervelden & Siegel, 1995).

Learning phonological awareness skills imposes significant demands on a learner's auditory processing and working memory. For example, in sound blending, learners must process the sounds in sequence, discriminate each sound accurately, and then hold these sounds in working memory in sequence long enough to blend them together to determine the target word. Some individuals with CCN may have particular difficulties with auditory processing and working memory (Larsson & Dahlgren Sandberg, 2008). Furthermore, they have limited access to the oral rehearsal that children typically use to shore up their working memory (e.g., oral repetition of the sounds in sequence). As a result, some individuals with CCN may benefit from the use of printed letters as visual supports during instruction in phonological awareness. For example, in a sound-blending activity, the instructor might point to each letter in sequence and say its sound slowly, extending each phoneme for 1–2 seconds; the learner then blends the sounds and indicates the target word. In this task, the learner is not required to know the letter–sound correspondences or produce them; the letters simply serve as a visual support as the instructor says the sounds. Using letters when teaching phonological awareness skills offers three potential advantages: 1) the letters provide concrete symbols for sounds that are transient and therefore difficult to grasp; 2) instruction reinforces knowledge of letter–sound correspondences as they are acquired; and 3) phonological awareness skills may transfer more effectively to reading and spelling tasks that ultimately require the integration of phonological awareness skills and knowledge of letter–sound correspondences (Ehri et al., 2001).

Letter–Sound Correspondences

In addition to phonological awareness skills, individuals who rely on AAC also need knowledge of letter–sound correspondences in order to learn to read and write. Specifically, letter–sound correspondences form the code that allows the translation of written language to spoken language and vice versa. Letter–sound correspondences include knowledge of the letters that represent the sounds of speech as well as knowledge of the sounds represented by letters. Knowledge of letter–sound correspondences relies on both phonological processing (i.e., detection and manipulation of the sound structures of speech) and orthographic processing (i.e., processing and identification of letters and letter patterns).

Adaptations to instruction in letter–sound correspondences to accommodate the needs and skills of individuals with CCN are relatively straightforward: 1) the instructor says a phoneme or sound, and 2) the learner selects the letter corresponding to this sound from an array of letters provided for the instructional task or from a keyboard. A number of researchers have investigated the effects of instruction on the acquisition of letter–sound correspondences by individuals with CCN (e.g., Blischak et al., 2004; Fallon et al., 2004; Johnston, Buchanan, & Davenport, 2009; Johnston, Davenport, Kanarowski, Rhodehouse, & McDonnell, 2009; Light & McNaughton, 2009a, 2011; Light, McNaughton, et al., 2008; Millar et al., 2004). Results of these studies suggest the following conclusions: 1) individuals of various ages who have a wide range of disabilities and rely on various types of AAC can successfully acquire letter–sound correspondences using these adapted procedures; and 2) the length of time required to acquire letter sounds varies, depending on a range of intrinsic and extrinsic factors. There is also some suggestion that learners benefit from instruction in which letters and sounds are introduced incrementally, one at a time; as learners master one letter sound, a new letter sound is introduced with regular review of the letter sounds previously acquired (e.g., Browder, Ahlgrim-Delzell, et al., 2008; Light & McNaughton, 2009a, 2011).

Light and McNaughton (2009a) proposed teaching letters and sounds according to the following sequence: *a, m, t, p, o, n, c, d, u, s, g, h, i, f, b, l, e, r, w, k, x, v, y, z, j, q.* This sequence, adapted from Carnine, Silbert, Kame'enui, and Tarver (1997), is designed to meet the following criteria: 1) lowercase letters are taught first because these letters occur more frequently in written texts; uppercase letters are taught later; 2) letters and sounds that occur more frequently in children's books are taught first so that learners are able to read more words earlier in instruction; 3) letters and sounds that are similar visually and/or aurally are separated in the instructional sequence to minimize confusion; 4) short vowels are taught before long vowels because words with short vowels (e.g., *cat, bus*) are more apt to follow simple decoding rules than are words with long vowels (e.g., *ride, eat*), which require application of more complex decoding rules; and 5) single letter–sound correspondences are taught before consonant clusters. Of course, this instructional sequence for letter–sound correspondences may be easily adapted to accommodate the needs, skills, interests, or preferences of individual learners.

Although, traditionally, letter names are introduced to children along with letter sounds, Light and McNaughton (2009a) suggested that, during initial instruction with individuals with CCN, it may be beneficial to focus primarily on the acquisition of letter sounds, rather than letter names. For some children, knowledge of letter names may actually interfere with the decoding process, rather than facilitate it. If a child looks at a word and recalls its letter name (rather than its sound), he or she will have difficulty decoding the word. For this reason, Light and McNaughton (2009a) suggested that early literacy instruction ought to focus on letter sounds; letter names can be taught later on, once the relationship between the letters and their sounds is firmly established.

Decoding Skills

Once an individual has acquired sound-blending skills and knows at least some letter–sound correspondences, he or she has the necessary skills to learn to decode written words. Single-word decoding skills are essential to the reading process because these skills allow individuals to read words that they may not have previously encountered or learned. Traditionally, literacy instruction for individuals with CCN has focused almost exclusively on sight word instruction (Browder, Wakeman, Spooner, Ahlgrim-Delzell, & Algozzine, 2006). Although this type of instruction may result in the successful acquisition of a small corpus of reading words, it does not adequately prepare individuals with CCN to develop true reading competence because they have few word-attack skills to learn to read new words and few skills to support the generation of written texts. Browder, Ahlgrim-Delzell, et al. (2008) investigated the relative effectiveness of a literacy curriculum that incorporated instruction in phonological awareness and decoding skills and one that used a traditional sight word approach with individuals with significant developmental disabilities and limited speech. Results indicated that the curriculum that incorporated phonological awareness and decoding was more effective than the traditional sight word approach.

In order to decode, a learner looks at the letters in a word in sequence, recalls the sound of each of the letters, blends the sounds together in sequence, and determines the target word. In most literacy curricula, students say the letter sounds aloud when decoding and then blend the sounds and say the target word orally. Instruction in decoding for individuals with CCN requires adaptations to bypass the need for oral responses. For example, a student may 1) look at the letters of the word in sequence; 2) recall the sounds of the letters and use subvocal rehearsal to blend the sounds together to determine the target word; and then 3) indicate the target word by signing it, using a speech approximation (if it can be understood by the instructor in context) or by selecting an AAC symbol (e.g., photograph, line drawing, or other aided symbol) from a group provided for the instructional task or from an aided AAC system (Light, McNaughton & Fallon, 2009a). Figure 12.3 provides an example of a symbol array that can be used for decoding instruction. In addition to decoding instruction that focuses on converting the individual letters in words into their corresponding sounds, students with CCN may also be introduced to frequently occurring letter combinations or word families (e.g., -at, -in, -up families of words; Hanser & Erickson, 2007).

A number of studies have investigated the effects of direct instruction on single word decoding and have yielded the following results: 1) individuals with CCN can successfully learn to decode words, despite their severe speech impairments; 2) many are able to generalize decoding skills to novel words that were not previously targeted in instruction; and 3) many are able to successfully apply decoding skills in the context of book reading activities (e.g., Coleman-Martin, Heller, Cihak, & Irvine, 2005; Fallon et al., 2004; Heller, Fredrick, Tumlin, & Brineman, 2002; Light & McNaughton, 2009a, 2011; Swinehart-Jones & Heller, 2009). These positive results extended to both instructor-mediated and computer-mediated instruction and have been demonstrated across word corpuses of various sizes (10 words to more than 100 words) and across participants of a wide range of ages (ages 3–22) with various disabilities (e.g., autism spectrum disorders, cerebral palsy, Down syndrome, childhood apraxia of speech).

Sight Word Recognition Skills

In order to become competent readers, individuals with CCN must be able to read both regular words (i.e., words that are made up of letters that can be decoded using knowledge of letter sounds and sound blending, such as *cat*) and irregular words (i.e., words that cannot easily be decoded using knowledge of letter sounds and sound blending, such as *light*). Thus, students need to develop sight word recognition skills in order to read words with irregular or complex spellings. Literacy intervention is most effective if instruction in sight word recognition is paired with instruction in phonological awareness and decoding skills (Browder, Ahlgrim-Delzell, et al., 2008). In addition to learning sight word recognition skills to read frequently occurring irregular words (e.g., *the, are*), individuals with CCN can also benefit from instruction in sight word recognition of high-interest words that are governed by more complex rules that they have not yet learned how to decode (e.g., *Darth Vader, dinosaur, friend*).

Bren has autism. He was 12 years old when he first started literacy instruction. He was very interested in YouTube. In order to build his motivation early in instruction, we introduced him to *youtube* as a sight word. He quickly learned to read the word *youtube* in personalized storybooks and is learning to type *youtube* to access this site on the Internet. We also adapted the sequence for teaching letter–sound correspondences and taught him first the letter sound of *y* at the start of a word because it was a preferred and highly motivating letter sound. View the Pennsylvania State University webcast *Improving Literacy Outcomes for Individuals with Autism Spectrum Disorders and Limited Speech* to learn more about Bren as he learned to read and type.

Numerous research studies have demonstrated that learners with CCN and those with moderate and severe cognitive impairments can learn to recognize sight words with appropriate instruction (e.g., Browder, Wakeman, Spooner, Ahlgrim-Delzell, &

Algozzine, 2006; Browder & Xin, 1998; Fossett & Mirenda, 2006; Hanser & Erickson, 2007; Light & McNaughton, 2009a, 2011; Light, McNaughton, et al., 2008). In general, the strongest evidence supports direct instruction in sight word recognition skills (incorporating systematic prompting and prompt fading) along with repeated opportunities to practice these skills (Browder et al., 2006). Instruction in sight word recognition skills typically relies on some form of paired associate learning whereby the individual learns to match the target written word to a picture, photograph, or other AAC symbol representing the word (Light & McNaughton, 2009a). Of course, some sight words are not easily imaged (e.g., *the, there*), and these words may be best taught in direct association with the spoken word. As with other skills, instruction in sight word recognition should continue until students are fluent and reading responses are automatic.

Application of Decoding and Sight Word Recognition Skills During Shared Reading

As recommended by the NRP (2000), in order to maximize literacy outcomes, direct instruction in basic literacy skills (e.g., phonological awareness skills, letter–sound correspondences, decoding, sight word recognition) should be combined with numerous opportunities to apply these skills in the context of meaningful, authentic literacy activities. As soon as individuals with CCN learn to read (i.e., decode or recognize by sight) a few words in isolation, they should have the opportunity to apply these skills during shared book reading activities. In shared book reading, a partner reads a story, pausing at key words that are targeted for the learner to decode or recognize by sight. For example, Figure 12.4 presents a page from a book about Halloween that was developed for shared reading. In this example, the partner reads the text, "I am a lady...," tracking the words with a finger, and then pauses at the target word, "bug," for the learner to decode it and then sign it, say it with a speech approximation (if it can be understood in context), or select an AAC symbol for the word from an array of options.

Shared reading activities are powerful teaching tools during the early stages of literacy instruction before the learner has acquired sufficient skills to read a book

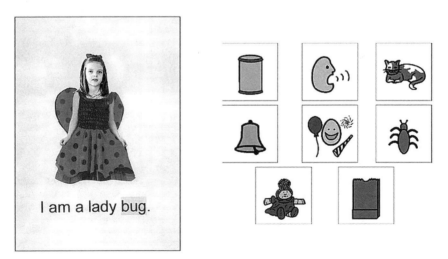

Figure 12.4.   A page from a Halloween book for shared reading. The instructor reads the text, "I am a lady," and pauses. The student decodes the target word, *bug,* and selects the appropriate AAC symbol from the communication display. Photo and symbols on the actual display should be in color. (*Source:* Light & McNaughton, 2009a; http://aacliteracy.psu.edu/. The Picture Communication Symbols ©1981–2012 by DynaVox Mayer-Johnson LLC. All Rights Reserved Worldwide. Used with permission.)

independently, or when reading an entire sentence is a highly effortful process. In shared reading activities, as the name suggests, the task of reading the text is shared between the partner and the learner, thus ensuring that the learner has numerous opportunities to practice reading skills in meaningful contexts without being overwhelmed. Shared reading offers numerous benefits: 1) it allows learners to actively participate in reading activities early in instruction, well before they are able to read full sentences or stories independently; 2) it provides opportunities for learners to apply basic literacy skills in meaningful and motivating reading activities, thus increasing motivation for learning; 3) it provides opportunities for additional practice in basic skills, thus building fluency; and 4) it promotes generalization of basic literacy skills across different reading materials and activities.

A variety of materials can be used for shared reading activities. For example, an instructor or parent can review simple books or magazines and highlight the words in the text that the learner is able to decode (or recognize by sight) using a highlighter pen. Commercially available books (e.g., the *I Spy* series) or magazines can be adapted so that the text includes words that can be decoded or recognized by sight by the learner. For example, the text of an *I Spy* book might be adapted to read, "I spy a *bus*," with the student expected to decode the highlighted word, *bus,* and then select the picture of the bus from the book. Simple books can also be easily created for individual learners, using photos of family events or motivating activities or using images of favorite book or TV characters from the Internet. The Pennsylvania State University web site for Literacy Instruction for Individuals with Autism, Cerebral Palsy, Down Syndrome and Other Disabilities has a Shared Reading web page with examples of books used for shared reading and of students participating in shared reading activities. The Tar Heel Reader collection provides free, easy-to-read, accessible books that can be downloaded in a variety of formats. The books can be speech enabled and accessed using multiple interfaces. Parents and professionals can write new books using their own pictures, and they can upload the books to the site to share with others.

Several researchers have investigated the generalization of decoding and/or sight word recognition skills to shared reading activities. Fallon et al. (2004) found that four of five participants were able to generalize single-word decoding skills that were learned in isolation and apply them successfully during shared reading activities. Light and McNaughton (2009a, 2011) investigated the effects of direct instruction in single-word decoding and sight word recognition skills paired with opportunities to apply these skills during shared reading and found that all of the participants successfully generalized these skills to a wide range of shared reading materials. As the students in this study demonstrated greater competence and fluency, the instructor targeted more words per page, gradually increasing the learning demands on the participants.

Reading and Understanding Simple Sentences and Stories

Once students are able to reliably and fluently decode and/or recognize by sight a range of words, they are ready to accept more responsibility for reading sentences and stories independently. Learning to read connected text is more complicated than simply decoding single words or recognizing single words by sight (Erickson et al., 1997). In order to read sentences and simple stories successfully, learners must 1) track through the words in the text in sequence from left to right, 2) decode or recognize by sight each word in the sentence, 3) recall the meaning of each word, and 4) process the words together to derive the meaning of the full text. Ultimately, learners must also be able to relate the text to their prior knowledge and experience to derive a full understanding. Learning to read connected text imposes greater demands on the learner's language skills than single-word decoding or sight word recognition skills. Specifically, the learner must have the vocabulary knowledge required to access the meaning of the words and the syntactic and morphological knowledge required to derive the meaning of the sentence (Adams, 1994).

Whereas typically developing children usually enter literacy instruction with a strong foundation in their receptive and expressive language skills, many individuals with CCN are at risk for deficits in their semantic, syntactic, and morphological skills due to limited expressive experiences and/or limited language input (Binger & Light, 2008; Light, 1997). They may therefore require focused instruction to successfully read and understand sentences and simple stories. Initially, such intervention should focus on ensuring basic literal comprehension skills; later more complex inference skills can be targeted. Light and McNaughton (2010) described a set of intervention procedures that are aimed at teaching a learner to read and comprehend simple sentences. First, the instructor presents three or more photographs, pictures, or illustrations from a story; the pictures include one that illustrates the meaning of a written sentence as well as several foils (i.e., incorrect responses) that are carefully selected to ensure that learners are reading the entire sentence accurately. The learner's task is to read the sentence independently and then select the picture that represents its complete meaning. Initial research suggests the efficacy of these adapted procedures in building basic comprehension skills.

As students develop accuracy and fluency at reading and understanding sentences, they can begin to read simple books independently. Reading simple stories requires learners not only to use basic literacy skills and semantic, syntactic, and morphological language skills, but also to draw on narrative skills to understand the relationships across sentences in order to build the meaning of the entire story (i.e., the situation, problem or complication, resolution, and denouement). Initially, instruction should focus on ensuring comprehension of each stage of the story before moving on to the next stage. As students face increased demands on reading comprehension, they will benefit from instruction in reading comprehension strategies (NRP, 2000). We discuss strategies for teaching more advanced reading comprehension strategies in a later section of this chapter.

Anna was 3 years old when she started literacy intervention. She had autism and had limited speech. She was using the Picture Exchange Communication System (PECS) to make simple requests but was limited in her expressive vocabulary and typically communicated in telegraphic single-word messages. Once Anna learned to decode or recognize by sight a wide range of words, we started to work on reading and understanding sentences. We focused on very simple sentences first (e.g., 2–3 word sentences), and we used familiar experiences to limit the cognitive and linguistic demands. We provided Anna with a range of photos of her family engaged in different activities (e.g., photos representing *mom naps, mom runs, dad naps*). We then presented Anna with a written sentence (e.g., *mom naps*). Anna had to read the sentence independently and then choose the photo that represented the meaning of the sentence. The response options provided were carefully selected so that Anna could not simply rely on reading and understanding a single word; rather, she had to read each word in the sentence and then derive the meaning of the full sentence. To learn more about Anna's success and to see videos of her literacy instruction, view the Pennsylvania State University webcast *Improving Literacy Outcomes for Individuals with Autism Spectrum Disorders and Limited Speech.*

Interventions to Teach Basic Writing Skills

Literacy skills encompass not only reading but also writing skills. Writing skills have assumed greater importance with society's increased reliance on electronic and wireless communication for education, employment, and social interaction (DeRuyter, McNaughton, Caves, Bryen, & Williams, 2007). Once individuals with CCN develop competence in written communication, they significantly expand the range and power of their communication. Unfortunately, writing instruction is frequently neglected for these individuals (Millar et al., 2004).

Learning to write depends on the integration of knowledge and skills across a variety of domains: 1) world knowledge and experience in order to have something to write about; 2) narrative skills to develop a cohesive story with a clear situation, problem, and resolution (or skills in another writing genre); 3) language skills (semantic, morphological, and syntactic knowledge) to express each part of the story clearly; 4) phoneme segmentation skills to break down the words in the sentences into their component sounds; 5) knowledge of letter–sound correspondences to know which letters represent these component sounds; 6) knowledge of the spellings of irregular frequently occurring words learned as sight words; and 7) skills in handwriting, keyboarding, or other access techniques to produce or locate and select the required letters and/or words (Light & McNaughton, 2009a). This process is more challenging than learning to read because it requires students to hold a significant amount of information in working memory (e.g., the story, the specific sentence within the story, the target word within that sentence, the letters to spell the target word) and at the same time encode text dynamically by selecting from a keyboard (or producing via handwriting) the required sequence of letters to form the words in each sentence of the story. The working memory demands are further increased for individuals who have motor impairments because the process of encoding (i.e., selecting letters from the keyboard or producing letters) may be slow and effortful for them (Millar et al., 2004). Obviously, concerted intervention is required to build writing skills with individuals with CCN. This intervention has two essential components: 1) access to appropriate writing tools and 2) appropriate and effective instruction in writing skills.

As individuals with CCN develop their literacy skills, written language can be used as a means not only to build further literacy skills but also to teach specific language skills, especially morphological/syntactic structures. Prior to literacy instruction, Jackson, a 4-year-old with Down syndrome, communicated telegraphically using speech and signs. As he learned to read simple sentences that included articles (e.g., *the, a*), he began to generalize use of these articles to his expressive communication as well. Similarly, Anna, mentioned in the previous case study, learned at age 4 to use the third-person singular present-tense verb ending (i.e., adding -s to the verb, as in *dad hugs*) through literacy activities. It was easier to teach Anna such abstract language structures through writing because the structure was presented not just orally but also visually. The written presentation of morphology/syntax was permanent, allowing Anna increased time to discern the relevant pattern, which facilitated learning. Visit the Pennsylvania State University Literacy Instruction for Young Children with Autism, Cerebral Palsy, Down Syndrome and Other Disabilities web site to view a video of Jackson as well as the Pennsylvania State University webcast *Improving Literacy Outcomes for Individuals with Autism Spectrum Disorders and Limited Speech* to view videos of Anna learning language through writing.

Access to Writing Tools

As discussed previously in this chapter, individuals with CCN require access to a range of writing tools early on during the emergent stage of literacy development (e.g., writing implements such as pencils and markers with adaptations to assist with grip as required, as well as keyboard access with letter sounds as output). As students with CCN transition to learning conventional literacy skills, they will benefit from consistent access to an appropriate keyboard(s) that meets their needs and skills, as well as to letter cards and a word wall or word banks of high-interest words that are difficult to spell (e.g., *Power Ranger, Tyrannosaurus rex*) and frequently occurring irregular words (e.g., *walk, friend, their;* Hanser & Erickson, 2007). Input from occupational or physical therapists and other members of the AAC team will be required to determine the most appropriate layout and configuration for the keyboard as well as the most appropriate access method (see Chapters 4 and 6). In addition to designing keyboards to facilitate access and accommodate visual and / or motor impairments, keyboards may also be adapted to facilitate early literacy learning. For example, Figure 12.5 presents an example of a standard keyboard adapted for an adolescent with autism. The keyboard presents the letters in lowercase and highlights the 11 letter sounds that the student has acquired; letters were added incrementally as the student acquired new letter sounds. Care should be taken to ensure that keyboard access is not overly taxing or it will detract from the learning of writing skills.

Bren, a 12-year-old with autism, started instruction in writing skills as soon as he had acquired some phoneme segmentation skills and knew about 6–7 letter–sound corre-spondences. The Pennsylvania State University webcast *Improving Literacy Outcomes for Individuals with Autism Spectrum Disorders and Limited Speech* includes a video of Bren learning to type his name with guided practice. In the video, Bren uses an adapted keyboard such as the one illustrated in Figure 12.5. As he acquires each new letter sound, it is highlighted on the adapted keyboard so that he can type more words and build his keyboard knowledge incrementally. As he learns uppercase letters, he will transition to a standard keyboard.

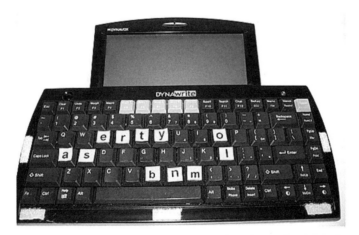

Figure 12.5.   An adapted keyboard designed for an adolescent with autism. The keyboard uses lowercase letters, with the 11 letter sounds that the student has acquired highlighted.

Instruction and Opportunities to Use Basic Writing Skills

Simply providing access to appropriate writing tools does not ensure the acquisition of effective writing skills; rather, focused instruction is required to build these skills. As with reading, instruction in writing should integrate two components: 1) direct instruction in basic writing skills (i.e., phoneme segmentation, letter–sound correspondences, single-word encoding/spelling skills) and 2) numerous opportunities to apply these skills in the context of meaningful authentic writing experiences (Millar et al., 2004; NRP, 2000).

The development of writing skills rests on phonological awareness skills (specifically phoneme segmentation skills) and knowledge of letter–sound correspondences, as discussed previously in this chapter. Once students have acquired phoneme segmentation skills and know some letter–sound correspondences, they are ready to learn to integrate these skills to encode or spell simple regular words. Typically, instruction in single-word encoding/spelling combines practice in phonological awareness skills and letter–sound correspondences with instruction in the integration of these skills to encode words (e.g., Blischak et al., 2004; Johnston, Davenport, et al., 2009). Light and McNaughton (2010) described adapted procedures for direct instruction in single word encoding/spelling as follows:

1. First, the instructor models single-word encoding skills by slowly saying a word out loud, extending each sound in the word, and selecting the corresponding letter for each sound as it is said.

2. Then, the instructor provides guided practice in encoding, saying the word slowly, and holding each of the sounds in the word while the student selects the corresponding letter from a keyboard (or from an array of letters).

3. Over time, the instructor gradually fades the oral scaffolding support (e.g., says the word in a quieter voice) as the student learns the skill.

4. As the student develops competence, he or she is given opportunities to practice encoding skills independently, without scaffolding support.

5. The instructor provides feedback to the student as appropriate.

Research supports the conclusion that, with appropriate instruction, students with CCN can demonstrate increases in the number of correct letter sequences and the number of words they spell correctly (e.g., Blischak et al., 2004; Johnston, Davenport, et al., 2009; Light & McNaughton, 2010; Millar et al., 2004). Often, instruction in encoding is organized around word families that end in the same letter combinations (e.g., the *-an* family includes words such as *can, man,* and *ran*) in order to promote generalization of spelling skills to new words that were not previously taught (Hanser & Erickson, 2007).

Individuals with CCN require numerous opportunities to apply basic encoding skills in the context of meaningful writing activities (Erickson & Koppenhaver, 1995; Foley & Wolter, 2010; Millar et al., 2004). Light, McNaughton, et al. (2008) cautioned that individuals with CCN can be easily overwhelmed by the multitude of demands during early writing activities, including demands on narrative skills; semantic, syntactic, and morphological skills; encoding/spelling skills; and/or keyboarding skills. They recommended exploring techniques such as the following to reduce demands in some of these areas as students acquire new skills: 1) reading books with repeated lines or story structures (e.g., *Brown Bear, Brown Bear, What Do You See?*) and having students use the repeated lines to structure and write their own stories, filling in their own content words (e.g., *Red pig, red pig, what do you see? I see a pink bug looking at me*);

2) using photos of highly motivating personal experiences as a basis for writing, thus providing familiar content and a familiar narrative structure as well as visual supports for generating content (i.e., a simple story with a beginning, middle, and end); 3) providing students with easily accessible models of high-frequency and high-interest words for use in their writing through a word wall or word bank (see Hanser & Erickson, 2007); and 4) using shared writing, wherein the instructor and student co-construct a story, with the student assuming responsibility for generating text and encoding regular words and the instructor providing scaffolding support to assist with encoding more complex and irregular words. As discussed earlier, students may benefit from modeling, guided practice (with scaffolding support from the instructor), and then independent practice in writing as they develop greater competence. The texts written by students can be printed as books and/or scanned into AAC technologies; the books can then be used for repeated readings with teachers, families, and peers.

The emphasis at this stage of development is the student's communication of meaning through written texts. The instructor recognizes the communicative intent of sound spellings and provides models of conventional spellings as appropriate (Foley & Wolter, 2010). Ultimately, students with CCN also require instruction in the conventional spellings of frequently occurring irregular words; these words may be introduced following the same sequence as the school curriculum. We discuss spelling instruction in a later section of this chapter.

Michael, a 4-year-old with autism, had been involved in literacy instruction for approximately 1 year. He had learned letter–sound correspondences, phoneme segmentation skills, decoding skills, and sight word recognition skills during this time. After reading a book about a robot dog, Michael wrote the following story using his newly acquired language and literacy skills:

   robot dog will fetch my gren powr ranger [Robot Dog will fetch my green Power Ranger.]
   robob dog is gowg to plae [Robot Dog is going to play.]
   robot dog haz tim ot becuz he duzut lisin [Robot Dog has time out because he doesn't listen.]

Visit the Student Success Stories section of the Pennsylvania State University web site for Literacy Instruction for Individuals with Autism, Cerebral Palsy, Down Syndrome and Other Disabilities to learn more about Michael's literacy journey.

TEACHING ADVANCED LITERACY SKILLS

Whereas the focus of the first 3 years of school is on learning to read and write, the focus of subsequent years of education is typically on reading and writing to learn (Graham & Perin, 2007; NRP, 2000). Literacy skills are the principal means by which students acquire new information and through which their learning is assessed (Foley & Wolter, 2010). This section of the chapter focuses on intervention to build more advanced literacy skills with individuals with CCN, with a specific focus on the development of reading comprehension and writing strategies. There has been limited published research investigating interventions to teach advanced literacy skills to individuals with CCN. Therefore, this section of the chapter draws heavily on the research on interventions for individuals who are at risk in the area of literacy development but who are able to use speech to communicate (e.g., Graham & Perin, 2007; NRP, 2000). Adaptations to these interventions are proposed to facilitate the participation of individuals with CCN and are based—at least in part—on anecdotal reports and case descriptions (e.g., Bedrosian, Lasker, Speidel, & Politsch, 2003; Blischak, 1995). Future research is urgently required to empirically validate these adapted interventions and to investigate the effectiveness of other interventions to build more advanced literacy skills with individuals with CCN.

Intervention to Build More Advanced Reading Skills

Ultimately, the goal of literacy instruction is for students to be able to understand and learn from a wide range of texts. The process of building reading comprehension skills should start early, during the stage of emergent literacy development, as parents or teachers read with children with CCN and discuss books to build the children's comprehension skills. As students develop greater competence in basic reading skills (i.e., decoding and sight word recognition), the focus can shift to ensuring that they are able to construct meaningful representations of the texts as they read, relate the texts to their own experiences and prior knowledge, and use the information they have read for a wide range of purposes (NRP, 2000). Building reading comprehension skills is a complex process that integrates competencies in four domains: 1) the ability to apply decoding and sight word recognition skills fluently; 2) the ability to understand the vocabulary, sentence structures, and text structures (e.g., narrative, expository, persuasive) that are read; 3) the ability to activate and apply world knowledge and domain-specific knowledge related to the text; and 4) the metacognitive skills to monitor comprehension and utilize appropriate comprehension strategies to ensure understanding (Copeland, 2007).

Building Fluency in Basic Reading Skills

At this stage of development, most students have learned to decode and recognize by sight a large corpus of words. They continue to build their decoding skills (e.g., learning to tackle more complex multisyllabic words), and they continue to expand the scope of their sight word recognition skills. With ongoing practice reading texts, students build fluency in decoding and sight word recognition skills, one of the key components of literacy instruction (NRP, 2000). Fluency and text comprehension are highly correlated (Fuchs, Fuchs, Hosp, & Jenkins, 2001). Students who are able to decode and recognize words by sight quickly and accurately are better able to devote their cognitive resources to understanding the text and relating it to their own experiences. Students who are not fluent in these tasks must devote significant effort to decoding and sight word recognition, leaving few cognitive resources available for reading comprehension.

A variety of techniques can be used to build fluency in decoding and sight word recognition skills, including 1) repeated readings of texts that are at the student's independent reading level, 2) reading along with audio recordings or multimedia presentations of texts, and 3) paired readings wherein fluent readers read aloud with less fluent readers (Foley & Wolter, 2010). Many students with CCN do not have sufficiently intelligible and fluent speech to participate in these oral/choral reading activities. Erickson and Koppenhaver (2007) recommended that students with CCN be encouraged to read silently during these activities, using subvocal speech (inner voice) as the group, partner, or tape reads the text aloud. These techniques all focus on providing repeated practice in basic skills in the context of meaningful reading activities and thus aid in the development of fluency. For students who have significant difficulty reading independently, assistive technologies or other supports (e.g., screen readers, digital texts, audiobooks) may be required to bypass reading demands and provide access to instructional content (see the section on assistive technologies for further discussion).

Building More Advanced Language Skills

Simply recognizing or decoding words fluently is not sufficient to ensure reading comprehension; in addition, students must also be able to understand the meanings of these words, the sentence structures, and the entire narrative or other written genre. Unfortunately, many students who rely on AAC may have limited language skills due to their restricted expressive language experiences and the reduced language input they may receive (Light, 1997). Concerted language intervention is required from an early age to build the semantic, syntactic, morphological, and narrative skills required to support reading comprehension (see Chapters 10 and 11 for further discussion). The language of written communication differs from that of conversation, using a wider range of vocabulary and more complex sentence structures. Ironically, the development of advanced language skills is enhanced through reading: The more students read, the more advanced their language skills become (Foley & Wolter, 2010). Reading books to individuals with CCN and discussing the texts provides an excellent opportunity to introduce new vocabulary and sentence structures systematically, in order to build the more advanced language skills required for reading comprehension. This broad-based intervention should be supplemented by focused instruction to teach specific vocabulary, sentence structures, or genres as required (Sturm & Clendon, 2004).

Developing World Knowledge and Domain-Specific Knowledge

In addition to language skills, students with CCN also require a well-developed base of world knowledge to bolster their comprehension of written texts. Relevant experiential and world knowledge allows students to use context to derive the meaning of unknown words, anticipate events and consequences, and quickly build understanding of texts. Unfortunately, many students with CCN have limited world knowledge due to architectural barriers, attitudinal barriers, health constraints, manipulation and mobility impairments, and limited communication opportunities. Without access to relevant prior knowledge, it is much more difficult and effortful to build understanding of written texts. Ironically, as with language skills, world knowledge and domain-specific knowledge are best built by reading a wide range of texts. In order to provide access to a greater range of books, individuals with CCN might benefit from access to audiobooks, multimedia presentations of texts, and screen readers as well as having teachers, parents, peers, and peer tutors read to them. It is important to note that simply listening to texts is not sufficient to build world knowledge; rather, students need to process text actively by talking with others and relating the new information to prior experiences. All of these activities will serve not only to expand their language skills but also to build their world knowledge and domain-specific knowledge.

Monitoring Comprehension and Utilizing Reading Comprehension Strategies

As students progress in their education, they encounter even greater reading demands: a greater number of books covering a wide range of topics, longer books that use more complex vocabulary and sentences, and books from a wide range of genres (e.g., expository, narrative, persuasive). These increased reading demands place greater demands on reading comprehension skills, especially for those students who may not have well-developed fluency, language skills, and/or world knowledge. The strain on reading comprehension skills may be further aggravated because many textbooks are poorly organized, contain extraneous content that detracts from key concepts, and assume wide-ranging prior knowledge (Boone & Higgins, 2007).

Students at all grade levels—especially those who are at risk in the area of reading comprehension, as students with CCN may be—benefit from instruction in reading comprehension strategies (Gersten, Fuchs, Williams, & Baker, 2001; NRP, 2000). Reading comprehension strategies are "specific cognitive procedures that guide students to become aware of how well they are comprehending as they attempt to read (and write)" (NRP, 2000, p. 40). Research suggests that students who use these strategies demonstrate significant gains in comprehension as a result (Gersten et al., 2001). Table 12.6 provides a list of evidence-based reading comprehension strategies that may benefit individuals who rely on AAC, along with adaptations to meet the specific needs of these students: comprehension monitoring, summarization, graphic and semantic organizers, question answering, question generation, and recognition of text structures (Armbruster, Lehr, & Osborn, 2001; NRP, 2000). Students with CCN benefit

Table 12.6. Strategies to support reading comprehension and adaptations for students with complex communication needs (CCN)

Reading comprehension strategy	Adaptations for individuals with CCN
Comprehension monitoring • Stop at regular intervals while reading • Check understanding of text	Use written words or augmentative and alternative communication (AAC) symbols as visual prompts to stop reading and check understanding
Summarization • Identify key ideas from text (e.g., who? did what?) • Eliminate irrelevant details	Use written words or AAC symbols as prompts to summarize the main idea Select the best summary from three or more summaries provided Put sentence strips in the correct sequence to summarize the story
Graphic and semantic organizers • Use organizational aids to map out the content of the text • Illustrate the structure of the text visually using a story map	Use software-based concept maps to illustrate story structure (provide assistance with navigation/formatting as required) Complete graphic organizer in collaboration with peer recorder
Question answering • Answer questions (both literal and inference) about the text • Receive immediate feedback on responses	Use AAC systems to generate responses to open-ended questions Use multiple-choice questions to increase efficiency and reduce fatigue Use question-and-answer matching
Question generation • Think about the topic prior to reading or while reading • Think of relevant questions about the text • Respond to questions while reading	Use AAC systems to generate questions Allow student to select questions of interest from an array of choices provided
Recognition of text structures • Determine the genre of the text (e.g., narrative, expository) • Determine the elements of the genre (e.g., setting, characters, problem, resolution)	Provide choices of written genres; program relevant vocabulary into AAC systems Preprogram question prompts for story elements into AAC systems (e.g., *Where does the story take place? What happens first?*) Use storyboards listing story elements

Sources: Bedrosian, Lasker, et al. (2003); Erickson (2003); Light and McNaughton (2009a, 2009b).

from learning multiple reading comprehension strategies because different strategies may be needed for different types of texts and different task requirements or assignments.

Learning to use reading comprehension strategies requires learners to integrate knowledge and skills in a multistep process to actively process information as they read, thus promoting comprehension and retention (Gersten et al., 2001). The University of Kansas Center for Research on Learning has developed a comprehensive, scientifically based model that can be used to teach reading comprehension strategies and that includes the following components (Deshler & Schumaker, 2006):

1. Conduct a pretest to determine the learner's use of the strategy prior to initiating instruction.

2. Obtain the learner's commitment to learning the strategy.

3. Describe the strategy and discuss its benefits.

4. Model or demonstrate use of the strategy, providing think-aloud explanations of the steps as they are performed.

5. Practice naming the steps of the strategy.

6. Provide the learner with guided practice in the use of the strategy with scaffolding support provided by the instructor as required to ensure the learner's success.

7. Fade support as the student learns the strategy.

8. Provide numerous opportunities for the student to practice the strategy independently with corrective feedback as required.

9. Provide practice in strategy use under increasingly more complex conditions (e.g., with more complex texts, in classroom conditions with various distractions).

10. Plan explicitly with the student to build generalization and maintenance of the strategy.

Gareth, a 5-year-old boy with severe cerebral palsy, learned to read before he started kindergarten. He was introduced to basic reading comprehension strategies early in his literacy instruction. As he read each page or section of a story independently, he stopped to answer questions to ensure comprehension before he went on to read the next section. We used multiple-choice questions (with carefully selected response options) so that Gareth could quickly and easily indicate his answer. For example, when reading a book about Clifford the dog, Gareth first read the text independently. Then he answered multiple-choice questions such as the following:

Why will Clifford win?

a) The dogs will race
b) Clifford is big and fast
c) Clifford is red
d) Clifford will win

This technique provided a quick check of Gareth's comprehension without making undue demands that would result in fatigue. This question-answering strategy also mirrored the demands that Gareth would face later on in many standardized tests. Questions that required both basic factual comprehension as well as inference skills could be quickly developed by Gareth's teacher or aide during the reading activity, thus minimizing demands for material preparation. Read more about Gareth and see videos of his use of this strategy in the Reading Comprehension section of the Pennsylvania State University web site for Literacy Instruction for Individuals with Autism, Cerebral Palsy, Down Syndrome and Other Disabilities.

Intervention to Build More Advanced Writing Skills

As students progress through school and consider future employment, they face increased writing demands. In third grade and thereafter, writing is the most common method used to communicate information and assess students' knowledge and learning. Writing not only allows students to convey information to others (e.g., tell stories, explain events, express opinions, persuade others) but also provides a mechanism to support student learning and understanding. As students write about a topic, they extend and deepen their knowledge (Graham & Perin, 2007). As the educational and vocational writing demands increase, students with CCN must be able to generate increasingly longer texts for a variety of purposes, using more complex vocabulary and sentence structures (Foley & Wolter, 2010). Meeting these writing demands requires well-developed knowledge and skills in 1) the conventions of writing, including spelling, punctuation, capitalization, and text production/keyboarding; and 2) the use of writing strategies to plan, write, and edit texts effectively across genres (e.g., narrative, expository, persuasive; Light & McNaughton, 2009b).

Although there are examples of individuals with CCN who have well-developed writing skills (e.g., Koppenhaver et al., 1991), many individuals who rely on AAC demonstrate difficulties with written communication. For example, Kelford Smith et al. (1989) investigated the written communication skills of six individuals (ages 13–22) who had cerebral palsy and relied on AAC. They reported that 1) the participants produced a limited amount of written communication in a one-week period; 2) the participants required significant amounts of time to plan, generate, and revise written texts; 3) the participants demonstrated difficulties with morphology; and 4) all but one participant demonstrated difficulties with sentence structures. Focused intervention is required to build advanced writing skills with individuals with CCN. This intervention should focus on instruction in the conventions of writing as well as instruction in the use of writing strategies.

Building Knowledge and Skills in Writing Conventions

In order to produce competent, intelligible written texts, students who rely on AAC need to develop skills in spelling (both regular and irregular words) as well as knowledge of the conventions of writing such as capitalization, punctuation, and paragraphing. Instruction in these skills should be ongoing, starting in the early stages of learning conventional literacy skills. As students acquire basic skills, the focus of instruction turns to the development of more complex spelling skills (e.g., long vowel patterns, multisyllabic words with prefixes and suffixes, homonyms) and word study skills (e.g., derivations of words, word meanings) as well as the acquisition of more advanced writing conventions (e.g., use of punctuation, paragraphs). As noted earlier, spelling skills rely heavily on phonological awareness skills and knowledge of letter–sound correspondences. Some individuals with severe speech impairments have difficulty applying their phonological awareness skills to spell words (Hart, Scherz, Apel, & Hodson, 2007); however, there is evidence that individuals who rely on AAC benefit from explicit instruction in spelling (McNaughton & Tawney, 1993; Schlosser, Blischak, Belfiore, Bartley, & Barnett, 1998). In addition, Blischak and Schlosser (2003) reviewed the effects of speech output (auditory feedback) on the spelling performance of individuals with autism who had limited speech. They found that speech output had a positive effect for at least some participants, leading the researchers to conclude that speech output should be considered as a support for writing instruction.

Along with the acquisition of more advanced skills in spelling and writing conventions, instruction should also focus on the development of fluency with writing conventions (e.g., spelling skills, punctuation, handwriting, keyboarding or other operational skills). If these skills remain effortful for individuals with CCN, they will have few cognitive resources available to support the actual writing process (i.e., the planning, drafting, and revising of written texts); instead, all of their attention and cognitive resources will be consumed by the conventions of spelling and selecting/producing letters to create written text. As noted earlier, fluency is built through practice. As these skills become more automatic, students who rely on AAC will be able to devote their attention and cognitive resources to the content of the writing process rather than the mechanics. Although all students benefit from numerous opportunities to produce written texts, it should be noted that for many individuals with CCN—especially those with significant motor, sensory/perceptual, and/or cognitive impairments—the process of producing written text can be especially challenging. As noted by Foley and Wolter (2010), these writers may fatigue easily and may have difficulty sustaining their attention to the writing task. For students who have significant difficulty producing text, assistive technologies may be required to provide scaffolding supports, enhance rate, and/or provide spelling and writing aids (see the section on assistive technologies for further discussion).

Learning to Use Writing Strategies

Skilled writing extends well beyond the simple mechanics of producing written text. In order to successfully produce longer, more complex texts, students must engage in an iterative writing process that includes reflection, production, and interpretation (Hayes, 2000). First, students plan and organize the text by reflecting on their ideas and experiences, as well as their goal or purpose; then, they translate their thoughts into written language and produce the text (by handwriting or keyboarding); and, finally, they review what they have written, reflect on their goal, and then revise accordingly. As with the development of more advanced reading skills and as writing demands increase, students benefit from the use of writing strategies to enhance their skills. Research demonstrates that learning writing strategies can result in positive gains in writing skills for middle school and high school students with and without disabilities (Graham & Perin, 2007). Typically, writing strategies provide multistep procedures to support each stage of the writing process—planning, writing the text, and editing (see Table 12.7 for examples of writing strategies at each of the stages). Like reading comprehension strategies, these types of writing strategies can be taught using a cognitive strategy instruction model (Deshler & Schumaker, 2006; Graham & Perin, 2007).

In addition to writing strategies, research suggests that collaborative writing also benefits students both with and without disabilities (Graham & Perin, 2007). Collaborative writing involves the development of "instructional arrangements whereby students work together to plan, draft," and revise their writing (Graham & Perin, 2007, p. 42). Conferencing with peers can serve to encourage students to assume greater responsibility for learning, increase learning of cognitive strategies (specifically writing strategies), provide feedback and supports during the writing process, and increase motivation through social interactions with peers (NRP, 2000). Bedrosian, Lasker, et al. (2003) described a writing intervention for an adolescent with autism who relied on AAC that involved instruction in writing strategies as well as collaborative writing with a speaking peer who had a mild cognitive impairment. Specifically, the intervention included the following components: 1) the provi-

Table 12.7.   Examples of writing strategies to support each stage of writing

Stage of the writing process	Writing strategy	Description
Planning stage	PLAN strategy (De La Paz, Owen, Harris, & Graham, 2000)	**P**ay attention to the writing prompt **L**ist the main ideas **A**dd supporting ideas **N**umber your ideas
Writing/drafting stage	WRITE strategy (De La Paz et al., 2000)	**W**ork from your plan to develop your thesis statement **R**emember your goals **I**nclude transition words for each paragraph **T**ry to use different kinds of sentences **E**xciting, interesting $10,000 words
Editing/revising stage	EDIT strategy (Hughes, Schumaker, McNaughton, Deshler, & Nolan, 2010)	**E**nter your first draft **D**o a spell check **I**nterrogate yourself about capitalization, overall appearance, punctuation, and substance **T**ype in corrections and run the spell checker again

sion of assistive technologies to support writing (i.e., an SGD, story grammar map, storyboards with relevant vocabulary and story starters, and story writing software); 2) explicit instruction in writing strategies; 3) modeling of writing by the instructor and the peer; 4) prompting; and 5) written support provided by peer scaffolding. Results suggested that the intervention had a positive impact on the writing of the adolescent with CCN; his postintervention story was longer and demonstrated more complete story grammar than his preintervention story. These improvements were noted not only in the writing completed collaboratively but also in writing completed independently. Future research is required to further investigate across a wide range of written genres the effects of intervention with individuals who rely on AAC.

From 2003 to 2011, 17 adults with CCN participated in the AAC-RERC (Rehabilitation Engineering Research Center on Communication Enhancement) Writers Brigade. They received coaching and instructional supports to develop effective writing skills. As part of the Writers Brigade, they published, in a wide range of magazines, newsletters, and online resources, more than 120 articles about current research and best practices in AAC. Visit the Writers Brigade web site for more information.

Building Writing Skills for Social Purposes

It is important to note that, as students grow, writing not only assumes increased importance educationally and vocationally but also assumes increased importance socially. For example, teenagers in the United States are now more likely to text friends than to speak with them on the phone, and half of teens send 50 or more text messages a day (Lenhart, Ling, Campbell, & Purcell, 2010). Using electronic communication media (e.g., texting, social networking sites such as Facebook) to build social relationships offers some unique advantages for individuals with CCN because these media allow them to communicate at their own rate and may free them from the negative social attitudes that often limit face-to-face interactions. Written communication via these social media, although often shorter and less formal than writing for educational and vocational purposes, imposes its own set of demands (e.g., use of an appropriate voice for the audience, use of Internet slang such as *LOL* [laugh out loud], *JK* [just kidding], and *IDK* [I don't know]). If students with CCN are to develop and negotiate successful social relationships, they will need to develop the written communication skills as well as the operational skills (e.g., skills to access and create web sites and blogs, skills to upload and download video and images) that allow them to participate effectively via these media as well.

ASSISTIVE TECHNOLOGIES TO SUPPORT LITERACY

In addition to requiring empirically based literacy instruction to develop reading and writing skills, individuals with CCN may also require access to a wide range of assistive technologies to support literacy development, including assistive technologies that provide 1) access to communication, 2) access to literacy instruction, and 3) supports to compensate for reading and writing difficulties. Decisions about assistive technologies should be made by the AAC team in conjunction with the individual and his or her family. Assistive technologies should be customized according to the needs and skills of the individual as well as the communication and literacy demands.

Assistive Technologies for Communication

Individuals with CCN require access to unaided and/or aided AAC systems to allow them to communicate and participate fully within literacy activities and instruction, from the early stage of emergent literacy development through the development of more advanced literacy skills. These AAC systems include those that support written communication (both conventional writing as well as early emergent writing activities) and telecommunication (e.g., texting, e-mail), as well as systems that support face-to-face communication during literacy activities and instruction (e.g., choosing topics, talking about books, answering comprehension questions, summarizing or retelling stories, asking questions about books, expressing opinions). AAC systems must include appropriate vocabulary to support communication during literacy activities and instruction. The communication demands of literacy activities and instruction differ from the functional communication demands in daily life. Individuals with CCN require access to AAC systems that incorporate the more formal semantics, syntax, and morphology of written language as well as the story grammar to structure narratives and build the language foundation that underpins literacy development (e.g., Bedrosian, Lasker, et al., 2003).

In addition to providing a means to support participation and discussion during literacy activities, AAC can also be used as an alternative mode to provide responses during literacy instruction. For example, Light and McNaughton (2009a, 2011) described adaptations that allowed individuals with CCN to use signs or graphic AAC symbols to respond effectively and efficiently during instruction in sound blending, phoneme segmentation, decoding, and/or sight word recognition.

Assistive Technologies for Instruction

In addition to communication, technologies can also be used to further literacy instruction, either in the delivery of computer-assisted instruction or through the provision of instructional supports for literacy learning. For example, Coleman-Martin et al. (2005) investigated the effects of computer-assisted instruction in word recognition skills and concluded that this approach may hold promise for individuals who rely on AAC. Furthermore, there are numerous software applications for computer and mobile technologies (e.g., iPad) that provide instructional activities or games to supplement instruction in letter–sound correspondences, decoding, and encoding activities. Before implementing these applications, it is critical to ensure that they address appropriate instructional goals, use appropriate instructional methods and materials, and are accessible for individuals with CCN who may have motor and/or sensory/perceptual impairments.

Assistive Technologies to Provide Support for Reading and Writing Difficulties

Finally, there are a wide range of technologies that provide the means for individuals with CCN to bypass specific literacy demands or compensate for specific skill deficits. For example, spell checkers can be used to compensate for spelling difficulties; on-screen dictionaries can be used to compensate for vocabulary limitations; linguistic prediction can be used to enhance rate or compensate for spelling limitations; screen readers can be used to compensate for reading difficulties; and software applications with graphic organizers and concept maps (e.g., Inspiration software) can provide visual supports for the planning and organization stage of the writing process. E-books and digital texts also offer a number of advantages for individuals with CCN: 1) text can be easily modified to accommodate visual impairments (e.g., use of larger font size, spacing, or color contrast); 2) text can be read aloud as a support to reading skills; 3) definitions and explanations can be provided for new concepts to support vocabulary development; 4) links can be provided to additional support materials to build world knowledge; and 5) electronic coaching that prompts students to use reading comprehension strategies can be built into the software (Anderson-Inman & Horney, 2007).

It is important to remember that simply providing assistive technology does not ensure successful literacy access for individuals with CCN. By reducing demands in one skill area, assistive technologies may actually increase demands in another. For example, access to texts through screen readers or other electronic media with speech output does not necessarily ensure successful comprehension of texts (Boone & Higgins, 2007). The provision of these assistive technologies simply shifts the comprehension demands from the visual graphic modality of written text to the auditory modality of spoken text. The challenges of vocabulary knowledge, world knowledge, and comprehension monitoring remain, regardless of the modality of presentation. Depending on the individual, this shift in modality may or may not facilitate comprehension and learning. Thus, it is important to ensure that assistive technologies and electronic texts are designed and implemented in ways that minimize the processing demands and maximize motivation and learning for the student (Anderson-Inman & Horney, 2007). As with other assistive technologies, applications of reading and writing technologies are most effective if they are implemented along with effective evidence-based instruction to support their successful use by individuals with CCN.

The CAST (formerly Center for Applied Special Technology) Universal Design for Learning (UDL) Book Builder provides free online tools to develop e-books with many features that are appropriate for students with CCN.

SUMMARY

The acquisition of literacy skills is fundamental to participation in today's society. Literacy skills support cognitive development, facilitate participation in education, increase employment opportunities, promote social relationships, enhance access to a wide range of technologies, and provide access to motivating leisure pursuits. Literacy skills provide even greater benefits for individuals with CCN who have limited access to speech: For these individuals, the acquisition of literacy skills expands communication options significantly, provides visual supports for language learning, enhances perceptions of competence, elevates expectations, and increases self-esteem.

Research has demonstrated that it is indeed possible to provide effective intervention to maximize literacy outcomes for individuals with CCN, starting by first developing emergent literacy skills, then transitioning to learning early conventional literacy skills, and ultimately building advanced literacy skills to support participation in educational, vocational, and community settings. Light and McNaughton (2011) argued that there are five key components to effective literacy intervention:

1. Providing sufficient time for literacy instruction
2. Targeting appropriate skills known to improve literacy outcomes
3. Using proven, effective instructional techniques
4. Providing appropriate instructional adaptations and supports to accommodate the needs and skills of individuals with CCN
5. Building positive rapport and ensuring student motivation for learning

The research discussed within this chapter provides the science that is essential to improve literacy outcomes for individuals with CCN: implementation of evidence-based practices, ongoing data collection, and performance monitoring to ensure the effectiveness of these practices for each individual. However, this science, although essential, is not sufficient on its own to ensure successful outcomes. Tied to this science must be the fundamental belief and commitment to the right of all individuals to have the opportunity to learn and to seek their full potential. Every individual can benefit from participation in literacy activities. Our society has vastly underestimated the learning potential of many individuals with CCN. There is a growing body of research-based evidence demonstrating that individuals who rely on AAC can learn to read and write if they are provided with appropriate instruction. When individuals with CCN can read and write, they have access to a whole new range of educational, vocational, and social opportunities. The acquisition of literacy skills empowers individuals with CCN to meet their life goals.

"I am thankful for one…gift I received early on in life which most people can take for granted: the gift of literacy—of reading and writing, of making sense of the world and having the reciprocal ability of letting the world make sense out of you and come to respect you for all that you have to offer and contribute. This to me is the true gift and power of literacy in each of our lives" (Bob Williams, 2000, p. 247).

QUESTIONS

12.1. What are some of the skills that good readers require? For one of these skills, describe the implication of a skill that is missing or insufficiently developed.

12.2. What are the key intrinsic factors that can impact literacy learning, and which of these factors may be of special concern for individuals with CCN? If an individual has a limitation or impairment related to one of these intrinsic factors, what are the implications for literacy instruction?

12.3. What are the key extrinsic factors that can impact literacy learning, and which of these factors may be of special concern for individuals with CCN? If an individual has a limitation or impairment related to one of these extrinsic factors, what are the implications for literacy instruction?

12.4. Describe the knowledge and skills that children typically acquire during the *emergent* literacy stage of development. What are some of the challenges in providing emergent literacy experiences for children with complex communication needs? Describe some interventions that have been demonstrated to have a positive impact in supporting the participation of children with CCN in emergent literacy activities.

12.5. What are the five key components of effective literacy instruction for children with CCN? For one of these components, describe a challenge commonly experienced by children with CCN, and suggest adaptations that would help to address the challenge.

12.6. What are the benefits of direct instruction for teaching basic literacy skills? What are the benefits of applying basic literacy skills in meaningful authentic literacy activities? What are the benefits of combining both approaches?

12.7. Identify the seven domains of knowledge and skills that are necessary for learning to write. What are the implications of an impairment or limitation in one of these domains, and how might intervention address this challenge?

12.8. Identify the four domains of competency that are necessary for building reading comprehension skills. What are the implications of an impairment or limitation in one of these domains, and how might intervention address this challenge?

CHAPTER 13

Educational Inclusion of Students with Complex Communication Needs

> Education is a specialized form of communication. Human beings have developed particular times and places in which the scripts of their cultures are to be communicated from one generation to the next. We have come to call the set of practices by which this communication of cultural scripts is accomplished "education." The communication that occurs in educational contexts happens in oral, written, verbal, and nonverbal modes....[Our] role is to facilitate the communication, thus the education, that occurs in the classroom. (Hoskins, 1990, p. 29)

Since the publication of the third edition of this book (Beukelman & Mirenda, 2005), three additional texts that are directly related to the education of students with complex communication needs (CCN) have also appeared in print. The first, *Practically Speaking: Language, Literacy, and Academic Development of Students with AAC Needs* (Soto & Zangari, 2009), focuses primarily on assessment and instruction directed at the communication, language, and literacy challenges faced by students who rely on augmentative and alternative communication (AAC) in school settings. The second, *The Beyond Access Model: Promoting Membership, Participation, and Learning for Students with Disabilities in the General Education Classroom* (Jorgensen, McSheehan, & Sonnenmeier, 2010), emphasizes the importance of AAC as a key practice that is required in order to include students with CCN in the general education curriculum. Finally, the third, *Transition Strategies for Adolescents and Young Adults Who Use AAC* (McNaughton & Beukelman, 2010), describes a number of important considerations that school personnel must consider as they prepare adolescents who rely on AAC for the transition from school to adult life.

All three of these books share a common assumption that also forms the basis for this chapter—namely, that "professionals must be committed to providing access to the general education curriculum for all students, regardless of their needs and abilities" (Soto & Zangari, 2009, p. x). At the same time, the authors emphasize that "merely attending a general education class does not automatically confer access to rigorous learning opportunities" (McNaughton & Beukelman, 2010, p. 73) and acknowledge "the challenge of how to make [inclusive education] happen in a meaningful way" (Soto & Zangari, 2009, p. x). Together, these three texts provide far richer and much more detailed information about inclusive education and how to accomplish it than we can possibly include in this single chapter. Rather, our goal is to provide guidelines for thinking about and planning for inclusive education for students with CCN, along with general strategies for how this might be accomplished.

WHAT IS INCLUSIVE EDUCATION?

We use the term *inclusive education* to refer to a number of practices and outcomes that take place primarily in a general education classroom that is populated by students of the same chronological age as the student with CCN. First, inclusive education requires the student to be a member of the class. Membership requires that the student has "access to valued social roles and the symbols of belonging...[that] reflect a vision of equity and reciprocity with classmates who do not have disabilities" (Jorgensen et al., 2010, p. 58). Table 13.1 displays some sample indicators of membership in the general education classroom.

Second, inclusive education requires that all students participate actively in the social and academic activities of the general education classroom. Participation in the social life of the classroom means, for example, that a student with CCN goes out to recess with his or her classmates; has a classroom job if everyone else has one; and attends assemblies, pep rallies, and school dances as often as other students do. Participation in the academic life of the classroom means that, with various types of supports, a student with CCN is engaged in large- and small-group learning activities, answers questions from the teacher, gives oral reports, and completes assignments that are aligned with the general academic curriculum provided to his or her classmates. Table 13.2 provides a summary of indicators of social and academic participation in the inclusive classroom.

Finally, inclusive education means that a student with CCN acquires skills that are meaningful and relevant, across all academic areas. In the United States, access to the general education curriculum for students with disabilities was mandated

Table 13.1. Sample indicators of student membership in the general education classroom

The student attends the school he or she would attend if he or she did not have a disability.

The student is a member of an age-appropriate general education class.

The student's name is on all class lists, lists of groups written on the board, job lists, and so forth.

Related services are delivered primarily through consultation in the classroom.

The student receives the same materials as students without disabilities, with supports (i.e., accommodations, adaptations) provided as necessary.

The student changes classes with other students, arriving and leaving at the same time.

The student has a locker or cubby alongside students without disabilities.

The student rides the same school bus as his or her peers without disabilities.

From Jorgensen, C., McSheehan, M., & Sonnenmeier, R. (2010). *The Beyond Access Model: Promoting membership, participation, and learning for students with disabilities in the general education classroom* (p. 60). Baltimore: Paul H. Brookes Publishing Co.; reprinted by permission.

Table 13.2. Sample indicators of student participation in general education classroom routines, activities, and lessons

The student participates in classroom and school routines (e.g., national anthem, lunch count, jobs, errands, lunch) in typical locations.

The student participates in school plays, field trips, and community service activities.

The student participates in classroom instruction in similar routines as students without disabilities (e.g., whole-class discussions, small groups, board work).

The student is called on to respond to teacher questions as often as students without disabilities are.

The student has a way to communicate the same academic messages that are expected of other students in instructional routines:

- *Whole-class discussions:* brainstorming, answering questions, sharing information when called on, engaging in social side talk, and so forth

- *At the board:* writing answers, drawing figures

- *In small groups:* commenting to classmates, sharing information, socializing, taking notes

The student completes assignments and other work products (with accommodations, as needed) that are the same as or similar to those completed by students without disabilities.

The student engages in outside-of-school, age-appropriate service and/or vocational activities that are similar to those of classmates without disabilities.

The student attends school dances, assemblies, pep rallies, and other extracurricular and social events as often as students without disabilities.

From Jorgensen, C., McSheehan, M., & Sonnenmeier, R. (2010). *The Beyond Access Model: Promoting membership, participation, and learning for students with disabilities in the general education classroom* (p. 63). Baltimore: Paul H. Brookes Publishing Co.; adapted by permission.

by the No Child Left Behind Act of 2001 (PL 107-110). This includes skills related to language arts and literacy (Browder & Spooner, 2006; Copeland & Keefe, 2007; Kluth & Chandler-Olcott, 2008), math (Browder, Spooner, Ahlgrim-Delzell, Harris, & Wakeman, 2008), science (Courtade, Spooner, & Browder, 2007), social studies, and relevant electives such as art, music, home economics, and drama, as appropriate (see Browder & Spooner, 2006). In this regard, annual goals related to content standards from the general education curriculum as well as functional skills that are needed for participation in school and community life are spelled out in a student's individualized education program (IEP).

Undoubtedly, accomplishing all of this is no small task and requires ongoing collaboration among general education teachers, school administrators, and all members of the AAC team (including the student with CCN and his or her family). Most importantly, because social and academic participation in the general education classroom requires many types of communication, effective AAC systems that are age and context appropriate serve as critical tools for success for students with CCN across the ability range. Unfortunately, it is not uncommon for these students to attend school for several years without having access to the communication, writing, reading, and drawing tools that are available to their fellow students. Students who cannot hold pencils or crayons may not have access to augmented writing or drawing systems. Students who cannot hold books, turn pages, or use their voices to sound out words and read may not be given adapted reading equipment or computers. Students who have difficulty answering questions in class, joining in discussions, and participating in conversations may not be provided with AAC systems that support information sharing and social interaction. Thus, it is not at all surprising that many of these students are unable to participate successfully in general education classrooms because their complex communication needs and the resources with which they have been provided place them at a distinct disadvantage for both academic and social learning. Sadly, when educational or social participation is not evident, these students are often deemed "inappropriate for inclusion" and assigned to self-contained special education classrooms, resource rooms, or other separate settings. In time, they find themselves increasingly isolated from general education classrooms and placed with same-age students without disabilities only during nonacademic classes such as music, art, or physical education. Long-term planning aimed at avoiding this outcome should begin when students with CCN are in preschool.

TRANSITION FROM PRESCHOOL TO SCHOOL

After they enter elementary school, many students with CCN spend months or even years engaging in assessment activities that are designed to provide them with appropriate AAC systems. A clear solution to this dilemma is to begin providing AAC services to children with CCN during their preschool years (Judge & Parette, 1998; Romski, Sevcik, & Forrest, 2001). Early AAC attention allows children to develop at least some of the linguistic, operational, and social competencies that are necessary to support participation in elementary school. In the United States, the Individuals with Disabilities Education Improvement Act of 2004 (PL 108-446) mandates publicly funded preschool education for children with disabilities who are older than 3 years of age and, together with Section 504 of the Rehabilitation Act of 1973 (PL 93-112), provides the legal basis for assistive technology supports, including those required for AAC. Preschool teams are challenged to design AAC interventions that meet the conversational and interactional needs of young children—communication for today—as well as the academic and social needs of the general education classroom—communication for tomorrow. The goal should be that, by the time children who rely on AAC reach first grade, they have the tools necessary for academic participation and instruction. These include augmented writing and reading supports (either electronic or nonelectronic), in addition to a communication system that is appropriate to meet their needs for social interaction (see Chapters 9–11). Of course, some children (e.g., those with physical and/or sensory impairments) will need a variety of other tools as well, such as mobility devices, vision aids, and so forth.

Ideally, the AAC team should begin planning for a child's elementary school (i.e., kindergarten) placement at least 1 year before the end of preschool so that the necessary adaptations and arrangements can be put in place (Sainato & Morrison, 2001). One way for AAC interventionists to facilitate a smooth transition to kindergarten is to visit the target entry-level classroom well before the beginning of the school year in order to gather information about the participation patterns of typically developing children in that setting. Some kindergarten settings are quite structured and academically oriented, whereas others emphasize building concepts through play, exploration, and cooperative learning. The nature and expectations of the kindergarten environment greatly influence the interactive requirements placed on the child, which will, in turn, influence the direction of intervention planning during the preschool years. Regardless of the type of classroom, kindergarten teachers themselves have identified a number of critical communication, social, and participation skills that they consider to be desirable for kindergarten entry. Examples of some of the most commonly cited kindergarten entry skills appear in Table 13.3.

Table 13.3. Expected kindergarten entry skills identified by teachers

Type of skill	Skill
Social	Cooperates, takes turns, and shares with other children
	Has self-control and is able to interact without aggression
	Is curious about and interested in unfamiliar events, activities
	Attends and listens to the teacher
	Is able to play independently with other children
Communication	Is able to express needs and feelings (e.g., asks for help, communicates wants and needs)
	Asks peers for information or assistance
	Initiates and maintains appropriate peer interactions
	Answers questions
Participation	Follows established classroom routines
	Uses playground and classroom equipment and materials appropriately
	Respects the property of others
	Follows group and individual directions
	Accepts positive and corrective feedback and changes behavior accordingly, as needed

Sources: Chandler (1992); Foulks and Morrow (1989); Hains, Fowler, Schwartz, Kottwitz, and Rosenkoetter (1989); Harradine and Clifford (1996); Johnson, Meyer, and Taylor (1996); Knudsen-Lindauer and Harris (1989); and Piotrkowski, Botsko, and Matthews (2001).

Pretransition visits also facilitate dialogue between the kindergarten teacher and the preschool AAC team concerning the child's needs and abilities as well as the supports necessary for accommodation. For example, the school may need to make architectural modifications to facilitate physical accessibility or may need to hire a part-time paraprofessional to assist the teacher to optimize the student's classroom participation. The speech-language pathologist and motor specialists in the new school may want to establish a proactive plan for learning to use the student's communication equipment or for sharing day-to-day management of the communication program. Family involvement in the transition and planning process is also critical because family members are likely to be the only people with whom the child has regular contact during the transition period. Thus, family members often play a crucial role in the transfer of information about AAC vocabulary (e.g., what manual signs does the student use and understand?), technology, interaction strategies, and other components of the child's communication program.

Several years ago, we received a card announcing Maria's graduation from high school. It was her way of saying thanks and caused us to remember her as a preschool child with few ways to communicate. Because of her cerebral palsy, she could not speak, walk, or eat independently. She had very expressive eyes, an infectious laugh, and quite a temper!

In just a few years, Maria made the transition from a home-based early childhood program, to an inclusive preschool, to kindergarten, to first grade. She arrived in first grade with an electronic AAC system and a powered wheelchair. She had not mastered using either, but she had the tools. With the help of her school district personnel and parents, she was able to keep up with her grade-level classmates and never needed to repeat a grade. Along the way, she participated in several summer school sessions to enhance her reading, writing, and communication interaction skills. Would she have been this successful if she hadn't received her communication and mobility equipment until she entered Grade 1 or Grade 2?

The specific kindergarten transition planning process depends on the school district and the individuals involved and is likely to vary widely. However, a few general guidelines can be applied. First, during the first several months after transition, the educators and staff in the new school need to pay careful attention to the child's needs in order to avoid reinventing the wheel by providing redundant or unnecessary AAC interventions. For example, the educational team should not modify the child's existing AAC system unnecessarily during the first year of school. If a child has been prepared well for school, drastic changes to the communication system should not be necessary; in fact, if the AAC team makes substantive changes, the child is at risk for falling behind the other students academically while he or she learns to use the revised system. Of course, if AAC preparation prior to entry into elementary school was inadequate, the elementary school AAC team faces a difficult problem and will need to intervene aggressively during the first few years, although this timing is not optimal.

Second, the elementary school AAC team needs to be up to speed with regard to the knowledge and skills required to facilitate the communication efforts of young children who rely on AAC. If team members must learn about an unfamiliar AAC system over the course of the school year, the student's ability to participate in the classroom will probably be affected adversely. We have found that one way to avoid this problem is for a paraprofessional to follow the student from preschool, to kindergarten, and then to elementary school, especially if his or her AAC system has sophisticated technical requirements. When this is not possible, providing facilitator training for the elementary school staff prior to the beginning of the academic year should be a priority component of transition planning.

"It is wise to choose a school that your neighborhood friends attend. I was no surprise to the majority of my classmates; they had known me and how I did things for many years before I became a fellow classmate. They also were able to explain about me to any new students who had never met me or had any exposure to a person with disabilities" (Victor Valentic, a man with cerebral palsy who uses AAC, in Valentic, 1991, p. 9).

THE PARTICIPATION MODEL: PLANNING CLASSWIDE ACCOMMODATIONS

The goal of inclusive education for students with CCN is meaningful academic and social engagement in the general education classroom. In order to accomplish this, students must have appropriate access to educational and social vocabulary to support both comprehension and production. This may require teachers to enhance the natural supports they already provide in the classroom, to support language understanding and student responding. For example, Mr. Thomas relied primarily on whole-class lectures and discussions to introduce new content during language arts, until Kalinda joined his Grade 3 classroom. Because Kalinda's AAC team knew that she learned best when verbal language was augmented with visual supports, they encouraged Mr. Thomas to incorporate tangible items, photographs, graphic organizers, and other visual media into his instructional presentations. It quickly became apparent that the other students in Grade 3 also benefited from these accommodations, so Mr. Thomas continued to use them even after Kalinda moved on to Grade 4.

Accommodations to support the active participation of students with CCN are almost always required as well. It is a real challenge to keep vocabulary in a student's AAC system current because the communication content in general education classrooms changes so rapidly. For example, Kalinda's science class studied dinosaurs for 2 weeks, then they completed a unit on the solar system, and this was followed by a unit on how the planet Earth has changed over time. For each of these units, Kalinda needed access to related vocabulary in her AAC system in order to participate in activities with her classmates. Unfortunately, there is a tendency to provide students who rely on AAC with communication systems that are primarily designed to address wants, needs, and social communication functions, rather than the information-sharing function that is integral to classroom participation. If this happens, students with CCN are often forced to be passive learners: They cannot ask or answer questions in class, deliver topical reports, or otherwise participate in subject-oriented discussions because they do not have the vocabulary to do so.

We use the Participation Model (see Figure 5.1) as a framework for instructional planning for students who rely on AAC in general education classrooms. The model begins with identification of participation patterns and communication needs, which, in this case, requires an assessment of the general education teacher's expectations with regard to student engagement in the classroom. It also requires examination of the strategies teachers already use to support student understanding and responding so that any barriers to participation can be identified and remediated. These variables should be assessed for each subject area individually (e.g., language arts, math, science, music, art, physical education) because most teachers tend to have different expectations and use different strategies across subject areas. Of course, as students get older, there is also the likelihood that each subject area will be taught by a different teacher in a different classroom, making such subject-by-subject assessment essential. Figure 13.1 provides a format that can be used for initial assessment while observing a classroom teacher as he or she teaches a class of typically developing students in each subject area. In the sections that follow, we review the four areas that require assessment—instructional arrangements, teacher expectations, existing supports for language comprehension, and existing vocabulary and response supports.

Instructional Arrangements

The most commonly used instructional arrangements are described in this section and are summarized in the first column of Figure 13.1.

Teacher-Led Whole-Class Instruction

Teacher-led whole-class instruction tends to predominate in most general education classrooms (Katz, Mirenda, & Auerbach, 2002). During whole-class instruction, teachers typically 1) control most interactions and have an established agenda about the information that they expect students to know and learn, 2) expect students to listen while they deliver topic-specific information, 3) expect students to ask questions about information that is important to the lesson at hand, and 4) expect student answers to be brief and provide relevant information (Sturm & Nelson, 1997). Given the highly structured and preplanned nature of most whole-class instruction, teachers can often be very effective informants regarding specialized vocabulary that is required. For example, Mr. Thomas, Kalinda's teacher,

Assessment of Existing Classroom Arrangements and Supports

Instructions: Observe the teacher and students during a typical lesson in a specific subject area. Check the types of instructional arrangements, student participation expectations, natural supports for comprehension, and natural supports for responding that are observed.

Teacher: _____   Grade: _____   Subject area: _____

Natural instructional arrangements	How students are expected to interact/participate	Natural supports provided for comprehension	Natural response options available to all students
☐ Teacher-led, whole-class	☐ Bid for response/question opportunities	☐ Tangible objects/manipulables	☐ Tangible objects/manipulables
☐ Teacher-led, small group	☐ Answer questions	☐ Photographs, pictures, maps	☐ Photographs, pictures, maps
☐ Teacher-led, sharing time	☐ Ask questions	☐ Video, DVD, YouTube	☐ Overhead transparencies
☐ Cooperative learning group	☐ Ask for help, clarification, or feedback	☐ Overhead transparencies	☐ Interactive whiteboard
☐ Learning centers/stations	☐ Make comments	☐ Interactive whiteboard	☐ Flipchart, blackboard
☐ Adult–student 1:1 instruction	☐ Brainstorm ideas, suggestions	☐ Flipchart, blackboard	☐ Graphic organizers
☐ Peer–peer 1:1 instruction	☐ Tell story/give oral report	☐ Graphic organizers	☐ Drawing
☐ Group or paired seat work	☐ Take notes/act as a recorder	☐ Visual schedules	☐ Writing (by hand or computer)
☐ Individual seat work	☐ Role play, act	☐ Computer images	☐ Universal response: multiple choice
☐ Individual test-taking	☐ Listen as teacher provides instruction	☐ Internet (WebQuest, etc.)	☐ Universal response: yes/no or true/false
☐ Other:	☐ Work quietly (no interaction)	☐ Role playing	☐ Other:
	☐ Other	☐ Other:	

Figure 13.1. Assessment of existing classroom arrangements and supports.

readily identified 10 key vocabulary words for each science unit (e.g., for the planet Earth unit, words such as *crust, mantle, inner core, outer core, volcano*). He provided the words to Kalinda's paraprofessional 1 week before each unit commenced, giving her plenty of time to locate appropriate symbols and program Kalinda's AAC device so that she had access to this vocabulary during the unit. If the required vocabulary is not made available in this way, whole-class discussions can be challenging for many students with CCN unless the teacher augments verbal information with visual and media supports.

Teacher-Led Small-Group Instruction

Usually, the purpose of small-group instruction is to develop language, literacy, problem-solving, and critical thinking skills, with an emphasis on comprehension of text material and verbal expression. Small-group interactions tend to be topical but conversationally based, with an emphasis on teacher-initiated questions and student responses. Individual students may interact by competing for turns or by being called on either randomly or sequentially. Katz et al. (2002) found that students with developmental disabilities in inclusive classrooms were more likely to be actively engaged when they were involved in small-group instruction (both teacher- and student-led) than when they were involved in any other grouping arrangement, including one-to-one instruction. Thus, small-group instruction appears to have advantages with regard to student participation. In addition, because the teacher tends to control both the topics discussed and the questions asked during small-group instruction, he or she can often act as an informant to guide the advance preparation of AAC communication displays for students who need them.

Teacher-Led Sharing Time

Teachers often employ a "sharing" format for current-event presentations, reports, and show-and-tell activities, especially in the primary grades. According to Duchan (1995), people use sharing contexts primarily to describe events in a logical and temporal sequence, usually in the past tense (e.g., *Last weekend, we went to visit my grandmother. We drove there in a car. We stopped for lunch at McDonald's. When we got there...*). Often, the teacher will comment following the completion of a student's narration and perhaps ask questions to expand or clarify the content. At times, the teacher encourages other students to ask questions. Thus, sharing interactions are very similar to the storytelling contexts described in Chapter 2, and AAC teams can design messages as described in that chapter.

Cooperative Learning Groups and Learning Stations or Centers

Putnam (1998) described several approaches to cooperative learning that vary considerably with regard to how groups and learning activities are structured. However, they all have a number of elements in common: 1) they involve a common task or activity that is suitable for small group work, 2) they emphasize cooperative behavior and positive interdependence, and 3) they include structures related to individual accountability. Learning stations or centers are often used in the context of cooperative learning. In this type of instructional arrangement, students are usually expected to move around the classroom from station to station and to engage in different cooperative learning activities related to an overall lesson theme at each.

Educators can use small, cooperative learning groups productively as contexts for instruction of students with CCN (Dugan et al., 1995; Hunt, Staub, Alwell,

& Goetz, 1994; Katz et al., 2002). The communication patterns among students in such groups tend to more closely resemble those that occur in peer conversational interactions than those that occur during teacher-led instruction (Katz et al., 2002), so the lesson-specific vocabulary requirements may be less predictable. In addition, for students who rely on AAC, mobility and increased task variability may become challenges when learning stations are employed. Nonetheless, many texts on inclusive education promote the use of cooperative learning groups for students across the range of age and ability because they are conducive to both active engagement and social participation (e.g., Downing, 2002; Jorgensen, 1998; Kluth, 2010; Putnam, 1998; Ryndak & Alper, 2003).

Seth communicated with a speech-generating device (SGD). He was assigned to a cooperative learning group to prepare a class report on tornadoes. Each member of the group was responsible for a different aspect of the report. With the help of his paraprofessional, Seth programmed the report into his AAC system. He gave the presentation, releasing the report one sentence at a time; he also participated in a panel discussion by asking preprogrammed questions of the other members in his group. He was able to answer yes/no questions from his classmates as well.

One-to-One Instruction

Simpson (1996) videotaped a series of students who relied on AAC in general education classrooms and observed that communication patterns varied considerably from one student to another. Some of the students communicated primarily on a one-to-one basis with the teacher; others distributed their interactions quite equally among the teacher, a paraprofessional, and their peers; and still others interacted almost exclusively with a paraprofessional in one-to-one teaching contexts (Simpson, Beukelman, & Sharpe, 2000). Of course, one-to-one instruction can be delivered both by adults and by peers (e.g., peer tutoring). Regardless, question-and-answer interactions tended to predominate, with fairly predictable words and phrases needed by the student with CCN.

Self-Directed Seat Work

In most classrooms, students spend some portion of instructional time each day completing worksheets or exercises, taking tests, writing in daily journals, and engaging in other types of self-directed seat work activities. During these activities, they may be expected to work in small groups, student pairs, or individually; regardless, interaction is usually neither required nor encouraged. For many students with CCN, seat work activities will need to be adapted so that they can be completed using specialized writing software or other alternative response modes such as pictures or graphic symbols. For example, during the planet Earth unit, Kalinda worked with a partner to complete a worksheet using symbols to show her understanding of the Earth's layers (Figure 13.2). Often, students with CCN have an easier time participating in meaningful ways in classrooms in which seat work is used minimally rather than regularly, because it is often quite time consuming for the teacher or paraprofessional to adapt seat work so that the student can complete it. When appropriate accommodations are not in place, students run the risk of either not participating at all or being assigned to activities that are separate from the rest of the class.

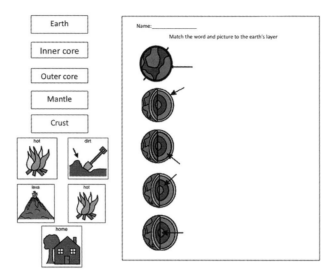

Figure 13.2. Adapted worksheet for a science unit on the Earth's layers. (The Picture Communication Symbols ©1981–2012 by DynaVox Mayer-Johnson LLC. All Rights Reserved Worldwide. Used with permission.)

Teacher Expectations

A second component of classroom instruction has to do with how teachers expect students to interact and participate in lessons or activities. In some classrooms, "silence is golden" is the rule; in others, students are encouraged to speak up and speak out regularly. Some teachers emphasize relatively predictable question-and-answer interactions over which they have control, whereas others prefer discussion-type interactions that are less structured and more student directed. Some teachers encourage students to read or respond individually, whereas others use whole-class response formats in which all students are expected to read or answer questions as a group. Classrooms also vary widely with respect to requirements related to sharing, storytelling, and reporting; participating in discussions; recording or note taking; following instructions; listening during teacher lectures; and so forth.

Instructional arrangements and expected interaction patterns often occur independent of one another, so both need to be assessed. For example, consider the difference between Ms. Evan's physical education (PE) class and Mr. Humphrey's social studies class, both of which are conducted predominantly through teacher-led whole-class instruction. In the PE class, students are expected to participate by listening to the teacher's instructions (e.g., related to a new game) and then following them. They are expected to ask Ms. Evan for help, clarification, or feedback as needed, but no other types of interaction are required, although students usually interact with each other as they play a game or engage in another activity. In the social studies class, on the other hand, Mr. Humphrey first asks students to discuss the chapter they read as homework (expectation: students will make comments), then engages in a question-and-answer session about the main ideas (expectation: students will answer questions), and finally presents a lecture about the information in the next chapter (expectation: students will listen quietly and ask for clarification as needed). Students are not encouraged to interact socially with one another; in fact, they are discouraged from doing so. It is clear that these two teacher-led whole-class lessons have very different interaction requirements, with very different implications for students who rely on AAC! The second column in Figure 13.1 can be used by the AAC team to identify the typical interaction and participation requirements expected of students in each subject area.

Natural Supports to Support Comprehension

Teachers often augment the meanings of instructional events by using objects, maps, drawings, photographs, videos or DVDs, interactive whiteboards, and other audiovisual media to augment spoken language, especially when they teach new information or unfamiliar concepts. In addition, they may write key words or longer passages on a blackboard, word wall, overhead transparency, or flipchart. For example, Mr. Zaidman uses illustrations; manipulables; and model squares, rectangles, and triangles when he teaches geometry concepts to his Grade 7 math class. He does this for two primary reasons: 1) to enhance students' attentiveness and thus decrease off-task behavior and 2) to enhance the likelihood that students will understand the target concepts, information, or instructions (i.e., to enhance language comprehension). For students with CCN, especially those with significant language delays or deficits, teachers' use of various types of instructional media is critically important to their ability to learn even basic information in a lesson. If teachers do not use such media regularly or in sufficient quantities, the AAC team may need to provide input and suggestions about how to include them, emphasizing that this is likely to enhance learning for all students, not just those with CCN. The third column of Figure 13.1 lists the natural supports that are most commonly used in classrooms to support comprehension.

Natural Response Options

Teachers also vary widely with regard to the options they provide for student responding during instructional interactions. As noted previously, some teachers support comprehension regularly with real objects, photos, illustrations, or written messages. These same teachers often pool potential response options by leaving tangible items, pictures, or words on display so that all students can use them as memory aids or point to them in response to questions. Such teachers often find it rather easy to include students with CCN when asking questions during whole-class and small-group instruction because these strategies apply to them as well. However, other teachers tend to remove tangible items or erase words once a lesson is completed and then require students to demonstrate what they have learned through writing or speech only. These teachers may need help to learn to use more effective response options that do not require students with CCN to rely almost entirely on their memories and on the vocabulary items available in their AAC systems.

In addition, some teachers may naturally use one or more response shortcuts, especially during whole-class question-and-answer activities. For example, Ms. Narang often uses a multiple-choice format to ask questions; she might say, *Did Marco Polo's book give Europeans their first information about Canada, Russia, or the Far East? If you think the correct answer is Canada, look up;* and so forth with the remaining options. Similarly, Mr. Yoshida uses a yes/no or true/false format during math class; for example, he might say *8 times 12 equals 86—true or false?* Because he uses this response option frequently, his students know to look at him if they think the answer is yes and to look at their desks if they think the answer is no. Such "universal response" strategies allow teachers to check the understanding of all students, including those who rely on AAC. Of course, questions and answers structured in this way can also be used to determine the knowledge of individual learners. In either case, from the perspective of the student with CCN, such strategies are vastly preferable to the more traditional "raise your hand if you know the answer" option that primarily rewards students who can move quickly and efficiently and who speak well. Furthermore, they make it easy for students with CCN to respond and participate without the need to have the answers on their personalized communication displays. The AAC team can use the fourth column in Figure 13.1 to identify the response options that are naturally available during instruction in each subject area.

Once existing, naturally available instructional and interaction arrangements, expectations, and support options have been identified, the AAC team can determine the need for various types of general classroom accommodations by asking a number of related questions:

- Which existing instructional arrangements enhance educational and social participation for the student with CCN? Which ones need to be adapted or replaced?
- Which natural interaction and participation expectations are readily achievable by the student, and which require adaptation?
- Which natural-language comprehension supports are appropriate for the student, and which require enhancement?
- Which naturally occurring response options are appropriate for the student, and which require enhancement?

Obviously, the AAC team should encourage the teacher to continue to use existing strategies that are appropriate and should also provide assurance that these strategies are likely to be as successful with a student who relies on AAC as they are with other students. On the other hand, if specific strategies are incompatible with a student's current communication and other abilities, the AAC team can provide suggestions to the teacher about how to modify or expand his or her repertoire accordingly. Figure 13.3 provides a checklist of instructional, comprehension, and response accommodations that can be added to those currently in place.

THE PARTICIPATION MODEL: PLANNING STUDENT-SPECIFIC ACCOMMODATIONS

Once classwide accommodations have been put in place, the Participation Model (see Figure 5.1) can also be used as a framework for planning and implementing a student's IEP. This requires several sequential steps that are linked together: constructing a student profile, developing an IEP, planning lessons that include all students, and identifying individualized accommodations, as needed. The process begins by identifying a student's current and desired participation and support patterns.

Develop a Student Profile

Especially when the general education teacher and/or key members of the AAC team change regularly, it is important to develop an annual strengths-based student profile that can be used to guide decision making and goal setting. This profile can be developed through informal interviews with family members and others who know the student well or through person-centered planning processes such as the

General Education Classroom Accommodation Planning Tool

Instructions: Check the accommodations that can be used to support instruction, comprehension, and responding in the general education classroom, to supplement those identified in the assessment of existing classroom arrangements and supports.

Teacher: _____ Grade: _____ Subject area: _____

Instructional arrangement accommodations	Instructional accommodations to support comprehension	Accommodations to support student participation and responding
☐ Adjust amount of whole-class instruction	☐ Make tangible objects/manipulables available	☐ Use switch and buzzer or light as an alternative to hand raising
☐ Adjust amount of small-group instruction	☐ Use photographs, pictures, maps, illustrations	☐ Use yes/no device for answering questions
☐ Adjust amount of sharing time	☐ Increase use of video, DVD, YouTube, etc.	☐ Use symbol vocabulary displays with key words for questions, comments, brainstorming
☐ Adjust amount of cooperative learning	☐ Write/draw on overhead transparencies	☐ Prerecord oral reports, stories, show-and-tell
☐ Adjust amount of learning centers/ stations	☐ Utilize interactive whiteboard, other interactive options	☐ Use visual displays for oral reports, stories, show-and-tell
☐ Adjust amount of adult 1:1 instruction	☐ Write/draw on flipchart, blackboard, word wall	☐ Record class notes on mp3 or other media
☐ Adjust amount of peer 1:1 instruction	☐ Increase use of graphic organizers	☐ Use role playing/acting
☐ Adjust amount of paired seat work	☐ Increase use of visual schedules	☐ Use tangible objects/manipulables
☐ Adjust how seat work is completed	☐ Increase use of computer images	☐ Use photographs, pictures, maps, illustrations
☐ Adapt tests or mode of learning assessment	☐ Increase use of Internet for WebQuest, etc.	☐ Use writing/drawings on transparencies, flip-chart, blackboard, word wall
☐ Other:	☐ Increase use of role playing	☐ Use interactive whiteboard and other interactive response options
	☐ Other:	☐ Use graphic organizers
		☐ Use universal response options (multiple choice, yes/no, true/false)
		☐ Other:

Figure 13.3. General education classroom accommodation planning tool.

Augmentative & Alternative Communication, Fourth Edition, by David R. Beukelman & Pat Mirenda

Social Networks inventory (Blackstone & Hunt Berg, 2003a, 2003b; see Chapter 9). Whatever process is used, some of the key questions to be answered include the following (Jorgensen, 2006):

- Who is this student, as a person? What are his or her preferences and/or affinities? What are his or her strengths and gifts? What are his or her goals and dreams? What the hopes and dreams of his or her parents or guardians?
- Who is this student, as a learner? How does he or she learn best? In what contexts is he or she challenged to learn?
- How does this student communicate? How does the student produce written work?
- What are the student's current literacy (i.e., reading, writing, spelling) abilities? numeracy and math abilities? social/emotional and behavioral abilities? language and communication abilities? daily living and personal hygiene skills?
- What are the student's challenges and needs?
- What are the priorities for learning for this school year, and what supports are needed to support this learning?

Table 13.4 summarizes the personal profile developed for Mitchell, a 16-year-old student with autism and CCN. It should be evident from this profile that Mitchell had a unique set of preferences, strengths, dreams, and challenges and that he was not performing at the academic level of his Grade 10 classmates.

Develop an Appropriate Individualized Education Program

It is important for the AAC team to determine priority goals for each student at least at the beginning of each school year (if not more frequently) so that meaningful educational programs can be designed and implemented. IEPs should include academic, social, and cross-curricular goals (e.g., in areas such as communication, daily living skills, and motor skills) as appropriate for each student, along with instructional and support strategies and criteria for determining whether each goal has been met. Unfortunately, a comprehensive discussion of how to identify appropriate goals and develop meaningful IEPs is beyond the scope of this book. However, Table 13.5 describes a number of resources that can be used in this regard. In addition, Jorgensen (2006) provided suggestions for writing standards-based IEPs. We provide an illustration of how to approach this task, using Mitchell as an example.

Step 1: Based on input from parents, the AAC team, and other key school support staff, identify priority goal areas for the student with CCN.

- *Example:* Mitchell will use his SGD to communicate topic-specific information during each unit or lesson.
- *Example:* Mitchell will increase his ability to write connected text on his SGD and on a computer.

Step 2: In each curriculum area (e.g., language arts, math, science), identify at least one grade-level general education standard that applies to all students. Determine the core skills (i.e., critical functions) that are inherent in the standards and develop annual goals that reflect the critical functions.

- *Example standard, science:* Students will demonstrate the ability to recognize parts of any object or system and understand how the parts interrelate in the operation of that object or system. *Critical function:* understanding how parts

Table 13.4.   Personal profile for Mitchell

Who is Mitchell?

- Age 16, entering Grade 10
- Has autism
- Lives at home with parents, brother
- Parents speak English and Spanish at home
- Attends his neighborhood school

Preferences, strengths, gifts

- Likes music, watching videos, looking at books
- Good at running, matching, drawing
- Fun to be around (happy) most of the time; good sense of humor

Hopes and dreams

- Likes being with other kids as "one of the gang" and seems to want more friends
- Would like more access to computers
- Enjoys working in small groups and would probably like to do more of this
- Parents want him to be more independent with personal hygiene skills
- Parents want to increase his literacy skills
- Parents want him to be more included in classroom activities

He learns best when

- Verbal instructions are supported visually (pictures, printed words)
- He is offered choices, even small ones
- He is praised frequently for effort as well as success
- He is given short breaks when he asks for them
- He is given sufficient time to process verbal directions (don't tell him over and over again!)
- He is encouraged to be independent and monitored from a distance

Current language/communication skills

- English is his first language; can say a few words and understand basic phrases and sentences in Spanish
- Follows one- or two-step directions in Spanish and English; understands more than people assume
- Can answer simple yes/no questions with head shakes, nods
- Started using a speech-generating device (SGD) last year; primarily uses it to make requests

Current literacy and numeracy skills

- Reads at a Grade 2 level with comprehension
- Writes on computer with Clicker 6 software support
- Can count to 100 and add and subtract simple numbers
- Knows basic concepts such as color, size, and so forth
- Can match anything to anything!

Current social/emotional skills

- Tries hard to please
- Tries to control behavior when confused or frustrated but has "meltdowns" two to three times per week
- Likes to watch for a while before trying new things

Current personal hygiene skills

- Is ambulatory
- Eats and uses toilet appropriately
- Needs help with dressing and fasteners
- Needs prompts to wash/dry hands

Table 13.5. Resources for developing individualized education programs (IEPs) for students who rely on augmentative and alternative communication in general education classrooms

Resource	Publisher
Adapting Curriculum and Instruction in Inclusive Classrooms (2nd ed.; Cole et al., 2000)	National Professional Resources
Choosing Options and Accommodations for Children: A Guide to Educational Planning for Students with Disabilities (3rd ed.; Giangreco, Cloninger, & Iverson, 2011)	Paul H. Brookes Publishing Co.
The Inclusion Facilitator's Guide (Jorgensen, Schuh, & Nisbet, 2006)	Paul H. Brookes Publishing Co.

of systems interrelate. *Annual goal:* Mitchell will demonstrate the ability to recognize parts of specific objects or systems and understand how the parts interrelate in the operation of those objects or systems.

- *Example standard, language arts:* Students will demonstrate the ability to communicate effectively through reading, writing, speaking, and listening. *Critical function:* effective communication. *Annual goal:* Mitchell will increase his ability to communicate effectively in writing and with his SGD.

Step 3: Identify classroom settings and activities in which each goal will be taught and the evaluation criteria that will be used to determine if the student has met the standard; these are the conditions, short-term objectives, and evaluation criteria that will be measured, respectively.

- *Example, science:* During units on the human body, Mitchell will give a class presentation on each system (e.g., circulatory, digestive, respiratory) and its function, using his SGD and models of the relevant organs.
- *Example, language arts:* Mitchell will contribute to weekly group book reports by producing at least three sentences with his SGD, with peer support.

Step 4: Determine the specific supports the student will need to achieve the goals and objectives; these are the accommodations.

- *Example, science:* Mitchell will need to have access to his SGD at all times, with 10–15 relevant vocabulary symbols programmed for each science unit by the paraprofessional; teacher will provide a list of key words for each unit.
- *Example, language arts:* Classmates will dictate sentences for Mitchell to write when preparing a group book report; key words will need to be added to the word lists in Mitchell's SGD by the paraprofessional.

It is important to emphasize that educational team members need to "think outside of the box" and adopt what Donnellan (1984) referred to as the "principle of the least dangerous assumption" when making decisions about educational goals and objectives that are appropriate for individual students. This principle states that, in the absence of conclusive data about a student's abilities, assuming competence has less dangerous consequences for the student than assuming incompetence, should the assumption ever be proven wrong. Failure to adhere to this principle often results in goals and objectives that are set too low and that limit both teacher expectations and student progress. Taking the risk of setting educational goals that are "too high," in the end, is less likely to negatively affect student progress than setting them too low (see Jorgensen et al., 2010). Table 13.6 displays some of IEP goals and objectives that were identified for Mitchell by his educational team based on the least dangerous assumption. Note that these goals and objectives articulate well with both the

Table 13.6.   Example individualized education program (IEP) goals and objectives for Mitchell, Grade 10

Science goal: Mitchell will demonstrate the ability to recognize parts of specific objects or systems and understand how the parts interrelate in the operation of those objects or systems.

Objectives:
- During units on the human body, Mitchell will give a class presentation on each system (e.g., circulatory digestive, respiratory) and its function, using his speech-generating device (SGD) and models of the relevant organs.
- During a unit on electricity, Mitchell will label devices that do and do not require electricity and materials that act as conductors or insulators. He will demonstrate the ability to plug in his SGD to charge it, turn on his SGD in the morning, and turn it off when not in use, daily for one month.
- During a unit on the solar system, Mitchell will work with classmates to complete a WebQuest worksheet on information about an assigned planet and will give a group-programmed presentation on the results using his SGD.

Language arts goal: Mitchell will increase his ability to communicate effectively in writing and with his SGD.

Objectives:
- Mitchell will contribute to weekly group book reports by producing at least three sentences with his SGD, with peer support.
- Mitchell will use his SGD to recite the lines of an assigned character in *Romeo and Juliet*.
- Mitchell will demonstrate his understanding of the setting, main characters, main plot elements, problem, and solution of *Romeo and Juliet* using drawings and printed words on a graphic organizer.
- During novel studies, Mitchell will use his SGD to read a prerecorded passage from each novel, sequencing the first part, the second part, and the conclusion of the story.

Social studies goal: Mitchell will demonstrate the ability to participate in the voting process.

Objectives:
- For the classwide vote on a weekly topic, Mitchell will distribute ballots, compile the results with the assistance of a classmate, and use his SGD to report the results.
- While working on a classmate's campaign for election to the student council, Mitchell will share three reasons to vote for his friend, using his SGD.
- Mitchell will vote in the student council election, assist the voting committee to count the ballots, and report the results at a school assembly, using his SGD.

priority goals identified for Mitchell and the critical functions of the general education curriculum identified in Steps 1 and 2.

> "We can, whenever and wherever we choose, successfully teach all children whose schooling is of interest to us. We already know more than we need in order to do this. Whether we do it must finally depend on how we feel about the fact that we haven't done it so far" (Edmonds, 1979, p. 29).

Use the Principles of Universal Design to Plan Units and Lessons

When applied to general education classrooms, the principles of universal design for learning (UDL) encourage teachers to set unit goals and design related activities that are inclusive from the outset (Bauer & Matuszek, 2001; Kame'enui & Simmons, 1999; Rose & Meyer, 2002). Universal design principles were originally developed with regard to physical accessibility for people with disabilities, based on the concept that it is less expensive and more efficient to build physical accessibility features into blueprints and community designs from the outset than to do so as an afterthought (Rose & Meyer, 2002). Thus, when new buildings are constructed following this principle, they automatically include features such as ramps, accessible washrooms, braille legends in elevators, and tactile stairs. When new communities are universally designed, they automatically include sidewalks with curb cuts, street intersections with both visual and audio signals, and so forth. Similarly, when classrooms are universally designed, they are likely to accommodate all students without the need for extensive (and usually time-consuming) accommodations.

When applied to general education classrooms, UDL involves three basic principles:

1. To support *recognition learning,* teachers should provide *multiple, flexible methods of presentation.*
2. To support *strategic learning,* teachers should provide *multiple, flexible methods of expression and apprenticeship.*
3. To support *affective learning,* teachers should *provide multiple, flexible options for engagement.*

When teachers use the three UDL principles to set goals and design instruction, all students—including but not limited to those with CCN—are likely to benefit (Rose & Meyer, 2002). For example, consider a language arts unit on *Romeo and Juliet* that was taught in Mitchell's Grade 10 classroom by Mrs. Johnson. Mrs. Johnson's original goal for the lesson was "Students will read the play *Romeo and Juliet* and write a five-page essay describing the key plot elements and character motivations"—a goal that made it virtually impossible for Mitchell to participate in any meaningful way, given his literacy and communication challenges. However, when Mrs. Johnson applied the principles of UDL to her lesson planning, she realized that using "multiple, flexible methods of expression and apprenticeship" meant that she should allow more flexibility with regard to how she assessed student learning. She also realized that providing "multiple, flexible methods of presentation" required her to employ strategies for comprehension that went beyond having students simply read the play, in order to accommodate not just Mitchell but also several other students in the class who also struggled with literacy. Finally, she understood that, in order to provide "multiple, flexible options for engagement," she would have to help students get past the challenges presented by Elizabethan English and become engaged in the play in a way that was relevant to their lives.

In light of these new understandings, Mrs. Johnson revised her goal for all students (including Mitchell) as follows: "Students will act out an abbreviated version of the play *Romeo and Juliet* and will be able to identify the setting, main characters, main plot elements, problem, and solution." Note that this goal does not specify *how* students will demonstrate their knowledge about the play, only what the content should be. In order to meet the goal, Mrs. Johnson assigned roles from *Romeo and Juliet* to each student in the class, including Mitchell (he played the part of the apothecary, who sold the poison to Romeo). The AAC team ensured that his speaking lines were programmed into his SGD so that he could practice them in class. Mrs. Johnson also added a new component of instruction because she knew that Mitchell, like many students with autism, was a visual learner. Thus, she had the class watch a portion of the Hollywood movie version of the play before they read each scene. For Mitchell's sake, she also had students work in small groups to practice their parts and complete a number of related activities; for example, during one week of the unit, students watched the movie *West Side Story,* a modern adaptation of *Romeo and Juliet.* Mrs. Johnson then provided a list of descriptors (e.g., *families, gangs, poison, guns, tragedy*) and a graphic organizer with three sections: "Romeo and Juliet," "West Side Story," and "Romeo and Juliet and West Side Story." The students had to sort the descriptors into the three categories to show their understanding of the similarities and differences between the two stories; in his group, Mitchell was able to participate by using Picture Communication Symbols that represented the descriptors (see Figure 13.4). As is typically the case when the principles of universal design are utilized creatively, the changes Mrs. Johnson made were of benefit to all of the Grade 10 students, not just Mitchell—so much so that she continued to teach the lesson the new way in subsequent school years, even after Mitchell was no longer in her class.

A number of web sites serve as excellent resources for information about and resources related to Universal Design for Learning. These include the web sites of CAST (formerly the Center for Applied Special Technology), ASCD (formerly the Association for Supervision and Curriculum Development), and Closing the Gap.

Identify Individualized Accommodations as Needed

Even when teachers incorporate classwide strategies to enhance comprehension and responding and combine these strategies with UDL principles to plan inclusive lessons, students with CCN often require individualized accommodations as well (Cole et al., 2000). A number of such accommodations, which can be used singly or in combination, are summarized in Table 13.7, with examples of each. As can be seen from this table, Mitchell required a few individualized accommodations in order to participate in the *Romeo and Juliet* unit.

Implement Instruction and Evaluate Outcomes

At this point, the AAC team has completed all of the necessary planning. They have assessed and made recommendations for classwide accommodations, completed a personal profile of the student who relies on AAC, and identified relevant goals and

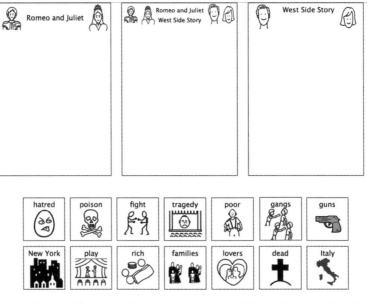

Figure 13.4. Graphic organizer for comparing *Romeo and Juliet* and *West Side Story*. (The Picture Communication Symbols ©1981–2012 by DynaVox Mayer-Johnson LLC. All Rights Reserved Worldwide. Used with permission.)

Table 13.7.   Types and examples of curriculum accommodations

Type	Definition	Examples
Size	Adjust the number of items a student is expected to learn or complete	• Seamus types using sip-and-puff Morse code to write. To accommodate his slow rate of text entry, his math test consists of five problems rather than ten. • Mitchell writes two sentences in his daily journal rather than the whole page expected of his classmates.
Time	Adjust the amount of time allotted for learning, task completion, or testing	• Stacy writes quite slowly when she uses her head mouse to compose text via her speech-generating device (SGD). In order to provide sufficient time for text composition, her social studies teacher asks her a question at the end of every class period. Stacy then prepares the answer at home in the evening and stores it in her SGD. The next day, when her teacher asks her the question, Stacy is able to quickly provide the answer in class. • Mitchell and his science group use additional study hall time to complete a science project on endangered species.
Level of support	Adjust the amount of personal assistance provided by peers or adults	• Jamie works with three of his classmates to complete a plaster relief map of Africa for a social studies project. • During the *Romeo and Juliet* unit, a paraprofessional programs the lines spoken by the apothecary into Mitchell's SGD and helps him practice activating them on cue.
Input	Adjust how instruction is delivered	• Mr. Hashman uses an interactive whiteboard to deliver instruction across all curricular areas to enhance learning for the students in his Grade 5 classroom. • Mrs. Johnson, Mitchell's teacher, uses an overhead projector to write key words and draw simple pictures during a whole-class discussion of *Romeo and Juliet*.
Output	Adjust how the student is expected to demonstrate learning	• In Foods class, Terry cuts out magazine pictures of the four food groups to show what he has learned, rather than taking a test. • Mitchell draws pictures and prints words on a story map to show what he has learned about *Romeo and Juliet*.
Difficulty	Adjust the skill level, problem type, or rules about how the learner approaches an activity	• Ramona combines adjectives and nouns using a shape grid to guide her selections. • Mitchell reads an adapted version of *Romeo and Juliet* that his educational assistant created using Boardmaker Plus.

Source: Cole et al. (2000).

objectives for the IEP. They have worked with the teacher to help him or her learn to design lessons based on the principles of UDL and have also identified individual accommodations that may be required. Finally—it is time to implement instruction and evaluate the student's progress!

Within the Participation Model (Figure 5.1) as it applies to inclusive educational environments, two main questions should be assessed for each curricular unit or activity:

1. Was the student able to actively participate in a meaningful way in this unit or lesson?

2. Did the student work on (and/or meet) one or more IEP goals?

Let's revisit Mitchell's Grade 10 language arts class as an example of how this can be accomplished. His class has successfully completed the *Romeo and Juliet* unit. With regard to participation, the primary lesson activities were 1) reading an abbreviated version of the play and discussing it in class, 2) participating in key scenes from the play, and 3) comparing the play with a modern version in the form of *West Side Story*. How did Mitchell participate? Along with his classmates, he watched scenes from the Hollywood movie version of the play before reading and acting out each scene. When Mitchell read the play, he used a symbol-supported, simplified version of the story that was adapted by his paraprofessional with the Symbolate tool in Boardmaker Plus (DynaVox Mayer-Johnson). Using his SGD, he recited the apothecary's lines during the class production, and when he was not in a scene, he was one of two "prop masters" who were responsible for making sure that the appropriate props were available on the "stage." He also watched *West Side Story* and completed several "compare and contrast" activities related to the two plays, including the graphic organizer activity depicted in Figure 13.4. Did Mitchell participate in meaningful ways? Clearly, yes!

The second issue to assess is, Did Mitchell make progress on or meet the IEP objectives related to this language arts unit? As displayed in Table 13.6, one of Mitchell's language arts objectives was "Mitchell will demonstrate his understanding of the setting, main characters, main plot elements, problem, and solution of *Romeo and Juliet* using drawings and printed words on a graphic organizer." This goal is consistent with the classwide goal Mrs. Johnson identified for all students: "Students will act out an abbreviated version of the play *Romeo and Juliet* and will be able to identify the setting, main characters, main plot elements, problem, and solution." As noted previously, Mitchell read an adapted version of the play. He also used his SGD to answer questions during the discussion that occurred in every class (e.g., *How did Romeo feel when Juliet died? How did Romeo die?*). Finally, he completed a graphic organizer using printed words and drawings to demonstrate his understanding of the play (see Figure 13.5). Did Mitchell meet his learning goals? Yes, again!

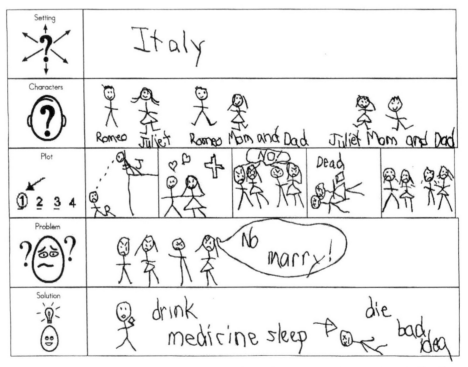

Figure 13.5. *Romeo and Juliet* story map completed with words and drawings by an adolescent with autism. (RYNDAK, DIANE LEA; ALPER, SANDRA K., CURRICULUM AND INSTRUCTION FOR STUDENTS WITH SIGNIFICANT DISABILITIES IN INCLUSIVE SETTINGS, 2nd,©2003. Printed and Electronically reproduced by permission of Pearson Education, Inc., Upper Saddle River, New Jersey.)

The planning process illustrated by Mitchell's story can be used to answer the two key outcome questions for students with CCN in general. If the answer to either question is no, the team should identify interfering factors and incorporate potential solutions into future lesson plans and activities, either for the entire class or for the individual student. Our experience is that, once this plan–implement–evaluate–revise cycle has occurred several times, the amount of time and effort required for each step decreases dramatically. As teams develop fluency around this process, both students with CCN and educational team members themselves are increasingly able to use UDL principles and other strategies to develop meaningful, inclusive lessons that benefit all learners. If you asked Mitchell, his family, or the members of his school team whether it was worth all the hard work and time, and whether inclusion really made a difference for Mitchell, there is no doubt that they would say yes. For Mitchell and for many other students at all academic levels who rely on AAC, inclusive education is not just here to stay—it is changing their lives.

QUESTIONS

13.1.   Define *inclusive education.*

13.2.   Describe at least four indicators of membership and of social and academic participation in a general education classroom.

13.3.   What are three key strategies for facilitating the transition of students with CCN from preschool to kindergarten?

13.4.   What are four common instructional arrangements in inclusive classrooms, and what are the implications of each for students with CCN?

13.5.   What are six natural supports that teachers often use to support comprehension in classrooms, and how can these be augmented for students with CCN?

13.6.   What are six natural response options that teachers often use in classrooms, and how can these be augmented for students with CCN?

13.7.   What is the purpose of a student profile, and what questions should be answered in compiling one?

13.8.   Describe a process for writing standards-based IEPs for students with CCN.

13.9.   What are the three principles of Universal Design for Learning, and what are their relevance to inclusive education for students with CCN?

13.10.   What two key questions can be asked to evaluate the extent to which the Participation Model (Figure 5.1) has been applied successfully to support inclusive education?

Augmentative and Alternative Communication Interventions for Individuals with Acquired Disabilities

CHAPTER 14

Adults with Acquired Physical Conditions

with Laura Ball

Sam had amyotrophic lateral sclerosis (ALS) for 6 years. For 4 of those years, he used mechanical, invasive ventilation and nutritional support. He was diagnosed with ALS after he noticed weakness in his arms and decided to see a neurologist. After about a year, his speaking rate began to slow. A speech-language pathologist from the ALS clinic monitored his speech performance, even though his speech was still intelligible, so that he would have time to choose, acquire, and learn to operate an augmentative and alternative communication (AAC) system before his speech deteriorated further. When Sam's speaking rate slowed to 120 words per minute (compared with 190 words per minute by typical adult speakers) on the Speech Intelligibility Test–Sentence Version (Yorkston, Beukelman, Hakel, & Dorsey, 2007), he completed an AAC assessment. Within a couple of months after his AAC assessment, he began to notice that listeners were straining to understand him in some situations. After that, his speech began to deteriorate very rapidly, and he was no longer understandable at all within 3 more months. Because an AAC assessment had been completed in a timely manner, his AAC technology arrived and he had time to learn how to operate it before he became unable to speak. He controlled a computer-based AAC technology using eye tracking to produce messages through spelling, word prediction, and message retrieval. He maintained an active social life by e-mailing and texting colleagues, friends, and family members. He also communicated over the telephone using his AAC technology and a speakerphone. He also used his device to access the Internet and read electronic books. In addition to his high-tech AAC system, Sam used an eye-linking low-tech strategy (see Chapter 4) when his eye-tracking technology was not available or convenient. He used his eye-tracking technology until a couple of weeks before his death. At that point he used eye linking to communicate with those around him.

This chapter summarizes assessment and intervention approaches to a number of acquired physical conditions, including ALS, multiple sclerosis (MS), Guillain-Barré syndrome (GBS), Parkinson's disease (PD), brainstem stroke, and others. Subsequent chapters discuss information related to the acquired disabilities of traumatic brain injury, aphasia, and dementia secondary to stroke.

AMYOTROPHIC LATERAL SCLEROSIS

ALS is a progressive, degenerative disease of unknown etiology involving the motor neurons of the brain and spinal cord (Mitchell & Borasio, 2007). It attacks nerve cells controlling voluntary muscles but does not affect sensation. Because 80% (Saunders, Walsh, & Smith, 1981) to 95% (Ball, Beukelman, & Pattee, 2003) of people with ALS are unable to speak by the time of their deaths, they require AAC support to meet their communication needs. Yorkston, Miller, Strand, and Britton (2012) report the mean age of onset for ALS as 56 years of age. The most common early symptom is weakness (Wijesekera & Leigh, 2009), with approximately one third of those affected reporting initial upper-extremity (arm and hand) weakness, one third reporting leg weakness, and one quarter presenting with bulbar (brainstem) weakness manifested by dysarthria and dysphagia. Extraocular muscles that control eye movements are usually unaffected, as is sphincter control. As the disease progresses, motor weakness may become pervasive, such that the individual requires assistance for personal care, mobility, and feeding as well as assistance in the form of respiratory support. The median survival rates are 32 months from onset of symptoms and 19 months from diagnosis (Yorkston et al., 2012); however, life expectancy can be significantly extended if those with ALS, supported by their families, choose mechanical ventilation for respiratory support.

For an extended discussion of AAC for people with ALS, see the webcast *AAC: A User's Perspective* by Colin Portnuff.

Communication Symptoms

Dysarthria, a motor speech disorder, results from the weakness and spasticity inherent in ALS. Dysarthria of the mixed flaccid-spastic type is almost universally present at some point (Duffy, 2005; Yorkston, Beukelman, Strand, & Hakel, 2010). People with predominantly bulbar (brainstem) involvement experience this speech disorder early in the disease process, and their speech and swallowing functions may deteriorate rapidly. Such individuals may be able to walk and even to drive, yet they are unable to speak. Individuals with predominantly spinal involvement, however, may retain normal or mildly dysarthric speech for a considerable period of time even as they experience extensive motor impairments in their extremities.

Although the progression of speech symptoms differs from individual to individual, nearly all people with ALS experience a severe communication disorder during the last portion of their lives. Laura Ball, Amy Nordness, David Beukelman, and Gary Pattee collaborated to develop and maintain the Nebraska ALS Database in which they recorded data from consecutive participants in ALS clinics sponsored by the Muscular Dystrophy Association and the ALS Association. As of 2009, data had been collected every 3 months from more than 300 people with ALS. Of that group, only 7% communicated using natural speech at the time of their deaths, and 93% relied on AAC strategies.

AAC interventionists must also be aware that cognitive changes do occur in some people with ALS. Research indicates that 40% to 50% of people with ALS experience some degree of dementia as determined by cognitive testing (Lomen-Hoerth et al., 2003; Yorkston et al., 2012). Yorkston et al. (2012) report that approximately 25% to 35% of individuals with ALS experience subtle changes in cognitive function, especially in the areas of executive functioning, reasoning, response generation, initiation, abstraction, planning and organization, new learning, verbal fluency, and picture recall; however, they do not exhibit overt dementia. Measures of cognitive functioning, along with some evidence from brain imaging, suggest a mild frontal dysfunction (Kiernan & Hudson, 1994; Lloyd, Richardson, Brooks, Al-Chalabi, & Leigh, 2000).

In addition, Montgomery and Erickson (1987) suggested that although neurological signs are usually absent in the early stages, overt dementia (i.e., frontotemporal dementia/ALS, or FTD/ALS) occurs in about 15% of individuals with ALS (Yorkston et al., 2012). Although relatively rare, FTD/ALS is characterized by profound personality changes and breakdowns in social conduct. Most individuals with FTD/ALS achieve low scores on tests of executive function and exhibit low abstraction, planning, and organizational skills. Together, these issues may impact individuals' acceptance of and ability to learn to use AAC systems.

Finally, aphasia may occasionally be associated with ALS (Bak & Hodges, 2001; Mitsuyama, Kogoh, & Ata, 1985; Tscuchiya et al., 2000). In a few rare cases, primary progressive aphasia appears to evolve into ALS. For example, Caselli et al. (1993) reported on seven individuals in whom articulatory and language impairment proceeded to rapidly progressive ALS. Duffy, Peach, and Strand (2007) described a series of cases in which progressive apraxia of speech ultimately was diagnosed as ALS. Researchers have also described a frontotemporal lobar dementia syndrome (FTLD) that has three categories: frontotemporal dementia (primarily involving personality changes), semantic dementia (e.g., fluent aphasia, which is characterized by fluent but often meaningless speech often with limited understanding of spoken or written words), and primary progressive aphasia (e.g., nonfluent aphasia with loss of spoken or written word meaning; Lomen-Hoerth, 2004, Lomen-Hoerth et al., 2003). FTLD has been reported to be more common among people with ALS who have bulbar symptoms, are somewhat older ($M = 65$ years), and have decreased functional vital capacity ($M = 66\%$ of predicted capacity).

A Model for Augmentative and Alternative Communication Intervention

AAC interventionists typically employ some version of the three-phase intervention model described by Ball, Beukelman, and Bardach (2007). The Early Phase (Monitor, Prepare, and Support) occurs during the period of time from initial diagnosis through referral for an AAC assessment. Speech-language pathologists monitor speech for changes and educate the people with ALS, as well as other decision makers, about possible changes in speech performance as well as other factors such as respiratory intervention options that will potentially influence future decisions about communication supports. The Middle Phase (Assess, Recommend, and Implement) refers to the time from the referral for AAC assessment until AAC strategies are selected and purchased and initial instruction is completed. The Late Phase (Adapt and Accommodate) involves the time after initial AAC intervention until the individual's death as modifications in AAC strategies are needed to deal with changes in communication needs and the individual's capabilities.

Early Phase: Monitor Speech Performance, Preserve Natural Speech Effectiveness, and Educate About Augmentative and Alternative Communication

The Early Phase begins at the time of the diagnosis, when the person with ALS often has natural speech that is functional to meet daily communication needs. If the person has spinal-onset ALS, changes in speech performance may not yet have begun. If the person has bulbar-onset ALS, mild changes in speaking rate may have begun.

An important activity in the Early Phase is to monitor speech performance on a systematic schedule to detect changes that signal the need for a timely referral for an AAC assessment. In the past, reduction is speech intelligibility (understandability) was used as the standard for determining when an AAC assessment should occur. However, once decreases in speech intelligibility are observed, such precipitous drops in intelligibility commonly occur that there is usually insufficient time to initiate and execute AAC assessment and intervention before the individual is unable to meet his or her communication needs through natural speech alone. Research has demonstrated that a progressive reduction in speaking rate precedes reduction in speech intelligibility (Ball, Beukelman, & Pattee, 2002; Yorkston, Klasner, et al., 2003).

Appropriate timing of AAC intervention requires systematic monitoring of speaking rate and intelligibility. Objective, rather than subjective, measures are essential because subjective estimates of intelligibility are often inaccurate. The authors use the Speech Intelligibility Test–Sentence Version (Yorkston et al., 2007) because it provides an objective measure of speaking rate and intelligibility. The speaking rate can be measured when the test is administered in the clinical setting so that the clinician can immediately provide rate information to the medical staff, the individual with ALS, and those who accompany the individual. This test produces a set of 11 sentences that are read aloud by the person with ALS. Speaking rate is calculated immediately, and the utterances are later transcribed to obtain measures of speech intelligibility.

Ball, Beukelman, and Pattee (2002) reported that people with ALS gradually reduce their speaking rate as ALS progresses. The relationship between speaking rate and speech intelligibility is illustrated in Figure 14.1. These authors recommend that an AAC assessment be recommended when the speaking rate reaches 125 words per minute. When speaking rate reaches approximately 125 words per minute, a rather dramatic decrease in speech intelligibility is expected within the next 2 months for some individuals and within 4 to 6 months for others. For a limited number of individuals, dysarthria of such severity that it reduces speech intelligibility occurs prior to significant rate reduction; in such cases, an AAC assessment is recommended when sentence intelligibility drops below 90%, regardless of speaking rate (Ball, Beukelman, & Bardach, 2007).

Speaking rate can be accurately monitored via conventional analog or digital telephone technology if an individual with ALS is unable to travel to a clinic due to distance, weather, health, or transportation difficulties. Measures of speaking rate are essentially identical for face-to-face and telephone monitoring (Ball, Beukelman, Ullman, Maassen, & Pattee, 2005). Of course, speech intelligibility scores are affected by telephone transmission and should not be evaluated at a distance over a telephone.

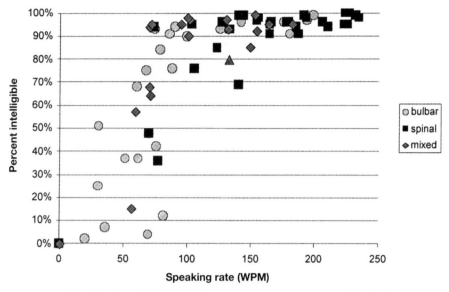

Figure 14.1. Speaking rate and intelligibility decline for people with amyotrophic lateral sclerosis (ALS). (*Key:* WPM, words per minute.)

A second activity in the Early Phase is to make a timely AAC referral so that there is sufficient time to complete the assessment, select AAC options, purchase the AAC technology, and instruct the person who will rely on AAC and his or her facilitators.

A third activity in the Early Phase is to assist the speaker with ALS to implement strategies that will preserve the communication effectiveness (see Form 9.5 in Beukelman, Garrett, & Yorkston, 2007) of their natural speech for as long as possible. By reducing speech effort and fatigue but amplifying residual speech, and by allocating speaking time for important social or informational exchanges during the day, the individual can conserve enough energy to communicate effectively, even though dysarthria might be apparent to listeners. For a limited number of individuals with specific velopharyngeal weakness that interferes with speech or oral breathing, a palatal lift may be recommended (Hanson, Yorkston, & Britton, 2011; Yorkston et al., 2010).

Toward the end of the Early Phase, some people with ALS use their remaining natural speech to prepare video or audio recordings for their loved ones. As Tom neared the time when he needed AAC to communicate, he arranged to prepare video-recorded messages for his wife, each of his children, and his children's spouses. He talked to each of them individually as he recalled important memories and shared experiences. He told them how much he appreciated and loved them. He talked about his disease and how much their care and respect meant to him. After completing the recordings, he selected pictures and had them incorporated into the video.

A fourth activity in the Early Phase is to educate the person with ALS and decision makers about AAC-related decisions. This education includes information about natural speech deterioration, timing of AAC assessment, low- and high-tech AAC options, and technology purchases as well as funding. The goal of this education is to prepare them to efficiently make AAC-related decisions when the time comes. We have observed that some people are very interested in this information and actually seek out additional information, whereas others express little or no interest and indicate that they will rely extensively on professionals to guide their decision making.

Middle Phase: Assess, Recommend, Implement

During assessment, four activities are stressed: 1) identifying participation patterns and associated communication needs; 2) assessing current and anticipated capabilities—physical, cognitive, language, visual, and hearing; 3) assessing social and personal care supports; and 4) selecting low- and high-tech AAC options that will meet current and future needs.

Identifying Participation Patterns and Communication Needs   Individuals who experience acquired physical disabilities that affect their ability to communicate often also experience other dramatic changes in their lives. Depending on the progression of the specific condition or disease, these changes may occur gradually (as with a degenerative disease) or more abruptly (as with trauma or stroke). Individuals' physical disabilities along with personal lifestyle preferences determine their communication needs and their participation roles and contexts (see Forms 9.8 and 11.1 in Beukelman, Garrett, & Yorkston, 2007). For example, some people with severe degenerative disabilities such as ALS prefer to center their lives within their home environment; Sam, described at the start of this chapter, was such an individual. These individuals find that it is more efficient and less demanding on their families to establish their homes as their primary work, social, and care setting rather than to continue to participate extensively in the larger community. Thus, they may work at home if they are active vocationally. Friends and family visit them at home, and they travel only for special events. Some use the Internet to maintain contact with their social and support networks. Eventually, they may go through numerous transitions involving their living situation (e.g., private home, assisted living, nursing home, hospice), which will have an impact on the available funding for AAC as well as necessitate changes to their AAC systems (Ball, 2003).

Continued employment plays an important role in the lives of some individuals with ALS (McNaughton, Light, & Groszyk, 2001). Jamie wished to continue working after she was diagnosed with bulbar ALS. She continued to work in her position as a data-entry specialist, using multimodal technologies for her daily communication supports. She used her computer with the keyboard to enter data, access the Internet, and send e-mail. She used her cell phone to send text messages to family and friends. Although she identified a more complex speech-generating device (SGD) to fully meet her communication needs, she purchased a mobile device (iPad) with an AAC application for communicating with people in meetings, socially, and on the telephone. She selected this as a temporary measure, knowing that she would require AAC technology with additional options in the future. She made the decision because although she was experiencing hand weakness and atrophy, she retained the ability to access devices with her hands. Interventions for people with ALS who wish to continue to work should include computer literacy and Internet training to provide options for furthering employment and accessing a range of supports. Expanded electronic communication options such as e-mail, the Internet, electronic conferencing, and cellular technology have resulted in expanded opportunities for employment, volunteering, distance learning, financial transactions, and commercial activity. Participation in virtual activity is of little interest to some people who use AAC technology; however, others participate regularly, both socially and vocationally, using the Internet.

Other individuals adopt a different participation strategy and attempt to stay active in the community as long as they possibly can. These individuals may continue to work outside the home, travel, and attend recreational activities, religious services and social events with friends and family. Tom, in the following case study, provides an example of this strategy.

> Tom and his family maintained a very externally focused lifestyle even after he was diagnosed with ALS. During the first 18 months following his diagnosis, Tom and his wife traveled extensively, at times with their children, at times with Tom's siblings, and often with friends. When he began to use a wheelchair and eventually rely on AAC technology, they scheduled "Time with Tom" at a local restaurant every Monday during the dinner hour. Friends, former colleagues, members of their church, neighbors, and relatives stopped by to participate at their convenience. Tom continued to attend athletic events and concerts. He telephoned family and friends to celebrate birthdays and anniversaries. Needless to say, Tom received considerable support and developed extensive AAC skills in order to participate in these extensive social interactions. (Rutz, 2005)

Decisions about patterns of participation substantially affect an individual's communication needs and corresponding AAC strategies. For example, an individual who communicates primarily at home or in a long-term acute care hospital may need AAC technology that can easily be moved to various rooms on a cart or on a computer stand with wheels, rather than an AAC device that attaches directly to a wheelchair. Individuals who participate actively in the community need communication systems that are self-contained, compact, and fully portable. Many prefer efficient Internet access via their AAC technology. Most require a means to use the telephone and e-mail. During assessment and intervention, it is important to consider the individual opinions and preferences of adults with acquired disabilities regarding their participation and lifestyle patterns.

It is also important to develop consensus among the person who uses AAC and the individuals who support him or her when developing a profile of the individual's communication needs and participation. One way to build consensus is to identify potential communication needs and assign each a level of importance. A review of the information provided previously about Jamie and Tom reveals that many of their communication needs were similar; however, their lifestyle choices dictated different communication solutions.

A detailed needs assessment has advantages for both the person with the disability and the members of his or her family and support networks. For example, it is not uncommon for adults with acquired communication disorders to insist that their AAC systems return to them (or maintain) all of the functions of natural speech. This insistence is natural because many people struggle to accept their disabilities and are often frustrated by their inability to communicate in the same way that was possible with natural speech. In the process of completing a communication needs inventory, these individuals are forced to go beyond the generic expectation of "being able to do everything that I could do before this happened" in order to identify *specific* communication needs and assign them priorities. In a study examining the purposes of AAC technology use for people with ALS as reported by their caregivers, Fried-Oken, Rau, Fox, Tulman, and Hindal (2004) found that the two most frequent and highly valued purposes involved regulating the behavior of others (for basic wants and needs) and staying connected (social closeness).

Assessment of Current and Anticipated Future Capabilities   As discussed in Chapter 6, AAC teams usually conduct assessments of cognitive, motor, language, and sensory capabilities with people who have acquired physical disabilities. One particularly important aspect of the assessment process for these individuals involves predicting the natural course of abilities. People with degenerative diseases will gradually lose some capabilities while other capabilities remain stable. For example, people in stable condition following a brainstem stroke or spinal cord injury may regain certain capabilities either naturally or with therapeutic intervention. Subsequent sections of this chapter discuss these issues in more detail with regard to specific disabilities.

Motor Skills   Individual patterns of motor control capability greatly affect the selection of an AAC system for individuals with ALS. These capabilities generally differ markedly depending on whether the person first experiences bulbar or spinal symptoms.

Bulbar ALS   For some time, people with predominantly bulbar (brainstem) symptoms are initially able to control AAC technology that they can carry and operate via direct selection using their hands or fingers. However, in time, they are often unable to access their AAC technology with their hands or fingers and must shift to a head- or eye-tracking access strategy. Of course, this is essentially always the case if they choose to use invasive ventilation for respiratory support.

For more information on AAC access for individuals with decreased motor capabilities, see the webcast *Supporting Communication of Individuals with Minimal Movement* by Susan Fager and David Beukelman.

Spinal ALS   People with ALS who exhibit predominantly spinal symptoms usually experience extensive trunk- and limb-related motor impairments before the time when they are unable to meet their communication needs through speech. For individuals with spinal ALS, the need for an augmented writing system often precedes the need for an augmented conversational system. Individuals with severe impairments related to limb control usually require a mounted system with either head- or eye-tracking access.

Assess Constraints   A variety of external constraints may affect AAC decisions in general, and some of these constraints are especially common for people with acquired communication disorders. As noted previously, the attitudes of family members and friends about the communication disorder in general and the acceptance of AAC technology in particular may influence decisions. For example, families of some adults with relatively stable medical conditions, such as aphasia from stroke, appear to have difficulty accepting the use of electronic communication techniques for a spouse or parent because they struggle with accepting their loved one's loss of speech or writing ability and wish to maintain the hope that functional speech will be restored. Typically, families of people with ALS accept AAC options because they realize that ALS is a degenerative disease.

Another constraint involves the availability of facilitators to learn about the operation and use of an electronic AAC system in order to assist the person who relies on AAC to learn and maintain it. In some locations, facilitators may not have access to adequate support for certain types of communication options. Another important external constraint involves the availability of funding for equipment and instruction.

Funding patterns for AAC systems vary dramatically in different parts of the world. Some countries, provinces, or states fund AAC systems for children who participate in educational programs but provide little financial support for adults. In the United States, Medicare, Medicaid, Tricare, and many insurance plans now fund AAC technology and instruction. It is impossible to outline such funding constraints in detail in this book because funding policies change frequently. The web site on AAC funding maintained by the AAC-RERC (Rehabilitation Engineering Research Center on Communication Enhancement) provides AAC funding information for the United States. Successful AAC interventions require that the AAC team assess constraints and focus on the remediation of these limitations as vigorously as they focus on the individual's communication needs and capabilities.

In addition, it is not uncommon for family members and friends who surround a person with an acquired physical disability to have differences of opinion regarding the person's communication needs as well as the use of assistive technologies. There is no way to predict what these differences will be, but it is important to try to achieve some degree of consensus among these people about the individual's communication needs or, if that is impossible, to at least clarify their differences of opinion and facilitate decision making. We discuss this issue with regard to specific disorders in subsequent sections of this chapter.

Evaluate Intervention Outcomes   There are three primary reasons for measuring the outcomes of interventions with adults who have acquired physical disabilities. The first is to identify the communication needs that have and have not been met. When an intervention approach succeeds in meeting certain communication needs, the AAC team should document the success for the sake of the individual and his or her family. If an initial intervention does not meet certain communication needs, the team should refine the approach and intervene accordingly. The second reason for measuring intervention outcomes is to document the effectiveness of the AAC agency providing the service. Agencies that provide funding for AAC interventions with adults usually demand this documentation for continued funding. The third reason for measuring intervention effectiveness is to document the overall AAC efforts of a particular center or agency, which may result in increased administrative support for AAC efforts over time.

Acceptance and Use of AAC by People with Amyotrophic Lateral Sclerosis and Their Families   Usually, individuals with ALS demonstrate relatively high acceptance of AAC technology. As AAC technology improves and is more common in society, acceptance rates continue to increase. Mathy, Yorkston, and Gutmann (2000) reviewed AAC use by people with ALS from numerous sources. They referred to data by Gutmann and Gryfe (1996), who evaluated trends in the use of AAC systems for 126 people seen at an assistive technology clinic in Toronto. Among these participants, 27% elected not to pursue AAC interventions. Gutmann, analyzing the same data, reported that "women preferred voice output systems twice as often as men (49% for women, 26% for men)" (1999, p. 211). In addition, "almost an equivalent number of men (27.8%) and women (26%) did not wish any AAC intervention" (Gutmann, 1999, p. 211).

Operational Competence   People with ALS, like most people who rely on AAC, require time and instruction in order to gain communicative competence with their AAC systems. Because ALS is predictably degenerative, these individuals are in the unique position of being able to select their AAC systems and learn to operate them while they can still use natural speech to meet at least their most basic communication needs. In fact, if an AAC system is selected and implemented after an individual is no longer able to speak, the AAC experience often becomes extremely frustrating.

Although rapid decline of speech function in ALS is certainly not inevitable, it occurs frequently enough that sound clinical management dictates early preparedness. In our experience, exploration of AAC options should begin when speech has slowed to about 125 words per minute and/or intelligibility is inconsistent in adverse listening situations.

Facilitator Support   People with ALS require ongoing support from AAC facilitators in order to use their AAC systems. This support may include instruction in technical or other skills that enable individuals to operate the technology efficiently and accurately. They may also need facilitator support to select and modify messages stored in their systems. In addition, as an individual's capabilities change with ALS progression, facilitators may need to change motor control options and the system position. Facilitators may also have to provide instruction in the social use of the AAC system. Ball, Schardt, and Beukelman (2005) surveyed 68 individuals with ALS who relied on AAC technology, and all reported the presence of a primary AAC facilitator. Nearly all facilitators (96%) were family members, most of them had nontechnical backgrounds, and 4% were professionals.

Late Phase: Adapt and Accommodate

The Late Phase begins after the implementation of AAC strategies recommended in the Middle Phase and continues until the individual's death. The objective of this phase is to provide effective communication options in response to changing communication needs, capabilities, and living situations. Generally, people with ALS are encouraged to and do make AAC decisions such that they make few changes in their SGD strategies. This enables them to become proficient with the technology while making slight changes to messages and access strategies as their communication needs and capabilities change.

In 2004, Ball, Beukelman, and Pattee reported on the AAC acceptance patterns of 50 individuals who were referred consecutively to an ALS clinic. Of the individuals with ALS in this study, 96% accepted AAC technology either immediately (90%) or after some delay (6%). Only 4% (i.e., two individuals) rejected AAC technology completely. In 2007, Ball, Anderson, et al. documented the duration of AAC use by people with ALS and reported average durations of 23.1 months for those with bulbar (brainstem) onset and 25.9 months for those with spinal onset. It should be noted that this sample included individuals with ALS who did and did not choose invasive mechanical ventilation support. Acceptance of mechanical ventilation (respirator or ventilator) extends the length of the individual's life and the duration of AAC use. Of course, invasive ventilation also extends the length of time that people with ALS must access their AAC options with minimal movement. None of the people with ALS in this study discontinued use of their AAC technology more than 2 months before their deaths. Families often report that within the last few weeks of life, people with ALS depend more and more on low-tech options, such as eye linking, eye gaze, or partner-assisted scanning to support the co-construction of messages with people who are very familiar with them. Roman, Quach, Coggiola, and Moore (2010) reported that people with ALS find eye linking to be faster and more preferred than an eye-pointing (e-tran) board or partner-assisted scanning. However, some individuals with ALS continue to have the strength and desire to use SGDs during the last days of their lives.

MULTIPLE SCLEROSIS

Multiple sclerosis (MS) is the most common neurological condition of young and middle-age adults. The cause of MS is unknown. It is an acquired, inflammatory, demyelinating disease of the central nervous system (Yorkston et al., 2012). Lesions are scattered in the central nervous system, and locations vary from person to person; therefore, symptom patterns also vary and must be considered when making AAC intervention decisions.

In the northern United States, the prevalence of MS is about 1 in 1,000; and in the southern states, the prevalence is about one third to one half of this figure. Approximately 95% of all cases begin between the ages of 10 and 50 years, with a median onset age of 27 years. Although MS is considered to be a disease of young people, it is not uncommon for an initial diagnosis to occur between 50 and 60 years of age. The female-to-male ratio of occurrence is 3:2 (Yorkston et al. 2012). Racially, people with MS are more likely to be white than African American and more likely to be African American than Asian.

The natural course of MS differs greatly from person to person. However, the typical relapsing-remitting pattern begins initially, and the progressive form of the disease occurs later. The average life expectancy of young males with MS is about 35 years following the onset of the disease. The prognosis is worse 1) in males than in females; 2) if the age at onset is greater than 35 years; or 3) if a chronic, progressive pattern appears at onset (Yorkston et al., 2012).

Communication Symptoms

Dysarthria is the most common communication problem associated with MS, but the study of large groups of individuals with MS has shown that dysarthria is not a universal characteristic of this disease. Darley, Brown, and Goldstein (1972) reported that 41% of their sample of individuals with MS demonstrated overall speech performance that was not "essentially normal" in terms of its impact on listeners. Nevertheless, when researchers utilized a self-reporting technique, only 23% of these individuals reported a "speech and/or communication disorder"; thus, a large percentage of this sample appeared to be unaware of the severity of their speech problems. Studies in which speech-language pathologists rated the adequacy of speech or performed a physical examination of the speech mechanism report a higher incidence of speech problems than studies using self-reports. Hartelius, Runmarker, and Andersen (2000) reported a rate of 51% in a cohort study in which individuals with MS diagnosed between 1950 and 1964 were followed for a mean of 37.5 years.

Augmentative and Alternative Communication Intervention for Multiple Sclerosis

A relatively small number of individuals with MS demonstrate such severe speech impairments that they require AAC systems. Beukelman, Kraft, and Freal (1985) reported that 4% of 656 survey respondents with MS indicated that their communication was so severely impaired that strangers were unable to understand them.

Early Phase Interventions

The Early Phase activities typically involved assistive technology other than traditional AAC strategies. Because the onset of MS occurs relatively early in life, individuals with MS are usually in educational programs or employed when they first experience symptoms. The intermittent and gradual onset of symptoms usually means that people with MS do not need to modify their lifestyles immediately, although some people with visual problems, which are quite common in MS, may require technological assistance to read computer screens or detailed printed materials. In time, however, impairments that are unrelated to verbal communication often prevent these individuals from attending school or working. For example, Kraft (1981) reported that arm and leg spasticity is an important reason why many people with MS drop out of employment. Loss of balance, loss of normal bladder control, and fatigue also interfere (Ford, Trigwell, & Johnson, 1998). In addition, a combination of weakness, spasticity, ataxia, and tremor may interfere with walking and necessitate the use of a wheelchair for mobility.

Specifically, vision problems require supports including font enlargement or speech output of printed messages. Keyboard control becomes difficult for some, so arm and hand supports as well as keyboard assists may be necessary to reduce nonproductive movement patterns (Yorkston & Beukelman, 2007). In particular, accessibility features included in the Apple and Microsoft computer operating systems can be helpful to those with vision and physical access limitations. Some people with MS also use memory and organizational supports found on many mobile electronic devices (Blake & Bodine, 2002).

Middle Phase Interventions

During the Middle Phase, compensatory support of natural speech is beneficial for those with speech intelligibility limitations. Alphabet supplementation involves identification of the first letter of each word by the speaker as the word is spoken. Typically, intelligibility of connected speech is improved by about 25% and intelligibility of single words by about 10% with alphabet supplementation (Hanson, Yorkston, & Beukelman, 2004).

Late Phase Interventions

For people with severe or profound dysarthria due to MS, in the Late Phase natural speech is no longer functional to meet all communication needs, and thus communication supports are required. Use of AAC supports can be difficult because vision problems, spasticity, ataxia, or intention tremor interfere with AAC access for these people. Therefore, AAC interventions tend to be very personalized, depending upon the communication need and capability profile of each person.

Identify Participation Patterns and Communication Needs

Most people with MS whose speech is so impaired that they require AAC systems are no longer able to attend school or work due to associated limitations in vision, fatigue, balance, and so forth (Yorkston et al., 2012); therefore, they rarely have communication needs related to these contexts. Furthermore, some individuals with severe speech impairments require personal care assistance beyond what their families can offer; and they may live in residential or nursing centers, which may limit their communication needs even further. Thus, the primary communication needs of many people with MS are conversational and care related, although some individuals may also require assistance with writing.

Assess Specific Capabilities

In this section, we describe the primary cognitive, language, sensory/perceptual, and motor capabilities that require assessment prior to AAC intervention.

Cognitive Skills

The cognitive limitations of individuals with MS have been poorly documented, but more than half of these individuals seem to display definite evidence of cognitive impairment (Rao, 1995; Yorkston et al., 2012). There is general consensus that cognitive changes are specific rather than global and can be described as a subcortical dementia with 1) the absence of aphasia; 2) memory retrieval impairment in the presence of relatively intact encoding and storage capability; 3) impaired conceptual reasoning in the context of near-typical intellect; 4) slowed information-processing time; and 5) personality disturbances including apathy, depression, or euphoria.

Language Skills

Although dysarthria is the most common communication problem associated with MS, aphasia has occasionally been reported. Several large studies of individuals with MS have noted no occurrence of aphasia (Olmos-Lau, Ginsberg, & Geller, 1977). However, Beukelman, Kraft, and Freal (1985) noted that other researchers reported the incidence of aphasia as ranging from 1% to 3% of people with MS. Yorkston, Klasner, and Swanson (2001) indicated that people with MS commonly report difficulty with word finding and changes in verbal or written organization. Murdock and Lethlean (2000) evaluated 60 people with MS and reported four potential subgroups: 1) those with pervasive language impairment (2%); 2) those with moderate to severe language impairment (13%); 3) those with mild to moderate language impairment (32%); and 4) those with essentially typical language abilities (53%).

Sensory/Perceptual Skills

Vision limitations are common in MS; in fact, 35% of people with MS experience optic neuritis, the acute or subacute loss of central vision in one eye with peripheral vision spared, as their first symptom (Wikstrom, Poser, & Ritter, 1980). Optic neuritis is often manifested initially by an inability to see text on a computer screen or to read small print in general. The visual limitations of MS cause particular problems in the context of AAC interventions because many AAC techniques require extensive visual capabilities. Many individuals with MS cannot use visual scanning arrays; instead, they may require auditory scanning systems such as the one described in a subsequent section of this chapter. Large-print text is a common requirement of people with MS, as is synthetic speech feedback that echoes the letters and words selected in typing or from a communication display. For example, an AAC system designed for a 30-year-old woman with MS consisted of an expanded keyboard with 1-inch square keys and speech feedback (Honsinger, 1989).

"[Here] is my list of lists: Long-term projects and obligations…daily tasks, projects, and obligations; spring cleaning tasks; items to be taken on overnight outings and trips,…personal care schedule; phone numbers; books on loan from the National Library Service for the Blind and Physically Handicapped and from Recordings for the Blind, Inc.; two lists of physical therapy exercises; names and phone numbers of friends and former clients; names and addresses of out-often friends and family; calendar; medical and surgical supplies that must be stocked; and fears and questions I have concerning life with a progressive disease. Some of my lists are on large sheets of braille paper, others are in a loose-leaf binder. All are on cassette tapes" (Denise Karuth, a woman who is blind as a result of MS, describing the lists she keeps as memory aids, in Karuth, 1985, p. 27).

Motor Skills

Individuals' motor control capabilities in MS vary considerably; therefore, careful motor assessment is an important aspect of all AAC interventions. According to Feys and colleagues (2001), intention tremor in the upper limb, which occurs during or is exaggerated by voluntary movement, is encountered in approximately one third of individuals with MS. The tremor often disrupts individuals' attempts to access assistive technology interfaces such as keyboards, computer mice, or switches. AAC teams can sometimes identify a way to stabilize the body part involved in access sufficiently so that the individual can make voluntary movements without excessive tremor. At other times, AAC teams may need to attach a switch to an individual's limb or hand so that the switch can move with the body part during tremor but still remain in position to be activated by a finger. Finally, specialized applications that provide motion-filtering software and support multiple interfaces have also been developed (Feys et al., 2001).

Often, the motor control problems and visual impairments of MS combine to limit AAC options severely. For example, Porter (1989) described an AAC intervention that was used near the end of a person's life. The individual's visual and motor control limitations were extensive, but he learned to control a simple call buzzer and auditory scanning system using a pressure switch that attached to a pillow beside his head.

Assess Constraints

Several characteristics of MS complicate many AAC interventions. First, symptom patterns vary considerably across individuals. Although the clinical course of MS follows five general patterns of progression, individual manifestations can be complex and vary over time. Obviously, changes in an AAC system may be needed to accommodate this variability. Second, as noted previously, visual impairments are common in MS and can make AAC interventions particularly challenging. Third, AAC interventions usually occur in conjunction with other efforts to compensate for the multiple impairments experienced by people with MS. Therefore, AAC teams must coordinate their interventions with other interventions in the context of changing symptom patterns.

GUILLAIN-BARRÉ SYNDROME

Guillain-Barré syndrome (GBS) results from progressive destruction and subsequent regeneration of the myelin sheath of peripheral nerve axons. Paralysis progresses from the lower extremities upward, and maximal paralysis usually occurs within 1–3 weeks of onset. As the myelin sheath slowly regenerates, nerve function and associated muscle strength gradually return. Typically, motor recovery begins with the structures of the head and face and progresses inferiorly. About 80% to 85% of people with GBS recover completely with no residual impairments (National Institute of Neurological Disorders and Stroke, 2009). Guillain-Barré syndrome affects 1 to 2 per 100,000 people in the United States and is equally common in men and women. Medical management includes ventilatory support, nutritional support and immunotherapy.

Communication Disorders

The weakness associated with GBS causes flaccid dysarthria and in many cases anarthria (complete loss of speech). In addition, severe weakness often requires ventilator support through oral intubation or tracheostomy. Language and cognition are usually unaffected.

Intervention Stages

The phases of progression of GBS require different types of AAC support, as described in the following sections.

Early Phase: Deterioration Phase, Loss of Speech

As noted previously, people with GBS experience maximal paralysis within 1–3 weeks of onset. Because weakness progresses upward from the lower extremities, the diagnosis usually is made before speech becomes impaired. Little time usually passes, however, between diagnosis and onset of severe speech impairment. Typically, individuals with GBS are hospitalized following their diagnosis so that medical personnel can monitor their symptom progression and provide appropriate supports and intervention. As part of this effort, medical teams should monitor these individuals' communication impairment so that AAC intervention can be provided at an appropriate time.

After a few weeks, the progress of symptoms stabilizes. Those people who require AAC intervention are usually unable to speak by this stage and receive respiratory support from a ventilator. Initially, AAC intervention consists of low-technology options, with emphasis on the establishment of a reliable yes/no system, followed by the development of an eye-pointing or eye-linking technique. AAC teams should develop communication boards that will support the individual's needs through partner-assisted visual and auditory scanning, yes/no responses, and eye linking or eye pointing. Communication boards typically include social messages, health-related messages, and letters and numbers for message construction.

Middle Phase: Prolonged
Speechlessness, Spontaneous Recovery of Speech

The time frame during which people with GBS are unable to speak varies from individual to individual. Some people experience weeks or months of using AAC systems to communicate with family, friends, and health care staff. Typically, these individuals continue to use low-tech strategies; however, electronic options may also be appropriate to provide greater independence and less reliance on knowledgeable, well-trained listeners. Usually, the extensive motor impairments of these individuals require them to use scanning AAC systems, often with a switch controlled by eyelid or head movement. Given the temporary nature of these individuals' AAC use, most learn to communicate with letter-by-letter spelling and retrieval of a limited number of messages.

Late in this phase, the individual with GBS makes the transition from speechlessness back to functional speech. Often, this transition takes several weeks or months. As muscle strength returns to the speech mechanism, the individual may still use a ventilator and a tracheostomy tube for breathing. Some speakers find an oral-type electrolarynx (see Chapter 17) very helpful at this point. By controlling the sound sources of the electrolarynx with a head switch, the sound can be turned on when the person wishes to speak and turned off when he or she wishes to listen or rest. While the muscles of the oral cavity remain weak, the individual may have imprecise articulation and reduced speech intelligibility. Some individuals find it helpful to first establish the communicative topic or context with their AAC system, then use their residual speech, and finally resolve communication breakdowns with their AAC system as necessary. As recovery progresses, medical personnel will remove ventilator support and the individual will again be able to speak independently. Usually, the individual requires no ongoing natural speech interventions.

Late Phase: Long-Term Residual Motor Speech Disorder

As mentioned previously, 85% of people with GBS experience complete recovery of motor control; the remaining 15% experience residual weakness. Of this residual group, only a few experience long-term motor speech disorders (i.e., dysarthria). For them, speech interventions to maximize the effectiveness of their natural speech are appropriate. We do not know of any individual with GBS who required long-term AAC support.

Garrett, Happ, Costello, and Fried-Oken (2007) provide an excellent chapter focusing on AAC for people in intensive and acute care units. This content is very informative for those who support the communication of people with GBS in the Middle Phase.

PARKINSON'S DISEASE

Parkinson's disease (PD) is a syndrome composed of a cluster of motor symptoms that include tremor at rest, rigidity, paucity (i.e., reduction in movement), and impaired postural reflexes. PD results from a loss of dopaminergic neurons in the basal ganglia (especially the substantia nigra) and the brainstem. The onset is typically insidious; in retrospect, many individuals recall stiffness and muscle aches that they first attributed to typical aging. The symptom that often initiates the first visit to a physician is tremor in a resting position (Yorkston et al., 2012).

Medical treatment since the 1970s has greatly altered the natural course of PD. Prior to the availability of existing medications, about one fourth of all individuals with PD died within the first 5 years following diagnosis, and 80% died after 10–14 years (Yorkston et al., 2010). Although the changes in mortality rate due to levodopamine (L-dopa) and other medications are not yet clear, these treatments have certainly altered the lifestyles of people with PD dramatically. Individuals with PD are able to move more freely and manage their lives much more independently with medication than without it. Surgical treatments have returned to favor for selected people with PD, as has deep brain stimulation.

For a more detailed discussion of medical and surgical interventions, see Yorkston et al. (2012). The pharmacologic management of PD continues to change. Readers are also referred to the web site of the Mayo Clinic for general information about drug and surgical management and the web site of the National Institute of Neurological Disorders and Stroke for information about clinical trials.

It should be noted that at the time this chapter was written, the impact of pharmacological, surgical, and deep brain stimulation interventions on the speech performance of individuals with PD was inconsistent and somewhat limited. During late stages of the disorder, responsiveness to medication decreases; thus, during the period when AAC intervention is needed, symptoms may be difficult to manage pharmacologically.

The average annual incidence of parkinsonism (excluding drug-induced cases) is 18.2 cases per 100,000 people. The prevalence is estimated to be between 66 and 187 cases per 100,000 people, with no significant difference in incidence between males and females. The incidence increases sharply above the age of 64, and peak incidence is between 75 and 84 years of age. There is a trend toward increased age at the time of diagnosis (Yorkston et al., 2010).

Although pharmocological treatment dramatically improves the performance of many people with PD, some side effects of the medication can interfere with the use of AAC approaches. There may be individual fluctuations in motor responses (also known as an on-off response), probably due to differences in medication absorption and dopamine receptor responsiveness. With long-term therapy, some people also experience involuntary movements that interfere with functional activities. These involuntary movements may cause emotional distress as well.

Communication Symptoms

Dysarthria is common in PD. Hartelius and Svensson (1994) surveyed 230 people with PD and noted that 70% of these individuals reported that speech and voice were worse than prior to the onset of the disease. Yorkston et al. (2012) and Duffy (2005) described the speech symptoms of people with PD in detail. Typically, symptoms include reduced pitch variability, reduced overall loudness, and decreased use of all vocal parameters for achieving stress and emphasis. Articulation is imprecise and is produced at variable rates. Voice quality is often harsh and sometimes breathy.

Nevertheless, speech disorders among people with PD are not uniform. Some speakers are difficult to understand, primarily because they speak excessively fast. Their speaking rates may exceed those of typical speakers or exceed those that are optimal for people with motor control disorders. Other speakers are difficult to understand because they speak with reduced intensity or loudness. Still others speak with such limited movement of their articulators that they have difficulty producing precise speech sounds. As PD progresses, many speakers demonstrate combinations of these speech patterns.

Clinical observations reveal a gradual process, with speech becoming increasingly difficult to understand. Most people with PD communicate with natural speech to a greater or lesser extent. Therefore, when they use AAC techniques, the techniques make up part of a multimodal communication system that includes natural speech.

"My ability to form thoughts and ideas into words and sentences is not impaired; the problem is translating those words and sentences into articulate speech. My lips, tongue, and jaw muscles simply won't cooperate. What words I do smuggle through the blockade can be heard, though not always comprehended. Try as I might, I can't inflect my speech to reflect my state of mind. And it's not like I can liven up my halting monotone with a raised eyebrow; my face, utterly expressionless, simply won't respond. Like Emmett Kelly, but without the greasepaint, I often appear sad on the outside while actually smiling, or at least smirking, on the inside" (Michael J. Fox, describing his PD symptoms in *Lucky Man* [Fox, 2002]).

Intervention Phases

Although the benefits of behavioral intervention to improve speech in people with PD are well documented in literature review articles (Spencer, Yorkston, & Duffy, 2003; Yorkston, Spencer, & Duffy, 2003), the following sections highlight AAC intervention options during the early, middle, and late phases of speech progression. For a more complete description of management of dysarthria in PD, see Yorkston et al. (2012).

Early Phase Intervention

Usually, AAC supports are not necessary to support communication during the Early Phase. However, assistance in computer control for employment, Internet use, and recreation may be necessary for some individuals with PD. A program for Internet training of people with PD is available (Stewart, Worrall, Egan, & Oxenham, 2004). Near the end of the Early Phase, people with PD often complete instruction in the Lee Silverman Voice Treatment in order to teach them how to maintain their speech performance as their PD progresses. Practice guidelines in the motor speech disorders field (Yorkston, Spencer, & Duffy, 2003) have documented the effectiveness of this behavioral intervention for people with PD.

Middle Phase Intervention

During the Middle Phase, assistive technology and AAC supports may be necessary to supplement natural speech. Delayed auditory feedback is used by some speakers with PD who need to control their speaking rate. This portable technology delays speech for a fraction of a second, thus slowing the person's speaking rate. A number of reports document successful use of this technology in hypokinetic dysarthria (Adams, 1994, 1997; Downie, Low, & Lindsay, 1981; Hanson & Metter, 1983). About 8% of people with PD benefit from delayed auditory feedback; however, there is little information about how to predict who will be successful, so trial intervention is needed to determine if this intervention will be effective.

In this phase, some with PD benefit from portable vocal amplifiers. Those with consistent voicing but reduced loudness levels are the best candidates. Amplification does not benefit those who cannot initiate phonation.

Late Phase Intervention

For those people with PD who become unable to meet their communication needs through residual natural speech, some choose to rely on AAC strategies to resolve communication breakdowns, communicate in adverse situations, or, in some cases, communicate most of their messages. Typically, they choose technology with speech synthesis output that can be accessed through letter-by-letter spelling. At the time of this writing, mobile technology with AAC applications is becoming available, but little information is available about the use of this technology by people with PD.

Identify Participation Patterns and Communication Needs

The communication needs of people with PD depend on two primary factors. Many people with PD are older adults, and most are retired. Therefore, their communication needs reflect, first of all, the social environments of their retirement. In addition, the range of physical impairments in PD varies greatly from person to person. Some people have such severe physical limitations that they require extensive physical assistance from attendants or family members. The level of assistance needed greatly influences each individual's communication needs.

Assess Specific Capabilities

In this section, we describe the primary cognitive/linguistic, sensory/perceptual, and motor capabilities that require assessment prior to AAC intervention for individuals with PD.

Cognitive/Linguistic Skills

People with PD acquire their disability late in life, so they usually have developed typical language skills. Therefore, they can spell and read at levels necessary to support most AAC interventions. Controversy exists as to whether dementia is a feature of PD (Bayles et al., 1996). During tests, examiners have found that some individuals have specific memory impairments, and some individuals complain of slowness in problem solving. The AAC team must consider whether such cognitive limitations are likely to interfere with AAC interventions. The team may provide additional instruction and practice in order to help the person compensate for learning or memory difficulties.

Sensory/Perceptual Skills

Disturbances in sensory function usually do not interfere with AAC interventions for people with PD.

Motor Skills

Clinical reports describe people who have successfully used direct selection AAC techniques such as alphabet boards, as discussed previously. Because researchers have reported few AAC interventions with PD speakers, the motor control problems that may influence such AAC interventions are not well documented. Thus, AAC teams may need to consider several potential motor control problems. Many individuals have reduced range and speed of movement due to the rigidity associated with PD. The AAC team will need to reduce the size of the selection display (e.g., on an alphabet board) for these individuals. Other individuals experience extensive tremors that are usually worse when they are at rest. Many can dampen the tremors if they can stabilize their hands on the surface of a communication board or device. A keyguard is often helpful with technology that has a keyboard. Some people experience hyperkinesia (excessive movement) as a side effect of the medication that controls their parkinsonian symptoms. These excessive movements may interfere with the fine motor control required for some AAC options.

"Micrographia is precisely what it sounds—tiny writing....Without drugs, my own penmanship becomes...microscopic. Combined with the stubborn refusal of my 'off' arm to move in a smooth, lateral, left-to-right direction, the result is a fractured column of miniature scribbles" (Michael J. Fox, describing his PD symptoms in *Lucky Man* [Fox, 2002]).

Assess Constraints

Two types of constraints are usually associated with AAC interventions for people with PD. First, because most people with PD are able to speak to some extent, they may display some resistance toward the need for an AAC intervention. Some may blame their listeners for their communication failures, even if this is not the case. Communication partners need to actively encourage these individuals to use AAC techniques. Second, many people with PD are older adults and have spouses and friends in the same age group. Therefore, the hearing limitations of their listeners may act as a significant barrier to effective communication.

BRAINSTEM STROKE

Strokes (i.e., cerebrovascular accidents) that disrupt the circulation serving the lower brainstem often cause severe dysarthria or anarthria (i.e., an inability to produce speech). Because the brainstem contains the nuclei of all the cranial nerves that activate the muscles of the face, mouth, and larynx, damage to this area of the brain may result in an inability or a reduced ability to control these muscles voluntarily or reflexively. The nerve tracts that activate the trunk and limbs via the spinal nerves also pass through the brainstem. Therefore, severe damage to the brainstem may impair motor control of the limbs as well as motor control of the face and mouth.

Communication Symptoms

Communication symptoms associated with brainstem stroke vary considerably with the level and extent of damage to the brainstem. Some people are dysarthric but can communicate partial or complete messages through speech. These individuals usually experience dysarthria of the predominantly flaccid type due to damage to the nerve nuclei of the cranial nerves. Other individuals may display a marked spastic component in addition to flaccidity. Many people with brainstem stroke are unable to speak because of the severity of their impairments. Nearly all of them require AAC support initially. Only about 25% regain some functional speech, and the rest require AAC support throughout the rest of their lives (Culp, Beukelman, & Fager, 2007).

Identify Participation Patterns and Communication Needs

Medical and lifestyle issues influence the communication needs of people who experience brainstem stroke, as does the extent of their communication disorders.

Following brainstem stroke, an individual may require extensive personal and medical care, depending on the severity of the stroke and subsequent health conditions. People who survive a brainstem stroke are usually unable to work. Some can be cared for at home, whereas others may live in settings that range from independent living to nursing care centers. Individuals who experience brainstem stroke are usually aware of the world around them and are able to exchange information and achieve social closeness through their message formulations. Thus, they may have extensive communication needs.

Intervention Phases

Typically, intervention to meet the communication needs of individuals who experience brainstem stroke is managed in three phases (Culp et al., 2007).

Early Phase

The Early Phase of intervention begins as soon as the referral is received when the individual enters a rehabilitation hospital or long-term care facility. The goal of this phase is to develop a functional yes/no response and the ability to access a call system. Early in this phase, the individual often has medical, attention, and fatigue issues that must be considered. Once a reliable yes/no response has been identified, communication partners must be aware that the accuracy of these responses can be influenced by fatigue (see Forms 3.5 and 3.6 in Beukelman, Garrett, & Yorkston, 2007). It is essential that all communication partners be aware of the yes/no response strategy, such as directing the eyes up for YES and directing the eyes down for NO, so that the individual partners do not attempt different strategies. This requires effective instruction of the care and therapy personnel as well as the family by posting specific strategies in the individual's room, on the wheelchair, and so forth. Once the yes/no response strategy has been implemented, it is common practice to post common care need questions in a yes/no form so that communication partners remember to use this form rather than other question forms, such as fill-in-the-blank, *what*, or *why* question forms.

Later in the Early Phase, the individual with brainstem impairment develops the ability to use a low-tech communication technique or techniques for functional communication (Culp et al., 2007). Depending on the individual's capability and preference, eye-linking, eye-gaze, or partner-assisted scanning strategies are considered (see Forms 3.7 and 3.8 in Beukelman, Garrett, & Yorkston, 2007). The selection of a strategy is dependent upon the accuracy with which the individual can communicate using a strategy and the willingness and capability of communication partners to implement it. Typically, in this phase the individual develops the capability to select specific messages, words, or letters (for letter-by-letter spelling) that are offered to him or her by a communication partner.

Middle Phase: Selection of AAC Technology

The Middle Phase begins with acceptance on the part of the individual with brainstem stroke and his or her important decision makers that a long-term AAC option will be needed because the individual's natural speech will not be restored sufficiently to meet his or her communication needs. Some resist this step because they feel that accepting AAC technology implies that they are giving up on the return of natural speech. They must be assured that all involved would be delighted if natural speech were restored, but until then, communication needs must be met.

During this phase, the individual with brainstem stroke undergoes formal AAC assessments to document his or her communication needs and residual capabilities so that a feature match can be completed to identify potential AAC options. The individual with AAC needs is then introduced to these options, and use trials are completed before AAC technology is selected and purchased.

The capability assessment involves cognitive, language, sensory/perceptual, and motor aspects. No accompanying cognitive limitations are expected if the stroke involves only the brainstem. If the stroke extends higher into the brain or is associated with a more extensive medical episode that interfered with the supply of oxygen to the brain, a wide variety of cognitive impairments may exist. These need to be assessed on an individual basis.

If brainstem stroke does not affect the cortical or subcortical structures associated with language functioning, language skills should not be impaired. Thus, the skills of people with brainstem stroke usually reflect their prestroke linguistic performances.

A high brainstem stroke may affect the cranial nerve nuclei that control muscles for eye and eyelid movement, whereas a middle or low brainstem stroke probably will not impair these muscles. Thus, visual functioning may or may not be impaired. In either case, brainstem stroke generally leaves hearing unimpaired but often impairs tactile and position senses.

People with severe dysarthria or anarthria following a brainstem stroke usually experience problems with motor control of their limbs as well as of their speech mechanisms. AAC specialists have reported interventions that employ eye or head pointing as the alternative access mode for individuals who experience motor control problems. For example, Beukelman, Kraft, and Freal (1985) reported case studies of two people with brainstem stroke who successfully used electronic AAC systems via optical pointers mounted on their eyeglasses. Both individuals were required to spend much time in bed for medical reasons and learned to operate their AAC systems while in their wheelchairs and also while lying supine. AAC teams designed special mounting systems to support their devices in bed.

Late Phase: Implementation of AAC Technology into Daily Life

Once AAC technology selected for an individual with brainstem stroke arrives, it is optimized for the individual in terms of mounting and access, message preparation, and message output. This step is followed by a period of intense instruction and practice to develop operational competence with the technology. Of course, AAC facilitators need to be instructed so that they can provide appropriate support. Finally, the person who relies on AAC needs to develop social competence with the technology to communicate effectively in different settings and with a range of communication partners.

Intervention Stages to Restore Natural Speech

As outlined in the previous section, some people with brainstem stroke require AAC to meet their communication needs immediately following the stroke and for the long term. Others recover natural speech to meet some or all of their communication needs. The following intervention stages are implemented for individuals who attempt to recover natural speech.

Stage 1: No Useful Speech

As discussed in the previous section, many people with brainstem stroke must rely on AAC for a period of time during the acute and early rehabilitation phases of their recovery. In an attempt to recover speech, these individuals typically focus on individual speech subsystems.

Stage 2: Reestablish Subsystem Control for Speech

During this stage, people unable to speak because of brainstem stroke work systematically to develop voluntary control of their respiratory, phonatory (vocal), velopharyngeal, and articulatory subsystems while they continue to use their AAC systems for communication interactions. Because weakness is a predominant symptom of brainstem stroke, intervention at this stage involves strengthening the muscles of the subsystem and coordinating actions of the subsystems during speechlike and speech behaviors. Early in this stage, the AAC system will be used to support the majority of communication interactions; however, late in this stage individuals will convey an increasing percentage of messages through natural speech. (For a complete description of these intervention strategies, see Yorkston, Beukelman, Strand, & Hakel, 2010.)

Stage 3: Independent Use of Natural Speech

During this stage, speech intervention focuses on speech intelligibility, with the goal of meeting all communication needs through natural speech. We have worked with several speakers who used alphabet supplementation early in this stage. In time, they relied on AAC only to resolve communication breakdowns, and finally, AAC became unnecessary for communication interaction, although writing was still difficult or required the use of AAC.

Stage 4: Maximizing Speech Naturalness and Efficiency

By this stage, the person with brainstem stroke will no longer need to use an AAC system. The goal is for the individual to speak as naturally as possible by learning to use appropriate breath groups and stress patterns.

Stage 5: No Detectable Speech Disorder

Few individuals who have sustained a brainstem stroke achieve typical speech patterns.

Locked-in Syndrome

Closely related to brainstem stroke is locked-in syndrome (LIS, also known as ventral pontine syndrome), which results in a conscious quadriplegic state in which the individual's only voluntary movement consists of vertical eye movements and perhaps eye blinks. The usual cause is a basilar artery stroke (occlusion or hemorrhage), a tumor, or trauma that results in damage to the upper pons or occasionally the midbrain.

In a follow-up study of 29 people with LIS, Katz, Haig, Clark, and DiPaola (1992) reported an 85% survival rate for 5 years, with survival ranging from 2 to 18 years. None of these individuals regained the ability to speak in full sentences, although one was able to utter single words consistently and four could produce single words occasionally. Low- and high-tech AAC strategies were used.

In another follow-up study, Culp and Ladtkow (1992) followed 16 people with LIS for at least 1 year. Fifteen of these individuals experienced LIS following stroke, and one experienced LIS following a blow to the occipital region. All remained non-ambulatory, and nearly half experienced sufficient visual difficulties to interfere with their AAC interventions. Eight eventually developed adequate vision and motor skills for direct selection AAC access, and nine relied on scanning access. Thirteen of the sixteen individuals chose high-tech AAC systems.

Finally, Soderholm, Meinander, and Alaranta (2001) followed the AAC use of 17 people with LIS. On average, these individuals were involved in rehabilitation for 3–4 months, during which they received computer-based AAC systems. Switch access sites included the head, mouth, fingers, and hands. AAC technology was used for communication, Internet access, e-mail, writing, telephone, games, and vocational duties. Through the years, AAC intervention evolved as these individuals' capabilities, living situations, and personal roles changed. Eventually, two of the seventeen individuals regained speech as their primary communication method.

In 1997, Jean-Dominique Bauby, a French man with LIS, completed a book entitled *Le Scaphandre et le Papillon [The Diving Bell and the Butterfly]*. After a stroke in 1995, Bauby required ventilator assistance to breathe and was fed via a gastric tube; he was unable to move except for blinking his eyes. He wrote the book with the help of an assistant, who repeatedly recited the alphabet arranged according to the frequency of letter use in the French language. Bauby used eye blinks to indicate to his assistant which letters to use to spell out words. At the end of the book, Bauby asked, "Is there a key out in the cosmos that can unlock my bubble? A currency valuable enough to buy my freedom? I have to look elsewhere. I'm going there" (Bauby, 1997, 131–132). Bauby died less than 72 hours later.

CONCLUSIONS

Numerous factors influence AAC interventions for people with severe communication disabilities due to acquired physical impairments. First, the diseases, conditions, and syndromes associated with the physical impairments usually require close medical monitoring. Therefore, frequent, detailed, and accurate communication with medical personnel is necessary.

Second, the medical and physical status of individuals with acquired physical impairments can affect their capability levels. Because fatigue is common for these individuals, interventionists should take care to provide them with AAC systems that they can control even when tired. In addition, these individuals' responses to medication can vary. For example, people with PD may experience a range of physical abilities, depending on their medication regimens. Those with physical impairments may be susceptible to health problems such as infections and respiratory disorders, both of which limit physical endurance.

Third, people with severe communication disabilities due to acquired physical impairments often experience additional disabilities in areas such as mobility, object manipulation, eating, and swallowing. Their communication needs are usually influenced by the nature and severity of these associated disabilities. In order to obtain appropriate services, they must request assistance, instruct caregivers and attendants, and interact with professional personnel regarding the range of their disabilities. Thus, AAC teams must plan their interventions to accommodate other assistive technologies, such as powered wheelchairs, electronically controlled beds, and respiratory support equipment.

Electronic communication options, such as e-mail, electronic chat rooms, closed electronic mailing lists, and web sites, provide people who use high-tech AAC systems important additional communication options. Several characteristics make these electronic communication options quite comfortable for people who communicate using AAC. For example, offline preparation of messages allows people with slow message preparation rates to take as much time during the process as they need. Also, individuals can access electronic communication options according to their personal schedules.

QUESTIONS

14.1. Your uncle has recently been diagnosed with ALS. What is the probability that he will maintain functional speech throughout the remainder of his life?

14.2. Your aunt has been diagnosed with spinal rather than bulbar (brainstem) ALS. How is that diagnosis likely to impact her walking, eating, and speaking?

14.3. What speech characteristic in an individual with ALS best predicts the need for an AAC assessment to take place in a timely manner? Does a diagnosis of spinal versus bulbar ALS affect the usefulness of that predictor?

14.4. What is an AAC facilitator? Do most individuals with ALS who rely on AAC need AAC facilitators? Who typically fills the facilitator role for people with ALS?

14.5. How do the goals of Early Phase, Middle Phase, and Late Phase AAC intervention for ALS differ?

14.6. Your neighbor has been diagnosed with Parkinson's disease. He asks if he will need "one of those talking machines." What do you tell him?

14.7. What percentage of people who experience brainstem stroke require long-term AAC supports?

14.8. What is the goal of Early Phase AAC intervention for someone with brainstem stroke?

14.9. What is meant by the term *locked-in syndrome*? What is the impact of this syndrome on communication options?

14.10. Your older brother has been diagnosed with multiple sclerosis. Do you expect that he will require AAC at some point in his life?

CHAPTER 15

Adults with Severe
Aphasia and Apraxia of Speech

Kathryn L. Garrett and Joanne P. Lasker

Aphasia is an impairment of the ability to interpret and formulate language resulting from brain injury. More than 1 million people live with aphasia in the United States (National Institute on Deafness and Other Communication Disorders, 2008). Although this is roughly equivalent to 1 in 300 Americans, the condition is relatively unfamiliar to the general public. Of the approximately 80,000 individuals who acquire aphasia each year, most do so as a result of a cerebrovascular accident (CVA, or stroke) in the left cerebral hemisphere. Other etiologies include brain injury related to accidents, tumors, or illnesses such as meningitis or epilepsy. Most people who have aphasia acquire it after the age of 60 years and a lifetime of communicating without difficulty. However, a substantial number of children and younger adults can also develop aphasia while in the prime of their school-age or working years.

In aphasia, the sequence of neurological steps required to communicate may be interrupted at any point—when comprehending what others say, creating ideas, retrieving words and sentence structures, or executing the motor movements to speak. Comprehension and manipulation of symbols (words, letters, sounds, numbers, pictures) is inaccurate or slow, which in turn impacts many activities that are ubiquitous for people in industrialized cultures: reading, writing, computing, e-mailing, using electronic devices and ATMs, listening in crowded or noisy venues, placing an order for tangible goods, asking and answering questions in face-to-face situations as well as by telephone, and more. Some people with aphasia demonstrate relatively intact intellectual ability; others demonstrate reductions in processing speed, attention, memory, executive functions, and/or problem solving that cannot be completely explained by the loss of language (Christensen & Wright, 2010; Erickson, Goldinger, & LaPointe, 1996; Helm-Estabrooks, 2002; Murray, Holland, & Beeson, 1997; Nicholas, Sinotte, & Helm-Estabrooks, 2011; Wright & Shisler, 2005).

Many people with aphasia continue to improve their communication, cognition, and language skills for months and years following onset (Jungblut, Suchanek, &

Gerhard, 2009; Rijntjes, 2006). However, many never communicate as efficiently or effectively as before the onset of aphasia. Language that once was swift, automatic, unconscious, and attuned to the dynamic challenges of communicating with others often remains awkward and effortful, even for those who regain natural speech. Even more urgently, up to 40% of all people with aphasia will experience chronic, severe language impairments across modalities (Collins, 1986; Helm-Estabrooks, 1984; Kurland et al., 2004; Martin et al., 2009).

Aphasia is a complex disorder that defies a straightforward, unitary treatment approach. In the early stages of recovery, speech-language pathologists should help those with aphasia to reestablish meaningful communication as rapidly as possible. Augmentative and alternative communication (AAC) strategies (particularly partner-supported AAC strategies—see the next section) can be extremely beneficial during this period, particularly if natural speech is slow to emerge and/or comprehension is severely impaired. During rehabilitation, interventionists begin to determine whether individuals are likely to regain natural speech and functional comprehension. Restorative therapy approaches are often emphasized in this phase. However, as individuals transition to home health, outpatient, or long-term care phases of treatment, AAC strategies and interventions may merit increased attention if aphasia continues to restrict an individual's ability to participate in important life activities.

AUGMENTATIVE AND ALTERNATIVE COMMUNICATION INTERVENTIONS FOR APHASIA

In our view, AAC strategies are essentially *external representations of meaning*. People with aphasia must refer to informational supports that are "outside of their heads"— that is, not part of the automatized network of memories, associations, and language that allowed them to communicate with minimal effort before onset of aphasia. AAC is also a broad collection of high- and low-technology supports that can serve many functions for people with aphasia, such as 1) enhancing the comprehension of individuals with auditory comprehension deficits; 2) providing a means of expressing preferences, needs, or basic personal information; 3) serving as a word or phrase bank for more elaborate topics; 4) serving as a comprehensive communication tool to generate both spoken and written language; or 5) offering a specific technique to enable some individuals to participate, with more independence, in an important life activity.

AAC approaches for aphasia typically involve multimodal communication strategies. Communicators with aphasia are encouraged to use natural communication modalities, such as residual speech, gestures, and writing, as well as externally represented messages, or AAC. In addition, a comprehensive view of AAC for aphasia incorporates communication partners as key contributors to many intervention techniques.

To aid in planning communication interventions for individuals with severe aphasia, a classification system was initially developed by Garrett and Beukelman (1992; 1998); it was revised in 2005 by the authors of this chapter and is discussed in detail by Lasker, Garrett, and Fox (2007). This system differentiates between individuals who can learn to communicate *independently* with AAC strategies and those who function best when AAC is used in *partner-supported* contexts. Within these two groupings, the AAC intervention varies depending on communicators' optimal participation levels, communication needs, or specific cognitive-linguistic competencies. Refer to Form 6.1 in Beukelman, Garrett, and Yorkston (2007) and the AAC-Aphasia

Categories of Communicators Checklist for an assessment tool that delineates the characteristics of each communicator category and subcategory.

The following categories of communicators constitute an ascending hierarchy of cognitive and linguistic competence, independence, and need. Clinicians can use this hierarchy as a rough guide when designing interventions. However, it should be noted that all of the strategies from each category may be useful at various times regardless of communicator type. The intermittency of aphasia and the dynamic nature of communication demand flexibility from clinicians and communicators alike.

Partner-Dependent AAC Communicators with Aphasia

Some communicators with aphasia will always require their communication partners to manage informational demands and provide communication choices within highly familiar contexts (Kagan, 1998; 2001). We describe three types of partner-dependent AAC communicators in an ascending hierarchy of communicative competence, along with corresponding intervention goals and strategies.

Emerging AAC Communicators

The emerging AAC communicator has a profound cognitive-linguistic disorder across modalities as a result of extensive brain injury from a single large CVA, multiple CVAs, trauma, or encephalopathy. The condition is often labeled with the term *global aphasia* or may be misidentified as dementia. Often, because of diminished arousal and comprehension skills, these people do not respond appropriately to the physician's or speech-language pathologist's initial screening questions in the acute medical setting. Many of these individuals are subsequently discharged to long-term care facilities after minimal or no rehabilitation. Some of these individuals are capable of responding immediately if partners adopt slightly different ways of communicating and engaging their attention. Others may experience increased attentional capacities months later, at which time additional therapy may be considered. A small proportion may eventually transition to more advanced levels of communication and even develop some speech, functional gestures, or ability to use moderately complex AAC strategies.

Emerging AAC communicators have extreme difficulties speaking, using symbols, and responding to conversational input. Apraxia of speech (i.e., speech production errors that are a result of breakdowns in motor planning and sequencing) may be profound and may occur at all levels of the motor planning system—oral motor, laryngeal, speech, gestural, even respiratory. Individuals with this condition seldom communicate purposefully; even fundamental nonverbal signals, such as pointing or nodding, are infrequent. They do not easily associate photos or line drawings of common objects with their referents, so providing prefabricated picture-symbol books to help them request wants and needs may be ineffective. They may not immediately be able to participate in typical linguistic treatment programs used in aphasia rehabilitation. For example, when answering a series of unrelated yes/no questions in a stimulation-type therapy session, these individuals often do not respond or will answer with vague, imprecise head nods. Communicators who have such limited linguistic ability may initially benefit from participating in contextual activities that elicit basic *referential* skills, such as pointing to request an item or looking in the direction of a mutually important item (e.g., out the window during a snowstorm), versus participating in highly linguistic question-and-answer tasks (Garrett & Huth, 2002; Ho, Weiss, Garrett, & Lloyd, 2005).

Low-tech AAC strategies can assist emerging AAC communicators to both comprehend and control their personal environment by making basic choices, symbolized with real objects, within the context of familiar routines such as dressing. To illustrate, the therapist or caregiver could point to the calendar, discuss the season or weather, and then indicate several items of clothing. After ensuring that the emerging AAC communicator has visually attended to the clothing items, the partner could verbally present the choices at a slow pace, encouraging the individual to choose or show preference by nodding, vocalizing, reaching, or showing changes in facial expression.

To encourage participation in familiar social activities such as selecting gift items for a family member, the therapist, caregiver, or family member could first show pictures of the individual for whom the gift is desired and discuss the occasion using props (e.g., for a birthday, present a calendar and a birthday card). Then, prior to asking choice questions, the partner could encourage the person with severe aphasia to look at pictures of gift choices presented in a simplified catalog (i.e., pictures cut apart, pasted on blank paper, and taped inside a real catalog) and to turn pages, if appropriate. After the person with aphasia chooses or shows preference for a gift, he or she can make other decisions regarding cost or color of the item if appropriate. Communicators should also be encouraged to "confirm" that a choice is desired as a preliminary step toward developing linguistic responses such as "yes" and "no."

Intervention Strategies   Treatment for the emerging AAC communicator focuses on developing the following foundational communication skills: turn taking,

Table 15.1.   Emerging AAC communicator: Intervention goals and strategies

Communicator strategies	Partner strategies
Choose items to meet needs during daily routines by pointing or reaching.	Develop contextual routines, life activities, and opportunities in which the individual can utilize choice-making, turn-taking, referential, acceptance, and rejection skills (e.g., choosing nail polish to match outfit, selecting gifts for spouse from a catalog).
Reference familiar photographs in photo album by pointing or by demonstrating appropriate facial expression when participating in a dyadic reminiscing activity.	Create a simple scrapbook or photo album (one or two pictures of important life events per page with key word labels).
Choose preferred items within the context of a functional activity (e.g., ordering garden seeds from a catalog; selecting coffee, tea, or hot chocolate).	Facilitate participation in simple, age-appropriate games (e.g., Tic-tac-toe, War) and activities (e.g., approving or rejecting antiques listed for sale on Craigslist).
Participate in turn taking within context of familiar visual games (e.g., Tic-tac-toe, War).	Provide contingent feedback for communicator's referential, joint attention, affirmation, and rejection signals (e.g., "Oh, you're looking at the pink nail polish...so that's what you want!").
Consistently signal affirmation/agreement (head nod) for preferred items during choice-making activities.	Utilize augmented input strategies: Supplement the emerging AAC communicator's comprehension of auditory information by pointing to referents, gesturing, or drawing key conversational points.
Consistently signal rejection (pushing away, head shake) for nonpreferred items during choice-making activities.	Include a humorous, nonpreferred choice in choice-making routines; tag yes/no questions with the phrase "Yes...or no?" using exaggerated intonation and corresponding head nod and head shake.
Demonstrate joint visual attention during interactions involving referential items (e.g., pictures, objects of interest).	Point to key elements within pictures or within personal space and engage the individual's visual attention simultaneously.

choice-making ability with tangible objects or photographs, referential skills, and clear signals for agreement and rejection (precursors to the linguistic "yes" and "no" signals). In addition, partners can benefit from instruction in how to provide choice-making opportunities throughout daily routines and reinforce the communicator's responses. Table 15.1 lists appropriate intervention objectives for both emerging AAC communicators and their communication partners.

Case Example and Therapy Outcomes   The following case study provides an example of AAC intervention and illustrates possible therapy outcomes for emerging AAC communicators.

James, an individual with an aphasia quotient of 6 out of 100 on the Western Aphasia Battery (Kertesz, 1982, 2006), fit the profile of an emerging AAC communicator. James unexpectedly sustained a large hemorrhagic left CVA when he was 51 years of age. He had experienced a lengthy hospitalization in an acute care facility, followed by several inpatient stays in rehabilitation facilities. With an attentive spouse and a generally sunny outlook on life, James experienced many bouts of pneumonia and other secondary illnesses in the 10-year period prior to his evaluation at a university outpatient clinic. At that time, James's verbal expression consisted of a single stereotypy, "wah-wah-wah-wah," produced with a variety of intonation patterns and facial expressions. He did not typically point to items that he wanted. Profound limb apraxia interfered with any ability to produce symbolic gestures. James had tremendous difficulty attending to communication partners and had no ability to recognize or use two-dimensional symbols as an alternate means of communication.

In the early phases of therapy, James was encouraged to listen to the clinician, inhibit his perseverative jargon, and pay attention to her referential communication (pointing) to other clients in the therapy group or to elements within photos associated with universally familiar news events. He also learned to visually attend to choices (initially objects, followed by photographs) that were presented within the context of a functional activity (see Figure 15.1). Next, he was encouraged to select a choice by reaching or pointing during an interrupted routine. For example, when

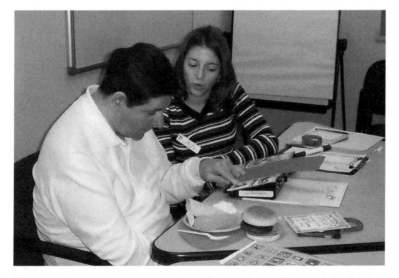

Figure 15.1.   An emerging AAC communicator (left), learning to point to symbolized choices to choose favorite foods on a digitized speech-generating device. Copyright © 2004 K.L. Garrett and J.P. Lasker, with permission of communicator and spouse, and student clinician. (Copyright © 2013 K.L. Garrett and J.P. Lasker.)

making coffee, the clinician completed one step of the activity (carrying the pot of coffee to the table), then stopped and offered James a choice of a mug or a fork. When James reached for an object, showed a preference for an item, or rejected an item, she provided contingent verbal feedback to increase his understanding that his communication effort conveyed meaning. James eventually learned to choose his favorite activities (e.g., listening to Frank Sinatra, playing cards or bingo, or watching old movies) by pointing to photographs or line drawings, after which he participated in the actual activity for a few minutes. When symbols representing nonpreferred activities (e.g., flossing teeth, smoking) were added to the set of choices, James quickly learned to scrutinize his choices before pointing to the desired symbol. He then learned to shift his attention from objects and symbols to other communicators in group therapy and ask them a question by pointing to them.

James ultimately developed a consistent ability to establish joint visual reference in individual and group activities, and to gain the attention of others and then point to props or drawings to indicate his focus of attention. He learned to purposefully inhibit his verbal jargon. He was approximately 80% accurate when making choices from a set of four items within a contextual activity, and he even began to proudly show his choices to other group members. His wife was elated when James took her by the arm, led her to the bathroom, and pointed to an overhead light bulb that needed to be replaced. On one notable occasion, he pointed to a newspaper ad for a seafood restaurant during a "Take your wife on a date" therapy activity. James eventually transitioned to the next category, contextual choice AAC communicator, after approximately 10 months of weekly individual and group therapy sessions.

Contextual Choice AAC Communicators

Contextual choice AAC communicators function more capably than emerging AAC communicators. They indicate basic needs by spontaneously pointing to objects and items. They easily recognize visual symbols such as photographs, labels, written names, and signs. They are aware of daily routines and schedules. During conversations, they may demonstrate partial awareness of some of the more predictable topics, questions, and comments. However, contextual choice AAC communicators do not have the linguistic ability to initiate or add to a conversation on their own. Thus, these individuals may be quite isolated socially. With assistance, however, they can participate in topical conversations when communication partners provide written or pictorial choices on a turn-by-turn basis. Most of these individuals also benefit from augmented input techniques to supplement their comprehension of others' auditory messages. Many individuals with aphasia syndromes such as global, severe Broca's, transcortical motor, or severe Wernicke's aphasia may function as contextual choice AAC communicators for the short or long term.

Intervention Strategies   AAC interventions for contextual choice AAC communicators are typically embedded within conversations about familiar topics. The primary expressive language goals involve teaching communicators with aphasia to consistently reference (point to) what they are talking about, understand the meaningfulness of graphic symbols, make choices to answer conversational questions, and begin to ask questions by pointing or using exaggerated intonation. Because these individuals are now participating more extensively in conversational exchanges, partners also help them understand specific messages and ideas that are being presented by using "augmented input" techniques (Garrett & Beukelman, 1998; Wood, Lasker, Siegel-Causey, Beukelman, & Ball, 1998). Strategies to support both expression and comprehension are listed in Table 15.2.

Table 15.2.   Contextual choice AAC communicator: Intervention goals and strategies

Communicator strategies	Partner strategies
Person with aphasia will point to one of the following to answer conversational *wh-* questions: • Written word choices • Points on a scale • Locations on a map	Implement written choice conversation strategy: • Identify interesting conversational topics. • Learn to generate consecutive, meaningful, conversational questions. • Learn to generate possible answers in the form of written word choices, scales, or locations on a map.
Answer partner's tagged yes/no questions with reliable gestures, head nods, or verbal responses.	Utilize tagged yes/no question format. Example: "Do you like Grace Kelly, the actress…yes [nod head up-and-down] or no [shake head side to side]?"
Point to communication partner or to items or photos to indicate interest or desire to find out more information (early questioning behavior).	Utilize augmented comprehension strategies when person with aphasia doesn't appear to understand incoming auditory messages: • Write or draw key words, new topics, family trees, or simple maps. • Gesture (e.g., hand over back = past tense). • Point to (reference) item being discussed.
Visually attend to partner's presentation of augmented input; confirm whether message was understood via head nods, yes/no responses, or vocalizations.	Respond to all modes of communication and interpret communication attempts of the person with aphasia.

Contextual Choice Conversation Strategies   A primary communication technique used with contextual choice AAC communicators is "written choice conversation" (Garrett & Beukelman, 1992, 1995). This technique requires the facilitator to generate written key-word choices pertinent to a conversational topic (Figure 15.2). The person with severe aphasia participates by pointing to the choices, thereby making his or her opinions and preferences known. Responses can be quite general, particularly when partners ask basic social questions (e.g., "Who visited this weekend?"). They also can be highly specific, particularly if the questions pertain to personal memories, beloved hobbies, or detailed knowledge associated with a past career. When partners present a sequence of related questions, interactions lengthen and communicators can discuss topics with relative depth.

In our clinical practices, many individuals with severe aphasia have demonstrated an ability to participate in interesting conversations when partners implement

Friend: Can you give me advice on what to make for the school bake sale tomorrow?

Person with aphasia (PWA):   [nods *yes*]

Friend: Should I take an angel food cake, brownies, or cookies? [writes choices vertically in notebook]

     • ANGEL FOOD CAKE
     • BROWNIES
     • COOKIES

PWA: [points to brownies]

Friend: Yes, those always sell fast [circles BROWNIES]. Should I make them from scratch or get a box mix? [writes choices]

     • SCRATCH
     • BOX MIX

PWA: [laughs and points to BOX MIX]

Friend: [laughs and circles BOX MIX] Yeah, it's hard to make them as good as Betty Crocker!

Figure 15.2.   Sample written choice conversation. (Copyright © 2013 K.L. Garrett and J.P. Lasker.)

the written choice conversation strategy—despite very limited reading comprehension test scores. Some have questioned whether people with low reading abilities on tests can truly understand the choices that partners write out for them. Several research studies have investigated this issue. Aphasic communicators with minimal reading ability on formal tests demonstrated more than 90% accuracy when responding to conversational questions by pointing to written choices, as long as the choices were presented within the context of a conversation and spoken aloud by the partner while she wrote them (Garrett, 1995). Accuracy was determined by having a family member verify whether the conversational choices selected by the communicator with aphasia were correct, or in the case of opinions, representative of the individual's typical opinions. In a more recent study (Smith, Garrett, & Lasker, 2007), the comprehension of six people with aphasia (three individuals with severe aphasia and three individuals with moderate aphasia/apraxia of speech) was assessed when text was presented in contextual conversation versus decontextualized text reading conditions. In experimental sessions, four response choices representing potential answers to conversational questions were presented auditorially and graphically in the contextual conversation condition; 10 unrelated questions and four corresponding response choices were administered via text only in the decontextualized text reading condition. Both sets of stimuli were of equal complexity. Results indicated that all six participants with moderate and severe aphasia scored significantly higher in the contextual conversation condition than in the decontextualized text reading condition. These studies suggest that some people with very severe aphasia can read well enough to recognize, comprehend, and consciously select vocabulary to represent personal facts and opinions during partner-supported communication interactions.

Variants of the written choice conversation approach include presenting choices in the form of points on a rating scale or locations on a map. These graphic options are particularly useful when communicators want to answer opinion questions (e.g., "How do you think the election's going…good…so-so…or bad?), quantitative questions (e.g., "How much should we spend on your birthday present…a lot…some… or a little?"), or questions about locations (e.g., "Where did your sister move…to New York…Texas…or Florida?"). (See Figures 15.3 and 15.4.) Lasker, Hux, Garrett, Moncrief, and Eischeid (1997) also determined that some individuals can respond to written choices that are not supplemented with the partner's spoken output, while others can answer verbal choice questions without the accompanying written words. Thus, the presentation of a pool of choices seems to be the critical requirement for

Friend: [Pause] what do you think about the kids' elementary school? Do you think they're getting a good
           education or a so-so one? [writes a rating scale on the page]

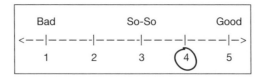

PWA: [hesitates, points to "4"]

Friend: [circles "4"] Yeah, we're pretty happy with the school district. Too bad the classes are so big,
           though!

PWA: [nods *yes*]

Figure 15.3.   Sample written choice conversation illustrating a communicator's response on a rating scale. (Copyright © 2013 K.L. Garrett and J.P. Lasker.)

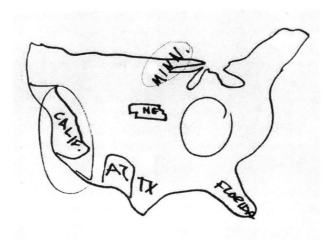

Figure 15.4. Map choices to answer the question "Where do you go on vacation?" (Copyright © 2013 K.L. Garrett and J.P. Lasker.)

contextual choice AAC communicators, but the optimal method of responding may be communicator specific.

The clinician's role is to introduce communicators to the written choice conversation strategy. Communicators can be encouraged to attend to the partner's questions, scan and comprehend the choices, and then respond thoughtfully by pointing. The clinician should also teach identified facilitators to use the strategy and then assist them to prepare simple notebooks to use in the supported interactions. An instruction card (Figure 15.5) can be placed on the cover of the notebook to explain the procedure to unfamiliar communication partners.

I HAVE HAD A STROKE. I WOULD LIKE TO TALK TO YOU, BUT I CANNOT SPEAK.

WE *CAN* CONVERSE IF YOU ASK ME A QUESTION AND OFFER ME WRITTEN CHOICES TO POINT TO. HERE'S HOW:

1. THINK OF A QUESTION YOU WOULD HAVE ASKED ME BEFORE MY STROKE. TRY TO FIND OUT MY OPINION, GET MY ADVICE, OR FIND OUT MY PREFERENCE.

    Example:
    "What crops have you gotten out of your garden so far?"
    "Who's going to win the football game Saturday?"
    "What do you think of the new tax law?"

2. ONCE YOU'VE ASKED THE QUESTION, THINK OF POSSIBLE ANSWERS OR CHOICES. WRITE THEM IN THIS NOTEBOOK. USE A DARK PEN OR MARKER. USE LARGE CAPITAL LETTERS. PUT A DOT IN FRONT OF EACH CHOICE. USE A SCALE FOR "HOW MUCH" QUESTIONS.

    Example:
    - (TOMATOES)
    - CUCUMBERS
    - BEANS

    _____

    - NEBRASKA
    - (PENN STATE)

    _____

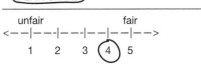

3. ENCOURAGE ME TO POINT. CIRCLE MY ANSWER. ASK PLENTY OF FOLLOW-UP QUESTIONS—I ENJOY CONVERSING!

Figure 15.5. Written choice communication notebook cover card. (Copyright © 2013 K.L. Garrett and J.P. Lasker.)

Yes/No Responses to Partner's Tagged Questions   Communicators with severe aphasia often have difficulty answering yes/no questions in a clear and unambiguous manner. Because of apraxia, they may have trouble coordinating their head movements to signify "yes" and "no." Or, they may not know how to answer the question because the grammatical structure of questions does not explicitly tell them to answer with "yes" or "no" versus a more specific word or phrase. Other times, communicators simply do not understand the question. The simple strategy of "tagging" the question can bypass the first two problems. Partners add the phrase "yes…or…no?" to the ends of their yes/no questions. They simultaneously model the head movements. This effectively provides the communicator with a narrow pool of choices for how to respond within the context of a conversation. See Figures 15.6 and 15.7 for examples of interactions in which the partner and communicator effectively organize their responses using the tagged yes/no strategy.

Augmented Comprehension (Input) Techniques   Often contextual choice AAC communicators have accompanying auditory processing difficulties that interfere with their ability to understand language, especially language that is complex or that shifts the conversational topic. These individuals will nod their heads to indicate that they understand, but in fact may be "holding their place" in the conversation instead of signaling true comprehension. Thus, they often experience significant confusion and communication breakdowns as a conversation progresses. At other times, these people withdraw completely from complex discussions.

To avoid communication breakdowns, communication partners can supplement their spoken language by gesturing, writing key words, or drawing. This set of strategies, called "augmented input" or "augmented comprehension" strategies (Garrett & Beukelman, 1992, 1998; Sevcik, Romski, & Wilkinson, 1991; Wood et al., 1998), can be implemented whenever the communicator with aphasia is having difficulty comprehending conversational questions, comments, or instructions. To provide augmented input, the communication partner first identifies that the communicator has misunderstood after carefully observing the person's blank facial expression, ambiguous head nods, or incorrect responses. The partner then reiterates the message while simultaneously pointing to the item being discussed; gesturing symbolically (e.g., throwing hand over shoulder to indicate "away from here"); pantomiming an event; showing photographs, drawings, or other diagrams; or writing key words and topics. Individuals with receptive aphasia can then use these visual representations to help them understand the conversational information (see Figure 15.8).

> We know of one man with profound aphasia due to bilateral CVAs whose wife had difficulty explaining where they needed to go before leaving the house. This resulted in confusion and combativeness. His wife printed photos of destinations using Internet images, collected them in a transportable envelope, and showed him the photos before going to each place. She reported that this technique successfully managed the confusion and resistance that he showed prior to transitioning from his house to the car and from place to place.

Partner: Robert, do you like omelettes…yes…or no? (nods head up and down while saying *yes* and shakes head side to side while saying *no*)

Robert: (tries to gesture thumbs up, then points down, then nods head *yes* after pausing to work out the movement sequence)

Partner: Yes?

Robert: (confirms *yes* by nodding his head up and down)

Figure 15.6.   Sample interaction with tagged yes/no question strategy. (Copyright © 2013 K.L. Garrett and J.P. Lasker.)

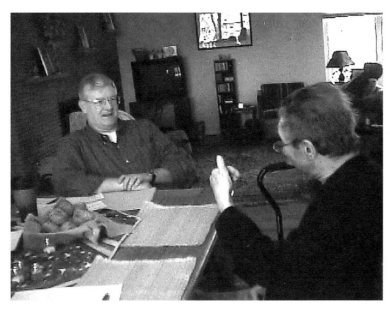

Figure 15.7.   Robert answering his brother-in-law's tagged yes/no question with a "thumbs up" signal. (Copyright © 2013 K.L. Garrett and J.P. Lasker.)

Augmented comprehension strategies are often used in conjunction with the written choice conversation technique described above. The technique of augmented input is similar in that it is completely partner supported, which means that communication partners must learn to resolve communication breakdowns by initiating the technique. The clinician can assist with this process by demonstrating the technique, providing a notebook with instructions on the cover to partners (Figure 15.9), and teaching the person with aphasia to signal when he or she is experiencing comprehension difficulties. Although a variety of individuals with severe aphasia may benefit from augmented comprehension techniques at some point in their recovery, people with global, Wernicke's, or transcortical sensory aphasia often require augmented input permanently. Other individuals with aphasia who demonstrate intermittent auditory processing problems may also benefit from this technique.

Case Example and Therapy Outcomes   In the following case study, Robert is an example of a contextual choice AAC communicator.

> Robert was a 61-year-old college-educated logistics engineer who sustained a sudden-onset, thrombotic left CVA in the region of the middle cerebral artery shortly after retiring. He participated in 1 month of inpatient rehabilitation, after which he returned

Partner: And so we went to the arboretum to see which trees grow best around here, and then we went to the nursery to pick out some varieties....

Charles: [raises hand to stop interaction, shakes head no]

Partner: Oh, I'm sorry—I was going too fast again. Here [writes *arboretum,* draws a picture of a tree].

We went to the arboretum [points to word and pauses to check for comprehension]...then we went to the *nursery* to get some plants [writes nursery and draws arrow from previous message] and then we took them home. Did I make sense?

Charles: [nods YES]

Figure 15.8.   Sample conversation in which augmentative and alternative communication (AAC) strategies are used. (Copyright © 2013 K.L. Garrett and J.P. Lasker, with permission of person with aphasia, spouse, and communication partner.)

Hello. I have had a stroke. Sometimes I'm not able to understand you. Can you...

Watch my face—if I look confused, I probably didn't understand you.

Signal topic changes like this...

"Now, I'd like to talk about something else...like baseball. Ready? Did you watch the *Pirates* baseball game on TV this weekend?"

For key words or concepts, it helps if you also:

- Gesture [e.g., swing bat for baseball]
- Write the important words in large print
          PIRATES???
- Draw maps, items, and so forth.

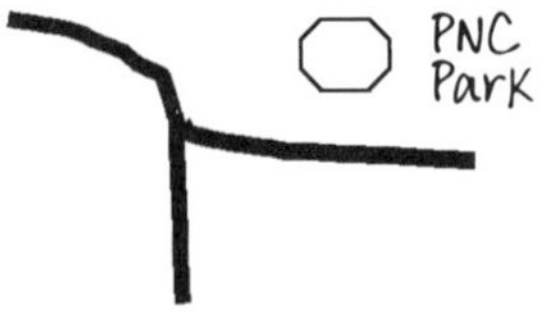

Figure 15.9.   Sample augmented input instruction card. (Copyright © 2013 K.L. Garrett and J.P. Lasker.)

to the home he shared with his wife. He attended five outpatient therapy sessions 2 months after onset. At that time, he was not able to produce speech because of profound apraxia of speech and severe aphasia. A high-technology AAC system was introduced, but Robert was unable to use it. Eight months after his stroke, he was reevaluated at a university outpatient clinic. He achieved an aphasia quotient of 9.2 of 100 possible, which corresponded with an impairment profile of global aphasia. However, his awareness of routines and response to the clinician's humorous comments indicated some communication competencies. He learned, within two treatment sessions, to point to written choices to answer conversational questions about his teapot collection, his political preferences, his children's travel adventures, and his feeble attempts to learn to play the bass guitar. He also gradually learned to answer conversational yes/no questions by nodding his head or using a "thumbs up" or "thumbs down" signal (Figure 15.7). He was much more accurate when the partner used the tagged yes/no question format; because of apraxia, however, he also required tactile cues and a model for approximately 2 months until he could produce consistent responses. Because of intermittent auditory comprehension breakdowns, the clinician frequently supplemented her spoken questions by writing or drawing key concepts. Robert then began participating in group therapy in addition to individual treatment sessions. Although he required initial hand-over-hand assistance to look at other participants and point at them to ask questions, he ultimately learned to initiate this simple request with only occasional cues. Interestingly, he also began to show other people his written choice responses in lieu of being able to announce them aloud, and used this strategy frequently to participate in group interactions.

Robert's wife confirmed that his written choices and yes/no responses were mostly accurate after 1 month of biweekly therapy sessions. Over the next year, Robert became more attentive, initiated more requests by gesturing symbolically and pointing, and learned to tease others. His reading comprehension increased. He also participated in traditional stimulation and motor speech therapy and developed an imitative spoken repertoire of more than 200 words. However, he never learned to use these spoken words consistently in real-life conversations. Therefore, his sons, brother-in-law, and wife learned to use partner-supported strategies, including written choice conversation, tagged yes/no question presentation, and augmented input.

Transitional AAC Communicators

Transitional AAC communicators demonstrate an ability to use external symbols and strategies to help them communicate. They may have fluent or nonfluent aphasia. Some gesture, draw, or speak to start an interaction with the communication partner. They may begin to search through their notebooks for written choices from prior conversations to find relevant information for the present discussion. They increasingly know the answers to questions before the partner even presents the choices. Communicators may, by this time, have communication notebooks or speech-generating devices (SGDs) containing message sets for common situations, such as telling about themselves or requesting snacks in the cafeteria. Some individuals even spell in combination with locating stored messages. In therapy, they may easily locate these messages and use them communicatively in structured interactions.

However, the hallmark of this category of communicators is that they typically *need cues from the partner to use an external strategy* to supplement their spoken communication. We have seen people with nonfluent aphasia who obviously have an idea and desire to convey it, and who are quite aware of their limitations in spoken language ability, but who can't think of *how* to communicate the answer in spontaneous communication contexts without cues. Other individuals, often those with comprehension deficits associated with fluent aphasia, may not perceive the need to supplement their unintelligible speech. These individuals may speak copiously but do not realize the inadequacy of their messages until a partner says, "I don't understand what you said." Thus, the "transitional AAC communicator" category represents a step between those communicators who need partner support to compose messages (i.e., emerging and contextual choice AAC communicators) and those who locate or generate messages on their own in everyday contexts (i.e., stored-message and generative AAC communicators).

Intervention Strategies

Intervention goals (Table 15.3) focus on teaching transitional AAC communicators to *initiate* AAC-supported conversations with as little cuing as possible. "Fading" cues is an important instructional technique. Specific AAC strategies provide the communicator with a means of conveying significant content without taxing cognitive and expressive language skills.

Introductions and Topic Setters   Transitional AAC communicators can introduce themselves using a prepared card or message on an SGD (e.g., I HAVE APHASIA FOLLOWING A STROKE. THEREFORE I HAVE DIFFICULTY THINKING OF WORDS AND SAYING THEM. I COMMUNICATE BY…). Scripted interactions and role playing may be helpful in teaching transitional AAC communicators what to do. They can learn to initiate a conversation by presenting a *remnant*, a tangible representation of an event considered noteworthy by the communicator (e.g., movie ticket stub, newspaper headline; Garrett & Huth, 2002; Ho, Weiss, Garrett, & Lloyd, 2005). If clinicians have not yet

Table 15.3.   Transitional AAC communicator: Intervention goals and strategies

Communicator strategies	Partner strategies
Call for assistance using a call bell or signal to a communication partner that he or she wishes to converse.	Provide suggestions, hints, or direct instructions to encourage the person with aphasia to use strategies in appropriate contextual situations.
Introduce self with a low- or high-tech augmentative and alternative communication (AAC) strategy (card, wallet, speech-generating device [SGD]).	Pause and expect communication.
Search for previous written choice responses to answer similar conversational questions.	Provide opportunities for communication of specific information within contextual, familiar conversations and routines. Example: "Tell me about your vacation."
Search for biographical info in a simple reminiscing book, scrapbook, or visual scene display to answer similar conversational questions.	Assist the person with aphasia to develop a scrapbook or communication wallet.
Answer predictable questions (e.g., autobiographical, topical) by searching for, selecting, and pointing to prestored messages on a simple SGD.	Assist the person with aphasia to store autobiographical or topical messages on an SGD prior to conversing.
Hand a potential communication partner a tangible topic setter or remnant to initiate a conversation.	Assist the person with aphasia to identify, collect, and present tangible topic setters (e.g., travel brochures) to potential communication partners.
Tell simple stories by activating sequential messages on an SGD (e.g., Step by Step Communicator, single-page sequential message display, visual scene display).	Assist the person with aphasia to identify favorite stories, then select and program the messages on an SGD.

Copyright © 2013 K.L. Garrett and J.P. Lasker.

assembled vocabulary within familiar topics (e.g., autobiographical information), it is appropriate to begin embedding these messages in notebooks or SGD levels to support these extended topical interactions.

Asking Questions   Transitional AAC communicators can become skilled conversational respondents when choices are pooled and presented in a contextual format. However, they may need additional intervention to initiate communication. One of the first strategies that can be implemented with transitional AAC communicators is to encourage them to point or gesture toward conversational partners to ask questions. In treatment, individuals may initially benefit from hand-over-hand assistance to point; later, a model cue may suffice. To prompt generalized use of this gestural strategy in conversations, it may be beneficial to remind the communicator that a question would be appropriate (e.g., "So…don't you want to know about my weekend?"). At other times, the clinician may introduce single-message SGDs or simple flip books (see Figure 15.10) and provide hand-over-hand assistance to teach communicators to initiate question asking within a conversational context.

Storytelling   Storytelling is another content-rich communication activity that matches the cognitive abilities of the transitional AAC communicator. When consecutive segments of the story are prestored in a communication book or SGD (typically in a left-to-right sequence if English is the primary language), the communicator simply has to point to the message square in the correct sequence to tell the story (Figure 15.11).

Visual Scenes   Visual scenes are another means of organizing both narrative information and potential comments and questions to extend an interaction about

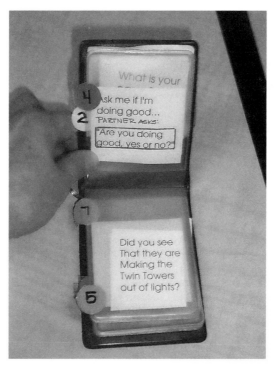

Figure 15.10. Sequentially organized communication wallet with introductions, topic setters, and questions for conversational partners. (Copyright © 2013 K.L. Garrett and J.P. Lasker.)

the topic. Action photographs of emotionally rich (personally relevant) events from the communicator's life are selected, and phrases that elicit conversation from partners (e.g., *This is our vacation in Hawaii; We tried boogie boarding; What do you think of Hawaii?*) are printed adjacent to the photograph. Communicators are encouraged to point to the phrases at appropriate moments in a conversation. In addition, a numeric scale (1–7) provides a means for communicators to convey opinions. This type of graphic support can provide transitional AAC communicators with the semantic content and shared visual context that they need to insert themselves into conversations. Visual scenes can be low-tech printouts, or they can be digital pages on a high-tech communication device (see Figure 4.3). Some devices allow hot spots within a digitally stored picture to be programmed with appropriate messages. Researchers have found that low-tech and high-tech visual scene displays help communicators relate personal stories and engage in reciprocal interactions by providing semantic

Guess what! We went gambling and I won $500! $$$	It's spent already— on a necklace for my wife and a lobster dinner for me.	I'm such a great guy! #1

Figure 15.11. Sample storytelling page for a digitized speech-generating device. (Copyright © 2013 K.L. Garrett and J.P. Lasker.)

and organizational support (McKelvey, Dietz, Hux, Weissling, & Beukelman, 2007; McKelvey, Hux, Dietz, & Beukelman, 2010).

Strategies for Transitional AAC Communicators

Table 15.3 summarizes potential strategies for transitional AAC communicators and their partners or clinicians.

Role Playing   Because of their history of needing instructions and cues, transitional AAC communicators benefit from practicing their strategies in structured role playing (e.g., introducing oneself to a bank teller, telling one's life story to a student clinician). Clinicians can set up an expectation for communication by repeating the role play and then pausing for the communicator to introduce him- or herself or answer a question using the target AAC strategy. Sometimes, it is helpful to embed the target strategies into a written script that the communicator can refer to during the role play. With transitional AAC communicators, therapists and conversational partners must wait to cue the individual until it is clear that he or she cannot figure out how to communicate without further instruction.

Case Example and Therapy Outcomes   The following example illustrates the use of AAC by a transitional AAC communicator.

> Beatrice was a 70-year-old woman who had sustained a thrombotic CVA while on vacation. She initially experienced very severe fluent aphasia (Wernicke's syndrome), with significant comprehension impairments and almost completely unintelligible jargon. She was discharged quickly to her home from a comprehensive rehabilitation facility because she was ambulatory, functional with regard to self-care and home activities (e.g., laundry, cooking), and continuously upset during all therapies. Home health therapy provided four visits, after which her husband enrolled her in specialized outpatient therapy for individuals with severe aphasia. Her initial therapy approach was augmented input to assist in managing comprehension deficits and providing feedback about her spoken output; Beatrice's daughter and husband were then taught this technique. She also worked on developing a consistent yes/no response in conjunction with augmented presentation of questions and the partner's use of a tagged yes/no question format. Following 6 months of therapy, she had decreased her jargon, increased the number of intelligible (though automatic) phrases, demonstrated the ability to repeat speech given printed text derived from augmented input interactions, and learned to pantomime to convey information about events and actions. She occasionally wrote single words with some spelling errors. Traditional restorative therapy also focused on decreasing her perseveration, improving her semantic comprehension skills, and increasing her ability to discriminate and produce words that contrasted phonologically. However, she still was unable to produce specific names or speak intelligibly enough to relate a narrative. Beatrice could not use a complex SGD. Instead, she and her husband described upcoming social situations that she was expected to participate in, for example, a high school reunion. She actively assisted in selecting phrases that would be helpful in these situations; messages were then represented with photos, line-drawing symbols, and text and were stored in a small flip notebook. Beatrice practiced using the phrases in role-playing scenarios and became adept at referencing them, particularly when the clinician suggested their use. However, after each of five events for which low-tech AAC systems had been constructed, she indicated that she had

not used the systems. When asked why, she indicated that she didn't think to pull them out of her purse, despite having practiced doing this in therapy. She continued to require cues to use her stored information systems in group interactions and community situations for the remainder of her time in therapy. However, she became adept at using pantomime, some natural speech, and retrieval of actual items to communicate her clearly held opinions and wishes with no assistance from others to initiate communication.

Goal of Partner-Supported Strategies for Transitional AAC Communicators

The aim of partner-supported AAC strategies is to establish a successful exchange of meaning between the person with severe aphasia and his or her partners as quickly as possible. Because AAC strategies provide visual supports to represent meaning (instead of auditory-verbal information alone), some individuals may demonstrate an ability to "latch on" to language and progress to higher levels of function. Partner-supported AAC strategies may thus have a role in the restoration of language while simultaneously serving to compensate for its loss, particularly for partner-dependent AAC communicators who have had limited access to communication opportunities when using natural speech alone.

Independent AAC Communicators with Aphasia

Transitional AAC communicators, described in the previous section, require the assistance of a communication partner to maximally participate in conversations and important life activities. In contrast, a number of people with severe aphasia have enough cognitive and linguistic competence to converse independently. These individuals comprehend most of what is said to them even when little contextual support is available. They can *intentionally* share their own ideas using a variety of strategies and modalities that they select themselves. These people can be termed *independent AAC communicators.*

However, without focused clinical intervention and implementation of AAC strategies, independent AAC communicators may experience frequent communication breakdowns. The connecting threads of conversation can dissolve when they try to communicate specific words (nouns, verbs, and/or function words) to clarify locations, details, names, cause-and-effect relationships, or event chronologies. Fortunately, independent AAC communicators can learn to utilize both natural communication strategies (e.g., speech, residual writing or drawing) and augmented strategies (e.g., pointing to elements of a picture to elaborate on a topic, finding messages stored in a multilevel SGD, spelling the first letter on an alphabet card) to communicate effectively in multiple environments with a variety of communication partners. Many of these individuals have aphasia patterns that correspond most closely with the traditional syndromes of anomic, moderate Broca's, conduction, or transcortical motor aphasia.

Stored-Message AAC Communicators

Stored-message AAC communicators can independently locate messages that have been stored in advance within their low- or high-tech AAC systems. They can learn to consistently access entire phrase or sentence messages in specific contexts. They may, for example, spontaneously activate a digitized SGD to offer a toast at a celebration or to order a double-thick strawberry milkshake at the ice cream store. Or, if they have extensive life needs, they may utilize a synthesized voice-output SGD with messages on multiple levels to greet, exchange small talk, and make predictions about the coming football season. They are initiators who use their systems to supplement or substitute for speech without prompting within familiar situations. They also may consciously intersperse some natural communication strategies (e.g., partially intelligible speech, symbolic gestures) after practice. However, they seldom generate enough novel information to participate in a discussion about an unusual topic because their spelling, speech, and AAC skills are not sufficient to participate independently in free-form conversations.

Intervention Strategies   Stored-message AAC communicators should work with clinicians and family members to create an inventory of messages and topics that they will need in specific situations in which they must communicate specifically and efficiently. They can assist in storing these messages in their low-tech communication notebooks or wallets or can help select locations and symbols for programming the messages onto a multilevel high-tech system. Lastly, they need to practice using their systems in role-playing or actual communication situations. Potential strategies for this group of communicators are listed in Table 15.4.

Clinicians may wish to conduct some intervention sessions with these individuals outside of the therapy room. For example, if an individual targets the post office as an environment for better communication, initial sessions could consist of identifying messages, storing them, and then practicing how to use both natural and AAC messages with a script (Figure 15.12). Later sessions may take place with a novel communication partner, such as another clinician or secretary, in a simulated post office scenario. If it is possible to conduct community outings, it would be beneficial to observe the communicator utilizing the strategies in the real situation. Finally, the clinician and communicator should evaluate the effectiveness of the interaction and make changes in message content, sequence of delivery, or use of natural communication strategies if needed.

Case Example and Therapy Outcomes   The case of Marco, a 44-year-old man with moderate-to-severe receptive and expressive aphasia and apraxia of speech (Lasker & Bedrosian, 2001), is summarized here to illustrate how a stored-message AAC communicator learned to use AAC.

Table 15.4.   Stored-message AAC communicator: Intervention goals and strategies

Communicator strategies
Participate in identification of specific situations, stories, or communication routines (e.g., restaurant, vacation, family stories, bank, returning an item to a store, asking spouse out on a date).
Participate in selection and storage of specific vocabulary for each situation.
Participate in selecting the representation of topics, messages, and referents as words, individual picture symbols, tangible items, or visual scenes on low- and/or high-tech systems.
Practice communicating in real-life situations and evaluate the following: • *Effectiveness:* Did I get my message across? • *Efficiency:* Was the partner fidgeting or uncomfortable? How many communication breakdowns did I have? • *Changes:* Was there anything I could have done to make this interaction go better?
Evaluate pros and cons of speech-generating devices versus low-tech communication options, make an informed decision, and develop the final system with the clinician.
Gradually use the system in more demanding situations (e.g., return an item to a store that has a difficult clerk with no knowledge of aphasia).

Clerk: Who's next?

PWA: (points to self)

Clerk: What do you need, sir?

PWA: (using SGD) I WANT TO PICK UP MY PACKAGE.

Clerk: What is that thing?

PWA: (goes to main level on SGD) I HAD A STROKE. IT IS HARD FOR ME TO SPEAK. I USE THIS MACHINE TO COMMUNICATE.

Clerk: OK, now what was that?

PWA: Patuj (returns to Post Office level on SGD; reactivates original message) I WANT TO PICK UP MY PACKAGE.

Clerk: Your name?

PWA: Chim...no...no... (returns to main level on SGD) MY NAME IS JAMES GREEN.

Clerk: Jim Green...OK sir, I'll check. Just a minute.

Figure 15.12.   Sample script for post office scenario. (*Key:* PWA, person with aphasia; SGD, speech-generating device.) (Copyright © 2013 K.L. Garrett and J.P. Lasker.)

Marco acquired aphasia as a result of a left CVA sustained 8 months before his evaluation. Prior to his stroke, he was employed as a mechanical press operator and was active in the community softball league and church. He had completed 2 years of college and earned an associate's degree. After his stroke, Marco was unable to work due to his residual physical disabilities and communication limitations. He lived at home with his wife, teenage son, and 3-year-old granddaughter. However, he continued to drive and conduct errands in the community. He also had some parenting responsibilities at home while his wife was at work.

Marco's motor speech and language problems interfered with his ability to participate in daily communication activities. His verbal output was limited to "yes," "no," and automatic speech sequences, although he often attempted to repeat verbal models. After 7 months of traditional "restoration" speech therapy with little improvement in speech production, Marco acquired a dynamic display voice-output device. He was unable to formulate novel messages using words or letters; however, he used the device extensively as a model for speech practice. In collaboration with Marco and his family, the clinician collected and stored messages for several communication contexts on several levels of Marco's electronic device. However, despite this individualized programming, Marco was unwilling to utilize his voice-output system in public. Marco did not require cues to access the messages on the system (as a transitional AAC communicator might). Rather, Marco communicated that he believed the device was "for the clinic" and "for practicing speech" but was not for "talking with friends...[or] strangers." When probed, Marco admitted that he was ashamed of using the machine in public and was afraid that people in the community would think he wasn't "normal."

To address the issue of AAC system acceptance, Marco's subsequent intervention program focused on selecting or spelling appropriate messages, practicing with written scripts, rehearsing via role plays with the clinician, and finally utilizing the system in community locations. Luckily, when Marco used his device for the first time in the post office, he received a favorable and interested response from the clerk. After his second experience communicating in public, Marco offered suggestions for his next community communication experience and also assisted in developing the practice script. In addition, he requested that the clinician maintain greater physical distance from him during his interaction with the clerk so that he could "do it himself." During his staged intervention program, Marco learned to access his stored-message system in a variety of locations. His ability to participate independently in public encounters increased with each experience, and he ultimately demonstrated acceptance of his system.

Generative AAC Communicators

Occasionally clinicians will encounter generative AAC communicators—speakers and/or writers with aphasia who can convey some novel information on their own. However, their generative communication skills are often too fragmented or inconsistent for effective communication to occur without some degree of conversational or AAC intervention. Breakdowns may occur in spoken communication and/or when writing. Apraxia of speech often obscures these individuals' linguistic competence when speaking because of sound substitutions or halting, effortful speech. Agrammatism (the inability to produce grammatically correct utterances, while retaining the ability to say single words), spelling, and word retrieval errors may interfere with functional writing.

Many generative AAC communicators maintain an independent lifestyle and wish to participate in conversations and transactional exchanges in many environments. Their semantic networks are usually more complete than those of stored-message AAC communicators, and they can generate some grammatically and semantically complex utterances. One individual with conduction aphasia and limited semantic specificity was an outstanding generative AAC communicator. She was able to manage the social aspects of communication quite well using verbal communication but required extensive support when she was asked to communicate specific information to her friends, her lawyer, her doctor, and the bus driver. Another individual with moderate anomic aphasia became a published writer with the assistance of augmentative writing software (King & Hux, 1995). General intervention strategies for generative speakers and writers are listed in Table 15.5.

Generative AAC Communicators: Intervention Strategies
AAC-based interventions for generative AAC communicators can be complex. In addition to identifying anticipated participation patterns, clarifying communication needs, and identifying topics of interest, the AAC specialist must also teach the individual to manage a variety of AAC techniques. For example, Beukelman, Yorkston, and Dowden (1985) described a man with Broca's aphasia who used a series of AAC approaches as he progressed through various phases of recovery. Initially, he communicated with a simple communication book that contained photographs of familiar people, places, and activities; his family provided additional picture albums identifying family members, interests, and experiences. This man later learned to expand his conversations by showing portfolios of his work as an interior designer. The portfolios helped him to establish a topic and provided pictorial support for specific words and ideas. Eventually, a multimodal AAC system was developed for him that included an electronic communication device with voice output, limited natural speech, gestures, a communication book, portfolios, books and posted blueprints in the design studio in his home, and a design assistant who also served as a facilitator.

An often overlooked but critical aspect of AAC interventions with generative AAC communicators is their need for substantial instruction and guided practice to teach them *when* to use the various AAC techniques provided. Garrett, Beukelman, and Low-Morrow (1989) described this process with a generative AAC communicator, as summarized in the following case study.

Ken used a low-tech AAC system that contained many different components, including stored messages for specific environments, lists of family names and sports teams, biographical history, maps, rating scales, a pocket for remnants, and blank

Table 15.5.   Generative AAC communicator: Intervention goals and strategies

Communicator strategies: Generative speakers

Initiate introduction of self *and* communication strategies

Communicate specific semantic info about a *variety* of topics via augmentative and alternative communication (AAC) strategies and natural communication modalities (e.g., presidential elections, stories from childhood, difficulties collecting Social Security, events from past weekend, bird watching highlights).

Establish topics prior to communicating complex conversational information using the following:
- Tangible topic setters
- Verbal introduction of topic
- Topic card (e.g., *I want to talk about…sports…family…etc.*)

Communicate in a variety of situations with familiar and unfamiliar (untrained and sometimes unsympathetic) communication partners. (e.g., with family; in stores, banks, video rental stores, bakery, Social Security office, bars, and social clubs; attending lectures; doing volunteer work).

Locate stored messages relevant to the topic on "hidden" pages in a communication book or "hidden" electronic levels in a high-tech speech-generating device (SGD).

Shift between accessing *stored* messages and creating *novel* messages to convey a complete idea.

Increase complexity of discourse by communicating relational semantic information via gestures, timelines, and some speech:
- *Temporal:* Past and present (motioning backward for "ago")
- *Spatial/locational:* Pointing to map to indicate "down the road"
- *Preferential:* Saying "the best" while making a thumbs-up gesture
- *Additive:* Finding a message about baseball, saying "and," and then finding a message about enjoying Steelers football
- *Actions:* Pantomiming doing the laundry, then saying "dryer"

Combine symbols to convey novel meanings:
- *Speech:* Saying "Big one" and "Warshendon" to mean "the President"
- *AAC messages:* Accessing PITTSBURGH and then finding BASEBALL on hobbies page to communicate "Pirates baseball team"
- *Combine writing and speech:* Writing "2" and then saying "boys" to indicate size of family

Ask questions of others:
- Combining key words, enhanced intonation, and gesturing (e.g., "Vacation…you?")
- Pointing to symbolized question forms in a communication notebook or on an SGD

Utilize specific, metacommunicative communication strategies to resolve communication breakdowns in conversation:
- Determine rule for number of times it's OK to repeat a message (e.g., no more than 2; then you have to try something else).
- Provide additional information or shift to a new strategy during communication breakdowns.
- Signal to partner that he or she has understood or has not understood.
- Manage conversational dynamics; make decisions about whether to continue or quit.

Work with clinician to assemble components of multimodal system or program and learn the operational requirements of high-tech systems.

Communicator strategies: Generative writers

Spell or write partial or complete words or phrases to generate novel messages using a low-tech system (e.g., pocket-sized notepad).

Learn to use word prediction or abbreviation/expansion high-tech strategies to supplement spelling.

Learn to use organizational templates (low-tech or computer-based) to generate written products such as letters, journal entries, summaries, and so forth.

paper for writing and drawing. In addition, Ken produced some partially intelligible key words and automatic phrases, and he could gesture symbolically part of the time to convey specific ideas. Over the course of 3 to 4 months, the clinician taught this man how to decide upon a specific AAC technique and then implement it in conversations. The clinician then developed the instructional sequence summarized in Figure 15.13, which Ken referred to when learning to choose the most effective communication strategy during intervention sessions. For example, Ken would first attempt to say a message using natural speech. If he experienced a communication breakdown, he would then attempt to gesture, write, or repeat the spoken message. If he was still unsuccessful, he would use his word notebook, display an alphabet card, or select a remnant to increase context for the communication partner. Finally, he would direct his listener to the clues or control phrases to manage the conversation from a metacognitive perspective if his initial communication attempts were unsuccessful. Following training, Ken greatly reduced the amount of effort he spent on resolving communication breakdowns because he became a conscious and strategic multimodal communicator.

Unfortunately, this essential training phase for generative AAC communicators may not receive enough attention in a multimodal intervention. Other common reasons that generative AAC communicators do not use their AAC systems effectively include the following: 1) the vocabulary and content of the AAC materials provided do not match specific opportunities in real-life communication situations; 2) important communication partners are not willing to accept augmented modes of communication; 3) teaching and training in naturalistic situations did not occur; 4) communication devices may be too large and unwieldy, or too small to be appropriate for the vision skills of the individual; and 5) the individual's social networks (Blackstone & Hunt Berg, 2003a, 2003b) have become so limited that the individual has few opportunities to communicate.

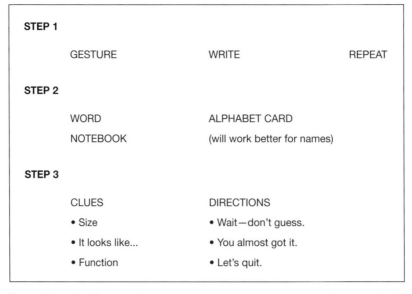

Figure 15.13. Modality instruction card for a generative AAC communicator. (Copyright © 2013 K.L. Garrett and J.P. Lasker.)

The role of technology in AAC interventions with this group of communicators continues to evolve (Fox & Fried-Oken, 1996; Jacobs, Drew, Ogletree, & Pierce, 2004; Koul & Harding, 1998; van de Sandt-Koenderman, 2004). Many of the high-tech AAC systems that have been developed for individuals with primarily physical impairments are not appropriate for communicators with aphasia. Their need for adaptive access is minimal, and some of the methods of accessing messages (e.g., abbreviation-expansion, recalling symbol sequences, complex level changes) are too difficult for most people with aphasia to use functionally. However, a variety of emerging technologies show promise for select generative AAC communicators who have the skills and the desire to use AAC. For example, some experimental software allows communicators to engage in small talk by accessing a category of communication messages stored by pragmatic function, such as "greetings" or "continuers" (Todman & Alm, 1997). Many dynamic screen devices can be programmed with messages that represent the continuum of speech acts needed to communicate in a given situation (i.e., from greetings to questions to responses). New methods of representing concepts visually—as scenes from episodic memory (e.g., photos of significant events), nodes on a flow chart (e.g., family tree), locations in a schematic layout, or points on a timeline—are increasingly possible with off-the-shelf technology (Hough & Johnson, 2009; Johnson, Strauss Hough, King, Vos, & Jeffs, 2008; Van de Sandt-Koenderman, Wiegers, Wielaert, Duivenvoorden, & Ribbers, 2007). Some promising technological approaches combine opportunities for speech practice with linguistic supports (Bartlett, Fink, Schwartz, & Linebarger, 2007; Linebarger, Romania, Fink, Bartlett, & Schwartz, 2008). Other communication technologies provide speech practice opportunities for clients with both aphasia and apraxia of speech (Cherney, Halper, Holland, & Cole, 2008; Lasker, Stierwalt, Hageman, & LaPointe, 2008).

Despite the advances that have been achieved in graphic interfaces, intelligibility of synthesized speech, and predictive capabilities of system software, there are few reports of truly independent, generative AAC communicators with aphasia. Discussions about the development of intuitive technologies continue—many clinicians dream of a system that can intelligently guess an individual's intended message given associational inputs (e.g., first letter, description, graphic outline on a touch tablet, word associations and paraphasic substitutions, even pantomime decoded by a smart videocamera). However, the great challenge for many communicators may not be technologic; rather, it is thinking to *use* AAC strategies to support residual communication skills in dynamic communication contexts (Garrett & Kimelman, 2000; Kraat, 1990).

Norman was a retired airport manager (Figure 15.14) with moderate expressive aphasia, apraxia of speech, and good comprehension who learned to use a portable dynamic screen communication device in combination with residual speech, partial word writing, and gestural communication (Fried-Oken et al., 2002). Norman lived independently, drove a truck, and maintained his own home. He was seen at a university clinic for an AAC evaluation 7 years after experiencing a stroke. At that time, he was already using a multimodal communication system consisting of residual speech, a small communication book, a notepad for word and letter writing, and various remnants. However, he required a voice-output system in order to participate more fully in all aspects of his life. He obtained a dynamic screen display device. Norman participated in several months of therapy to program his system with appropriate messages so that he could socialize and conduct business

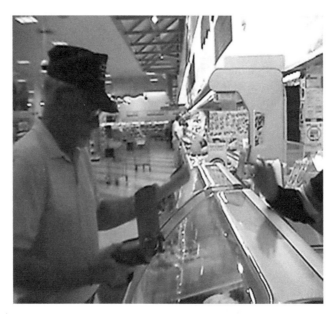

Figure 15.14.   Norman ordering deli foods with his portable speech-generating device, natural speech, and gestures. (Copyright © 2013 K.L. Garrett and J.P. Lasker; used by permission of person with aphasia.)

in the community. Many messages were stored as an entire phrase or sentence on multiple levels, but Norman also demonstrated the ability to spell out single words of messages using the keyboard level. He often typed in the first letter of words to augment his speech attempt, to help the communication partner guess the word, or to access a number of pictured word-prediction choices. He also learned to integrate natural communication modalities with AAC access. During role plays that gradually increased in difficulty, he learned to repair communication breakdowns by rephrasing, locating additional messages on his device, writing, or using conversational control messages such as you're way off. At last report, he independently used his system in the community on a daily basis whenever he believed it would enhance his communication effectiveness.

Generative AAC Writers: Intervention Strategies   Although writing may not be the first communication function that people with aphasia wish to target following a stroke, it can become an important focus for those individuals who previously wrote extensively to communicate with others or to convey specific information at work. Some individuals with mild aphasia write for the first time to tell of their recovery from a devastating illness. Because many of the symptoms of aphasia are manifested in the written modality as well as in speaking and understanding, writers with aphasia are frequently frustrated by difficulties with word retrieval, spelling, and syntactic formulation. King and Hux (1995) described the written output of an individual with mild aphasia who ultimately used AAC software to both select specific words and correct the spelling errors as he wrote. His software ran in the background of standard word-processing packages and allowed him to choose specific words from a list when he was not able to encode selected words into the correctly spelled form. He also learned to use standard spell checker and grammar checker functions to accurately write his text. Both of the authors of this chapter have assisted individuals with aphasia to use prediction software that was built into their high-tech AAC devices or word-processing programs to generate written notes. Sohlberg, Fickas, Ehlhardt, and Todis (2005) have incorporated prediction, choices, and prefabricated sentences into a simplified e-mail program (CogLink) for generative AAC writers who cannot manage the processing demands of a regular e-mail interface (see description in the section on specific-need AAC communicators below). Jackson-Waite, Robson, and Pring (2003) incorporated a Lightwriter communication device into intervention as a practice tool to improve written spelling by a client with jargon aphasia.

People with very severe aphasia, on the other hand, cannot write independently. Their linguistic impairments prevent them from meeting the composition, semantic, syntactic, and spelling demands of independent writing. However, to address the specific need of writing personal letters, some individuals with severe aphasia and agraphia have used a low-tech approach that is addressed in the section on specific-need AAC communicators.

Specific-Need AAC Communicators

Some communicators may not wish (and do not need) to use AAC as a primary communication method to meet their specific communication needs. For them, speech and gestures may be adequate, and indeed optimal, for most social situations. However, some communication situations require high degrees of specificity, clarity, or efficiency. For example, an individual with aphasia might want to communicate on the telephone, place bets at the racetrack, pick up a prescription, write a personal letter, organize ideas to manage a meeting, or give a toast at a wedding. Any person with aphasia could have such well-defined, specific communication needs related to either speaking or writing. Individuals who live in settings that require some independence generally need this type of AAC technique on an intermittent basis. Clinicians can ask the fundamental question, "Is there anything in your life that you would like to participate in more fully?" to identify these individuals and their desired participation contexts.

Intervention Strategies
AAC interventions for specific-need AAC communicators are usually limited in scope because these individuals can often manage much of their communication through gestures and limited speech. When planning an intervention, it is first necessary to analyze the requirements of the specific communication task and the person's capabilities for managing that task. For example, an individual may need help setting up a system to allow verbal communication over the telephone. This might be managed by placing a digitized SGD by the telephone, preprogrammed with a message such as HI—THIS IS SERENA. PLEASE ASK ME QUESTIONS THAT CAN BE ANSWERED YES OR NO. SPEAK SLOWLY AND CLEARLY. Another common need is to communicate specific messages in places such as a noisy cafeteria or bank. Often, a small communication card can be prepared with a restricted set of the messages that are needed in the situation. Another example of a specific need was expressed by one woman with mild expressive aphasia but severe agraphia. She was frustrated by her inability to recall the items she needed to purchase after arriving at the grocery store. Because she could not easily write items she needed on a list before shopping, she had to rely on her memory and frequently forgot important items. A grocery list (Figure 15.15) was created for her so she could simply circle items instead of writing them. Another individual used speech in most situations but was unable

Date _____

We need to buy:

FOOD

Basic Foods
  Bread
  Cheese
  Margarine
  Ketchup
  Mustard
  Mayonnaise
  Salt
  Pepper
  Lettuce
  Potatoes
  Rice
  Macaroni
  Spaghetti
  • Sauce
  • Noodles
  • Mushrooms

Meats
  Hamburger
  Chicken breast
  Bacon
  Tuna
  Rib eye
  Delmonico steak

DRINKS
  Milk
  Coffee
  Tea
  Juice
  • Orange
  • Grapefruit
  Pop
  • Pepsi
  • Coke
  • 7Up

CLEANING SUPPLIES
  Bath soap
  Soft soap
  Toilet paper
  Ajax
  Bleach
  Scouring pads
  Paper towels

COSMETICS
  Shampoo
  Deodorant
  Band-Aids
  Shaving cream
  Razors

Figure 15.15.   Sample grocery list. (Copyright © 2013 K.L. Garrett and J.P. Lasker.)

to order items by telephone because of frequent semantic and phonemic paraphasias that interfered with saying the names of numbers. A list of numbers, 0 through 100, was printed for him (Figure 6.7 in Beukelman, Garrett, & Yorkston, 2007). The number words (e.g., *forty*) were written next to the number, which successfully cued him to state a transportation pickup time or his address correctly over the telephone.

People with severe agraphia who wish to write letters may benefit from a scaffolded letter-writing format (Garrett, Staab, & Agocs, 1996). In this augmented writing approach, individuals who have difficulty writing a letter without assistance can choose phrases from a list and copy them into the partially completed sentences on a letter format (Figures 15.16 and 15.17). One woman known to the authors wrote 50 letters in a 2-week period after initial instruction with the letter format. Other individuals have progressed from this partner-supported approach to independent letter generation with additional therapy. The use of scaffolded formats has also been useful in helping people with aphasia write e-mail messages. As mentioned above, CogLink, an e-mail program designed specifically for people with cognitive and language impairments, provides support in the form of letter templates, picture association to select e-mail recipients, a spell checker, word choices, and a simplified visual format (Sohlberg et al., 2005). The program can be used independently, or an assistant can input letter templates and vocabulary banks in advance. The successful completion and mailing of a letter, the generation of a life story, or the sending of an e-mail message to a friend or family member is another illustration of how the Participation Model, described in Chapter 5 and pictured in Figure 5.1, can be applied to all types of communication activities for people with aphasia.

The specific-need AAC communicator may also benefit from situational communication instruction similar to that described above. If, for example, the person with aphasia needs to use a simple voice-output device for telephone communica-

```
1. _____  _____, 201_


Dear 2. _____

3. _____ ! How 4. _____?

I am 5. _____. This month we

6. _____. We really

7. _____.

So, tell me about 8. _____.

I hope you are 9. _____.

Please 10. _____.

11. _____,


_____
```

Figure 15.16.   Blank letter format. (Copyright © 2013 K.L. Garrett and J.P. Lasker.)

tion, he or she may benefit from multiple opportunities to role play the situation. If the specific-need AAC communicator is using a letter-writing format, it may be important to draft a few letters in a therapy session so that the clinician can provide some initial cues before the individual completes the activity independently. Table 15.6 lists a few examples of possible goals for specific-need AAC communicators; specific strategies are limited only by the needs of the communicators and the creativity of the clinicians.

1.	Jan	Feb	March	April	May	June	July	Aug	Sept	Oct	Nov	Dec
	1	2	3	4	5	6	7	8	9	10	11	12	13	14	15	16
	17	18	19	20	21	22	23	24	25	26	27	28	29	30	31

2. (write in names of possible letter recipients here)

3. Hello!   Hi!   Howdy!   Greetings!

4. . . . are you?   . . . is it going?   . . . is your family?

5. fine   OK   pretty good   terrific   a little tired

6. stayed at home   visited the family   worked around the yard
   vacationed in _____   had the grandkids for a week

7. had a great time   enjoyed ourselves   were glad for Fall

8. your vacation   your family   school   your job   your friends

9. fine   keeping busy   taking it easy   enjoying your grandkids

10. write soon   call me sometime   come visit   take care

11. Sincerely,   Fondly,   With best wishes,   Love,

Figure 15.17.   Multiple choice letter format. (Copyright © 2013 K.L. Garrett and J.P. Lasker.)

Table 15.6. Specific-need AAC communicator: Intervention goals and strategies

Communicator strategies (examples)
Utilize single-message speech-generating devices (SGDs) to communicate info by telephone or in community situations (e.g., I HAVE APHASIA—GIVE ME TIME TO COMMUNICATE) or to participate in rituals (e.g., prayer).
Present phrase cards to communicate specific needs in specific situations (e.g., place bets at the race-track, explain upcoming bus stop, place bridge bets, ask grandchildren about school and sports, request specific hairstyle at salon).
Use a complex SGD to convey a sequence of messages to complete a community transaction or tele-phone call (e.g., to set up a doctor's appointment).
Write letters or personal journal entries using the scaffolded letter-writing templates and word or phrase choices.

Partners of specific-need AAC communicators can contribute significantly by identifying situations at home or in the community that require highly precise communication on the part of the person with aphasia. Their continued participation in the message inventory process and role-playing activities is also very beneficial.

Case Examples and Therapy Outcomes   The following case studies illustrate the use of AAC with specific-need AAC communicators.

Elizabeth, a 55-year-old woman with moderate-to-severe Broca's aphasia and apraxia of speech, participated independently in most activities 10 years after experiencing a stroke. Her use of telegraphic speech, gestures, and partially spelled words helped her manage most interactions. Elizabeth also relied on a caregiver to speak for her at times. She had seen her social network dwindle in the 10 years since her CVA, but she indicated she had always been a bit of a loner. However, she was frustrated by her inability to contact the local transportation system for people with disabilities when her caregiver was not available, particularly on weekends. Her complex SGD was mounted on her power wheelchair. She worked with the speech-language pathologist to devise a page that allowed her to convey her desired pickup times, destinations, and return times to the transportation operator by speakerphone (see Figure 15.18). These transactions were predictable in terms of their message sequence, so Elizabeth could efficiently access messages when they were arranged in a corresponding visual sequence on her device display. She eventually developed the confidence and capability to schedule a ride without assistance.

Jane, a 53-year-old geography professor with aphasia, had been employed by a university for more than 20 years prior to onset of a left CVA. One year after the stroke, an evaluation revealed an aphasia quotient of 79.1 on the Western Aphasia Battery (Kertesz, 1982), which was most consistent with a diagnosis of anomic aphasia. She scored 80 out of 100 on the reading subtest and 75 out of 100 on the writing subtest. Jane was determined to return to work as a college professor. She communicated in most daily situations using natural speech but required AAC support to lecture on specific topics in her classes. Jane obtained a voice-output device through a combination of vocational rehabilitation and university resources. She used her computer-based voice-output system to deliver class lectures that she had typed in advance using software that allowed her to spell whole words or select predicted programs. The software then allowed her to "speak" her lecture sentence by sentence through a

THIS IS KATHY GARRETT.	I NEED A PICKUP AT:	I'D LIKE TO SCHEDULE THE PICKUP FOR:	I WANT TO SCHEDULE A RETURN TRIP FOR:	I AM GOING BACK TO MY APARTMENT.
MY ACCESS CODE IS 5 - 1 - 2 - 5	MY APARTMENT AT 111 HAM AVENUE	9:00 A.M.	1:00 P.M.	I AM GOING SOMEWHERE ELSE. ASK ME TO TELL YOU WHERE.
I AM USING THIS MACHINE TO TALK.	DR. MCHENRY'S OFFICE, 444 BROCA'S PLACE.	10:00 A.M.	2:00 P.M.	DO YOU HAVE ANOTHER TIME SLOT AVAILABLE?
PLEASE ASK ME TO REPEAT IF YOU DON'T UNDERSTAND ME.	GIANT BIRD GROCERY STORE AT SQUIRREL ST.	11:00 A.M.	3:00 P.M.	THAT'S NOT CORRECT. LET'S TRY AGAIN.
EXCUSE ME, CAN YOU CHECK? MY RIDE HASN'T SHOWN UP YET.	SPEECH THERAPY AT 1401 FORBES AVENUE.	NOON	4:00 P.M.	THANK YOU FOR YOUR ASSISTANCE.

Figure 15.18.   Stored-message display for a specific-need AAC communicator to schedule transportation. (Copyright © 2013 K.L. Garrett and J.P. Lasker.)

speech synthesizer; she also learned to augment these prestored messages with her natural telegraphic speech. Her teaching evaluations have been excellent since she began to utilize this teaching approach to compensate for acquired aphasia (Lasker, LaPointe, & Kodras, 2005).

Speech-Generating Device Choices for Independent AAC Communicators

There are no prescriptive formulas for selecting an optimal communication device for independent AAC communicators. Some available devices are specifically designed for people with aphasia (e.g., Lingraphica, SentenceShaper). Some of these devices are actually intended to be used as speech practice systems, whereas others are meant to augment communication. Some standard SGDs now contain additional features that were developed for people with aphasia, including DynaVox products with visual scene displays. We must emphasize that each person with aphasia has a unique profile of skills, needs, and preferences, so it is impossible to determine whether someone can or will use a device without first conducting an extensive trial of the system.

Decision making regarding SGDs for independent AAC communicators is quite different than for partner-dependent AAC communicators. Most of the low-tech strategies recommended for partner-dependent AAC communicators can and should be implemented immediately. The skills of independent AAC communicators, however, typically evolve over periods ranging from several months to many years. For that reason, we do not generally recommend procurement of complex, high-tech AAC devices for independent AAC communicators until they have settled into a reasonably consistent living situation or until a support network has been identified. Communicators can learn many skills by borrowing devices and using them for designated time periods; clinicians can also support these individuals in the relative structure of the clinical environment. It is only when the right combination of ability, support, and opportunity converge that an appropriate "system match" can be identified. We recommend that clinicians provide many tangible opportunities for practice and home use of devices before finalizing a high-tech AAC decision for independent AAC communicators. The following assessment protocol is also highly recommended as an aid in AAC decision making for people with aphasia.

ASSESSMENT

Because aphasia is not a motor impairment, the AAC assessment and intervention paradigms developed for people with physical disabilities are not appropriate. Instead, clinicians need a clear understanding of the cognitive and linguistic competencies possessed by the communicator with aphasia and required by a specific AAC intervention to achieve optimal improvement in communication (Garrett & Kimelman, 2000). Sensory, motor, representational, and communicative competencies must also be evaluated. In addition, clinicians also need systematic methods for evaluating communication needs and participation contexts prior to selecting AAC interventions.

Identifying Communicator Profiles

Throughout the assessment process, the clinician seeks to answer the questions in Table 15.7 as part of a complete AAC skills assessment for a communicator with aphasia. To provide answers to these questions, clinicians may employ multiple assessment tasks. The individual's performance on these assessment activities can help clinicians identify which category of communicator best describes the individual with aphasia.

The following AAC aphasia assessment tools, discussed here in logical order of administration, can facilitate AAC decisions by providing opportunities for clinicians to answer the five basic assessment questions presented in Table 15.7. This process may aid the clinician to make overall decisions about the nature of the primary AAC intervention based on the category in which the individual best fits at the time of the initial assessment as well as the individual's demonstrated potential to learn additional strategies with teaching and cues.

Table 15.7. Aphasia augmentative and alternative communication assessment tools and questions

Tool	Questions
Unaided modalities	Does the person with aphasia use strategies (such as residual natural speech, writing, gesture, or drawing) to augment or substitute for ineffective spoken messages? If not, can he or she be taught to do so?
Partner-supported techniques	To reestablish a communication exchange, does the person with aphasia benefit from partner-supported communication strategies, such as augmented input and the written choice conversation strategy? Can the person with aphasia learn to use tangible supports, such as pictures or objects, in predictable conversational routines? If the person with aphasia does not currently use these strategies, can he or she be taught to do so?
External stored information	Does the person with aphasia demonstrate the ability to respond to questions by accessing messages represented by symbols, such as pictures in a communication book, on a simple speech-generating device, or on a letter board? Does the individual need cues to do so?
Stored messages through voice-output systems	Does the person with aphasia utilize prestored whole messages, such as those created ahead of time on a digitized or synthesized voice-output device by a facilitator, to communicate? If not, can he or she be taught to do so?
Generative messages through voice-output systems	Does the person with aphasia generate novel communicative messages using letters, photographs, pictures, or symbols? If not, can he or she be taught to do so?

Garrett and Beukelman's (1992) AAC categorical assessment for communicators with aphasia, revised by Garrett and Lasker in 2004 (available as Form 6.1 in Beukelman, Garrett, & Yorkston, 2007; also available on the Barkley AAC web site), provides the clinician with a checklist of present or emerging communication competencies. This observational checklist is designed to help clinicians match AAC strategies with a person's capabilities. Clinicians can document competencies and challenges observed within conversational contexts, during unsupported interactions, and during AAC strategy trials with trained conversational partners. When the majority of communication behaviors appear within a single category (e.g., contextual choice AAC communicator), it is likely that the person is functioning primarily within that category. It is also important to determine if skills in the next category seem to be emerging; therapeutic goals can then be developed to move the individual along the continuum from partner-dependent to independent AAC communicator, or at least to the next category within each group.

Baseline Modality Assessment

A modified PACE (Promoting Aphasics' Communicative Effectiveness) procedure (Davis & Wilcox, 1985) elicits a communication exchange between a message sender with aphasia and a receiving communication partner; clinicians can explore the natural tendencies of the person with aphasia to use alternate modalities or whether it appears that the person can be taught to use them. The clinician selects an action picture from a commercially available set of picture cards or any other informal source such as magazines or photographs. Pictures can depict a person completing a simple action (e.g., a woman cutting a cake) or represent a story or scene. Using a barrier task format, the person with aphasia is asked to communicate ideas about the picture to a partner who cannot see the picture. The clinician documents the overall success of the communication (i.e., does the partner eventually understand what is happening in the picture?) and also the methods used by the person with aphasia to communicate. Does the person with aphasia attempt to communicate primarily with speech? When speech is not effective at communicating the message to the partner, does the person with aphasia attempt to use other natural strategies, such as gesture, drawing, or writing? If not, when the clinician cues or models the use of these strategies, can the person with aphasia implement them successfully to convey the information to the partner?

This semistructured exercise allows the clinician to document how the person with aphasia utilizes residual speech skills, how natural it is for him or her to use strategies other than speech, how well gesture or pantomime is used, and how he or she makes use of retained writing skills (i.e., using air writing, initial letters, word fragments, alphabet boards; see Form 6.3 in Beukelman, Garrett, & Yorkston, 2007).

Conversational Strategy Trials

Clinicians should also assess expressive and receptive linguistic skills in a *conversational context*, both with and without AAC or contextual supports. This may include a general "getting to know you" conversation. In this portion of evaluation, the clinician selects a personally relevant conversational topic (e.g., past work, hometown memories, a hobby or pastime, family, growing up, courting, getting into trouble in school) and introduces it to the person with aphasia while simultaneously modeling partner-supported communication strategies. In particular, the clinician may wish to explore the following partner-supported conversation strategies: written choice conversation, augmented input, cued question asking, photo or visual scene referencing, and tagged yes/no responses. These techniques are described in greater detail in previous sections of this chapter. As part of the assessment process, the clinician should record data on the accuracy of the responses. For example, when using written choice conversation or tagged yes/no responses, the clinician should confirm accuracy with family members or significant others. In addition, the clinician should document how much cuing (e.g., none, minimal, moderate, maximal) was necessary to teach the strategy to the person with aphasia. Finally, it is important to tally whether a topic or message was communicated successfully to the partner.

Multimodal Communication Screening Task for Persons with Aphasia

Multimodal Communication Screening Task for Persons with Aphasia (MCST-A; Garrett & Lasker, 2004; Lasker & Garrett, 2006) reveals how a communicator answers situational questions (i.e., "How would you tell me you went to California in July?") by gesturing, spelling, pointing to locations on a map, or locating pictorial symbols throughout the eight-page booklet used in the screening. It also provides information on the person's ability to categorize and to point referentially when telling a story. The MCST-A stimulus book contains the following pages: 1) concrete concepts represented with pictures, photos, and words (e.g., *eat, lamp*); 2) three categories represented with an incomplete series of visual symbols—the person with aphasia chooses from a row of six additional symbols to complete the categories; 3) graphic symbols representing descriptors (e.g., *open, cold*); 4) slightly more abstract concepts that can be combined with other items to represent complex meanings (e.g., grandchildren, money, monthly calendar); 5) two sets of written words and phrases, one for communicating in a pharmacy and another for conversing with grandchildren; 6) a set of photographs representing a story sequence for a storytelling/retelling task; 7) an outline map of the United States to represent locations of children's homes or favorite vacations; and 8) an alphabet board to communicate highly specific names (e.g., towns, restaurants) by spelling or pointing to the first letter. The scoring form documents the accuracy of message transmission via use of the symbols in the stimulus book, as well as the types of cues that the clinician uses to help the communicator achieve communication success.

 The MCST-A booklet and scoring instructions are available on the Barkley AAC web site.

Clinical experience (Lasker & Garrett, 2006) suggests that the MCST-A effectively distinguishes between communicators who require partner support to indicate choices and stored-message AAC communicators who can independently search through the booklet to locate symbols. Data on the amount and type of cuing can help determine whether the communicator falls into the category of partner dependent (i.e., consistently requires cues to locate a symbolized message) or independent (i.e., needs no cues or minimal cues to locate symbols to convey a message). It is also relatively easy to identify generative AAC communicators. Clinicians can ask the person with aphasia to communicate a complex message (e.g., "How would you communicate that your grandchildren are going to Disney World next month if they have enough money?") and then observe if the person can successfully communicate this idea by pointing to a logical sequence of pictures, words, letters, or locations on the map. In addition, observing this diagnostic activity may assist some family members to better understand why a clinician may suggest low-tech instead of high-tech options for an individual with aphasia.

Speech-Generating Device Trials: Transactional Role Play

To evaluate how effectively a communicator can access stored messages on a voice-output system in an actual communication situation, clinicians can develop scripted scenarios representing a community transaction and program the communicator's SGD with relevant messages. Digitized voice systems for stored messages or synthesized speech output systems (for those people with aphasia who have potential spelling capability) may be used. When selecting a sample conversational scenario, clinicians should consider such factors as time constraints (how quickly the information must be delivered), information specificity, length and complexity of response, predictability (whether messages can be stored in advance and retrieved), communication functions expressed (social closeness versus basic needs), familiarity (with the conversation content and with the partner), and personal relevance (how important the information is to the individual). For example, a consumer-based transaction in which the communicator orders a cup of coffee from a vendor may be considered an "easier" conversation than one in which the communicator discusses the nature of his or her disability with a medical practitioner.

After a situation has been scripted, the clinician prepares representative types of voice-output communication devices. Clinicians may utilize a digitized device with a static overlay (and perhaps multiple levels) or a synthesized device with dynamic screen technology; however, at this stage of system trials, the person with aphasia is not asked to switch levels or pages. Basing the choices on preliminary estimates, the clinician selects devices with the most appropriate size and arrangement of message squares and number of messages per page. In general, a sequence of four to eight pre-stored messages on a digitized device may be used. Then, the clinician should program necessary vocabulary. For example, the following messages might be included in a scenario related to handling car trouble.

- MY NAME IS BILL RYAN.
- I'M HAVING TROUBLE WITH MY CAR.
- CAN YOU CALL A TOW TRUCK FOR ME?
- MY CURRENT LOCATION IS AT THE INTERSECTION OF PARK ST. AND 3RD AVENUE.
- THANK YOU.

In another example, a coffee-ordering scenario might be scripted to combine speech, gesture (shown in brackets), and device use as follows:

Clinician (in the role of a coffee vendor):	Hi, how are you today?
Person with aphasia:	Fine/good/okay.
Clinician:	What can I get you?
Person with aphasia:	I'D LIKE A CUP OF COFFEE.
Clinician:	Okay. For here or to go?
Person with aphasia:	[To go].
Clinician:	What size?
Person with aphasia:	MEDIUM.

Clinician:	How do you take it?
Person with aphasia:	CREAM AND SUGAR.
Clinician:	Here you go. That will be $1.25.
Person with aphasia:	Okay. [hands over money]
Clinician:	Have a good day.
Person with aphasia:	[Bye].

Each communication attempt during the role play is scored based on response adequacy, mode of response (gesture, speech, AAC system), timing, and amount of clinician cuing. Clinicians can use a cuing hierarchy described by Light and Binger (1998) for teaching AAC technology. The clinician first waits and creates an expectation that a message will be generated, points to the individual or the AAC tool, and then models the communication behavior. The blank data collection form is available as Form 6.4 in Beukelman, Garrett, and Yorkston (2007).

Advanced Systems Trials: Combining Stored and Generative Messages

The clinician may occasionally observe that a person with aphasia is a candidate for a generative AAC system because he or she used combinations of two or three symbols on the MCST-A, scored highly on reading and writing subtests on standardized tests, or used writing to convey information during PACE picture description tasks. In this situation, a more demanding role play that requires the communicator to use a combination of generative and stored-message strategies can be implemented. In a process similar to the basic system trials, the clinician creates a scenario that requires the person with aphasia to demonstrate both message retrieval and message formulation behaviors. In addition, the clinician notes whether the person with aphasia can repair communication breakdowns with natural modalities (gestures, speech, spelling/writing), can combine unaided strategies with aided strategies, and can initiate messages. For dynamic display or multilevel devices, the clinician may choose to program a situation related to planning a trip, buying a car, or having a "getting to know you" conversation on at least two to three levels. A trip-planning scenario could be introduced with the following preamble: *You are going to plan a vacation trip with a travel agent who will book all of the arrangements. You will use anything you can to communicate with the travel agent. You will need to arrange all of the details—where you are going, how you will get there, where you will stay.* For this scenario, the clinician can create a main page with some phrase or sentence messages and links to a second page that contains days of the week, money topics, and preferred vacation activities. After the clinician briefly introduces the system and available messages, the trials proceed at first without extensive instruction regarding AAC approaches. Once the initial trial is completed, the communication behaviors are scored, and then instruction and modeling occurs. Following instruction, the role play is then repeated and scored again.

In addition to documenting communication behaviors during the role play, the clinician should note the degree of cuing required for the person with aphasia to perform various operational functions of the device, such as attending to several screens of information, locating messages successfully, navigating among pages, changing various output features of the device, turning the device on and off, utilizing rate enhancement strategies such as word prediction, and storing new messages.

It is also important to consider the nature of the message retrieval formulation techniques employed by different AAC devices. Some SGDs may offer a combination of spelling, picture symbol message access, and word prediction. Others require communicators to locate and string together symbols or icons to create messages. Symbols and images may be contained in folders, on grids, on hidden levels, or on paper pages. Still other SGDs enable people with aphasia to access elements of visual scenes to communicate specific messages (Dietz, McKelvey, & Beukelman, 2006). These choices should be considered in light of the communicator's preferences and ability to retrieve messages in these formats.

Assessing Other Capabilities

Traditional assessment procedures for aphasia typically identify the cognitive, linguistic, and perceptual skills of an individual with aphasia.

Residual Language Skills

Often, language testing has been conducted prior to AAC assessment, and selected information from these tools can contribute to the selection of AAC strategies. First, a standard aphasia battery such as the Western Aphasia Battery–Revised (Kertesz, 1982, 2006), the short form of the Boston Diagnostic Aphasia Exam–Revised (Goodglass & Kaplan, 1983; Goodglass, Kaplan, & Barresi, 2000), or the Boston Assessment of Severe Aphasia (Helm-Estabrooks, Ramsberger, Morgan, & Nicholas, 1989) will measure the extent of the receptive and expressive language impairment when no external AAC strategy or partner support is available. Communicators with nonfluent aphasia typically exhibit difficulties with syntactic encoding. Therefore, AAC strategies that require using symbol combinations to communicate a single message may frustrate these individuals. Even spelling, a more "natural" communication skill, is a type of encoding that requires sequential selection and sequencing of arbitrary symbols to represent sounds and meanings. Because successful spelling requires many repetitions of this procedure, it is often extremely difficult for people with aphasia. Therefore, providing people with aphasia with a typewriter or computer keyboard may be more frustrating than therapeutic. People with aphasia may benefit when clinicians consider how the language demands imposed by particular AAC systems mesh with the skills of communicators (Garrett & Kimelman, 2000; Lasker, 2008).

Cognition

Several aphasiologists (Helm-Estabrooks, 2002; Nicholas, Sinotte, Helm-Estabrooks, 2005; Purdy & Koch, 2006) have suggested that clinicians can gain predictive information on an individual's potential to independently communicate with AAC systems by administering cognitive assessment batteries. The Cognitive Linguistic Quick Test (Helm-Estabrooks, 2001) contains several subtests that assess attention, memory, and reasoning without taxing linguistic ability. Helm-Estabrooks (2002) suggested that several nonverbal reasoning tasks (e.g., trail making) may be useful in identifying individuals with adequate cognitive ability to use high-tech, symbol-based AAC systems. Research is still needed to correlate subtest performance with AAC user ability.

Arranging messages in leveled communication systems may impose significant processing challenges for many people with aphasia who demonstrate problems recalling the location of stored messages and symbols. They must also demonstrate sufficient working memory to complete the steps involved in accessing the messages before forgetting their intent or losing their partner's interest. Several individuals we have worked with shifted from being partner-dependent AAC communicators with leveled high-tech AAC systems to independent AAC communicators after their messages were stored on single cards within a simple binder or low-tech system of cards on a ring.

Individuals with aphasia should also be observed to determine their awareness of their own communicative ability. Are they able to explain their novel communication strategies to unfamiliar partners? Do they know when their natural language is not adequate for a particular situation? Can they use their strategies in a dynamic manner, for example, using speech and writing when able to do so and then shifting to an AAC strategy when they experience communication breakdowns? In addition, the clinician should informally observe the individual's initiative and tenacity to convey a message to a partner despite frequent communication breakdowns. Ken, described earlier in this chapter, initially spent almost half of his communication efforts on resolving breakdowns. However, after he was instructed to shift to a different strategy (e.g., rewording, locating information in his communication notebook) instead of simply repeating the words over and over, the percentage of communication turns used to resolve communication breakdowns decreased from 46% to 11% (Garrett et al., 1989).

Representational Skills

People with aphasia often understand many of the visual images that are used to represent the world. For example, they recognize various icons of geography, such as maps, and icons of events, such as logos and signs. They also usually retain the ability to identify photographs and drawings that relate to people and places. Many people with aphasia retain knowledge about the relative relationships of size, shape, goodness, and importance among objects and experiences. For example, an individual with aphasia may refer to another adult by gesturing to indicate his or her taller height as compared with a child. However, these skills should be probed. Asking an individual to tell about his or her family or childhood during a reminiscing conversation in which a scrapbook is used will allow the clinician to informally observe these skills.

Motor Skills

Individuals with aphasia following a stroke usually retain the ability to control their limbs on at least one side of the body (usually the left). Therefore, they can typically gesture, turn pages, or point to communication choices in a direct selection mode. However, they may experience difficulties when asked to complete a complex sequence of motor movements (e.g., locating words on multiple pages of a book or multiple levels of an electronic communication device) because of limb apraxia or cognitive deficits. They may also have some difficulty physically carrying or manipulating heavy communication devices or using the on/off buttons of those systems. Consultation with an occupational or physical therapist may be appropriate when deciding upon a portable communication device or system.

Hearing

Standard hearing screening procedures can be used to identify hearing impairments (either the communicator's or the partner's) that may interfere with successful communication.

Operational Skills

If they use SGDs to augment their communication, communicators may have to learn new operational skills such as turning the device on and off, comprehending synthesized or digitized speech, locating messages stored on invisible levels, using flow-chart operational menus, keyboarding, and charging the device.

Life Experiences and Vocabulary

The experiences and life history of an individual are particularly relevant as clinicians co-construct AAC interventions with them. Most individuals with aphasia have lived for a considerable period of time and have experienced relatively typical, routine lifestyles, so their knowledge about the world is extensive. To gather "fuel" for upcoming AAC interactions, it may be helpful to informally assess interests, topics, and autobiographical information through interviews with family members prior to beginning an AAC intervention. Forms 6.5 and 6.6 in Beukelman, Garrett, and Yorkston (2007) may be used to structure these interviews.

Partner Skills

Because communication partners are so important in communication interactions with people who have severe aphasia, it is useful to assess their capabilities as well. This assessment usually cannot be formally conducted, so information about the communication skills of partners is obtained from observing their interactions with the individual with aphasia. It is also important to determine if the partner is able to learn or is interested in learning new ways of communicating with the person with severe aphasia. The clinician can also evaluate the potential communication partner's speaking style and understandability, handwriting legibility, reading skills, hearing, and vision.

Assessing Communication Needs in Real-Life Contexts

Guidelines for developing the content of AAC systems generally starts with a discussion of the individual's *needs,* by which we mean the environments and activities in which the person wishes to participate, as well as the specific messages required to communicate in those contexts. Families and friends of people with severe aphasia often play a vital role in identifying these communication needs. For clinicians who are conducting a formal evaluation with an individual who has severe aphasia, the following procedures may be helpful.

Needs Assessment Interview

First, during an initial interview to assess an individual's needs, the clinician can simply ask the communicator, the communicator's family, and significant others to list communication situations that are particularly challenging or difficult for the individual with aphasia. Next, the clinician should ask the interviewees to imagine situations in which they foresee opportunities for meaningful communication. Initially, families may often list situations in which physical needs are communicated (e.g., seeing the doctor, getting dressed). Additional urging to think of situations in which the individual had an important life role prior to stroke may be necessary; providing the family with examples such as betting at the racetrack, saying the dinner prayer at Thanksgiving, attending sports events of grandchildren, and having coffee with a friend also may be helpful. The Aphasia Needs Assessment (Garrett & Lasker, 2004), available as Form 6.2 in Beukelman, Garrett, and Yorkston (2007) and on the Barkley AAC web site, may also assist clinicians to obtain some of this information in a systematic manner. For communicators who cannot verbally express the answers to these questions without supports, the written choice conversation strategy described previously may be useful. Providing the communicator with written word choices (representing situations) and scales for rating the relative importance of the activity can provide a window onto the communicator's perceptions of important communication needs.

Fox, Ginley, and Poulsen (2004) described how real-life communication needs were elicited from a group of people with aphasia and their significant others who attended a weeklong "communication camp" experience. She asked these individuals to describe communication situations that had specifically challenged them and to share strategies that had been particularly effective in those situations. For example, one man told about the difficulties he encountered when trying to order menu items in a fast-food restaurant. He developed an ingenious strategy—shining a red light from a laser pointer on the menu items posted behind the counter—to communicate his food order. Fox and colleagues encouraged participants to develop and incorporate strategies such as the laser pointing technique in their own "communication strategy toolbelt." This "toolbelt" suggestion is an excellent example of how clinicians can assist communicators with aphasia to identify important communication needs in a variety of life situations.

Topic Sorting

Fox, Sohlberg, and Fried-Oken (2001) encouraged research participants with aphasia to sort topics into *preferred* and *nonpreferred* categories prior to engaging in conversational training. They learned that one individual, of the three that participated in their study, communicated much more extensively about topics that he had selected than those that had been chosen for him. This topic-sorting task may be a useful means of identifying important topics and situations, particularly for individuals who cannot verbally express them.

Social Networks

In addition to communication topics and situations, it can be helpful to identify specific communication partners with whom the individual wishes to communicate. With one client, we used the assessment tool known as Social Networks: A Communication Inventory for Individuals with Complex Communication Needs and Their Communication Partners (Blackstone & Hunt Berg, 2003a, 2003b). This tool diagrams the social network of the communicator by using a series of concentric circles to denote level of involvement. For example, the individual communicator is at the center of the circles, those who are identified as life partners are included in the first circle, those identified as close friends are in the second circle, and so forth. The authors of this chapter have modified the tool by creating a large visual diagram to interview communicators about their social networks before and after onset of aphasia (see Figure 15.19). We also use partner-supported communication strategies and photos to facilitate the individual's participation in the interview. Communication partners and social networks from before the onset of aphasia were compared with currently available partners. Treatment goals were then designed to improve interactions with the partners who were currently most important to the communicator.

If it is not possible to conduct a face-to-face interview to identify social networks, clinicians can indirectly estimate communication needs by assessing *peer participation patterns.* Peers can be individuals of the same age or culture as the person with apha-

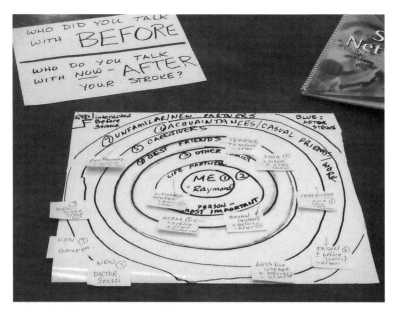

Figure 15.19.   Chart showing circles of communication partners used as part of the Social Networks Inventory (Blackstone & Hunt-Berg, 2003a) to assess a client with aphasia. (Copyright © 2013 K.L. Garrett and J.P. Lasker.)

sia or can be individuals who have similar interests. For example, if a person with aphasia used to socialize at a veterans' club in town, the clinician could observe or ask others about the types of messages or communication needs that would arise in that situation. It may be helpful to ask the communicator to envision the sequence of communication events within each of these situations so that a comprehensive message inventory also can be created.

INTERVENTION ISSUES

"The most difficult thing for us is actually thinking of when to use the [AAC system]— including it in our daily routines" (wife of a communicator with aphasia, personal communication, October 25, 2004).

Several issues may impact the successfulness of an AAC intervention. They include, but are not limited to, the individual's or family's continued desire to work on speech alone, difficulty with acceptance of AAC alternatives, adherence to a medical model of treatment versus a participation model in available intervention centers, discontinuation of treatment, inappropriate match of system features to the communicator's capabilities, limited availability of personalized messages, lack of practice in contextual situations, lack of available communication partners for partner-supported communicators, a limited support network to assist in message development for generative AAC communicators, and/or a lack of communication opportunities because needs are met and anticipated by others (Garrett & Kimelman, 2000; Purdy & Dietz, 2010; Scherer, Sax, Vanbiervliet, Cushman, & Scherer, 2005).

The following interaction with the spouse of a contextual choice AAC communicator) reflects some of the attitudinal barriers that family members may initially project when discussing AAC strategy implementation at home:

Clinician:	So how has it been going at home?
Spouse:	Oh, it's much easier to communicate with Robert now. He really seems to know what's going on.
Clinician:	Are you and your sons comfortable with talking more slowly, making sure he understands? Can he clearly tell you "yes" and "no"?
Spouse:	Yes, although sometimes he laughs if we go too slowly...he'll even make fun of us. But we're doing well there. He really thinks about how he's nodding his head. And he points to what he wants now...that really helps.
Clinician:	Have you been able to talk about more complicated topics? Like what to get the kids for the holidays...or opinions on what's happening in the news?
Spouse:	No, not really...mostly we just talk about what he needs.
Clinician:	Have you tried to use the written choice technique we practiced?
Spouse:	No, I'm glad I haven't had to resort to that yet...

To promote acceptance of AAC strategies, clinicians may find it helpful to acknowledge communicators' and partners' hesitations about communicating using these somewhat unusual alternatives to speech. Many of the spouses of communicators in the authors' clinics have gradually accepted some level of AAC after several months of simultaneously working on recovery of speech and gradually incorporating AAC strategies into conversations. Group therapy is another positive means of illustrating how AAC and natural communication modalities can blend. Watching other, more "senior" participants converse about old movies or introduce themselves in a simulated social club may be more convincing than academic explanations about the benefits of AAC strategies.

It is also essential that the *content* of an AAC system remain dynamic. As changes occur in the situations and contexts of an individual's life, the AAC system must reflect these changes; otherwise, motivation and interest in using the system will quickly diminish. Continual modification of the content of an AAC system requires that one or more facilitators, usually family members or caregivers, be trained to monitor and adjust the AAC system. Facilitators must also be able to train new people who enter the life of the person with aphasia (e.g., a new son- or daughter-in-law or a new neighbor) so that they, too, can become effective communication partners. Failure to identify and adequately prepare facilitators is a common reason for unsuccessful AAC intervention among people with severe aphasia.

Clearly, the success of an AAC intervention depends as well on flexibility and continuity of service delivery as the individual with aphasia transitions from setting to setting. Professionals, family members, and people with aphasia may wish to work as a team to create better solutions for management of long-term aphasia. Options could include increasing the emphasis on training partners to use immediate communication strategies early in the individual's recovery, with more intensive involvement of the speech-language pathologist later in the rehabilitation process. It may be useful to schedule clients with aphasia for routine follow-up visits each year. Some people with aphasia may benefit from weekly group therapy sessions rather than individual treatment sessions only. Still others may benefit from home visits by the speech-language pathologist as well as other health care professionals because some communication challenges may be visible only in the individual's home environment. With careful planning and extended clinical support, AAC interventions can enrich the communication options for individuals and their communication partners at all stages of adjustment to life with aphasia.

QUESTIONS

15.1.   List five general functions of AAC (low-tech and high-tech) for people with aphasia or apraxia of speech.

15.2.   What are the two broad categories of communicators with aphasia? Describe how they differ.

15.3.   What fundamental communication skills would you work on with an emerging AAC communicator? List two communication contexts, or interactive scenarios, that you would develop to support teaching these strategies.

15.4.   Describe two strategies to use augmented input to enhance comprehension for people with severe aphasia.

15.5.   How would you design an intervention program to teach communication partners how to alter their communication style to converse with a person who is a contextual choice AAC communicator?

15.6.   What is the primary communication skill that transitional AAC communicators do not have? Describe one teaching activity in which you might facilitate the development of this skill.

15.7.   How do stored-message and generative AAC communicators differ? How would this difference influence your selection of a low-tech or high-tech communication strategy?

15.8.   How would you select messages and vocabulary for an independent AAC communicator's AAC system?

15.9.   Describe one teaching activity in which you would facilitate an independent AAC communicator's competent use of both AAC and natural speech communication in a real-life context.

15.10.   Describe one low-tech activity you could use to support functional writing for an independent AAC communicator with significant language formulation difficulties.

15.11.   Describe some high-tech approaches that can be used for scaffolding the generative writing of a person with aphasia who has moderate difficulty with spelling errors, word selection, use of pronouns, omission of verbs of being, and morphologic errors.

15.12.   List some examples of specific-need AAC communicators' AAC strategies or systems.

15.13.   Describe how you would assess the *capabilities* of an individual with aphasia who cannot meet all of his or her communication needs through verbal communication.

15.14.   Describe at least two types of interviewing activities that you might use to identify the communication *needs* and changes in *participation patterns* of an individual with severe aphasia.

CHAPTER 16

Adults with Degenerative Cognitive and Linguistic Disorders

with Elizabeth Hanson

The gradual deterioration of communication effectiveness is a commonly reported symptom of various types of degenerative cognitive and linguistic conditions. The exact pattern of communication deterioration varies in that some people experience cognitive symptoms such as memory loss with accompanying impaired judgment, reduced problem solving, or visuospatial orientation before changes in their language are observed. Others demonstrate a gradual deterioration of language as an early symptom. During the past decade, augmentative and alternative communication (AAC) strategies have been implemented to enhance the receptive and expressive communication effectiveness of people with degenerative language and cognitive disorders such as primary progressive aphasia (King, Alarcon, & Rogers, 2007), dementia (Bourgeois & Hickey, 2007), and Huntington disease (Yorkston & Beukelman, 2007).

PRIMARY PROGRESSIVE APHASIA

Primary progressive aphasia (PPA) is recognized as a distinct clinical condition characterized by language impairment (aphasia) that is caused by a neurodegenerative disease (progressive) and is the most salient (primary) aspect of the condition (Mesulam, 2007). Duffy (2000) reported that the mean age of onset is 60.5 years with about a 2:1 ratio of men to women. PPA is considered the fifth most common type of dementia. There is no known cause of PPA, although about half of patients with PPA have a family history of dementia and research into a genetic component in PPA is ongoing (Mandell, 2002; Mesulam, 2001).

After experiencing a history of language symptoms, some individuals with PPA eventually demonstrate other cognitive impairments consistent with a diagnosis of dementia. In 1999, Rogers and Alarcon reviewed 57 articles that described the course of 147 individuals with PPA. Of these individuals, 25% demonstrated symptoms of fluent aphasia, 60% had symptoms of nonfluent aphasia, and 15% had indeterminate symptoms. Twenty-seven percent of the fluent group, 37% of the nonfluent group, and 77% of the indeterminate group eventually demonstrated symptoms of dementia. Although the initial symptoms of PPA vary among individuals, anomia (i.e., trouble thinking of specific words) is the most commonly reported language symptom. Another common symptom, particularly in the nonfluent group, is slow, hesitant speech with long pauses.

> For further information, see the AAC-RERC (Rehabilitation Engineering Research Center on Communication Enhancement) webcast *AAC for Persons with Primary Progressive Aphasia* by Melanie Fried-Oken.

Stages of Intervention

King et al. (2007) recommended the implementation of a proactive intervention plan. In anticipation of future declines in language function, intervention that focuses on early incorporation of AAC strategies into everyday communication is recommended. Form 7.7 in Beukelman, Garrett, and Yorkston (2007) contains extensive information to guide communication partners when interacting with people who have PPA.

Early Stage

During the early stages of PPA, affected individuals continue to use speech to interact with others. However, in order maintain independence in communication, they need assistance to manage communication breakdowns and need to develop strategies that they will probably need in the future, such as help in word finding (i.e., recall of specific words) with drawing, writing, print, and picture support for commonly used but difficult words. Intervention techniques involve many of the strategies identified in the section on specific-need AAC communicators in Chapter 15. These strategies include booklets or cards with specific information, prepared questions for difficult situations, and gestures (yes, no, left, right, past, and future) to resolve communication breakdowns. The techniques should be introduced gradually and early so that people with PPA and their listeners can become familiar with them and accept this type of communication support. Form 7.1 in Beukelman, Garrett, and Yorkston (2007) offers an intake profile for people with PPA.

Middle Stage

People with PPA in the middle stage are considered to be *generative* or *transitional AAC communicators* (see Chapter 15) in that they need AAC support in most communication contexts. In addition to communication notebooks and cards, these individuals often benefit from photographs of scenes that are familiar to them (Fried-Oken, Rowland, & Gibbon, 2010). Some also benefit from drawing scenes to communicate or clarify messages. For others, spatial representations such as maps, calendars, family trees, and floor plans are helpful to communicate specific content (Cress & King, 1999). Individuals in this stage often need augmented input strategies to enhance their comprehension of spoken information as well. Such strategies may include key words (printed), photos, gestures, drawings, or line drawings.

Late Stage

The severe communication limitations associated with late-stage PPA are often quite similar to the needs of contextual choice AAC communicators, as described in Chapter 15. These individuals need help both to communicate and to comprehend information about basic needs and routines. Early in this stage, they may continue to use the materials developed in the early and middle stages. However, as they progress further into the late stage, they become *emerging AAC communicators* (see Chapter 15), in that they need to be presented with very limited choices in order to communicate about their needs, preferences, and routines. In this phase, they are partner-dependent AAC communicators, in that partner education and supports are essential to ensure that the individual with PPA receives effective communication support (King et al., 2007).

Development and Use of Communication Notebooks

Communication notebooks are usually small, easy-to-carry binders that contain information that supports the communication efforts of people with complex communication needs. The content and form of the notebooks is personalized. For example, these notebooks may contain pictures for individuals who are unable to read or may contain considerable printed information if the individuals can read but have difficulty remembering the names of people, places, and activities. People with PPA usually begin the notebooks early so that they can participate in the selection of content and in the organization of the notebook. King et al. (2007) presented an excellent discussion of the preparation and maintenance of communication notebooks for people with PPA, including guidelines to enhance the long-term usefulness of such books. These include the following:

- The communication notebook must reflect the person with PPA; it must be personalized.
- The person with PPA must take a lead role in determining its content early in the course of the disease.
- The communication notebook and opportunities to use it must be available consistently throughout the course of PPA.
- The communication notebook is never finished; it must be dynamic so that it reflects the changing needs and experiences of the person with PPA and his or her social network.

Figure 16.1 provides an example of a communication page described by Cress and King (1999).

"It is important to begin communication supports (AAC strategies) as soon as possible for people with PPA because familiarity and context seem to influence the use and retention of AAC strategies. [These individuals] demonstrate...their most effective communication using strategies that they...generate...themselves....If we can provide early guidance and information to facilitate these self-generating strategies, then further intervention can concentrate on maintaining and modifying those strategies or techniques, and providing additional facilitator training as needed" (Cress & King, 1999, pp. 254–255).

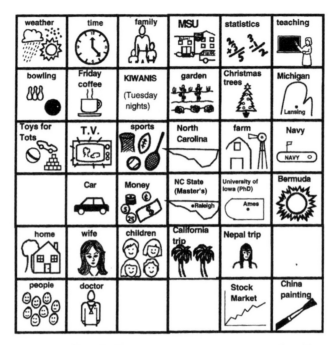

Figure 16.1. Example of a communication page. (From Cress, C., & King, J. [1999]. AAC strategies for people with primary progressive aphasia without dementia: Two case studies. *Augmentative and Alternative Communication, 15,* 248–259; reprinted by permission of Informa Healthcare.)

Summary

In summary, PPA is a progressive condition characterized by language impairment at least 2 years prior to the occurrence of other cognitive impairments, which typically lead to dementia. AAC interventions can help individuals with PPA to enhance both expressive and receptive language. AAC strategies should be introduced early in the course of the disease to allow the person with PPA to contribute to the design and content, and to help both the person with PPA and their communication partners to learn how to use the strategies.

DEMENTIA

Dementia is a medical syndrome characterized by an acquired, chronic cognitive impairment. A diagnosis of dementia requires that the cognitive impairment involve memory and related changes in another cognitive domain, such as language, abstract thinking, judgment, or executive or frontal lobe functions (Bourgeois & Hickey, 2007, 2009). Dementia is a relatively common syndrome, affecting about 28 million people around the world, which results in $156 billion in direct care costs each year (Wimo, Jonsson, & Winblad, 2006). The prevalence of dementia is 1% of the population for people age 65 and almost 50% for individuals aged 90 years and older (Jorm & Jolly, 1998). Alzheimer's disease is the most common form of dementia. The Alzheimer's Association (2001) estimates that between 2.4 and 5.1 million people in the United States have Alzheimer's disease, and if the trend continues it is estimated that 13 million Americans will have Alzheimer's disease by the year 2050 (Herbert, Scherr, Bienias, Bennet, & Evans, 2003).

Memory Strengths and Impairments

Dementia involves the impairment of the ability to transfer information from working or short-term memory to long-term memory, which presents serious problems for the people who develop it as well as for their families and caregivers. Memory impairments in dementia affect various memory domains in different ways.

Episodic memory about recent events is often impaired quite early in the progression of the syndrome. Thus, memory loss in the early stages includes an inability to recall information such as who has visited, where items were left, what was eaten for breakfast, and so forth. Bourgeois and Hickey (2009) suggests that recent episodic memory limitations reflect a reduced ability to transfer information from short-term (working) to long-term memory.

Semantic memory involves factual information and general, organized knowledge. Impairments may be evidenced in an inability to remember facts such as the name of the leader of one's country, that bananas are yellow, or that both cats and dogs are animals. Semantic memories are usually stored much earlier than episodic memories and typically are retained longer. Therefore, semantic memory impairments are typically observed later in the course of dementia than impairments in episodic memory.

Procedural memory is often the best preserved of the memory domains. Procedural memory involves retaining the ability to complete common procedures such as shaving, dressing, writing checks, and so forth.

Recognition memory may remain a strength for people with dementia for longer than other types of memory. Examples of recognition memory include people realizing that they know someone when they see him or her, recognizing that a familiar item is out of place, selecting a specific item from among a choice of items, and recognizing a favorite TV show when they see it.

Recall memory, on the other hand, relies on one's ability to retrieve "invisible" information that is not concretely represented in some way, such as a person's name, the code for a digital door lock, or the TV channel for a favorite show. Typically, people with memory impairments due to dementia perform better when using recognition memory than when using recall memory.

Memory and Communication

Memory plays a very important role in human communication. It helps to maintain the thread of a conversation, it ensures that topics are fully discussed, and it allows new topics to be introduced at appropriate times. Impaired transfer of information from short-term to long-term memory can therefore have a severe impact on a person's conversations, resulting in topics being repeatedly introduced and giving the appearance that the person is not listening. This can be very disturbing and frustrating for the conversation partner, and can in turn have a negative effect on the person as he or she becomes aware of a partner's negative emotions but does not understand how they have come about.

Stages of Intervention

The purpose of dementia care is to maintain the personhood of the individual in spite of the individual's cognitive decline. Kitwood (1997) maintains that a specific set of psychological needs must be addressed to sustain the individual's mental health.

These include needs for comfort, identity, inclusion, occupation, and attachment. Although relative strength and impairment profiles differ widely among people with dementia, there are overall patterns of strengths and impairments that occur with each stage of the condition. Building on communication strengths and addressing psychological needs may be the foundation of interventions for people with dementia throughout the course of the disease. Communication strengths and impairments by stage are summarized in Table 16.1.

In the early stage of dementia, caregivers and communication partners need to learn how to support communication interaction by reducing the challenge of remembering specific words or events by redirecting conversations as needed and providing compensatory strategies for information that needs to be remembered. During this stage, the individual with dementia is aware of memory limitations, and the focus of this stage is to maintain the individual's dignity and self-respect. This stage is also an opportunity for proactive involvement of the person with dementia in designing memory tools that he or she will use later on. Some predict that early involvement in the process will increase the likelihood that people will accept the technology (Lehoux & Blume, 2000).

Table 16.1. Communication strengths and impairments of people with dementia by stage

Stage	Strengths	Impairments
Early stage	Language comprehension	Diminished reading comprehension
	Grammar	Difficulty with written expression
	Syntax	Difficulty with word finding
	Ability to express needs independently	Reduced verbal output
	Ability to hold conversations	Pragmatic deficits
	Ability to answer multiple choice and yes/no questions	Distractibility
		Difficulty concentrating
		Confusion
		Disorientation
		Problems managing activities of daily living
Middle stage	Grammar	Difficulty with pragmatics: topic changes, discourse cohesion and coherence
	Syntax	Significantly diminished reading and writing skills
	Reading comprehension for single words	Reduced verbal output
	Ability to express needs with help	
	Ability to follow two-step commands	
	Gestural input helps	
	Recognition memory	
Late stage	Some meaningful words	Need for partner support
	Possible ability to read single words	No relevant language
	Social communication (greetings)	
	Ability to attend to pleasant stimuli	

In the middle stages, people with dementia lose awareness of their cognitive and communication problems. Communication partners need to support interaction that maintains social closeness. To do this, the partner needs to take more control or leadership of interactions. At the end stage of the disease, communication partners and caregivers increasingly learn to communicate for the person with dementia to provide comfort and familiarity (Bourgeois & Hickey, 2007). Personal communication technology such as multimedia memory biographies may become important tools to provide comfort and a sense of personhood through the guided reminiscences that they offer.

Communication Strengths and Impairments

The primary focus of intervention for individuals with dementia is to enhance their residual strengths at each stage rather than to attempt to remediate their impairments. Thus, materials and training should target frequent communication partners so that they can support people with dementia to use their strengths and allow them to compensate for their particular pattern of impairments. For example, if a person with dementia experiences impairments in recent episodic memory (i.e., remembering what happened yesterday), intervention might consist of providing him or her with a concrete reminder, such as a memento of a recent event in the form of a remnant or a photograph. Training activities designed to strengthen episodic memory are generally not indicated. The following intervention guidelines and strategies focus on the cognitive and communicative strengths of people with dementia:

*   *Reduce memory demands.* Because impairments of recall memory in particular are so common in dementia, AAC interventions should be designed to reduce demands on recall memory and processing capacity. Bourgeois, Dijkstra, Burgio, and Allen-Burge (2001) described a "memory book" with pages that each contain one sentence or one item, such as an illustration, to provide graphic information. The memory books typically include autobiographical information, daily schedules, and problem resolution information. Providing information in the form of memory books builds on recognition memory, which takes less effort than recall tasks (Bayles & Kim, 2003). Figure 16.2 shows memory cards that were created for

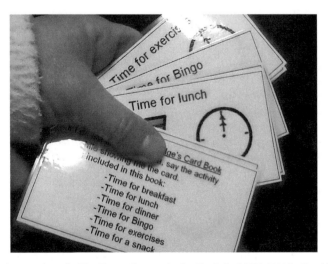

Figure 16.2.   Sample memory cards. (The Picture Communication Symbols ©1981–2012 by DynaVox Mayer-Johnson LLC. All Rights Reserved Worldwide. Used with permission.)

a man with dementia who lived in a nursing facility as a result of staff requests for better ways to help him understand what was happening throughout the day.

- *Reduce distractions.* People with dementia often experience difficulty processing information and interacting in environments that contain distractions. Therefore, their communication partners, including family and caregivers, need to be trained to position themselves in a way that minimizes distractions and optimizes performance.

- *Chunk information.* Organizing information into manageable "chunks" often enhances the communication effectiveness of people with dementia. This can be done using a variety of AAC strategies. For example, if listeners use augmented communication in the form of identifying topics of conversation using pictures, the associated information will often be understood better than if the person with dementia is engaged in a free-flowing conversation that moves from topic to topic without clear demarcation of content.

- *Provide information in alternative forms.* Provision of alternative forms of information allows for redundancy, thereby reducing the information-processing load. Consider the perceptual and cognitive complexity of a family reunion. Photographs of family groupings will allow a person with dementia to remember more clearly who is related to whom. In addition, a written schedule of activities will allow the person to understand the flow of activities better than verbal descriptions alone, provided that the listing is not excessively complex.

Behavioral Communication Therapy for Dementia

In a study that included 25 participants with dementia, Bourgeois et al. (2003) examined the effectiveness of two training approaches, spaced retrieval and a modified cuing hierarchy, to teach individuals with dementia strategies to remember to use external aids such as memory books and memory wallets. Spaced retrieval involves learning to remember information by recalling it over increasingly longer durations of time. For example, a goal of looking in the memory book to remind oneself when lunch is would be addressed by talking about the need to remember and cuing the person to look in the book. After the person does so, the clinician would engage in small talk for 30 seconds, and then ask the person how they know what time lunch is served. If the person responds by looking in or showing the memory book, the small talk would continue, this time for 60 seconds, doubling each time the person correctly remembers the procedure. At the point when the person forgets, the clinician shows him or her what to do and reduces the retrieval time to the last successful duration. The results demonstrated that both approaches resulted in the participants' ability to learn new strategies that generally lasted for 4 months after the intervention. However, the spaced retrieval approach yielded better performance overall than the modified cuing hierarchy approach did. This research demonstrates that, contrary to widely held views, new learning that targets procedural and recognition memory is possible for some individuals with dementia.

Represent Language Symbolically

With regard to AAC strategies and options, Fried-Oken, Rau, and Oken (2000) direct clinicians to address both language representation and organization. Messages communicated to and by a person with dementia can be represented visually using several levels of symbolization, depending on the person's capabilities. Simple print can be read by many individuals with mild, moderate, and (occasionally) severe dementia. Printed words can be used to label the locations of items, provide memory support, clarify spoken messages, and act as reminders of tasks to be completed. As dementia progresses, printed words can be accompanied by photographs and pictures. For some, objects eventually become the most effective way to represent information. If printed words become ineffective, drawings or photographs may be used to represent language concepts. Once the language symbolization level of a person with dementia is determined, the range of language content to be represented needs to be identified. Usually, this is a team effort by the person with dementia, caregivers, family members, and others. The content will depend on the person's lifestyle, the settings in which he or she participates, and the supports that are available.

Use a Variety of Augmentative and Alternative Communication Strategies

The incorporation of language representation techniques into the lives of people with dementia and the members of their social networks (e.g., caregivers, family, friends, members of the public) can be managed using a number of common AAC strategies. For example, written choice techniques (see Chapter 15), originally developed for people with aphasia, can be used with print or pictures to provide communication choices that represent the preferences and needs of people with dementia. Communication notebooks or small wallets are also useful in many cases, particularly when they include information represented using digital photography techniques that allow editing, enhancement, sizing, and manipulation of images to support communication. Figure 16.3 shows a communication card from a set developed for an older adult with Alzheimer's disease whose wedding anniversaries were an event in the long-term care facility in which he spent his final years. This type of information can emphasize the personhood (Kitwood, 1997) of individuals who have to leave so much behind in order to maintain their health and safety in the care of others when they can no longer live at home.

Communication cards and labels throughout a home may support the person in identifying various rooms of the house or the contents behind closed cupboard

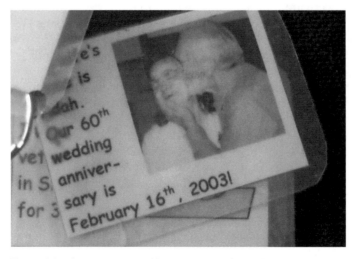

Figure 16.3. Communication card for man with Alzheimer's disease.

doors, following the steps to complete an activity such as flushing the toilet after use or washing hands, or remembering to take medicine.

As noted previously, memory books have probably been the most investigated AAC intervention for people with dementia. Bourgeois and colleagues (Bourgeois, 1990, 1992, 1993, 1996; Bourgeois et al., 2001) reported that the quality of conversational interactions for people with mild and moderate dementia improved significantly when they used personalized memory wallets or books. Improvements included increases in the overall number of utterances as well as the number of positive statements and informative utterances from the person with dementia in conversations. The nursing aides in the study used more facilitative comments when talking to the residents.

A trend that builds on the autobiographical focus of memory books while taking advantage of the burgeoning affordability and availability of digital photos, videos, and audio technologies is to provide multimedia biographies in the form of digitally edited picture videos complete with music and narration (Alm, Astell, Ellis, Dye, Gowans, & Campbell, 2004; Cohen, 2000; Smith, Crete-Nishihata, Damioanakis, Baecker, & Marziali, 2009; Yasuda, Kuwabara, Kuwahara, Abe, & Tetsutani, 2009). Cohen (2000) developed such a tool using digitized photos with slow movement and transitions between pictures, music from the appropriate era, and well-told story narratives to support photos in the biography. Old home movies and videos may also be digitally converted and incorporated. Cohen found that such multimedia presentations increased positive engagement and decreased agitation in the people with dementia for whom the displays were developed, as well as providing caregivers and visitors with a focus for interactions. Yasuda et al. (2009) measured the attention of participants to personalized reminiscence photo videos compared with a popular TV variety show and a news program. Eighty percent of the participants showed greater attention to their personalized photo videos. Alm et al. (2004) measured increased attention in participants with dementia and increased enjoyment of the interactions in their communication partners when using a multimedia reminiscence presentation. Smith, Crete-Nishihata, et al. (2009) are working to develop a streamlined procedure to help long-term care staff, family members, and volunteers create customized multimedia biographies that are cost effective and time efficient.

The technologies to produce such multimedia biographies evolve too rapidly to realistically try to provide a list of software or hardware here. However, most computers now come with straightforward photo- and video-editing programs, and newer digitized photo picture frames found in the rooms of many nursing facility residents now support audio as well as remote uploads of photos via Internet connections.

Not all high-tech strategies work for people with dementia. Fried-Oken et al. (2009) studied the impact of digitized voice output (one-or two-word utterances) on two-person conversations of people with Alzheimer's disease and their communication partners. The authors concluded that AAC technologies with digitized output depressed conversational performance and actually distracted people with moderate Alzheimer's disease, as compared with communication performance without digitized voice output. The researchers acknowledged that the voice output might have been less distracting if the participants with Alzheimer's disease had been introduced to it early in the progression of the disease.

Train Communication Partners

As evidenced in the studies by Andrews-Salvia, Roy, and Cameron (2003) and Bourgeois et al. (2001), communication intervention for people with dementia must target both the person and his or her communication partners (Hopper, 2003). The degenerative nature of this condition means that the responsibility shared between two communication partners will increasingly fall to the partner without impairment as the capability of the person with dementia decreases. A screening protocol for people with dementia is provided as Form 8.3 in Beukelman, Garrett, and Yorkston (2007). Therefore, the partner must learn strategies to enhance communication as the disease progresses. Caregivers, family members, professionals, and friends make up the social networks of most people with dementia, and most of these individuals are used to communicating primarily through speech. Ongoing training must teach them new, more effective ways to communicate with individuals with dementia by shifting their communication patterns to include AAC techniques such as memory aids. Small, Gutman, Makela, and Hillhouse (2003) studied communication strategies used by 18 married couples that included one spouse with Alzheimer's disease as the dyads communicated about various activities of daily living. The researchers observed the couples and documented the effectiveness or ineffectiveness of 10 strategies that are commonly recommended to increase communicative success for people with dementia. Table 16.2 lists the strategies and illustrates their effectiveness.

The researchers also asked the spouses, who did not have impairment, to rate how often they used the strategies and the effectiveness of the resulting interactions. Some of the results were quite surprising. Of the 10 strategies documented, only 3 were found to decrease communication breakdowns: eliminating distractions, speaking in simple sentences, and using yes/no questions. One strategy, using slower speech, appeared to be related to increased communication breakdowns; however, the investigators found that some spouses were not slowing their speaking rate even when they thought they were. In other cases in which the rate was slower but still not effective, the researchers postulated that the longer duration of the message increased the burden on the already limited working memory capacities of the spouses with Alzheimer's disease, consistent with previous research (Bayles & Kim, 2003; Small, Kemper, & Lyons, 1997; Tomoeda, Bayles, Boone, Kaszniak, & Slauson, 1990). Overall, the spouses reported a higher level of communicative effectiveness than was supported by the objective data on communication breakdowns. This study

Table 16.2. Communication strategies commonly recommended for people who care for individuals with Alzheimer's disease and their effectiveness

Strategy	Did the strategy decrease communication breakdowns?
Eliminate distractions	Yes
Approach from front slowly; give eye contact	No clear difference
Use short, simple sentences	Yes
Speak slowly	No
Offer one question or instruction at a time	No clear difference
Use yes/no rather than open-ended questions	Yes
Repeat verbatim	No clear difference
Repeat using paraphrase	No clear difference
Avoid interrupting; allow time to respond	No clear difference
Encourage person to describe word, if word finding is a problem	No clear difference

emphasizes the critical need for interventions that target the communication partners of people with dementia.

Summary

In summary, dementia is a syndrome characterized by progressive memory impairment that affects communication and other cognitive domains. Distinct communicative strengths and weaknesses are associated with each stage of the syndrome. People with dementia may benefit from AAC strategies that are designed to support and enhance communication strengths rather than remediate communication impairments. Personalized memory books and multimedia biographies, which enhance communicative interactions, have received much of the research attention as an AAC strategy for dementia. Memory books can serve as alternate forms of communication input, enhance procedural memory for completing daily care activities, and support the communicative intent of a person with dementia who is experiencing expressive language difficulty. A growing body of research confirms the effectiveness of partner training in AAC interventions for dementia. Partner training is critical to the success of AAC interventions, and new investigations are determining which communicative strategies used by partners are actually effective. A memory aid form is provided as Form 8.7 in Beukelman, Garrett, and Yorkston (2007).

Figure 16.4 shows a low-tech communication system developed by researchers in Europe (Ferm, Sahlin, Sundin, & Hartelius, 2010; Murphy, Tester, Hubbard, Downs, & McDonald, 2005) to help nursing facility residents communicate about their likes and dislikes. Talking Mats use picture symbols representing topics, options related to each topic, and a visual scale to help residents communicate their general

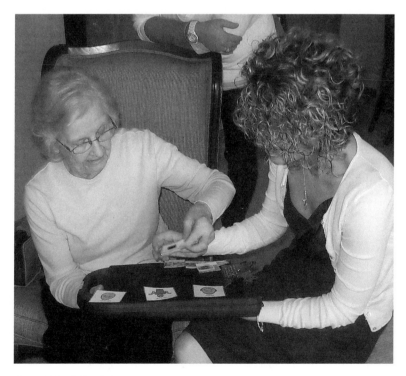

Figure 16.4.   Talking Mats.

feeling about each item. Residents can move symbols for activities to the visual scale in order to communicate their preferences. A digital photo of the display serves as documentation in the person's chart. Over time, consistency of responses may validate the communicative intent of the symbol choices.

HUNTINGTON DISEASE

The communication limitations associated with Huntington disease (HD) are challenging because they reflect a complex interaction of impairment of motor function (dysarthria) and disruptive change in cognitive-linguistic skills (Klasner & Yorkston, 2000). Therefore, AAC systems must meet the needs of the individual, be easy to use, and be adaptable to the progressions of the disease (Yorkston & Beukelman, 2007). HD is an inherited autosomal dominant degenerative disease, which means that people who have one parent with the disease have a 50% chance of inheriting it. The symptoms of HD typically appear in the fourth decade of life, with death occurring 15 to 17 years after onset. People with HD are often unable to speak functionally by the end stages of the disease (Folstein, 1990).

The primary symptoms of HD include chorea (involuntary, irregular spasmodic movements of the limbs or facial muscles), emotional disturbance, and hyperkinetic dysarthria. Early cognitive changes include impaired attention, memory, and cognitive functions with full dementia developing in some patients in later stages (Murray, 2000). The communication impairments associated with HD vary considerably from person to person. Language comprehension impairments associated with HD include high-level processing difficulties with metaphoric or ambiguous sentences or sentences containing implied information or complex grammar. Expressive language impairments include shorter, less complex, and less grammatical utterances (Murray, 2000). For some, atypical motor movements may be restricted primarily to the lower extremities without obvious speech disorder. For others, speech is so impaired that AAC strategies are required (Klasner & Yorkston, 2000).

Klasner and Yorkston (2001) documented a case report in which linguistic and cognitive supplementation strategies were employed to support the communication of a 44-year-old man with HD. Linguistic supplementation through scripting "home to work" conversations involved a notebook in which regular daily activities were described in two or three short sentences. Cognitive supplementation using task lists on tagboard sheets was used to support his completion of household activities such as caring for the family pet.

Early-Phase Augmentative and Alternative Communication Intervention

Strategies to guide communication interactions are often helpful even when dysarthria is mild. Kennedy, Meyer, Knowles, and Shukla (2000) suggested the use of "memory organization packets" that outline the initiation, maintenance, and termination of conversations. Topic scenes consisting of verbal scripts can be used to organize a set of utterances. The use of these external prompts has shown some potential to assist those with HD to maintain communication by participating in conversations (Klasner & Yorkston, 2001). Index cards with the topic and utterance on one side and the key word on the other side have been used to rehearse these scripts. Some with HD can generate the utterance simply by looking at the key word (Klasner & Yorkston, 2001). Those with moderate dysarthria need support to resolve communication breakdowns. These strategies must be developed on an individual basis depending upon the residual capability of the individual and the willingness of regular communication partners to provide this support.

Middle-Phase Augmentative and Alternative Communication Intervention

By the middle phase of intervention, cognitive problems typically prevent individuals with HD from participating fully in activities for daily living. They have difficulty remembering to initiate an activity and completing all of the steps. Klasner and Yorkston (2001) describe "cognitive supplementation" options to break down tasks, such as feeding a cat, into manageable steps.

Late-Phase Augmentative and Alternative Communication Intervention

In late-phase intervention, the communication partner must assume a greater and greater role in supporting communication. This stage of intervention focuses primarily on those who regularly interact or care for the individual with HD, and the strategies used are very similar to those described in the section on dementia in this chapter.

QUESTIONS

16.1. In what ways should treatment for PPA reflect interventions for nonprogressive aphasia? Explain your answer.

16.2. In what ways should treatment for PPA and nonprogressive aphasia not be the same? Explain your answer.

16.3. What is the rationale for starting intervention early in the course of PPA rather than waiting until the communication impairment is more apparent?

16.4. What are the benefits of beginning dementia intervention, such as developing a memory book, in the early stages of the condition?

16.5. Can you think of multimedia software or web sites that you could use to construct a multimedia biography similar to those described in this chapter?

16.6. Describe two strategies to use augmented input to enhance comprehension for people with dementia.

16.7. How would you design an intervention program to teach communication partners how to alter their communication style to meet the needs of a person with dementia?

CHAPTER 17

Individuals with Traumatic Brain Injury

with Susan Fager

Augmentative and alternative communication (AAC) interventions for people who have experienced traumatic brain injury (TBI) have changed dramatically through the years. Until the mid-1990s, AAC interventions occurred primarily with individuals who experienced severe, persistent anarthria or dysarthria following TBI. It was not uncommon for teams to delay AAC interventions until the individual's associated communication disorders "stabilized"; consequently, many people with TBI were unable to communicate functionally for months or even years after their accidents. The justification for this conservative approach had three bases. First, cognitive limitations during early stages of recovery make it difficult for many people with TBI to operate complex AAC technology. Second, because the cognitive and motor performance of a person with TBI changes over time, an appropriate long-term AAC system is difficult to select. Third, clinical observations indicate that some individuals with TBI do recover functional speech and thus do not require long-term AAC systems. With this view, AAC teams often felt that the most conservative approach was the "safest" when recommending an intervention.

Currently, the goal of an AAC team is to provide communication assistance so that people with TBI can participate effectively in a rehabilitation program and are able to communicate their ongoing needs. Thus, the focus of intervention has shifted from providing a single AAC system for long-term use to providing a series of AAC systems designed to meet short-term communication needs while continuing efforts to reestablish natural speech. For example, begin with understandable yes/no responses, provide a communication board for immediate wants and needs, develop a way to call for attention, develop communication supports to share information, support written communication, focus on the development of natural speech, and provide instruction in the use of multimodal communication that integrates residual natural speech and AAC strategies (Light, Beesley, & Collier, 1988).

This chapter outlines the general approaches to AAC intervention for individuals with TBI. However, because individuals with brain injuries recover over an extended period of time, it is beyond the scope of this book to detail the extensive AAC intervention concepts, techniques, and strategies developed for these individuals. Fager, Doyle, and Karantounis (2007) have written in depth about such information.

PREVALENCE AND ETIOLOGY

Injuries to the head that result in temporary or permanent brain damage are quite common. It is difficult to estimate the number of these injuries that occur each year because many go unreported. Individuals who do not lose consciousness or do so only briefly are rarely admitted to the hospital and may not even go to an emergency room. According to the Centers for Disease Control and Prevention (2010), approximately 1.7 million people sustain TBI annually. Of them, 52,000 die, 275,000 are hospitalized, and 1.365 million are treated and released from emergency departments. Of the individuals who sustain TBI in the United States each year, 80,000 to 90,000 survive with impairments that are so severe that they interfere with independent living. One of six individuals is unable to return to school or work when discharged from the hospital or from rehabilitation. Children younger than the age of 5 years, teenagers, and adults older than 65 years are the most likely to sustain TBI (Centers for Disease Control and Prevention, 2010; Thurman, Alverson, Dunn, Guerrero, & Sniezek, 1999).

Individuals with TBI do not represent a random sample of the total population. More than twice as many males as females are injured. Male children between the ages of 0 and 4 have the highest rates of emergency room visits, hospitalizations, and deaths related to TBI (Centers for Disease Control and Prevention, 2010).

The causes of TBI are varied. Falls are the most common cause (35.2%). Among all age groups, motor vehicle traffic crashes were the second leading cause of TBI (17.3%). Other causes include assaults and "struck by/against" events that include colliding with moving or stationary objects (Centers for Disease Control and Prevention, 2010; Hux, 2011).

As people with TBI recover, they usually progress through a continuum of care that begins in a trauma unit and may include time in a variety of different living situations. Fager (2003) described the experiences of a 36-year-old man who relies on AAC technology to communicate all messages except a few greetings. In the 15 years since his TBI, he has lived in 11 different settings including an acute care hospital, a rehabilitation center, an assisted living center, his parents' home, and an independent living situation with attendant care. He has successfully used AAC strategies in each of these settings. However, not all individuals with TBI have adequate support to use AAC technologies consistently. Fager, Hux, Karantounis, and Beukelman (2004) documented long-term AAC use patterns by 25 people with TBI and reported that two of these individuals discontinued use of their AAC systems because they did not receive adequate support and/or AAC facilitators in their living situations. The facilitator support received by people with TBI who successfully use AAC is often extensive. Thus, intervention efforts must focus on facilitator training as these individuals transition through the multiple living situations that they are likely to experience.

Cognitive/Linguistic and Communication Disorders

Several categorical scales have been developed in an effort to describe people with severe TBI. The Rancho Levels of Cognitive Functioning Scale (Hagen, 1984), which describes cognitive and associated language behaviors that occur during recovery, is presented in Table 17.1. AAC teams use scales such as this to design AAC and other interventions appropriate to each stage.

In general, the communication disorders associated with TBI are the result of impairments in three areas. First, some of the language characteristics of people with TBI are a consequence of cognitive impairments, as summarized in Table 17.1. The level of linguistic performance can vary depending on the individual's cognitive level. Second, language disorders may occur because of damage to specific language processing areas of the brain. Sarno, Buonaguro, and Levita (1986) evaluated 125 individuals with TBI using the Battery of Language Test and reported that 29% of these individuals exhibited classic symptoms associated with acquired aphasia. An additional 36% exhibited subclinical aphasia, which the researchers defined as "linguistic processing deficits on testing in the absence of clinical manifestations of linguistic impairment" (p. 404).

Third, some communication disorders in TBI are caused by damage to the motor control networks and pathways of the brain that occurred at the time of injury. Dysarthria has often been reported as one of the long-term sequelae of TBI. Oliver, Ponford, and Curren (1996) reported that motor speech disorders were present in 34% of their sample 5 years after injury. Yorkston, Honsinger, Mitsuda, and Hammen (1989) surveyed 151 people following TBI and found that prevalence changed as a function of time after onset. Of those in acute rehabilitation, 45% reported mild to moderate dysarthria and 20% reported severe dysarthria. In outpatient settings, 12% demonstrated mild to moderate dysarthria and 10% demonstrated severe dysarthria. For children, Ylvisaker (1986) reported that 10% of children and 8% of adolescents continued to produce unintelligible speech during follow-up studies. Several different types of dysarthria have been observed following TBI, including ataxic, flaccid, spastic, and combinations (Yorkston, Beukelman, Strand, & Bell, 1999).

"[Judy] tried to talk several times during the day. Much of it sounded unintelligible, but occasionally we heard a 'Where am I?' or other words we could understand. We could not tell if she knew us, or understood anything we said. Then a few days later….Judy started trying to answer.…We spent the rest of the day hanging over her bed admiring her, as you might hang over the crib of a newborn baby.…The next day she responded less. This turned out to be a pattern. Nearly every day on which she showed definite improvement was followed by one of passivity or even apparent regression. It kept us on an emotional roller coaster" (D. Thatch, recounting the first few days in the hospital after her daughter Judy's severe TBI, in Weiss, Thatch, & Thatch, 1987, p. 17).

Recovery from Severe Communication Disorders

Communication disorders of individuals with TBI can change dramatically over the course of their recovery. Limited longitudinal research describes the patterns of these changes; however, some authors have provided insight about the course of recovery.

Ladtkow and Culp (1992) followed 138 people with TBI over an 18-month period. They reported that 29 of these individuals (21%) were judged unable to speak at some point in their recovery. Of these 29, 16 individuals (55%) regained functional speech

Table 17.1.   Levels of cognitive functioning and associated language behaviors

General behaviors	Language behaviors
I. No response	
Patient appears to be in a deep sleep and is completely unresponsive to any stimuli.	Receptive and expressive: No evidence of processing or verbal or gestural expression.
II. Generalized response	
Patient reacts inconsistently and non-purposefully to stimuli in a nonspecific manner. Responses are limited and often the same, regardless of stimulus presented. Responses may be physiologic changes, gross body movements, or vocalization.	Receptive and expressive: No evidence of processing or verbal or gestural expression.
III. Localized response	
Patient reacts specifically, but inconsistently, to stimuli. Responses are directly related to the type of stimulus presented. May follow simple commands such as "Close your eyes" or "Squeeze my hand" in an inconsistent, delayed manner.	Language begins to emerge. Receptively: Patient progresses from localizing to processing and following simple commands that elicit automatic responses in a delayed and inconsistent manner. Limited reading emerges. Expressively: Automatic verbal and gestural responses emerge in response to direct elicitation. Negative head nods emerge before positive head nods. Utterances are single words serving as "holophrastic" responses.
IV. Confused-agitated	
Behavior is bizarre and nonpurposeful relative to immediate environment. Does not discriminate among persons or objects; is unable to cooperate directly with treatment efforts; verbalizations are frequently incoherent or inappropriate to the environment; confabulation may be present. Gross attention to environment is very short, and selective attention is often nonexistent. Patient lacks short-term recall.	Severe disruption of frontal–temporal lobes, with the resultant confusion apparent. Receptively: Marked disruption in auditory and visual processing, including inability to order phonemic events, monitor rate, and attend to, retain, categorize, and associate stimuli. Disinhibition interferes with comprehension and ability to inhibit responses to self-generated mental activity. Expressively: Marked disruption of phonologic, semantic, syntactic, and suprasegmental features. Output is bizarre, unrelated to environment, and incoherent. Literal, verbal, and neologistic paraphasias appear with disturbance of logico-sequential features and incompleteness of thought. Monitoring of pitch, rate, intensity, and suprasegmentals is severely impaired.
V. Confused, inappropriate, nonagitated	
Patient is able to respond to simple commands fairly consistently. However, with increased complexity of commands or lack of any external structure, responses are nonpurposeful, random, or fragmented. Has gross attention to the environment but is highly distractible and lacks ability to focus attention on a specific task; with structure, may be able to converse on a social-automatic level for short periods; verbalization is often inappropriate and confabulatory; memory is severely impaired; often shows inappropriate use of subjects; individual may perform previously learned tasks with structure but is unable to learn new information.	Linguistic fluctuations are in accordance with the degree of external structure and familiarity-predictability of linguistic events. Receptively: Processing has improved, with increased ability to retain temporal order of phonemic events, but semantic and syntactic confusions persist. Only phrases or short sentences are retained. Rate, accuracy, and quality remain significantly reduced. Expressively: Persistence of phonologic, semantic, syntactic and prosodic processes. Disturbances in logicosequential features result in irrelevances, incompleteness, tangents, circumlocutions, and confabulations. Literal paraphasias subside, while neologisms and verbal paraphasias continue. Utterances may be expansive or telegraphic, depending on inhibition–disinhibition factors. Responses are stimulus bound. Word retrieval deficits are characterized by delays, generalizations, descriptions, semantic associations, or circumlocutions. Disruptions in syntactic features are present beyond concrete levels of expression or with increased length of output. Written output is severely limited. Gestures are incomplete.

General behaviors	Language behaviors
VI. Confused-appropriate	
Patient shows goal-directed behavior but depends on external input for direction; follows simple directions consistently and shows carryover for relearned tasks with little or no carryover for new tasks; responses may be incorrect due to memory problems but appropriate to the situation; past memories show more depth and detail than recent memory.	Receptively: Processing remains delayed, with difficulty in retaining, analyzing, and synthesizing. Auditory processing is present for compound sentences, while reading comprehension is present for simple sentences. Self-monitoring capacity emerges. Expressively: Internal confusion-disorganization is reflected in expression, but appropriateness is maintained. Language is confused relative to impaired new learning and displaced temporal and situational contexts, but confabulation is no longer present. Social–automatic conversation is intact but remains stimulus bound. Tangential and irrelevant responses are present only in open-ended situations requiring referential language. Neologisms are extinguished, with literal paraphasias present only in conjunction with an apraxia. Word retrieval errors occur in conversation but seldom in confrontation naming. Length of utterance reflects inhibitory–initiation mechanisms. Written and gestural expression increases. Prosodic features reflect the "voice of confusion," characterized by monopitch, monostress, and monoloudness.
VII. Automatic-appropriate	
Patient appears appropriate and oriented within hospital and home settings, goes through daily routine automatically, but is frequently robotlike with minimal-to-absent confusion; has shallow recall of activities; shows carryover for new learning but at a decreased rate; with structure, is able to initiate social or recreational activities; judgment remains impaired.	Linguistic behaviors appear "normal" within familiar, predictable, structured settings, but deficits emerge in open-ended communication and less structured settings. Receptively: Reductions persist in auditory processing and reading comprehension relative to length, complexity, and presence of competing stimuli. Retention has improved to short paragraphs but without the abilities to identify salient features, organize, integrate input, order, and retain detail. Expressively: Automatic level of language is apparent in referential communication. Reasoning is concrete and self-oriented. Expression becomes tangential and irrelevant when abstract linguistic concepts are attempted. Word retrieval errors are minimal. Length of utterance and gestures approximately normal. Writing is disorganized and simple at a paragraph level. Prosodic features may remain aberrant. Pragmatic features of ritualizing and referencing are present, while other components remain disrupted.
VIII. Purposeful and appropriate	
Patient is able to recall and integrate past and recent events and is aware of and responsive to the environment, shows carryover for new learning and needs no supervision once activities are learned; may continue to show a decreased ability relative to premorbid abilities in language, abstract reasoning, tolerance for stress, and judgment in emergencies or unusual circumstances.	Language capacities may fall within normal limits. Otherwise, problems persist in competitive situations and in response to fatigue, stress, and emotionality, characterized in reduced effectiveness, efficiency, and quality of performance. Receptively: Rate of processing remains reduced but unremarkable on testing. Retention span remains limited at paragraph level but improved with use of retrieval—organization strategies. Analysis, organization, and integration are reduced in rate and quality. Expressively: Syntactic and semantic features fall within normal limits, while verbal reasoning and abstraction remain reduced. Written expression may fall below premorbid level. Prosodic features are essentially normal. Pragmatic features of referencing, presuppositions, topic maintenance, turn taking, and use of paralinguistic features in context remain impaired.

From Hagen, C. (1984). Language Disorders in Head Trauma *Note.* From *Language Disorders in Adults* (pp. 257-258), by A. Holland (Ed.), 1984, Austin, TX: PRO-ED. Copyright 1984 by PRO-ED, Inc. Reprinted with permission.

during the middle stage of recovery (i.e., Rancho Levels of Cognitive Functioning IV and V in Table 17.1). Thirteen individuals (45%) did not regain functional speech; unfortunately, the description of the cognitive recovery of those who did not regain functional speech is incomplete. The authors merely indicated that only three people (10%) reached the late stage of recovery, corresponding to Levels VI, VII, and VIII.

In a similar study, Dongilli, Hakel, and Beukelman (1992) investigated the recovery of 27 people who were unable to speak on admission to inpatient rehabilitation following TBI. Of these, 16 individuals (59%) became functional natural speakers during inpatient rehabilitation, whereas the other 11 (41%) did not. All individuals who became functional speakers did so at Rancho Level of Cognitive Functioning V or VI (see Table 17.1). Of the 11 individuals who left inpatient rehabilitation unable to speak, one achieved functional natural speech almost 24 months post injury, and another was making substantial progress toward becoming a functional speaker 48 months post injury.

As the Dongilli et al. (1992) study shows, people with TBI may experience severe communication disorders for cognitive as well as motor-related reasons. Jordan and Murdoch (1990) described a 7-year-old girl who was mute for 10 months subsequent to coma. Following her mutism, the girl demonstrated rapid and unexpected recovery of functional communication skills, although she continued to experience higher-level language impairments. In a 4-year follow-up report, her speech intelligibility was within normal limits, and she exhibited improvements in her cognitive/linguistic abilities (Jordan & Murdoch, 1994).

Adding to this limited information base regarding recovery from communication disorders are two interesting case studies. In one, Workinger and Netsell (1988) described a man who recovered intelligible speech 13 years after injury and used various AAC systems during the intervening years. In addition, Light et al. (1988) described the transitions of an adolescent girl with TBI through approximately 3 years of multiple AAC systems before she became a functional natural speaker. Enderby and Crow (1990), who followed four people with severe bulbar dysfunction due to TBI, reported similar outcomes. They reported that although the individuals made few gains within the first 18 months after injury, they made substantial improvements as much as 48 months post injury.

During the past decade the medical treatment for TBI has changed considerably. Swelling of the brain and pressure on the brain from being enclosed in the skull have been reduced through medications and opening of the skull to relieve pressure. For example, removing sections of the skull (called a bone flap) soon after TBI allows the brain to swell outside of the confines of the skull. Once swelling has subsided and the individual is medically stable, the bone flap is typically replaced. Therefore, the authors are seeing fewer and fewer individuals with TBI who, while retaining or regaining considerable cognitive function, experience severe speech limitations because of damage to the brainstem due to the interruption of blood flow in the brainstem. Rather, many TBI patients with sustained inability to communicate using their natural speech often also experience considerable cognitive limitations. The multiple capability limitations of these individuals must be considered when selecting AAC options for them.

NATURAL-ABILITY INTERVENTIONS RELATED TO SPEECH

As noted in the previous discussion, some individuals with TBI recover natural speech following injury, whereas others do not. Predicting the path of natural speech recovery for individuals with TBI is difficult. Therefore, individuals who experience TBI, their families, and their rehabilitation teams must address natural speech recovery on an individual basis.

Some individuals may be able to produce a number of intelligible words, although they may not develop completely functional speech in all situations. Family members, friends, and team members should encourage the use and improvement of these words if they allow the individuals to manage certain aspects of communication interactions. Others with dysarthria following TBI can say many words, but their words are unintelligible because of impaired motor control. They may use AAC techniques to augment the intelligibility of their natural speech. In fact, most individuals with TBI use multiple modes of communication at every stage of recovery. Rehabilitation that emphasizes reestablishing natural speech only or using AAC only may not meet all the communication needs of a person with TBI.

Topic Supplementation

If a person's speech is marginally intelligible, his or her message can often be understood if the listener is aware of the semantic context or topic. Communication boards containing lists of frequently occurring topics can be used to establish context at the beginning of an interaction or to resolve communication breakdowns. Hanson, Yorkston, and Beukelman (2004) reviewed the literature on topic supplementation for speakers with various types of dysarthria. They reported that topic supplementation increased word intelligibility by an average of 28% and sentence intelligibility by 10.7%. Use of topic supplementation should be considered after assessment with the technique documents that 1) the individual with TBI can learn to implement it in conversational interactions and 2) the technique has a positive impact on speech intelligibility. In a study involving only individuals with TBI, Beukelman, Fager, Ullman, Hanson, and Logemann (2002) reported intelligibility gains of more than 50% for some speakers and as low as 2.4% for others.

Alphabet Supplementation

Beukelman and Yorkston (1977) reported that a supplemented speech strategy substantially improved the speech intelligibility of speakers with dysarthria. In alphabet supplementation, the speaker identifies the first letter of each word on an alphabet board or other type of AAC display while saying the word. This procedure provides listeners with information that allows them to restrict their word retrieval to words that begin with the letter indicated. In the same study, Beukelman and Yorkston described the impact of alphabet supplementation on the speech of a young man who had sustained TBI. His habitual sentence intelligibility was 33%, compared with 66% when he used alphabet supplementation. Hanson et al. (2004) reported that, across speakers with various types of dysarthria, alphabet supplementation increased sentence intelligibility by 25.5% and single-word intelligibility by 10%. Use of alphabet supplementation should be considered if an assessment confirms that 1) the individual with TBI can learn to implement it in conversational interactions and 2) the technique has a positive impact on speech intelligibility. In a study involving only people with TBI, Beukelman et al. (2002) reported intelligibility gains of up to 69% for some speakers (see Figure 17.1).

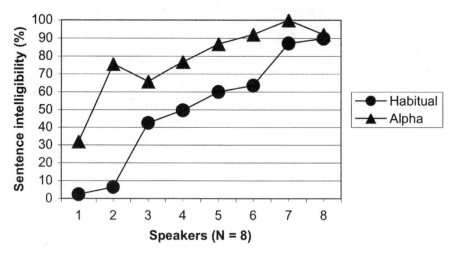

Figure 17.1. Habitual and alphabet-supplemented speech intelligibility for eight speakers with dysarthria due to traumatic brain injury. (*Source:* Beukelman & Fager et al., 2002.)

Portable Voice Amplification

Some people with dysarthria following TBI speak so quietly that their speech is difficult to hear, especially in groups of people or in noisy environments. These individuals may find it useful to increase the loudness of their speech with a portable speech amplifier (see Chapter 14 for a more extensive discussion of this approach).

AUGMENTATIVE AND ALTERNATIVE COMMUNICATION ACCEPTANCE AND USE PATTERNS

Outcome studies have described AAC recommendations for individuals with TBI. DeRuyter and Lafontaine (1987) collected data on 63 individuals who were referred to the Non-oral Center at Rancho Los Amigos Medical Center for AAC assessment. AAC recommendations included communication boards ($n = 37$); simple systems other than communication boards, such as yes/no systems, gestures, or writing ($n = 11$); dedicated communication devices ($n = 12$); and no communication system ($n = 3$).

Fager et al. (2004) described the AAC acceptance and use patterns of 25 individuals with TBI. Following AAC assessment, 17 high-tech and 8 low-tech AAC systems were recommended. Fifteen of the seventeen individuals for whom high-tech AAC was recommended received AAC technology. One individual rejected the recommendation, and one did not receive an AAC device due to funding constraints. Thirteen of the fifteen individuals who received a high-tech AAC device continued to use their devices for an extended period of time, for an overall acceptance rate of 87%. Two individuals discontinued use of their high-tech AAC systems due to loss of ongoing facilitator support. All individuals for whom low-tech AAC was recommended accepted the recommendation. Three of these individuals discontinued use of their systems due to recovery of natural speech. These individuals formulated their messages primarily through letter-by-letter spelling, unless they experienced a preexisting language disorder. Few used encoding strategies. Only one used alpha encoding extensively.

ACCESS ASSESSMENT AND INTERVENTION

AAC teams should base their intervention approaches with people who have TBI on individual levels of cognitive recovery (DeRuyter & Kennedy, 1991; Fager et al., 2007; Fager & Karantounis, 2011; Ladtkow & Culp, 1992). AAC approaches have been described for three general stages of recovery: 1) the early stage, which involves Rancho Levels of Cognitive Functioning I, II, and III (see Table 17.1); 2) the middle stage, which includes Levels IV and V; and 3) the late stage, which includes Levels VI, VII, and VIII.

Early Stage (Rancho Levels of Cognitive Functioning I, II, and III)

Assessment

It is almost impossible in the early stage of recovery to assess cognitive, language, or motor control capabilities because the individual may be unable to stay awake or pay attention for any significant amount of time. Thus, at this stage AAC teams attempt very little formal assessment. Instead, team members document systematic observations to identify changes in the individual's response patterns and to identify functional movements that the individual may use in a subsequent AAC program. Family members, friends, and other communication partners can also observe and chart such information if they spend a large amount of time with the individual. Because they know the person well, they are in a good position to document changes and responses. Form 5.1 in Beukelman, Garrett, and Yorkston (2007) provides a strategy to document response modes and consistency (Fager et al., 2007).

As individuals with TBI become more alert, they gradually become able to differentiate between two or more people or objects. This is a positive sign because it is often a precursor to the development of a yes/no response. The response mode for differentiation varies from person to person and may include eye pointing, moving a body part, or activating a beeper. The stimuli to which people recovering from TBI are able to respond must be presented in a careful and controlled manner. Family members and communication partners can usually be trained in this approach. They can also provide information about the interests and preinjury activities of the individual with TBI so that medical and rehabilitation personnel can provide the person with interesting and meaningful stimulation.

Augmentative and Alternative Communication Intervention

During the early stages of recovery, people with TBI are unable to speak functionally because of cognitive impairments. Some people may have language or motor control impairments that further contribute to their communication disorder. Fager et al. (2007) suggest that the goals of AAC in the early stages of recovery are to increase the consistency of responses and to shape these responses into meaningful communication. Form 5.2 in Beukelman, Garrett, and Yorkston (2007) provides instructions on various ways of shaping responses.

AAC techniques used at this point vary considerably depending on the individual's overall neurological involvement. For example, consider the individual who is functioning in the range of Rancho Levels of Cognitive Functioning I to III and who also has considerable motor control impairment. This individual might be unable to respond to stimuli consistently not only because of cognitive problems but also because of motor weakness, spasticity, or lack of coordination. An AAC intervention for such a person might provide an alternative access mode, such as a single switch (Garrett,

Schutz-Muehling, & Morrow, 1990). Then, as the individual begins to respond to various stimuli by making purposeful movements, facilitators can encourage contingency awareness or cause and effect (Lancioni, Bosco, et al., 2010; Lancioni, Singh, O'Reilly, Sigafoos, Oliva, et al., 2010; Lancioni, Singh, O'Reilly, Sigafoos, Signorino, et al., 2010). For example, facilitators might encourage the individual to operate a CD/DVD player or an mp3 player with a single switch to play favorite music, listen to recorded messages from family members or friends, or play short video clips of personal relevance. In addition, a single switch with a control unit can be used to activate electrical appliances such as fans, radios, and lamps. As the individual becomes more purposeful, he or she may activate single-message communication technology containing basic greetings and other social phrases with a single switch (see Chapter 10 for additional suggestions). Then, if motor control permits, facilitators can connect two or more switches to different audio devices so that the individual can choose among different musical selections, messages, or videos. During the early stage of recovery, a limited number of symbols (e.g., one to four) might represent choices. Symbols should be brightly colored or exaggerated (Fried-Oken & Doyle, 1992). AAC teams should take care to understand the visual capabilities of individuals following TBI because impairments can range from double vision to cortical blindness. Stimuli (e.g., music, voices, video, pictures) should be motivating and personally relevant. Family members and friends can provide guidance in the development of these stimulus options.

Keenan and Barnhart (1993) documented the return of yes/no responses in 82 individuals with severe TBI: 49% signaled yes/no with head nods, 26% with motor responses of upper and lower extremities, 15% with eye gaze, and 9% with speech. Individuals with primarily cognitive or hemiplegic impairments developed yes/no responses earlier than those with flexor withdrawal or high or low muscle tone. Twenty-nine percent of the individuals regained yes/no responses within 3 months of onset; 66%, within 6 months; and 84%, within 9 months.

Middle Stage (Rancho Levels of Cognitive Functioning IV and V)

In the middle stage of recovery, the individual may respond consistently to stimuli while still showing evidence of considerable performance and communication impairments due to attention and memory impairments. Individuals who do not have specific language impairments or severe motor control impairments usually begin to speak functionally during these stages, although they may produce somewhat confused messages (Dongilli et al., 1992; Ladtkow & Culp, 1992). In addition, people with TBI generally begin to indicate their basic needs at this point. These may include comfort messages related to being hot, cold, hurt, or hungry. Individuals may also be able to communicate messages related to their location, the time of day, and other personal information. Family members and friends can assist with the selection of topics that are particularly important to people in the middle stage of recovery.

Early in the middle stage of recovery, people with TBI often experience agitation and poor awareness of their communication deficits. Therefore, they may initially have difficulty accepting AAC interventions. This may be reflected in limited willingness to participate in some aspects of AAC assessment.

Assessment

The aim of assessment in the middle stage is to identify residual capabilities that the individual with TBI can utilize to achieve the specific communication goals mentioned previously. Examples are provided by Fager et al. (2007); see Form 5.6 in Beukelman, Garrett, and Yorkston (2007). Most of the procedures for this assessment are nonstandardized and informal. The initial assessment often focuses on seating and postural issues, which team members should coordinate with AAC concerns. Proper seating and positioning help to minimize reflex activity, excessive tone, and other movements that may interfere with verbal communication or AAC system usage (DeRuyter & Kennedy, 1991). Specifically, "the overall seating and positioning goals during [this] stage should be to provide for a structurally appropriate and functional position in which minimal or no pain is encountered" (DeRuyter & Kennedy, 1991, p. 342).

The AAC-RERC (Rehabilitation Engineering Research Center on Communication Enhancement) webcast *Seating and Positioning for Individuals Who Use AT* by Aileen Costigan discusses seating and positioning for individuals who use AAC.

Assessment of motor control capability is important to determine the individual's direct selection or scanning options. As discussed in Chapter 7, assessors should consider various access sites in terms of accuracy, efficiency, reliability, and endurance. A survey form by Fager et al. (2007) is provided as Form 5.8 in Beukelman, Garrett, and Yorkston (2007). This assessment may be difficult in some cases because people with TBI may require orthopedic surgical procedures that interfere, either temporarily or permanently, with their ability to use specific motor access sites (DeRuyter & Kennedy, 1991). Thus, it is important for AAC specialists to coordinate communication interventions with medical procedures by working closely with the medical team responsible for the individual's overall care. Assessment should also focus on the memory and attention capabilities of people with TBI. Complex scanning patterns (row–column or group–item) may be too demanding, so AAC teams should limit the individual's early scanning experiences to circular or linear scanning.

People with TBI often experience visual-perceptual and visual acuity disturbances, and these should also be considered in AAC assessment. At lower cognitive levels, assessors can usually determine visual functioning by observing the individual's ocular response to threat, gross focus movements of the eyes, and ability to follow a bright object or familiar face (DeRuyter & Kennedy, 1991). At higher cognitive levels, many visual disturbances can be detected through standard ophthalmologic examinations. A member of the AAC team should accompany the individual to such assessments to encourage the examiner to consider AAC-related issues, such as the optimal size for symbols and the array and the optimal distance between the individual and the display.

Augmentative and Alternative Communication Intervention

Depending on the nature of the brain injury, AAC teams should choose one or two major communication goals for the middle stage of recovery. The goal may be to help the person compensate for attention and memory impairments. This is particularly relevant for individuals with TBI who begin to speak during this stage because they often need communication techniques to help them remember, for example, the names of important people and their schedule of activities. A second goal of intervention in the middle stage applies specifically to individuals who have sustained damage to language or motor control areas of the brain. These individuals probably will not develop natural speech at this point in their recovery. Thus, AAC interventions should seek to provide these individuals with techniques that support conversational interaction. In Levels IV and V, messages that relate to wants, needs, and information sharing are more important to most individuals than messages that support social closeness and social etiquette (DeRuyter & Kennedy, 1991).

Most AAC interventions during the middle stage of recovery are either with nonelectronic (i.e., alphabet boards, pictures, word boards, yes/no techniques, and partner-assisted scanning) or with a single or limited number of simple displays on a speech-generating device. In an effort to reduce the complexity of communication, AAC teams may elect to use context-specific activity displays at this stage. For example, specific boards might facilitate participation in cognitive rehabilitation activities, recreational events, or daily living routines. Depending on the linguistic capabilities of the individual, photographs, line drawings, or printed words and phrases may symbolize the messages on the activity displays. Interventionists should remember that people in this stage of recovery may experience difficulty visually discriminating similar symbols or symbols with several elements. Individuals might use alphabetic displays, but encoding is almost always too difficult at this stage of recovery (Fried-Oken & Doyle, 1992). To control the complexity of the AAC system, teams may choose small activity displays with specific content, rather than large, complex boards containing multiple areas of content. For individuals with extensive attention and memory limitations, interventionists might consider written choice strategies (see Chapter 15). During the middle stage, the individual might also use single switches to activate call buzzers or appliances or to run CD/DVD or mp3 players. Depending on the physical capabilities of the individual, such switch control activities may serve as training for the operation of a long-term environmental control device.

Communication partners play an important role in structuring communication interactions during the middle stage. Fager et al. (2007) provided strategies to support communication (see Form 5.10 in Beukelman, Garrett, & Yorkston, 2007). For example, partners may need to introduce topics for conversation, suggest the augmentative mode that can be used most productively at a particular time, assist with resolving communication breakdowns, and create motivating communication opportunities. Communication partners should actively help to structure interactions, but they should also be very patient and allow ample time for people with TBI to prepare, clarify, and repair their messages. Perhaps one of the most common partner errors is to rush or offer excessive encouragement during this stage by making multiple suggestions of how to formulate or complete a message. This can be very distracting and frustrating to the individual with TBI, who must concentrate very hard in order to think, plan, compose, and finally produce a communicative utterance. At times, partners will also need to learn to provide systematic cuing in order for the person in the middle stage to use his or her communication system effectively. In time, individuals with TBI should attempt to phase out partner cuing.

DeRuyter and Donoghue (1989) described in detail the AAC interventions over a 28-week period for a man who was unable to speak functionally due to TBI. During the first weeks of intervention (8 months post injury), he established a reliable yes/no response by nodding his head, and he began to learn the visual-perceptual and upper-extremity skills necessary for eventual use of a communication board. In addition, his AAC team initiated interventions designed to encourage the development of natural speech during this time. By the 10th week of intervention, he was able to use a simple alphabet board with approximately 2-inch letters. Initially, he exhibited "extreme frustration" (p. 52) with the board because of his motor planning deficits. By the 26th week of intervention, however, this man exhibited "no hesitation in using his alphabet board when he was unable to communicate effectively verbally or gesturally" (p. 53). His team introduced electronic AAC technology with voice output. With very little training on the device, he was able to communicate at a rate of up to eight words per minute. At the time of his discharge from the inpatient rehabilitation facility, he communicated via limited speech, a sophisticated gesturing system, an alphabet board, and an AAC device with an expanded membrane keyboard.

Late Stage (Rancho Levels of Cognitive Functioning VI, VII, and VIII)

By the late stage of recovery, most individuals have regained the cognitive capability to become natural speakers, and those who remain unable to speak usually experience severe specific language or motor control disorders.

Assessment

AAC teams can implement the Participation Model (see Figure 5.1) for effective assessment and intervention planning in the late stage of recovery. Analysis of the participation patterns of individuals with TBI and their families forms a particularly important part of this process. When people with TBI move from acute rehabilitation to outpatient rehabilitation, to independent living, and to employment, their patterns and expectations of participation change dramatically. These expectations greatly affect the nature and extent of their communication needs. It is also important to assess opportunity barriers, in much the same manner as is discussed in Chapter 5. For people with TBI in late-stage recovery, AAC teams often identify communication needs, assess specific capabilities and constraints, and match these to AAC technology interventions (DeRuyter & Kennedy, 1991; Ladtkow & Culp, 1992).

Augmentative and Alternative Communication Intervention

In the late stage of recovery, individuals with TBI are generally oriented and able to demonstrate goal-directed, socially appropriate behavior. However, they may still have difficulties learning new information due to residual cognitive impairments. Some individuals may become natural speakers during Level VI, but by Levels VII and VIII, most individuals who are likely to become natural speakers without extensive intervention have already done so (Dongilli et al., 1992). Thus, by the late stage of recovery, many people with TBI can interact and converse with their families and friends through natural speech. Nevertheless, even those individuals who regain speech may require augmented writing systems for an extended period. In addition, people with residual language and motor control impairments will continue to require long-term communication systems to meet their specific interaction needs. Individuals have many interaction needs at this point, including those related to communicating wants and needs, sharing information, achieving social closeness, and participating in social routines (DeRuyter & Kennedy, 1991).

During the late stage of cognitive recovery, traditional AAC techniques that resemble those used with other individuals who experience physical and cognitive impairments are often appropriate. Although people with TBI who cannot speak usually experience a high incidence of physical problems, one study found that approximately 78% were able to successfully utilize direct selection AAC techniques (DeRuyter & Lafontaine, 1987). Almost 75% of the individuals who used direct selection in DeRuyter and Lafontaine's database operated their technology with their fingers or hands, whereas the remainder used eye pointing, headlight pointing, or chin pointing; 16% utilized partner-assisted and unassisted scanning, and the remainder used other or no AAC techniques.

As social support for health care and rehabilitation decreases in some countries, people with TBI are spending less and less time in intensive rehabilitation programs in which AAC services may be available. It is important that people with TBI and their families educate themselves early in the recovery process about available AAC services and how to gain access to such services when they are needed.

It might be assumed that because of the cognitive impairments associated with TBI, individuals with TBI will require AAC systems that contain pictorial or other non-orthographic symbols. However, this is often not the case. It is important to remember that even late in the recovery process, cognitive impairments may mask considerable residual skills. One of the most important skills that many people with TBI retain is the ability to read and spell. Thus, many individuals with TBI can utilize AAC systems that employ orthographic symbols, including letters, words, and sentences (Fager et al., 2004; Fried-Oken & Doyle, 1992). In fact in one review, Doyle, Kennedy, Jausalaitis, and Phillips (2000) reported that the majority of adults with TBI eventually are candidates for spelling-based systems. AAC teams should take care when introducing encoding strategies because some people, even in the late stage of recovery, may have difficulty learning and implementing these strategies efficiently (Beukelman, Fager, Ball, & Dietz, 2007). If coding strategies are used, they need to be relatively concrete rather than abstract (Doyle et al., 2000). Doyle et al. (2000) provided a summary of the impact of cognitive limitations on AAC interventions with TBI survivors.

Those who assist people with TBI during the recovery process may be well aware that new learning can be difficult and require considerable time and practice. This is an important consideration for individuals who require long-term communication systems because some AAC approaches require extensive training for operation. Examples of such methods are those that are technically complex to operate or that require the individual to learn a large number of messages using sequences of alphabetic or iconic codes. The AAC team should exercise caution when introducing such techniques and should be careful not to make frequent changes in a system once the individual has learned it.

QUESTIONS

17.1.   What communication problems are often associated with a severe TBI?

17.2.   If an individual is unable to speak following a severe TBI, how likely is it that the individual will recover functional natural speech?

17.3.   What is alphabet supplementation, and how does it affect speech intelligibility of a dysarthric speaker?

17.4.   What are the goals of the early stage of intervention following TBI?

17.5.   How do the goals of the early stage differ from the middle and late stages of intervention for individuals with TBI?

17.6.   How might the cognitive and learning problems experienced by some individuals with TBI interfere with AAC use?

Augmentative and Alternative Communication in Intensive, Acute, and Long-Term Acute Medical Settings

In 2010, the Joint Commission published *Advancing Effective Communication, Cultural Competence, and Patient- and Family-Centered Care: A Roadmap for Hospitals*, which states the following:

> No longer considered to be simply a patient's right, effective communication is now accepted as an essential component of quality care and patient safety [5,6]....Effective communication [is t]he successful joint establishment of meaning wherein patients and health care providers exchange information, enabling patients to participate actively in their care from admission through discharge, and ensuring that the responsibilities of both patients and providers are understood. To be truly effective, communication requires a two-way process (expressive and receptive) in which messages are negotiated until the information is correctly understood by both parties. Successful communication takes place only when providers understand and integrate the information gleaned from patients, and when patients comprehend accurate, timely, complete, and unambiguous message from providers in a way that enables them to participate responsibly in their care. (2010, p. 1)

Acute medical units, intensive care units (ICUs), and long-term acute medical care hospital (LTACH) units serve a wide range of individuals who are unable to communicate using natural speech, either temporarily or permanently. Such communication problems occur as a result of primary medical conditions, such as traumatic brain injury, stroke, myasthenia gravis, oral-laryngeal cancer, and Guillain-Barré syndrome, or as a side effect of interventions such as surgery, intubation, and/or tracheostomy. Because these individuals are under direct medical care, we will refer to them as *patients* in this chapter. Thirty-six percent of ICU patients require mechanical ventilation (Garrett, Happ, Costello, & Fried-Oken, 2007). Following a review of 30 outcome studies, Eskildsen (2007) reported that slightly more than a quarter of patients discharged from ICU into LTACH units required ventilator assistance to breathe, whereas 34% to 65% of patients, depending on the study, stopped requiring ventilator assistance while in the LTACH setting. For many individuals, knowledge of acute medical experiences is based on visits to friends or family in the hospital or on television documentaries. As a result, people often think that most individuals in these settings are passive regarding their own care and are "having things done to them." This perception logically leads to the belief that, because acutely ill patients are so ill and so passive, they do not need to communicate. This is not at all the case. Most people in acute medical settings need to communicate regularly with hospital staff, including nurses, assistants, doctors, respiratory therapists, and so forth in order to participate in their own medical and personal care, and they report an urgent need to communicate with family members at these uncertain and frightening times in their lives. Depending on the length of stay, it may also be necessary for them to communicate about family finances, the operation of a business, the care of dependent children, and other personal matters. When one considers the different patients served in acute medical as well as short- and long-term (LTACH) units, the need for augmentative and alternative communication (AAC) strategies to support a wide range of communication needs becomes apparent. This chapter is only an introduction to communication supports for these patients. Professionals who provide regular communication support in these environments are referred to 1) the chapter by Garrett et al. (2007), "AAC in the Intensive Care Unit," and 2) the book by Hurtig

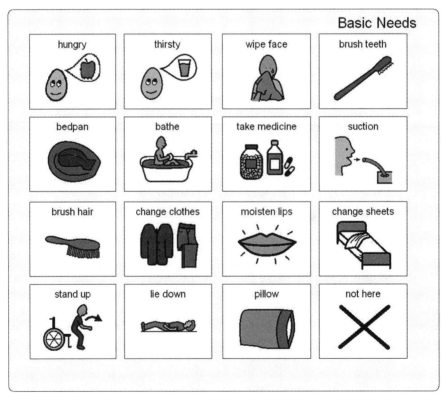

Figure 18.1. Communication board, basic needs. (From Hurtig, R., & Downey, D. [2009]. *Augmentative and alternative communication in acute and critical care settings.* San Diego: Plural; reprinted by permission. The Picture Communication Symbols ©1981–2012 by DynaVox Mayer-Johnson LLC. All Rights Reserved Worldwide. Used with permission.)

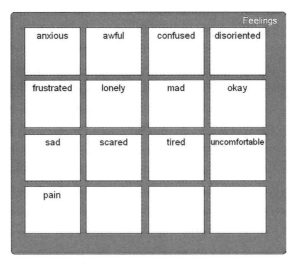

Figure 18.2. Communication board, feelings. (From Hurtig, R., & Downey, D. [2009]. *Augmentative and alternative communication in acute and critical care settings.* San Diego: Plural; reprinted by permission.)

and Downey (2009), *Augmentative and Alternative Communication in Acute and Critical Care Settings.* These authors provide CD-ROMs containing electronic files of low-tech AAC materials designed for use in acute medical settings. Examples of these communication support materials are provided in Figures 18.1 to 18.5.

For most people in acute medical settings who are unable to use their natural speech to communicate, and for their families, a severe communication impairment is a new and unfamiliar condition. Typically, they are unaware of AAC approaches. Other individuals—for example, those with progressive disorders such as amyotrophic lateral sclerosis—will have used AAC systems prior to entering the hospital, and both they and their families may be familiar with a wide range of AAC options. In either case, however, hospital staff are unlikely to be knowledgeable about the particular communication needs of the individual or the AAC strategies in use and will need to learn about these strategies rather quickly. ICU communication needs and a screening protocol are provided as Forms 2.1 and 2.2 in Beukelman, Garrett, and Yorkston (2007).

"It [AAC] allowed him to vent his anger. Every time we would do a procedure he would say 'I hate you,' and 'This sucks,' and it would make him feel better. I was glad to hear it every time he pushed the buttons because at least he was clearly expressing how he felt, which makes him feel better" (the mother of a child in an ICU, in Costello, 2000).

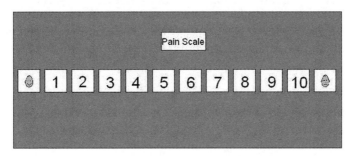

Figure 18.3. Communication board, pain scale. (From Hurtig, R., & Downey, D. [2009]. *Augmentative and alternative communication in acute and critical care settings.* San Diego: Plural; reprinted by permission. The Picture Communication Symbols ©1981–2012 by DynaVox Mayer-Johnson LLC. All Rights Reserved Worldwide. Used with permission.)

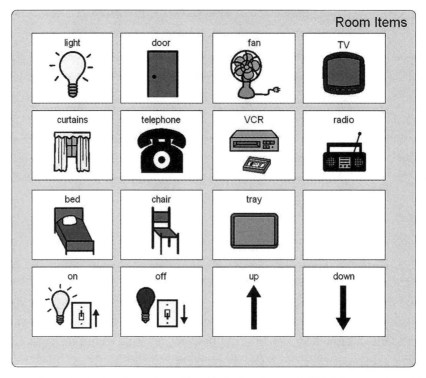

Figure 18.4.   Communication board, room items. (From Hurtig, R., & Downey, D. [2009]. *Augmentative and alternative communication in acute and critical care settings.* San Diego: Plural; reprinted by permission. The Picture Communication Symbols ©1981–2012 by DynaVox Mayer-Johnson LLC. All Rights Reserved Worldwide. Used with permission.)

Hurtig and Downey (2006) surveyed 135 nurses. One hundred percent reported that they were serving patients for whom communication was difficult. They further reported that 95% of them were serving patients who would benefit from AAC support, and 99% of the nurses reported that they had used AAC strategies with their patients.

CAUSES OF COMMUNICATION DISORDERS IN ACUTE MEDICAL SETTINGS

Communication disorders in acute medical settings can occur as a result of both primary causes (i.e., those directly related to an individual's illness or condition) and secondary causes (i.e., those related to an individual's need for temporary respiratory support). The primary neurological causes of complex communication needs are discussed throughout this book and will not be reviewed here. Patients with head and neck cancer typically require communication support during the days and weeks following surgical intervention. Some regain the use of natural speech in time, others supplement their residual natural speech with AAC strategies, and some rely extensively on low- or high-tech AAC strategies to meet their communication needs.

Individuals with a number of different medical conditions may require respiratory support, either temporarily or permanently. Such respiratory support often interferes with communication processes and a person's ability to speak. This is particularly true if endotracheal intubation or tracheostomy is required.

Endotracheal Intubation

An endotracheal tube (see Figure 18.6) is designed to transport air from a ventilator to an individual's respiratory system. Endotracheal tubes are usually passed in emergency situations through the person's mouth, pharynx, and larynx into the trachea (i.e., the airway below the larynx). Oral intubation interferes with communication in several ways. First, because the endotracheal tube passes through the oral cavity, it is impossible to articulate speech accurately. Second, because the endotracheal tube passes between the vocal folds, which are located in the larynx, it is impossible to produce sound (i.e., phonation). Thus, people who are orally intubated are unable to communicate using natural speech.

"When they put the tubes in, you get to the point of being helpless and you feel a need to communicate and talk to someone. You can't move. And you can't talk. And you want to say things. And you think, 'Now I'd like to ask some more questions. You explained to me what's going on. But no, I want to know more now. What's going to happen?' And all you can really do is just lay there. That's when you really, really get spooked the most" (Mike S., a 46-year-old man who had Guillain-Barré syndrome, in Fried-Oken, Howard, & Stewart, 1991, p. 43).

An endotracheal tube may also pass through the nasal cavity into the trachea. Although in this case the tube does not interfere with articulation as occurs when it passes through the mouth, the endotracheal tube does pass between the vocal folds. Therefore, an individual is still unable to produce vocal sounds, and efforts to communicate are limited to mouthing messages with the lips.

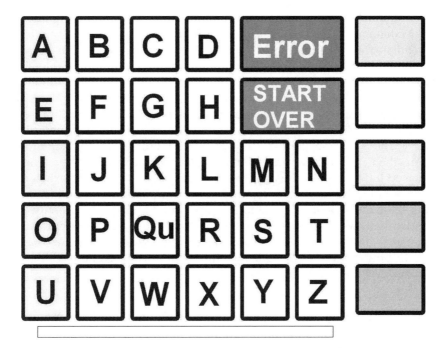

Figure 18.5.   Communication board, letters game. (From Hurtig, R., & Downey, D. [2009]. *Augmentative and alternative communication in acute and critical care settings.* San Diego: Plural; reprinted by permission.)

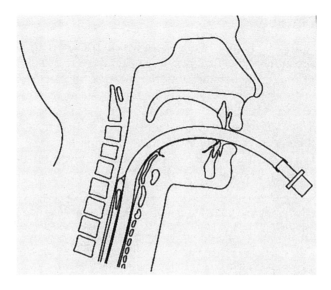

Figure 18.6.   Lateral view of an endotracheal tube.

Tracheostomy

A tracheostomy is another way to transport air from a ventilator to an individual's re-spiratory system. It is a surgical opening from the front wall of the lower neck into the trachea (i.e., the airway below the larynx). Tracheostomies are usually performed at the level of the second or third tracheal ring. Generally, the opening of the tracheostomy is maintained by inserting a tube or button through the neck wall into the trachea. As illustrated in Figure 18.7, the tracheostomy tube curves to extend down into the trachea to keep it open for the movement of air. The ventilator attaches to the portion of the tube that extends anterior to the neck. An individual with a tracheostomy tube who uses a ventilator often has limited natural speech because air passes from the ventilator through the tube, rather than through the oral cavity and past the vocal folds.

When the individual no longer needs ventilator support, tracheostomy tubes may remain in place to maintain an open airway or to permit suction of respiratory secretions. Nonetheless, air passes in and out of the trachea via the tracheostomy tube, bypassing the vocal folds. Thus, no phonation is possible, and messages must be mouthed. However, depending on the respiratory problem, some individuals who do not breathe with ventilator assistance are able to inhale through the tracheostomy tube, then occlude the tube with their fingers or an external valve and exhale through the larynx and the oral cavity. In this way, air moves past the vocal folds on exhala-tion, and these individuals are able to produce sound and speak naturally. In other cases, individuals who can breathe on their own may be fitted with a tracheal button that maintains the tracheostomy through the neck wall. These individuals can inhale through the button and then occlude the button with their finger or a valve to direct air past the vocal folds and produce speech.

AUGMENTATIVE AND ALTERNATIVE COMMUNICATION SERVICE DELIVERY IN ACUTE MEDICAL SETTINGS

"[His] messages were short but effective....I remember some of them clearly: Where am I, When, What happened, Move me up/down, Bedpan, More pillow, Get Nurse.... It was clear that the perceptions of others were influenced by his communication performance....The portable typewriter [Lightwriter] with voice output was essential in changing the way people talked to Barry and asked him questions" (Melanie Fried-Oken, 2001, writing about her husband's use of AAC in an ICU following a severe bicycling accident, in Fried-Oken, 2001, p. 139).

Because acute medical settings are so organizationally complex, on-site professionals usually provide the most effective ongoing AAC services. It is much more difficult for a consultant to come intermittently to a hospital to provide AAC services because the individual who requires the services may be unavailable, too ill, resting, or receiving other medical treatments that take priority at the time of the consultant's visit. The core AAC team generally includes a speech-language pathologist, a nurse, and, depending on the patient, a physical therapist or an occupational therapist. In addition to their roles on the AAC team for a particular patient, these professionals also may be responsible for other care and therapy needs of these individuals. They may consult with personnel from a regional AAC center or with a local AAC specialist.

The delivery of AAC services in acute medical settings is structured differently from delivery of AAC services in typical rehabilitation or educational settings. A successful AAC program in any given setting must accommodate factors specific to the setting in order to be accepted and used by patients and medical personnel.

Patient Issues

Individuals in acute medical settings have serious medical needs that are critical to their survival. The delivery of AAC services simply cannot interfere with the delivery of medical care. Communication support services must be integrated into the overall care plan for the individual.

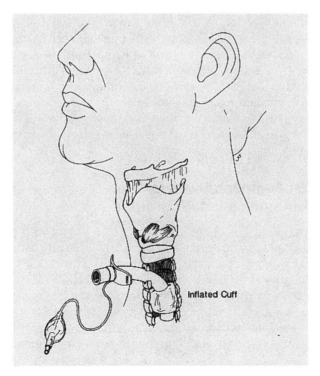

Inflated Cuff

Figure 18.7.   Lateral view of a cuffed tracheostomy tube with the cuff inflated.

The intensity of medical care affects the AAC program in a variety of ways. Medical staff are responsible for establishing and delivering an overall medical plan in which communication intervention plays an integral role. Thus, the AAC staff cannot provide services without a request or referral from the medical team. The AAC team members must clearly communicate the types of services they can deliver. They must consult with the medical team before and during AAC interventions to ensure that efforts coordinate well with and support the overall medical plan. If communication specialists do not follow these guidelines, they may fail to meet individuals' AAC needs.

Because individuals in acute medical settings receive such extensive medical support, it is common for as many as 10–25 different professionals as well as visiting family members and friends to have contact with each person during a 24-hour period. Thus, a variety of individuals must be able to understand AAC interventions. Signs on the walls, written messages, or verbal instructions must provide instructions for all these people. AAC interventions must be minimally complex and require minimal training and learning to be successful.

Medical Team Issues

Because nursing personnel are generally responsible for carrying out many day-to-day activities in the medical care plan, they have extensive contact with both individuals with complex communication needs and their family members. Thus, nurses are in an excellent position to assist the AAC team by monitoring an individual's status, coordinating AAC interventions with the medical care plan, documenting the individual's communication needs, and keeping family members informed of changes in the communication plan. The nursing coordinator often assumes the role of patient advocate during communication intervention and actively encourages physicians to request AAC services.

Respiratory therapists deal with a high proportion of the people in acute care units. These therapists are generally responsible for day-to-day management of individuals' respiratory status, including that of people with endotracheal or tracheostomy tubes. The AAC team must cooperate closely with respiratory therapists for successful intervention. Ongoing physician education is also important, especially in training hospitals in which the staff consists of interns and residents as well as senior medical personnel. The AAC team members may be invited to present their plan directly to the medical team. Instruction about AAC services, however, usually occurs in the context of ongoing service delivery.

Establishing an Augmentative and Alternative Communication Program

It is beyond the scope of this chapter to provide an extensive discussion regarding how to develop an AAC program in an intensive or acute care medical setting (see Costello, 2000; Garrett, et al., 2007; and Hurtig & Downey, 2009, for a detailed descriptions of this process). Garrett et al. (2007) noted that AAC teams should pay careful attention to individuals' equipment needs in acute care settings as well as to administrative, organizational, and personnel training issues. They suggested that the following equipment and materials form the basis for many AAC interventions in acute medical settings: 1) a lightweight neck-type electrolarynx (i.e., one that is positioned against the neck and vibrates the air column within the vocal tract); 2) an oral-type electrolarynx (i.e., one that delivers sound into the oral cavity through a tube); 3) materials to construct alphabet boards, word boards, and picture boards; 4) several magic slates (these are generally sold as toys and consist of a sheet of plastic over a piece of coated board that can be written on; when the plastic is lifted, written messages disappear); 5) very occasionally, a speech-generating device (SGD) with speech output for some individuals in LTACH units; and 6) a portable mounting system on wheels to hold cardboard message boards or eye-pointing displays. These minimal equipment needs reflect the previously stated philosophy of simplifying AAC interventions in this area and are echoed by Dowden, Beukelman, and Lossing:

> Clinicians with very few communication augmentation systems can nonetheless serve ICU patients quite well….The majority of our patients were served with electrolarynges or…modified natural speech approaches. With additional access to the least expensive communication systems (Plexiglas boards for eye-gaze,…paper and pencil, [and a few small text-to-speech typing systems]), we were able to serve all but a few of our patients. This means that even the smallest clinical program should consider serving patients in intensive care units. (1986, p. 43)

It is quite common for the AAC team to prepare a set of AAC materials for the ICU or acute care unit in the hospital so that the staff has access to these materials as needed. Garrett et al. (2007) provide a list of basic AAC-ICU equipment (see Table 18.1). More extensive electronic AAC devices may be necessary for people who remain in long-term acute care settings. Typically, this technology is purchased or rented by the patient depending upon financial support options, life expectancy, and anticipated course of the medical condition.

AUGMENTATIVE AND ALTERNATIVE COMMUNICATION INTERVENTION MODEL

Identify Participation Patterns and Communication Needs

The Participation Model (see Figure 5.1) supports the overall delivery of AAC services to people in acute care environments. Interventionists can expect restricted participation patterns because individuals are in essentially only one communication environment, have limited face-to-face contact with people in their social networks, and are not working. However, communication over a telephone remains an option for some, as does Internet communication in an increasing number of LTACH units (including electronic face-to-face communication at a distance).

> Olinda uses a ventilator to breathe as a result of amyotrophic lateral sclerosis (Fager & Beukelman, 2009). She communicates, reads, and controls her environment with an eye-tracking AAC technology. She e-mailed the AAC clinic and asked for help in learning how to use her technology to communicate using Skype (a face-to-face video calling application) so that she could communicate in a new way with her son and daughter-in-law who live across the country from her. Her daughter-in-law was pregnant, and Olinda wanted to be ready to see and interact with her first grandchild (Susan Fager, personal communication, October 2010).

Table 18.1.   Basic equipment list for augmentative and alternative communication (AAC) in intensive care units

Writing kits

- Spiral bound notebooks or brightly colored clipboards and tablets (look for clipboards that hook over the bed rails)
- Felt-tip pens
- Long strips of Velcro to attach pens (affix one end to clip, attach other to pen cap)
- Flexible pencil grips or orthotic writing aids
- Universal elastic cuff

Written choice communication notebooks

- Cover card
- Outline of U.S. map
- Preprinted scales

Communication boards

- Yes/no boards
- Needs/emotions boards
- Alphabet boards (various sizes)
- Symbol set(s) and posterboard for family-made communication boards

Partner-assisted scanning notebooks

- Cover sheet with instructions
- Topic list
- Message pages
- Alphabet page
- Eye-gaze communication board set
- Blank overlay
- Alphabet/number overlay
- Choice overlay
- Yes/no overlay
- Clear Plexiglas display board (optional)
- Erasable markers
- Adhesive notes for novel choices
- Metal rings to hold or store overlays
- Posterboard for encoded message chart display

Electrolarynx with oral adapter

- Select one with audible quality and volume control
- Select one with a relatively moistureproof housing and disposable oral tubes

Simple (digitized voice output) speech-generating devices (SGDs)

- Computer screen preferred versus paper displays
- Bright screen display preferred
- Sealed housing preferred, or purchase a waterproof "skin" for a specific device

Complex, multilevel SGDs with visual and auditory scanning capability

- Bright screen display
- Lightweight
- Durable
- Moistureproof screen
- Easy to program
- Handheld electronic spelling device or spelling-based AAC device

Switches (see Chapter 4)

- Large, medium, and small touch-plate switches
- Lever switches
- Light touch
- Piezoelectric and/or infrared switches
- Pillow switches
- Squeeze switches
- Sip-and-puff switches

Switch and device mounting equipment

Weighted poles for hanging low-tech and/or lightweight high-tech devices

Communication information posters

- Patient's signal chart
- Gesture dictionaries

Miscellaneous supplies

- Velcro
- Metal recloseable rings, various sizes
- Plastic page sleeves for communication boards and overlays
- Posterboard and markers
- Clear plastic mailing tape for affixing labels
- Ties for attaching items to IV poles, triangle pulls, or bed rails

John experienced chronic Guillain-Barré syndrome. Due to his respiratory needs, we assisted him while he was in the LTACH unit. His communication was limited in several ways. Using head-tracking AAC technology, John was able to interact with staff and family. To communicate at a distance, he used his AAC technology to speak on the telephone, but most distance communication with his family, friends, and a long-term, personal physician was by e-mail. He also used his head-tracking skills to access information from the Internet and to play electronic games.

Assess Opportunity Barriers and Supports

Individuals in acute medical settings deserve to have access to AAC services to meet their communication needs, and a lack of availability of AAC services can be considered to be an opportunity barrier. Few hospitals appear to have actual policies against AAC services; even so, AAC teams must deal with a number of practice or knowledge barriers. These barriers may include 1) medical teams that do not refer individuals for AAC services; 2) personnel who prefer not to be burdened with additional work in an already busy (and, perhaps, understaffed) workplace; and 3) speech-language pathologists and other professionals who are not familiar with conducting AAC interventions in these settings, or staffing patterns that result in the speech-language pathologists working in acute and intensive care settings having little or no AAC experience while AAC specialists serve the inpatient and outpatient rehabilitation programs.

Assess Access Barriers and Capabilities

As with other AAC assessments, those that occur in acute care settings require considerations of specific access barriers and capabilities.

Assess Specific Capabilities: Preliminary Screening

Many individuals in acute medical settings are unable to participate in extensive assessment procedures. The AAC team should conduct a preliminary screening as the first step of an assessment to determine what capabilities are available to support communication. Garrett et al. (2007) identified a series of communicative tasks that might be considered. *Natural communication signals* should be identified and evaluated to determine if the medical staff can accurately interpret them. These signals might include licking the lips to signal the need for lip moisturizer, "wrinkling" the face to signal pain or itchiness, protruding the tongue to signal the need for a urinal, or closing the eyes to signal the desire to be left alone. *Yes/no signals* are essential to early communication in ICU settings. Affirmation or negation can be signaled with hand squeezes, eye movement (up for YES and down for NO), or thumb movement (up for YES and down or sideways for NO). Of course, these codes should be noted on a sign (or whiteboard) posted on a wall in the room, recorded in the medical chart, and shared at team meetings. The AAC team should provide sensory aids by making sure that the need for glasses and hearing aids is identified and that these aids are routinely provided. *Comprehension and attention strategies* that are effective for each patient should be identified. After all, the ICU is an unfamiliar environment to most individuals. It is typically noisy with a range of technology and alarm systems in operation, and it is busy with many different staff coming and going. At times, two or more staff members will be in the room at once, with multiple people attempting to communicate with the patient. Therefore, it is important to identify strategies that effectively get the attention of the patient before questions are asked or instructions are given. Also, Garrett et al. recommended a strategy in which staff "establish and maintain eye gaze with the patient when trying to communicate with them" (2007, p. 32). If patients require augmented input or augmented comprehension support, comprehension of information is often assisted by providing visual information in the form of print, drawings, or pictures in addition to the spoken message. Finally, communication is typically improved if the patient is given a description of more complex procedures before the procedure is begun, rather than not describing the procedure at all or trying to describe it as the procedure is being implemented.

People with Sufficient Oral-Motor Control for Speech

Many individuals in acute medical settings have sufficient motor control for speech, provided that they have an adequate sound source for voicing. Thus, the first step in evaluation should be assessment of oral-motor capabilities. If these are adequate to support speech, assessors should explore oral communication options. If oral-motor control is inadequate, assessors must explore other communication options.

Voicing Capabilities   Many individuals who have adequate oral-motor control for speech are unable to produce sound (i.e., voice) for one of several reasons. Some lack airflow past their vocal folds because of a tracheostomy but are able to produce vocal sounds if this airflow can be reestablished temporarily. Other individuals may experience severe respiratory problems or require ventilator supports that preclude any airflow past the vocal folds. We discuss interventions options related to these two conditions later in this chapter.

Still other people may not have the motor control necessary to produce voicing. For these individuals, one of two types of electrolarynges often serves as an effective intervention device. The first, a "neck-type" electrolarynx, is positioned against the exterior neck wall and vibrates the air column within the vocal tract. Mouthing of words then produces audible speech. The second, an oral-type electrolarynx, delivers sound into the oral cavity through a tube or a catheter. The oral-type electrolarynx is useful for individuals who cannot use a neck-type electrolarynx due to extensive tissue damage, swelling, or surgical tenderness in the neck area or because they must wear cervical collars that obscure their necks. The electrolarynx is commonly used by individuals with complex communication needs due to laryngeal cancer, but it is also used by those who cannot produce phonation to support speech.

Reestablishing the Airflow for Voicing   The first step in initiating an intervention to reestablish the flow of air past the vocal folds is to determine if the individual requires a cuffed tracheostomy tube and whether the cuff must be inflated. (A cuffed tracheostomy tube is shown in Figure 18.7.) The air supply for respiration passes through the cuffed tube into the lungs. The cuff around the tube inflates against the wall of the trachea to prevent air from escaping from the ventilator and lungs through the mouth and to prevent food or liquid from moving through the mouth and pharynx into the respiratory system. Many individuals require the cuff to be inflated at all times. Some devices, however, allow the airflow to be directed through the vocal folds on exhalation although the cuffed tracheostomy tube is in place. An external valve that directs the air stream usually operates these "talking tracheostomy" products. Individuals who can tolerate the deflation of their tracheostomy cuffs for brief periods may achieve phonation by allowing air to escape from the respiratory system past the deflated cuff and vocal folds. They are able to produce natural speech in this way.

Another option is to use a tracheostomy tube that does not involve a cuff. This option may be appropriate for someone who requires a tracheostomy to maintain an open airway because of swelling or trauma to the neck area but who does not require ventilator assistance to breathe. In this case, the individual can direct air past the vocal folds by 1) learning to occlude the tube with a finger during exhalation, 2) utilizing a fenestrated tracheostomy tube that has an opening on the top in the trachea, or 3) using a one-way valve that permits inhalation through the tube and exhalation through the vocal tract.

Individuals with Insufficient Oral-Motor Control for Speech

Some people have insufficient oral-motor control for speech. If this is the case, individuals may require communication systems that use writing, direct selection, and/or scanning, as discussed in the following sections.

Writing Options   Handwriting can serve as an effective communication mode because many people are comfortable and familiar with this mode of communication. Some individuals prefer to use a pencil and tablet so that as they write and save messages, they can begin to construct their own communication book. Then, rather than writing the same message again and again, they can simply refer to a question or a comment they have communicated previously. Others prefer to use a magic slate so that they can erase messages when they are finished and thus maintain privacy.

"I think that board [a magic slate] was my preference over everything. You could communicate quickly and say what you wanted to say. You can write your letters and separate your words, like in normal writing. And it was much quicker and easier to understand by other people. I think they probably like it the best, too. So the magic board was the best one, once I could start using my hands again. When I was unable to use my hands, of course the alphabet board [for partner-assisted scanning] was the best, assuming that the other person understood how to use it, which many didn't" (Alec K., a 35-year-old man who had Guillain-Barré syndrome, in Fried-Oken et al., 1991, p. 47).

Options for People Who Cannot Write   Some individuals are unable to write by hand, but they can point accurately with their hands, eyes, or head. AAC teams generally encourage these individuals to use a direct selection communication system. The direct selection system can be as simple as an alphabet board with some words or phrases on it. Other individuals may prefer a small typing system. Usually, individuals in acute medical settings do not have the time or motivation to use an encoding strategy. Therefore, some prefer to type their messages.

If available, voice output may be preferred by some individuals. Costello (2000) described the use of "voice banking" for children scheduled in advance for major surgical procedures such as facial reconstruction. Prior to their surgeries, the children recorded messages that were later transferred to simple AAC technologies that they used in the ICU. Thus, the children were able to use their own voices to "talk" during this difficult and stressful time. Small, portable, digitized SGDs that contain 30–60 easily accessible messages are convenient for this purpose. If the individual has insufficient hand or arm control to use these options, he or she may use a headlight pointer to indicate words or letters on a wall- or ceiling-mounted chart or on a communication board placed on a mounting stand.

George was unable to communicate, except to move his head slightly side to side to signal NO and to point with his eyes. With a diagnosis of severe myasthenia gravis, he faced an extended hospital stay. An observant nurse informed us that he could move his right foot a bit, so we mounted a laser pointer on his big toe and a communication device at the foot of his bed. With his head propped up slightly so that he could see the device, George spelled his messages by moving his foot. Six weeks later, he recovered sufficiently to return home, speaking once again.

Some individuals may be limited to eye pointing in one of two forms. The first form is conventional eye pointing, in which the individual selects and gazes at a message on a display that is mounted on a transparent plastic board. The communication partner then interprets the direction of the individual's eye gaze and reads the related message. The second form, a technique known as eye linking (see Chapter 4), may be used. In eye linking, the individual looks at the desired message, and the partner (who is positioned opposite the individual on the other side of the transparent communication board) moves the board until his or her eyes are "linked" directly across from the individual's. At that point, the message that the individual wants to convey lies between the two people. Many individuals find this strategy to be easier than eye pointing.

Options for People Who Cannot Use Direct Selection   Some individuals do not have the motor capability to engage in direct selection communication. If they have other reliable, consistent motor responses, these individuals may be able to successfully use a scanning communication option. Many families can learn to use partner-assisted scanning, in which an array of letters or messages is displayed on a communication board. The communication partner points to various message options, and the individual signals when a desired message is reached by making a gesture, blinking the eyes, or activating a beeper with a switch. Unassisted (i.e., electronic) scanning is more difficult to implement in these settings, and, as noted previously, this difficulty may cause a low rate of success with this option (Dowden et al., 1986). Most individuals generally are unfamiliar with this type of communication, and the learning requirements for scanning are often too great for effective application of this option in acute medical environments.

Assess Constraints

A common constraint that affects AAC interventions is related to listener instruction. The short-term acute medical environment imposes extensive learning constraints. First, individuals are very ill and under a considerable amount of stress. Many individuals in these settings demonstrate little ability or tolerance for learning. Second, many professionals and others interact with these individuals over the course of their stay. Thus, the most effective AAC interventions are those that require minimal listener training. As noted previously, individuals and their medical teams tend not to use complicated AAC systems in short-term acute medical environments.

QUESTIONS

18.1.   What are the differences between ICU and LTACH medical units?

18.2.   How commonly do nursing staff in ICU and LTACH settings interact with patients who have AAC needs?

18.3.   Why do patients with a tracheostomy require AAC support?

18.4.   Why is it useful to identify the communication needs of patients in an LTACH unit as part of an AAC intervention?

18.5.   If you were responsible for the selection of yes/no eye signals to be used in an ICU, what signals would you propose, and why? Would you insist that all staff use the same yes/no eye signals or allow each staff member to select the signal that he or she preferred? Why?

18.6.   If you were responsible for the selection of AAC support materials for an ICU, what items would you select, and why would you select them?

18.7.   A patient who cannot speak or write can only communicate using her eyes. However, her spouse has difficulty interpreting her eye pointing, so you decide to teach him eye linking. How would you introduce this strategy to him?

References

Adams, M.J. (1990). *Beginning to read: Thinking and learning about print.* Cambridge, MA: MIT Press.

Adams, S.G. (1994). Accelerating speech in a case of hypokinetic dysarthria: Descriptions and treatment. In J.A. Till, K.M. Yorkston, & D.R. Beukelman (Eds.), *Motor speech disorders: Advances in assessment and treatment* (pp. 213–228). Baltimore: Paul H. Brookes Publishing Co.

Adams, S.G. (1997). Hypokinetic dysarthria in Parkinson's disease. In M.R. McNeil (Ed.), *Clinical management of sensorimotor speech disorders* (pp. 261–285). New York: Thieme.

Adamson, L., & Dunbar, B. (1991). Communication development of young children with tracheostomies. *Augmentative and Alternative Communication, 7,* 275–283.

Alant, E. (1999). Students with little or no functional speech in schools for students with mental retardation in South Africa. *Augmentative and Alternative Communication, 15,* 83–94.

Alant, E., & Lloyd, L.L. (Eds.). (2005). *Augmentative and alternative communication: Beyond poverty.* London: Whurr.

Alm, N., Astell, A., Ellis, M., Dye, R., Gowans, G., & Campbell, J. (2004). A cognitive prosthesis and communication support for people with dementia. *Neuropsychological Rehabilitation, 14,* 117–134.

Almeida, M., Piza, M., & LaMonica, D. (2005). Adaptações do sistema de comunicação por troca de figuras no contexto escolar [Adaptation of the Picture Exchange Communication System in a school context]. *Pró-Fono Revista de Atualização Científica, 17,* 233–240.

Alsop, L. (2004). *Competencies for training intervenors to work with children and students with deafblindness.* Logan: SKI-HI Institute, Utah State University.

Alsop, L., Blaha, R., & Kloos, E. (2000). *The intervenor in early intervention and educational settings for children and youth with deafblindness.* Monmouth, OR: National Technical Assistance Consortium for Children and Young Adults Who Are Deaf-Blind.

Alzheimer's Association. (2001). *An overview of Alzheimer's disease and related dementias.* Retrieved from http://www.alz.org

American Speech-Language-Hearing Association. (2004). Roles and responsibilities of speech-language pathologists with respect to augmentative and alternative communication: Technical report. *ASHA Supplement, 24,* 1–17.

American Speech-Language-Hearing Association. (2005). *Roles and responsibilities of speech-language pathologists with respect to augmentative and alternative communication: Position statement.* doi:10.1044/policy.PS2005-00113

American Speech-Language-Hearing Association. (2007). *Childhood apraxia of speech* [Technical report]. Retrieved from http://www.asha.org/policy

Americans with Disabilities Act of 1990, PL 101-336, 42 U.S.C. §§ 12101 *et seq.*

Anderson-Inman, L., & Horney, M.A. (2007). Supported eText: Assistive technology through text transformations. *Reading Research Quarterly, 42,* 153–160.

Andrews-Salvia, M., Roy, N., & Cameron, R.M. (2003). Evaluating the effects of memory books for individuals with severe dementia. *Journal of Medical Speech-Language Pathology, 11*(1), 51–59.

Angell, M., Stoner, J., & Fulk, B. (2010). Advice from adults with physical disabilities on fostering self-determination during the school years. *Teaching Exceptional Children, 42,* 64–75.

Angelo, J. (1987). *A comparison of three coding methods for abbreviation expansion in acceleration vocabularies* (Unpublished doctoral dissertation). University of Wisconsin–Madison.

Angermeier, K., Schooley, K., Harasymowycz, U., & Schlosser, R. (2010). The role of finger-spelled self-cues during spelling with a speech generating device by a child with autism: A brief report. *Journal of Developmental and Physical Disabilities, 22,* 197–200.

Archer, A.L., & Hughes, C.A. (2010). *Explicit instruction: Effective and efficient teaching.* New York: Guilford Press.

Armbruster, B.B., Lehr, F., & Osborn, J. (2001). *Put reading first: The research building blocks for teaching children to read: Kindergarten through grade 3.* Washington, DC: National Institute for Literacy.

Arnold, A. (2007). Living at home and my thoughts for the future. In R.V. Conti & T.J. McGrath (Eds.), *Proceedings of the Eleventh Biennial Pittsburgh Employment Conference for Augmented Communicators* (pp. 94–96). Pittsburgh: Shout Press.

Arnott, J., & Javed, M. (1992). Probabilistic character disambiguation for reduced keyboards using small text samples. *Augmentative and Alternative Communication, 8,* 215–223.

Ashwal, S., Russman, B.S., Blasco, P.A., Miller, G., Sandler, A., Shevell, M., & Stevenson, R. (2004). Practice parameter: Diagnostic assessment of the child with cerebral palsy: Report of the Quality Standards Subcommittee of the American Academy of Neurology and the Practice Committee of the Child Neurology Society. *Neurology, 62,* 851–863.

Assistive Technology Act Amendments of 2004, PL 108-364, 29 U.S.C. §§ 3001 *et seq.*

Aston, M.C. (2001). *The other half of Asperger syndrome: A guide to living in an intimate relationship with a partner who has Asperger syndrome.* London: National Autistic Society.

Aston, M.C. (2003). *Aspergers in love: Couple relationships and family affairs.* London: Jessica Kingsley.

Bailey, B., & Downing, J. (1994). Using visual accents to enhance attending to communication symbols for students with severe multiple disabilities. *RE:view, 26*(3), 101–118.

Bailey, R.L., Parette, H.P., Jr., Stoner, J.B., Angell, M.E., & Carroll, K. (2006). Family members' perceptions of augmentative and alternative communication device use. *Language, Speech, and Hearing Services in Schools, 37,* 50–60.

Bak, T.H., & Hodges, J.R. (2001). Motor neuron disease, dementia and aphasia: Coincidence, co-occurrence or continuum? *Journal of Neurology, 248,* 260–270.

Baker, B. (1982, September). Minspeak: A semantic compaction system that makes self-expression easier for communicatively disabled individuals. *Byte, 7,* 186–202.

Baker, B. (1986). Using images to generate speech. *Byte, 11,* 160–168.

Balandin, S., & Iacono, T. (1998a). A few well-chosen words. *Augmentative and Alternative Communication, 14,* 147–161.

Balandin, S., & Iacono, T. (1998b). Topics of meal-break conversations. *Augmentative and Alternative Communication, 14,* 131–146.

Balandin, S., & Iacono, T. (1999). Crews, wusses, and whoppas: Core and fringe vocabularies of Australian meal-break conversations in the workplace. *Augmentative and Alternative Communication, 15,* 95–105.

Balandin, S., & Morgan, J. (2001). Preparing for the future: Aging and augmentative and alternative communication. *Augmentative and Alternative Communication, 17,* 99–108.

Ball, L. (2003). AAC transition for adults: Maximizing communication and participation. *ASHA Leader, 8,* 141.

Ball, L. (2008). Childhood apraxia of speech: Augmentative & alternative communication strategies. In J. Wambaugh, N. Alarcon, L. Shuster, & L. Ball (Eds.), *Traditional and AAC approaches for apraxia of speech in adults and children.* Miniseminar presented at the American Speech-Language-Hearing Association annual conference, Chicago.

Ball, L.D., Anderson, E., Bilyeu, D., Pattee, G., Beukelman, D., & Robertson, J. (2007). Duration of AAC technology use by persons with ALS. *Journal of Medical Speech Language Pathology, 15,* 371–381.

Ball, L., Beukelman, D., & Bardach, L. (2007). AAC intervention for ALS. In D.R. Beukelman, K.L. Garrett, & K.M. Yorkston (Eds.), *Augmentative communication strategies for adults with acute or chronic medical conditions* (pp. 287–316). Baltimore: Paul H. Brookes Publishing Co.

Ball, L., Beukelman, D.R., & Pattee, G. (2002). Timing of speech deterioration in people with amyotrophic lateral sclerosis. *Journal of Medical Speech-Language Pathology, 10,* 231–235.

Ball, L., Beukelman, D.R., & Pattee, G. (2003, November). *AAC transitions for adults I: Maximizing communication and participation (AAC transitions for persons with ALS).* Presentation at the annual convention of the American Speech-Language-Hearing Association, Chicago.

Ball, L., Beukelman, D.R., & Pattee, G. (2004). Acceptance of augmentative and alternative communication technology by persons with amyotrophic lateral sclerosis. *Augmentative and Alternative Communication, 20,* 113–122.

Ball, L., Beukelman, D., Ullman, C., Maassen, M., & Pattee, G. (2005). Monitoring speaking rate by telephone with amyotrophic lateral sclerosis. *Journal of Medical Speech Language Pathology, 13,* 233–240.

Ball, L., Fager, S., Nordness, A., Kersch, K., Mohr, B., Pattee, G., & Beukelman, D. (2010). Eyegaze access of AAC technology for persons with amyotrophic lateral sclerosis. *Journal of Medical Speech Language Pathology, 18,* 11–23.

Ball, L., Marvin, C., Beukelman, D.R., Lasker, J., & Rupp, D. (1999). "Generic small talk" use by preschool children. *Augmentative and Alternative Communication, 15,* 145–155.

Ball, L., Schardt, K., & Beukelman, D. (2005). Primary communication facilitators. *Augmentative Communication News, 17,* 6–7.

Ball, L.J., & Stading, K.L. (2006, November). *Functional communication strategies for children with apraxia of speech.* Seminar presentation at the annual convention of the American Speech-Language-Hearing Association, Miami, FL.

Bambara, L., & Kern, L. (2005). *Individualized supports for students with problem behaviors.* New York: Guilford Press.

Bambara, L., Spiegel-McGill, P., Shores, R., & Fox, J. (1984). A comparison of reactive and non-reactive toys on severely handicapped children's manipulative play. *Journal of the Association for Persons with Severe Handicaps, 9,* 142–149.

Banajee, M., Dicarlo, C., & Stricklin, S. (2003). Core vocabulary determination for toddlers. *Augmentative and Alternative Communication, 19,* 67–73.

Barrera, R., Lobato-Barrera, D., & Sulzer-Azaroff, B. (1980). A simultaneous treatment comparison of three expressive language training programs with a mute autistic child. *Journal of Autism and Developmental Disorders, 10,* 21–38.

Barritt, L., & Kroll, B. (1978). Some implications of cognitive developmental psychology for research in composing. In C. Cooper & L. Odell (Eds.), *Research on composing: Points of departure* (pp. 49–57). Urbana, IL: National Council of Teachers of English.

Bartlett, M.R., Fink, R.B., Schwartz, M. F., & Linebarger, M. (2007). Informativeness ratings of messages created on an AAC processing prosthesis. *Aphasiology, 21*(5), 475–498.

Basil, C. (1992). Social interaction and learned helplessness in severely disabled children. *Augmentative and Alternative Communication, 8,* 188–199.

Basil, C., & Soro-Camats, E. (1996). Supporting graphic language acquisition by a girl with multiple impairments. In S. von Tetzchner & M.H. Jensen (Eds.), *Augmentative and alternative communication: European perspectives* (pp. 270–291). London: Whurr.

Basson, M., & Alant, E. (2005). The iconicity and ease of learning of picture communication symbols: A study with Afrikaans-speaking children. *South African Journal of Communication Disorders, 52,* 4–12.

Batshaw, M.L., & Shapiro, B. (2002). Mental retardation. In M.L. Batshaw (Ed.), *Children with disabilities* (5th ed., pp. 287–305). Baltimore: Paul H. Brookes Publishing Co.

Bauby, J.-D. (1997). *The diving bell and the butterfly* (Jeremy Leggatt, Trans.). New York: Alfred A. Knopf.

Bauer, A.M., & Matuszek, K. (2001). Designing and evaluating accommodations and adaptations. In A.M. Bauer & G.M. Brown (Eds.), *Adolescents and inclusion: Transforming secondary schools* (pp. 139–166). Baltimore: Paul H. Brookes Publishing Co.

Bayles, K.A., & Kim, E.S. (2003). Improving the functioning of individuals with Alzheimer's disease: Emergence of behavioral interventions. *Journal of Communication Disorders, 36,* 327–343.

Bayles, K., Tomoeda, C., Wood, J., Montgomery, E., Cruz, R., Azuma, T., & McGeagh, A. (1996). Changes in cognitive function in idiopathic Parkinson's disease. *Archives of Neurology, 53,* 1140–1146.

Beck, A., Bock, S., Thompson, J., & Kosuwan, K. (2002). Influence of communicative competence and augmentative and alternative communication technique on children's attitudes toward a peer who uses AAC. *Augmentative and Alternative Communication, 18,* 217–227.

Beck, A., & Dennis, M. (1996). Attitudes of children toward a similar-aged child who uses augmentative communication. *Augmentative and Alternative Communication, 12,* 78–87.

Beck, A., & Fritz, H. (1998). Can people with aphasia learn iconic codes? *Augmentative and Alternative Communication, 14,* 184–195.

Beck, A., Fritz, H., Keller, A., & Dennis, M. (2000). Attitudes of school-aged children toward their peers who use AAC. *Augmentative and Alternative Communication, 16,* 13–26.

Beck, A., & Fritz-Verticchio, H. (2003). The influence of information and role-playing experiences on children's attitudes toward peers who use AAC. *American Journal of Speech-Language Pathology, 12,* 51–60.

Beck, A., Kingsbury, K., Neff, A., & Dennis, M. (2000). Influence of length of augmented message on children's attitudes towards peers who use augmentative and alternative communication. *Augmentative and Alternative Communication, 16,* 239–249.

Beck, A., Stoner, J., & Dennis, M. (2009). An investigation of aided language stimulation: Does it increase AAC use with adults with developmental disabilities and complex communication needs? *Augmentative and Alternative Communication, 25,* 42–54.

Beck, A., Thompson, J., & Clay, S. (2000). The effect of icon prediction on college students' recall of icon codes. *Journal of Special Education Technology, 15,* 17–23.

Beck, A.R., Thompson, J.R., Kosuwan, K., & Prochnow, J.M. (2010). The development and utilization of a scale to measure adolescents' attitudes toward peers who use augmentative and alternative communication (AAC) devices. *Journal of Speech, Language, and Hearing Research, 53,* 572–587.

Beckman, P., & Kohl, F. (1984). The effects of social and isolated toys on the interactions and play of integrated and nonintegrated groups of preschoolers. *Education and Training of the Mentally Retarded, 19,* 169–174.

Bedrosian, J. (1999). AAC efficacy research: Challenges for the new century. *Augmentative and Alternative Communication, 15,* 2–3.

Bedrosian, J., Hoag, L., Calculator, S., & Molineux, B. (1992). Variables influencing perceptions of the communicative competence of an adult augmentative and alternative communication system user. *Journal of Speech and Hearing Research, 35,* 1105–1113.

Bedrosian, J., Hoag, L., Johnson, D., & Calculator, S. (1998). Communicative competence as perceived by adults with severe speech impairments associated with cerebral palsy. *Journal of Speech, Language, and Hearing Research, 41,* 667–675.

Bedrosian, J., Hoag, L., & McCoy, K. (2003). Relevance and speed of message delivery tradeoffs in augmentative and alternative communication. *Journal of Speech, Language, and Hearing Research, 46,* 800–817.

Bedrosian, J., Lasker, J., Speidel, K., & Politsch, A. (2003). Enhancing the written narrative skills of an AAC student with autism: Evidence-based research issues. *Topics in Language Disorders, 23,* 305–324.

Bellon-Harn, M., & Harn, W. (2008). Scaffolding strategies during repeated storybook reading: An extension using a voice output communication aid. *Focus on Autism and Other Developmental Disabilities, 23,* 112–124.

Bellugi, U., & Fischer, S. (1972). A comparison of sign language and spoken language. *Cognition, 1,* 173–200.

Benigno, J., Bennett, J., McCarthy, J., & Smith, J. (2011). Situational and psychosocial factors mediating coordinated joint attention with augmentative and alternative communication systems with beginning communicators without disabilities. *Augmentative and Alternative Communication, 27,* 67–76.

Berlowitz, C. (1991, January 13). Ana begins to speak. *This World,* 16.

Berninger, V., & Gans, B. (1986). Language profiles in nonspeaking individuals of normal intelligence with severe cerebral palsy. *Augmentative and Alternative Communication, 2,* 45–50.

Beukelman, D.R. (1987). When you have a hammer, everything looks like a nail. *Augmentative and Alternative Communication, 3,* 94–95.

Beukelman, D.R. (1991). Magic and cost of communicative competence. *Augmentative and Alternative Communication, 7,* 2–10.

Beukelman, D. (2005). Tom's AAC system. *Augmentative Communication News,* 5–6.

Beukelman, D., Ball, L., & Fager, S. (2008). An AAC personnel framework: Adults with acquired complex communication needs. *Augmentative and Alternative Communication, 24,* 255–267.

Beukelman, D., Fager, S., Ball, L., & Dietz, A. (2007). AAC for adults with acquired neurological conditions: A review. *Augmentative and Alternative Communication, 23,* 230–242.

Beukelman, D.R., Fager, S., Ullman, C., Hanson, E., & Logemann, J. (2002). The impact of speech supplementation and clear speech on the intelligibility and speaking rate of people with traumatic brain injury. *Journal of Medical Speech-Language Pathology, 10,* 237–242.

Beukelman, D.R., & Garrett, K. (1988). Augmentative and alternative communication for adults with acquired severe communication disorders. *Augmentative and Alternative Communication, 4,* 104–121.

Beukelman, D.R., Garrett, K.L., & Yorkston, K.M. (2007). *Augmentative communication strategies for adults with acute or chronic medical conditions.* Baltimore: Paul H. Brookes Publishing Co.

Beukelman, D.R., Jones, R., & Rowan, M. (1989). Frequency of word usage by nondisabled peers in integrated preschool classrooms. *Augmentative and Alternative Communication, 5,* 243–248.

Beukelman, D.R., Kraft, G., & Freal, J. (1985). Expressive communication disorders in persons with multiple sclerosis: A survey. *Archives of Physical Medicine and Rehabilitation, 66,* 675–677.

Beukelman, D.R., & Mirenda, P. (1988). Communication options for persons who cannot speak: Assessment and evaluation. In C.A. Coston (Ed.), *Proceedings of the National Planners Conference on Assistive Device Service Delivery* (pp. 151–165). Washington, DC: Association for the Advancement of Rehabilitation Technology.

Beukelman, D.R., & Mirenda, P. (2005). *Augmentative and alternative communication: Supporting children and adults with complex communication needs* (3rd ed.). Baltimore: Paul H. Brookes Publishing Co.

Beukelman, D.R., & Ray, P. (2010). Communication supports in pediatric rehabilitation. *Journal of Pediatric Rehabilitation Medicine, 3,* 279–288.

Beukelman, D.R., & Yorkston, K. (1977). A communication system for the severely dysarthric speaker with an intact language system. *Journal of Speech and Hearing Disorders, 42,* 265–270.

Beukelman, D.R., & Yorkston, K. (1984). Computer enhancement of message formulation and presentation for communication augmentation system users. *Seminars in Speech and Language, 5,* 1–10.

Beukelman, D.R., Yorkston, K., & Dowden, P. (1985). *Communication augmentation: A casebook of clinical management.* Austin, TX: PRO-ED.

Beukelman, D.R., Yorkston, K., Poblete, M., & Naranjo, C. (1984). Frequency of word occurrence in communication samples produced by adult communication aid users. *Journal of Speech and Hearing Disorders, 49,* 360–367.

Bevan-Brown, J. (2001). Evaluating special education services for learners from ethnically diverse groups: Getting it right. *Journal of the Association for Persons with Severe Handicaps, 26,* 138–147.

Biklen, D. (1990). Communication unbound: Autism and praxis. *Harvard Educational Review, 60,* 291–314.

Biklen, D. (1992). *Schooling without labels.* Philadelphia: Temple University Press.

Binger, C. (2008a). Classroom-based language goals and intervention for children who use AAC: Back to basics. *Perspectives on Augmentative and Alternative Communication, 17,* 20–26.

Binger, C. (2008b). Grammatical morpheme intervention issues for students who use AAC. *Perspectives on Augmentative and Alternative Communication, 17,* 62–68.

Binger, C., Kent-Walsh, J., Berens, J., del Campo, S., & Rivera, D. (2008). Teaching Latino parents to support the multi-symbol message productions of their children who require AAC. *Augmentative and Alternative Communication, 24,* 323–338.

Binger, C., Kent-Walsh, J., Ewing, C., & Taylor, S. (2010). Teaching educational assistants to facilitate the multisymbol message productions of young students who require augmentative and alternative communication. *American Journal of Speech-Language Pathology, 19,* 108–120.

Binger, C., & Light, J. (2007). The effect of aided AAC modeling on the expression of multi-symbol messages by preschoolers who use AAC. *Augmentative and Alternative Communication, 23,* 30–43.

Binger, C., & Light, J. (2008). The morphology and syntax of individuals who use AAC: Research review and implications for effective practice. *Augmentative and Alternative Communication, 24,* 123–138.

Binger, C., Maguire-Marshall, M., & Kent-Walsh, J. (2011). Using aided AAC models, recasts, and contrastive targets to teach grammatical morphemes to children who use AAC. *Journal of Speech, Language, and Hearing Research, 54,* 160–176.

Bird, F., Dores, P., Moniz, D., & Robinson, J. (1989). Reducing severe aggressive and self-injurious behaviors with functional communication training. *American Journal on Mental Retardation, 94,* 37–48.

Bishop, D. (2003). *Test for Reception of Grammar–Version 2 (TROG-2).* San Antonio, TX: Harcourt Assessment.

Bishop, K., Rankin, J., & Mirenda, P. (1994). Impact of graphic symbol use on reading acquisition. *Augmentative and Alternative Communication, 10,* 113–125.

Blackstien-Adler, S. (2003). *Training school teams to use the Participation Model: Evaluation of a train-the-trainer model* (Unpublished master's thesis). Ontario Institute for the Study of Education, University of Toronto.

Blackstone, S. (1989). The 3 R's: Reading, writing, and reasoning. *Augmentative Communication News, 2*(1), 1–6, 8.

Blackstone, S. (1990). Populations and practices in AAC. *Augmentative Communication News, 3*(4), 1–3.

Blackstone, S. (1993). Cultural sensitivity and AAC services. *Augmentative Communication News, 6*(2), 3–5.

Blackstone, S. (1994). Auditory scanning. *Augmentative Communication News, 7*(2), 6–7.

Blackstone, S. (2004). Clinical news: Visual scene displays. *Augmentative Communication News, 16*(2), 1–8.

Blackstone, S.W., Cassatt-James, E.L., & Bruskin, D. (Eds.). (1988). *Augmentative communication: Implementation strategies.* Rockville, MD: American Speech-Language-Hearing Association.

Blackstone, S., & Hunt Berg, M. (2003a). *Social Networks: A Communication Inventory for Individuals with Complex Communication Needs and Their Communication Partners—Inventory Booklet.* Monterey, CA: Augmentative Communication, Inc.

Blackstone, S., & Hunt Berg, M. (2003b). *Social Networks: A Communication Inventory for Individuals with Complex Communication Needs and Their Communication Partners—Manual.* Monterey, CA: Augmentative Communication, Inc.

Blackstone, S., & Pressman, H. (1995). *Outcomes in AAC conference report: Alliance '95.* Monterey, CA: Augmentative Communication.

Blackstone, S., & Wilkins, D. (2009). Exploring the importance of emotional competence in children with complex communication needs. *Perspectives on Augmentative and Alternative Communication, 18,* 78–87.

Blackstone, S., Williams, M., & Joyce, M. (2002). Future AAC technology needs: Consumer perspectives. *Assistive Technology, 14,* 3–16.

Blake, D.J., & Bodine, C. (2002). An overview of assistive technology for persons with multiple sclerosis. *Journal of Rehabilitation Research and Development, 39*(2), 299–312.

Blischak, D.M. (1995). Thomas the writer: Case study of a child with severe speech and physical impairments. *Language, Speech, and Hearing Services in Schools, 25,* 11–20.

Blischak, D.M. (1999). Increases in natural speech production following experience with synthetic speech. *Journal of Special Education Technology, 14,* 44–53.

Blischak, D., Lombardino, L., & Dyson, A. (2003). Use of speech generating devices: In support of natural speech. *Augmentative and Alternative Communication, 19,* 29–36.

Blischak, D.M., & Schlosser, R.W. (2003). Use of technology to support independent spelling by students with autism. *Topics in Language Disorders, 23,* 293–304.

Blischak, D.M., Shah, S.D., Lombardino, L.J., & Chiarella, K. (2004). Effects of phonemic awareness instruction on the encoding skills of children with severe speech impairment. *Disability & Rehabilitation, 26,* 1295–1304.

Blissymbolics Communication International. (2012). *Why Bliss?* Retrieved March 1, 2012, from http://www.blissymbolics.org/pfw/index.php?option=com_content&view=article&id=5&Itemid=6

Blockberger, S., Armstrong, R., & O'Connor, A. (1993). Children's attitudes toward a nonspeaking child using various augmentative and alternative communication techniques. *Augmentative and Alternative Communication, 9,* 243–250.

Blockberger, S., & Johnston, J. (2003). Grammatical morphology acquisition by children with complex communication needs. *Augmentative and Alternative Communication, 19,* 207–221.

Blockberger, S., & Kamp, L. (1990). The use of voice output communication aids (VOCAs) by ambulatory children. *Augmentative and Alternative Communication, 6,* 127–128.

Blockberger, S., & Sutton, A. (2003). Toward linguistic competence: Language experiences and knowledge of children with extremely limited speech. In J.C. Light, D.R. Beukelman, & J. Reichle (Eds.), *Communicative competence for individuals who use AAC: From research to effective practice* (pp. 63–106). Baltimore: Paul H. Brookes Publishing Co.

Bloom, L., & Lahey, M. (1978). *Language development and language disorders.* New York: Wiley.

Bloomberg, K. (1996). *PrAACtically speaking* [Videotape]. Melbourne, Australia: Yooralla Society.

Bloomberg, K., & Johnson, H. (1990). A statewide demographic survey of people with severe communication impairments. *Augmentative and Alternative Communication, 6,* 50–60.

Bloomberg, K., Karlan, G., & Lloyd, L. (1990). The comparative translucency of initial lexical items represented by five graphic symbol systems and sets. *Journal of Speech and Hearing Research, 33,* 717–725.

Bloomberg, K., West, D., Johnson, H., & Caithness, T. (2004). *InterAACtion Strategies for intentional and unintentional communicators* [DVD]. St. Kilda, Victoria, Australia: Scope Communication Resource Centre.

Bloomberg, K., West, D., Johnson, H., & Iacono, T. (2009). *The Triple C: Checklist of Communication Competencies–Revised.* Victoria, Australia: Scope Communication Resource Centre.

Bock, S.J., Stoner, J.B., Beck, A.R., Hanley, L., & Prochnow, J. (2005). Increasing functional communication in non-speaking preschool children: Comparison of PECS and VOCA. *Education and Training in Developmental Disabilities, 40,* 264–278.

Boden, D., & Bielby, D. (1983). The way it was: Topical organization in elderly conversation. *Language and Communication, 6*(1/2), 73–79.

Bölte, S., & Poutska, F. (2002). The relation between general cognitive level and adaptive behavior domains in individuals with autism with and without co-morbid mental retardation. *Child Psychiatry & Human Development, 33,* 165–172.

Bolton, S., & Dashiell, S. (1991). *Interaction Checklist for Augmentative Communication–Revised edition.* Austin, TX: PRO-ED.

Bondy, A., & Frost, L. (2001). *A picture's worth: PECS and other visual communication strategies in autism.* Bethesda, MD: Woodbine.

Bondy, A., & Frost, L. (2009). The Picture Exchange Communication System: Clinical and research applications. In P. Mirenda & T. Iacono (Eds.), *Autism spectrum disorders and AAC* (pp. 279–302). Baltimore: Paul H. Brookes Publishing Co.

Bonvillian, J., & Nelson, K. (1978). Development of sign language in autistic children and other language-handicapped individuals. In P. Siple (Ed.), *Understanding language through sign language research* (pp. 187–209). New York: Academic Press.

Bonvillian, J., & Siedlecki, T., Jr. (1996). Young children's acquisition of the location aspect of American Sign Language: Parental report findings. *Journal of Communication Disorders, 29,* 13–35.

Bonvillian, J., & Siedlecki, T., Jr. (1998). Young children's acquisition of the movement aspect of American Sign Language: Parental report findings. *Journal of Speech, Language, and Hearing Research, 41,* 588–602.

Boone, R., & Higgins, K. (2007). The role of instructional design in assistive technology research and development. *Reading Research Quarterly, 42,* 135–140.

Bopp, K., Brown, K., & Mirenda, P. (2004). Speech-language pathologists' roles in the delivery of positive behavior support for individuals with developmental disabilities. *American Journal of Speech-Language Pathology, 13,* 5–19.

Bornman, J., Alant, E., & Meiring, E. (2001). The use of a digital voice output device to facilitate language development in a child with developmental apraxia of speech: A case study. *Disability and Rehabilitation, 23,* 623–634.

Bornstein, H. (1990). Signed English. In H. Bornstein (Ed.), *Manual communication: Implications for education* (pp. 128–138). Washington, DC: Gallaudet University Press.

Bourgeois, M. (1990). Caregiver training, generalization, and maintenance of communicative behaviors in patients with Alzheimer's disease: Treatment efficacy research in communication disorders. *Asha, 32,* 65.

Bourgeois, M.S. (1992). Evaluating memory wallets in conversation with persons with dementia. *Journal of Speech and Hearing Research, 35*(6), 1344–1357.

Bourgeois, M.S. (1993). Effects of memory aids on the dyadic conversation of individuals with dementia. *Journal of Applied Behavior Analysis, 26,* 77–87.

Bourgeois, M.S. (1996). Memory wallet intervention in an adult day-care setting. *Behavioral Interventions, 11*(1), 3–18.

Bourgeois, M.S., Camp, C., Rose, M., White, B., Malone, M., Carr, J., & Rovine, M. (2003). A comparison of training strategies to enhance use of external aids by persons with dementia. *Journal of Communication Disorders, 36,* 361–378.

Bourgeois, M.S., Dijkstra, K., Burgio, L., & Allen-Burge, R. (2001). Memory aids as an augmentative and alternative communication strategy for nursing home residents with dementia. *Augmentative and Alternative Communication, 17,* 196–209.

Bourgeois, M., & Hickey, E. (2007). Dementia. In D.R. Beukelman, K.L. Garrett, & K.M. Yorkston (Eds.), *Augmentative communication strategies for adults with acute or chronic medical conditions* (pp. 243–286). Baltimore: Paul H. Brookes Publishing Co.

Bourgeois, M., & Hickey, E. (2009). *Dementia: From diagnosis to management—a functional approach.* Mahwah, NJ: Lawrence Erlbaum.

Bracken, B.A., & McCallum, R.S. (1998). *Universal Nonverbal Intelligence Test (UNIT).* Itasca, IL: Riverside.

Bracken, B.A. (1998). *Bracken Basic Concept Scale–Revised.* San Antonio, TX: Harcourt Assessment.

Brady, D., & Smouse, A. (1978). A simultaneous comparison of three methods for language training with an autistic child: An experimental single case analysis. *Journal of Autism and Childhood Schizophrenia, 8,* 271–279.

Brady, N.C., & Halle, J.W. (2002). Breakdowns and repairs in conversations between beginning AAC users and their partners. In J. Reichle, D.R. Beukelman, & J.C. Light (Eds.), *Exemplary practices for beginning communicators: Implications for AAC* (pp. 323–351). Baltimore: Paul H. Brookes Publishing Co.

Braille Authority of North America. (2002). *English Braille—American Edition*. Louisville, KY: American Printing House for the Blind.

Brandenberg, S., & Vanderheiden, G. (1988). Communication board design and vocabulary selection. In L. Bernstein (Ed.), *The vocally impaired: Clinical practice and research* (3rd ed., pp. 84–135). Needham Heights, MA: Allyn & Bacon.

Branson, D., & Demchak, M. (2009). The use of augmentative and alternative communication methods with infants and toddlers with disabilities: A research review. *Augmentative and Alternative Communication, 25,* 274–286.

Brault, M. (2008, December). *Americans with Disabilities: 2005, Household Economic Studies* (Current Population Reports P70-117). Washington, DC: U.S. Census Bureau, U.S. Department of Commerce, Economics and Statistics Administration.

Bridges, S. (2000, May). Delivery of AAC services to a rural American Indian community. *ASHA Special Interest Division 12 Newsletter, 9*(2), 6–9.

Bridges, S.J. (2004). Multicultural issues in augmentative and alternative communication and language research to practice. *Topics in Language Disorders, 24,* 62–75.

Bristow, D., & Fristoe, M. (1984, November). *Systematic evaluation of the nonspeaking child.* Miniseminar presented at the annual convention of the American Speech-Language-Hearing Association, San Francisco.

Bristow, D., & Fristoe, M. (1987, November). *Effects of test adaptations on test performance.* Paper presented at the annual convention of the American Speech-Language-Hearing Association, New Orleans.

Brodin, J. (1991). *Att tolka barns signaler. Gravt utvecklingsstörda flerhandikappade barns lek och kommunikation* [To interpret children's signals: Play and communication in profoundly mentally retarded and multiply handicapped children] (Doctoral dissertation). Stockholm University, Department of Education.

Brophy, J.E. (2010). *Motivating students to learn* (3rd ed.). New York: Routledge.

Browder, D.M., Ahlgrim-Delzell, L., Courtade, G., Gibbs, S.L., & Flowers, C. (2008). Evaluation of the effectiveness of an early literacy program for students with significant developmental disabilities. *Exceptional Children, 75,* 33–52.

Browder, D.M., Mims, P.J., Spooner, F., Ahlgrim-Delzell, L., & Lee, A. (2008). Teaching elementary students with multiple disabilities to participate in shared stories. *Research and Practice for Persons with Severe Disabilities, 33,* 3–12.

Browder, D., & Spooner, F. (Eds.). (2006). *Teaching language arts, math, and science to students with significant cognitive disabilities.* Baltimore: Paul H. Brookes Publishing Co.

Browder, D., Spooner, F., Ahlgrim-Delzell, L., Harris, A., & Wakeman, S. (2008). A meta-analysis on teaching mathematics to students with significant cognitive disabilities. *Exceptional Children, 74,* 407–432.

Browder, D.M., Wakeman, S., Spooner, F., Ahlgrim-Delzell, L., & Algozzine, B. (2006). Research on reading for students with significant cognitive disabilities. *Exceptional Children, 72,* 392–408.

Browder, D.M., & Xin, Y.P. (1998). A meta-analysis and review of sight word research and its implications for teaching functional reading to individuals with moderate and severe disabilities. *Journal of Special Education, 32,* 130–153.

Brown, C. (1954). *My left foot.* London: Secker & Warburg.

Brown, F. (1991). Creative daily scheduling: A nonintrusive approach to challenging behaviors in community residences. *Journal of the Association for Persons with Severe Handicaps, 16,* 75–84.

Brown, K.A., Wacker, D.P., Derby, K.M., Peck, S.M., Richman, D.M., Sasso, G.M.,...Harding, J.W. (2000). Evaluating the effects of functional communication training in the presence and absence of establishing operations. *Journal of Applied Behavior Analysis, 33,* 53–71.

Brown, L., Sherbenou, R.J., & Johnsen, S.K. (2010). *Test of Nonverbal Intelligence–Fourth Edition (TONI-4).* San Antonio, TX: Pearson Assessments.

Brown, R. (1977, May–June). *Why are signed languages easier to learn than spoken languages?* Keynote address at the National Association of the Deaf Symposium on Sign Language Research and Teaching, Chicago.

Brown, V., Hammill, D., & Wiederholt, J.L. (1995). *Test of Reading Comprehension--Third Edition (TORC-3).* Austin, TX: PRO-ED.

Bruce, S.M. (2005). The impact of congenital deafblindness on the struggle to symbolism. *International Journal of Disability, Development and Education, 52,* 233–251.

Bruno, J. (2005). *Test of Aided-Communication Symbol Performance (TASP).* Pittsburgh: DynaVox Mayer-Johnson.

Bruno, J., & Dribbon, M. (1998). Outcomes in AAC: Evaluating the effectiveness of a parent training program. *Augmentative and Alternative Communication, 14,* 59–70.

Bruno, J., & Trembath, D. (2006). Use of aided language stimulation to improve syntactic performance during a weeklong intervention program. *Augmentative and Alternative Communication, 22,* 300–313.

Bryen, D.N. (2008). Vocabulary to support socially-valued adult roles. *Augmentative and Alternative Communication, 24,* 294–301.

Bryen, D., Carey, A., & Frantz, B. (2003). Ending the silence: Adults who use augmentative communication and their experiences as victims of crimes. *Augmentative and Alternative Communication, 19,* 125–134.

Bryen, D., & Joyce, D. (1985). Language intervention with the severely handicapped: A decade of research. *Journal of Special Education, 19,* 7–39.

Bus, A.G., van IJzendoorn, M.H., & Pellegrini, A.D. (1995). Joint book reading makes for success in learning to read: A meta-analysis on intergenerational transmission of literacy. *Review of Educational Research, 65,* 1–21.

Buzolich, M., King, J., & Baroody, S. (1991). Acquisition of the commenting function among system users. *Augmentative and Alternative Communication, 7,* 88–99.

Buzolich, M., & Lunger, J. (1995). Empowering system users in peer training. *Augmentative and Alternative Communication, 11,* 37–48.

Cafiero, J. (1998). Communication power for individuals with autism. *Focus on Autism and Other Developmental Disabilities, 13,* 113–121.

Cafiero, J. (2001). The effect of an augmentative communication intervention on the communication, behavior, and academic program of an adolescent with autism. *Focus on Autism and Other Developmental Disabilities, 16,* 179–189.

Calculator, S. (1999). AAC outcomes for children and youths with severe disabilities: When seeing is believing. *Augmentative and Alternative Communication, 15,* 4, 12.

Calculator, S. (2002). Use of enhanced natural gestures to foster interactions between children with Angelman syndrome and their parents. *American Journal of Speech-Language Pathology, 11,* 340–355.

Calculator, S. (2009). Augmentative and alternative communication (AAC) and inclusive education for students with the most severe disabilities. *International Journal of Inclusive Education, 13,* 93–113.

Calculator, S., & Bedrosian, J. (1988). *Communication assessment and intervention for adults with mental retardation.* San Diego: College-Hill Press.

Calculator, S., & Black, T. (2009). Validation of an inventory of best practices in the provision of augmentative and alternative communication services to students with severe disabilities in general education classrooms. *American Journal of Speech-Language Pathology, 18,* 329–342.

Calculator, S., & Dollaghan, C. (1982). The use of communication boards in a residential setting. *Journal of Speech and Hearing Disorders, 14,* 281–287.

Callaghan, T. (1999). Early understanding and production of graphic symbols. *Child Development, 70,* 1314–1324.

Camarata, S.M., & Nelson, K.E. (2006). Conversational recast intervention with preschool and older children. In R.J. McCauley & M.E. Fey (Eds.), *Treatment of language disorders in children* (pp. 237–264). Baltimore: Paul H. Brookes Publishing Co.

Cambridge, P., & Forrester-Jones, R. (2003). Using individualized communication for interviewing people with intellectual disability: A case study of user-centred research. *Journal of Intellectual and Developmental Disability, 28,* 5–23.

Canella-Malone, H.I., DeBar, R.M., & Sigafoos, J. (2009). An examination of preference for augmentative and alternative communication devices with two boys with significant intellectual disabilities. *Augmentative and Alternative Communication, 25,* 262–273.

Canfield, H., & Locke, P. (1997). *A book of possibilities: Activities using simple technology.* Minneapolis, MN: AbleNet.

Card, R., & Dodd, B. (2006). The phonological awareness abilities of children with cerebral palsy who do not speak. *Augmentative and Alternative Communication, 22,* 149–159.

Cardona, G.W. (2000). Spaghetti talk. In M. Fried-Oken & H.A. Bersani, A.. (Eds.), *Speaking up and spelling it out: Personal essays on augmentative and alternative communication* (pp. 237–244). Baltimore: Paul H. Brookes Publishing Co.

Carey, S. (1978). The child as word learner. In M. Halle, J. Bresnan, & G. Miller (Eds.), *Linguistic theory and psychological reality* (pp. 264–293). Cambridge, MA: MIT Press.

Carey, S., & Bartlett, E. (1978). Acquiring a single new word. *Papers and Reports on Child Language Development, 15,* 17–29.

Carlson, F. (1981). A format for selecting vocabulary for the nonspeaking child. *Language, Speech, and Hearing Services in Schools, 12,* 140–145.

Carnine, D., Silbert, J., Kame'enui, E., & Tarver, S. (1997). *Direct instruction reading.* Upper Saddle River, NJ: Pearson.

Carpenter, M., Nagell, K., & Tomasello, M. (1998). Social cognition, joint attention, and communicative competence from 9 to 15 months of age. *Monographs of the Society for Research in Child Development, 63*(4, Serial No. 255).

Carr, E. (1982). Sign language. In R. Koegel, A. Rincover, & A. Egel (Eds.), *Educating and understanding autistic children* (pp. 142–157). San Diego: College-Hill Press.

Carr, E., Binkoff, J., Kologinsky, E., & Eddy, M. (1978). Acquisition of sign language by autistic children: I. Expressive labeling. *Journal of Applied Behavior Analysis, 11,* 459–501.

Carr, E., & Dores, P. (1981). Patterns of language acquisition following simultaneous communication with autistic children. *Analysis and Intervention in Developmental Disabilities, 1,* 1–15.

Carr, E.G., Levin, L., McConnachie, G., Carlson, J.I., Kemp, D.C., & Smith, C.E. (1994). *Communication-based intervention for problem behavior: A user's guide for producing positive change.* Baltimore: Paul H. Brookes Publishing Co.

Carr, E., Pridal, C., & Dores, P. (1984). Speech versus sign comprehension in autistic children: Analysis and prediction. *Journal of Experimental Child Psychology, 37,* 587–597.

Carr, E., Robinson, S., & Palumbo, L. (1990). The wrong issue: Aversive versus nonaversive treatment. The right issue: Functional versus nonfunctional treatment. In A. Repp & N. Singh (Eds.), *Perspectives on the use of nonaversive and aversive interventions for persons with developmental disabilities* (pp. 361–380). Sycamore, IL: Sycamore.

Carrow-Woolfolk, E. (1999). *Test for Auditory Comprehension of Language–Third Edition (TACL-3).* Austin, TX: PRO-ED.

Carter, M. (2003a). Communicative spontaneity of children with high support needs who use augmentative and alternative communication systems I: Classroom spontaneity, mode, and function. *Augmentative and Alternative Communication, 19,* 141–154.

Carter, M. (2003b). Communicative spontaneity of children with high support needs who use augmentative and alternative communication systems II: Antecedents and effectiveness of communication. *Augmentative and Alternative Communication, 19,* 155–169.

Carter, M., & Grunsell, J. (2001). The behavior chain interruption strategy: A review of research and discussion of future directions. *Journal of the Association for Persons with Severe Handicaps, 26,* 37–49.

Carter, M., & Iacono, T. (2002). Professional judgments of the intentionality of communicative acts. *Augmentative and Alternative Communication, 18,* 177–191.

Caselli, R.J., Windebank, A.J., Petersen, R.C., Komori, T., Parisi, J.E., Okazaki, H.,…Stein, S.D. (1993). Rapidly progressive aphasic dementia and motor neuron disease. *Annals of Neurology, 33*(2), 200–207.

Casey, L. (1978). Development of communicative behavior in autistic children: A parent program using manual signs. *Journal of Autism and Childhood Schizophrenia, 8,* 45–59.

Centers for Disease Control and Prevention. (2012). Prevalence of autism spectrum disorders: Autism and Developmental Disabilities Monitoring Network, 14 sites, United States, 2008. *Morbidity and Mortality Weekly Report, 61,* 1–19.

Centers for Disease Control and Prevention. (2010). Injury prevention & control: Traumatic brain injury. Retrieved from http://www.cdc.gov/TraumaticBrainInjury/statistics.html

Chadsey-Rusch, J., Drasgow, E., Reinoehl, B., Halle, J., & Collet-Klingenberg, L. (1993). Using general-case instruction to teach spontaneous and generalized requests for assistance to learners with severe disabilities. *Journal of the Association for Persons with Severe Handicaps, 18,* 177–187.

Chadsey-Rusch, J., & Halle, J. (1992). The application of general-case instruction to the requesting repertoires of learners with severe disabilities. *Journal of the Association for Persons with Severe Handicaps, 17,* 121–132.

Chambers, M., & Rehfeldt, R. (2003). Assessing the acquisition and generalization of two mand forms with adults with severe developmental disabilities. *Research in Developmental Disabilities, 24*, 265–280.

Chandler, L. (1992). Promoting children's social/survival skills as a strategy for transition to mainstreamed kindergarten programs. In S. Odom, S. McConnell, & M. McEvoy (Eds.), *Social competence of young children with disabilities: Issues and strategies for intervention* (pp. 245–276). Baltimore: Paul H. Brookes Publishing Co.

Chapple, D. (2000). Empowerment. In M. Fried-Oken & H.A. Bersani, Jr. (Eds.), *Speaking up and spelling it out: Personal essays on augmentative and alternative communication* (pp. 153–159). Baltimore: Paul H. Brookes Publishing Co.

Chen, D. (1999). Beginning communication with infants. In D. Chen (Ed.), *Essential elements in early intervention: Visual impairment and multiple disabilities* (pp. 337–377). New York: AFB Press.

Cherney, L.R., Halper, A.S., Holland, A.L., & Cole, R. (2008, February). Computerized script training for aphasia: Preliminary results. *American Journal of Speech-Language Pathology, 1*, 19–34.

Cheslock, M., Barton-Hulsey, A., Romski, M.A., & Sevcik, R. (2008). Using a speech-generating device to enhance communicative abilities for an adult with moderate intellectual disability. *Intellectual and Developmental Disabilities, 46*, 376–386.

Choe, Y.-K., Azuma, T., Mathy, P., Liss, J.M., & Edgar, J. (2007). The effect of home computer practice on naming in individuals with nonfluent aphasia and verbal apraxia. *Journal of Medical Speech-Language Pathology, 15*, 407–421.

Choi, H., O'Reilly, M., Sigafoos, J., & Lancioni, G. (2010). Teaching requesting and rejecting sequences to four children with developmental disabilities using augmentative and alternative communication. *Research in Developmental Disabilities, 31*, 560–567.

Christensen, S.C., & Wright, H.H. (2010). Verbal and non-verbal working memory in aphasia: What three n-back tasks reveal. *Aphasiology, 24*(6–8), 752–762.

Cipani, E. (1988). The missing item format. *Teaching Exceptional Children, 21*, 25–27.

Clibbens, J., Powell, G., & Atkinson, E. (2002). Strategies for achieving joint attention when signing to children with Down's syndrome. *International Journal of Language and Communication Disorders, 37*, 309–323.

Cline, D., Hofstetter, H., & Griffin, J. (1980). *Dictionary of visual science* (3rd ed.). Radnor, PA: Chilton.

Cohen, C., & Light, J. (2000). Use of electronic communication to develop mentor-protégé relationships between adolescent and adult users: Pilot study. *Augmentative and Alternative Communication, 16*, 227–238.

Cohen, C., & Palin, M. (1986). Speech syntheses and speech recognition devices. In M. Grossfeld & C. Grossfeld (Eds.), *Microcomputer applications in rehabilitation of communication disorders* (pp. 183–211). Rockville, MD: Aspen.

Cohen, G.D. (2000). Two new intergenerational interventions for Alzheimer's disease patients and families. *American Journal of Alzheimer's Disease, 15*(3), 137–142.

Cole, S., Horvath, B., Chapman, C., Deschenes, C., Ebeling, D., & Sprague, J. (2000). *Adapting curriculum and instruction in inclusive classrooms* (2nd ed.). Port Chester, NY: National Professional Resources.

Coleman-Martin, M.B., Heller, K.W., Cihak, D.F., & Irvine, K.L. (2005). Using computer-assisted instruction and the nonverbal reading approach to teach word identification. *Focus on Autism and Other Developmental Disabilities, 20*, 80–90.

Collier, B.M. (2000). *See what we say: Situational vocabulary for adults who use augmentative and alternative communication*. Baltimore: Paul H. Brookes Publishing Co.

Collier, B., McGhie-Richmond, D., Odette, F., & Pyne, J. (2006). Reducing the risk of people who use augmentative and alternative communication. *Augmentative and Alternative Communication, 22*, 62–75.

Collier, B., McGhie-Richmond, D., & Self, H. (2010). Exploring communication assistants as an option for increasing communication access to communities for people who use augmentative communication. *Augmentative and Alternative Communication, 26*, 48–59.

Collier, B., & Self, H. (2010). Preparing youth who use AAC to communicate with their personal assistants. In D.B. McNaughton & D.R. Beukelman (Eds.), *Transition strategies for adolescents and young adults who use AAC* (pp. 163–180). Baltimore: Paul H. Brookes Publishing Co.

Collins, M. (1986). *Diagnosis and treatment of global aphasia*. San Diego: College-Hill Press.

Collins, S. (1996). Referring expressions in conversations between aided and natural speakers. In S. von Tetzchner & M.H. Jensen (Eds.), *Augmentative and alternative communication: European perspectives* (pp. 89–100). London: Whurr.

Cook, A.M., & Polgar, J.M. (2008). *Cook and Hussey's assistive technologies: Principles and practice* (3rd ed.). St. Louis, MO: Mosby.

Copeland, S.R. (2007). Reading comprehension. In S.R. Copeland & E.B. Keefe (Eds.), *Effective literacy instruction for students with moderate or severe disabilities* (pp. 79–94). Baltimore: Paul H. Brookes Publishing Co.

Copeland, S.R., & Keefe, E.B. (2007). *Effective literacy instruction for students with moderate or severe disabilities.* Baltimore: Paul H. Brookes Publishing Co.

Cossette, L., & Duclos, E. (2003). *A profile of disability in Canada, 2001.* Ottawa: Statistics Canada.

Costello, J. (2000). Intervention in the intensive care unit: The Children's Hospital Boston model. *Augmentative and Alternative Communication, 16,* 137–153.

Costello, J., & Shane, H. (1994, November). *Augmentative communication assessment and the feature matching process.* Miniseminar presented at the annual convention of the American Speech-Language-Hearing Association, New Orleans.

Courtade, G., Spooner, F., & Browder, D. (2007). Review of studies with students with significant cognitive disabilities which link to science standards. *Research and Practice for Persons with Severe Disabilities, 32,* 43–49.

Cowan, R., & Allen, K. (2007). Using naturalistic procedures to enhance learning in individuals with autism: A focus on generalized teaching within the school setting. *Psychology in the Schools, 44,* 701–715.

Creech, R., Kissick, L., Koski, M., & Musselwhite, C. (1988). Paravocal communicators speak out: Strategies for encouraging communication aid use. *Augmentative and Alternative Communication, 4,* 168.

Creedon, M. (1973, March). *Language development in nonverbal autistic children using a simultaneous communication system.* Paper presented at the meeting of the Society for Research in Child Development, Philadelphia.

Cress, C. (1997, November). *AAC service delivery with children: Twenty frequently asked questions.* Paper presented at the American Speech-Language-Hearing Association conference, Boston.

Cress, C., & King, J. (1999). AAC strategies for people with primary progressive aphasia without dementia: Two case studies. *Augmentative and Alternative Communication, 15,* 248–259.

Cress, C., & Marvin, C. (2003). Common questions about AAC services in early intervention. *Augmentative and Alternative Communication, 19,* 254–272.

Croen, L.A., Grether, J.K., & Selvin, S. (2001). The epidemiology of mental retardation of unknown cause. *Pediatrics, 107,* 86–90.

Crone, D., & Horner, R.J. (2003). *Building positive behavior support systems in schools.* New York: Guilford Press.

Crystal, D. (1987). Teaching vocabulary: The case for a semantic curriculum. *Child Language Teaching and Therapy, 3,* 40–56.

Culp, D. (1989). Developmental apraxia and augmentative or alternative communication: A case example. *Augmentative and Alternative Communication, 5,* 27–34.

Culp, D., Beukelman, D., & Fager, S. (2007). Brainstem impairment. In D.R. Beukelman, K.L. Garrett, & K.M. Yorkston (Eds.), *Augmentative communication strategies for adults with acute or chronic medical conditions* (pp. 59–90). Baltimore: Paul H. Brookes Publishing Co.

Culp, D., & Carlisle, M. (1988). *PACT: Partners in augmentative communication training.* Tucson, AZ: Communication Skill Builders.

Culp, D., & Ladtkow, M. (1992). Locked-in syndrome and augmentative communication. In K. Yorkston (Ed.), *Augmentative communication in the medical setting* (pp. 59–138). San Antonio, TX: Harcourt Assessment.

Cumley, G. (1997). *Introduction of augmentative and alternative modality: Effects on the quality and quantity of communication interactions of children with severe phonological disorders* (Unpublished doctoral dissertation). University of Nebraska–Lincoln.

Cumley, G., & Swanson, S. (1999). Augmentative and alternative communication options for children with developmental apraxia of speech: Three case studies. *Augmentative and Alternative Communication, 15,* 110–125.

Curcio, F. (1978). Sensorimotor functioning and communication in mute autistic children. *Journal of Autism and Childhood Schizophrenia, 8,* 181–189.

Dada, S., & Alant, E. (2009). The effect of aided language stimulation on vocabulary acquisition in children with little or no functional speech. *American Journal of Speech-Language Pathology, 18,* 50–64.

Dahlgren Sandberg, A. (1998). Reading and spelling among nonvocal children with cerebral palsy: Influence of home and school literacy environment. *Reading and Writing, 10,* 23–50.

Dahlgren Sandberg, A. (2001). Reading and spelling, phonological awareness, and working memory in children with severe speech impairments: A longitudinal study. *Augmentative and Alternative Communication, 17,* 11–25.

Dahlgren Sandberg, A. (2006). Reading and spelling abilities in children with severe speech impairments and cerebral palsy at 6, 9, and 12 years of age in relation to cognitive development: A longitudinal study. *Developmental Medicine & Child Neurology, 48,* 629–634.

Dahlgren Sandberg, A., & Hjelmquist, E. (1996a). A comparative, descriptive study of reading and writing skills among non-speaking children: A preliminary study. *European Journal of Disorders of Communication, 31,* 289–308.

Dahlgren Sandberg, A., & Hjelmquist, E. (1996b). Phonologic awareness and literacy abilities in nonspeaking preschool children with cerebral palsy. *Augmentative and Alternative Communication, 12,* 138–154.

Dalby, D.M., Hirdes, J.P., Stolee, P., Strong, J., Poss, J., Tjam, E.Y.,…Ashworth, M. (2009). Characteristics of individuals with congenital and acquired deafblindness. *Journal of Visual Impairment & Blindness, 103,* 93–102.

Daniloff, J., Lloyd, L., & Fristoe, M. (1983). Amer-Ind transparency. *Journal of Speech and Hearing Disorders, 48,* 103–110.

Darley, F., Brown, J., & Goldstein, N. (1972). Dysarthria in multiple sclerosis. *Journal of Speech and Hearing Research, 15,* 229–245.

Dattilo, J., Benedek-Wood, E., & McLeod, L. (2010). Activity brings community back into our lives: Recreation, leisure, and community participation for individuals who use AAC. In D.B. McNaughton & D.R. Beukelman (Eds.), *Transition strategies for adolescents and young adults who use AAC* (pp. 131–144). Baltimore: Paul H. Brookes Publishing Co.

Dattilo, J., & Camarata, S. (1991). Facilitating conversation through self-initiated augmentative communication treatment. *Journal of Applied Behavior Analysis, 24,* 369–378.

Dattilo, J., Estrella, G., Estrella, L., Light, J., McNaughton, D., & Seabury, M. (2008). "I have chosen to live life abundantly": Perceptions of leisure by adults who use augmentative and alternative communication. *Augmentative and Alternative Communication, 24,* 16–28.

Davis, G.A., & Wilcox, M.J. (1985). *Adult aphasia rehabilitation: Applied pragmatics.* San Diego: College-Hill Press.

Day, H.M., Horner, R., & O'Neill, R. (1994). Multiple functions of problem behaviors: Assessment and intervention. *Journal of Applied Behavior Analysis, 27,* 279–290.

DeCoste, D.C. (1997). Augmentative and alternative communication assessment strategies: Motor access and visual considerations. In S.L. Glennen & D.C. DeCoste (Eds.), *The handbook of augmentative and alternative communication* (pp. 243–282). San Diego: Singular.

Delange, F. (2000). The role of iodine in brain development. *Proceedings of the Nutrition Society, 59*(1), 75–79.

De La Paz, S., Owen, B., Harris, K.R., & Graham, S. (2000). Riding Elvis' motorcycle: Using self-regulated strategy development to PLAN and WRITE for a state writing exam. *Learning Disabilities Research & Practice, 15,* 101–109.

Dell, A., Newton, D.A., & Petroff, J.G. (2008). *Assistive technology in the classroom.* Upper Saddle River, NJ: Pearson Education.

DeLoache, J., Miller, K., & Rosengren, K. (1997). The credible shrinking room: Very young children's performance with symbolic and nonsymbolic relations. *Psychological Science, 8,* 308–313.

DeLoache, J., Pierroutsakos, S., & Troseth, G. (1997). The three 'R's' of pictorial competence. In R. Vasta (Ed.), *Annals of child development: A research annual* (Vol. 12, pp. 1–48). Philadelphia: Jessica Kingsley.

DeLoache, J., Pierroutsakos, S., & Uttal, D. (2003). The origins of pictorial competence. *Current Directions in Psychological Science, 12,* 114–118.

Demers, L., Weiss-Lambrou, R., & Ska, B. (2002). The Quebec User Evaluation of Satisfaction with Assistive Technology (QUEST 2.0): An overview and recent progress. *Technology and Disability, 14,* 101–105.

DePaepe, P., Reichle, J., & O'Neill, R. (1993). Applying general-case instructional strategies when teaching communicative alternatives to challenging behavior. In J. Reichle & D.P.

Wacker (Eds.), *Communicative alternatives to challenging behavior: Integrating functional assessment and intervention strategies* (pp. 237–262). Baltimore: Paul H. Brookes Publishing Co.

DePaul, R., & Yoder, D.E. (1986). Iconicity in manual sign systems for the augmentative communication user: Is that all there is? *Augmentative and Alternative Communication, 2,* 1–10.

DeRuyter, F. (1995). Only the lead dog sees the scenery? In S. Blackstone & H. Pressman (Eds.), *Outcomes in AAC conference report: Alliance '95* (pp. 13–14). Monterey, CA: Augmentative Communication.

DeRuyter, F., & Donoghue, K. (1989). Communication and traumatic brain injury: A case study. *Augmentative and Alternative Communication, 5,* 49–54.

DeRuyter, F., & Kennedy, M. (1991). Augmentative communication following traumatic brain injury. In D.R. Beukelman & K. Yorkston (Eds.), *Communication disorders following traumatic brain injury: Management of cognitive, language, and motor impairments* (pp. 317–365). Austin, TX: PRO-ED.

DeRuyter, F., & Lafontaine, L. (1987). The nonspeaking brain injured: A clinical and demographic database report. *Augmentative and Alternative Communication, 3,* 18–25.

DeRuyter, F., McNaughton, D., Caves, K., Bryen, D., & Williams, M. (2007). Enhancing AAC connections to the world. *Augmentative and Alternative Communication, 23,* 258–270.

Deshler, D.D., & Schumaker, J.B. (2006). *Teaching adolescents with disabilities: Accessing the general education curriculum.* Thousand Oaks, CA: Corwin Press.

DeThorne, K., & Schaefer, B. (2004). A guide to child nonverbal IQ measures. *American Journal of Speech-Language Pathology, 13,* 275–290.

DeThorne, L.S., Johnson, C.J., Walder, L., & Mahurin-Smith, J. (2009). When "Simon Says" doesn't work: Alternatives to imitation for facilitating early speech development. *American Journal of Speech-Language Pathology, 18,* 133–145.

Diamanti, T. (2000). Get to know me. In M. Williams & C. Krezman (Eds.), *Beneath the surface: Creative expressions of augmented communicators* (pp. 98–99). Toronto: ISAAC Press.

Didden, R., Korzilius, H., Duker, P., & Curfs, L.M. G. (2004). Communicative functioning in individuals with Angelman syndrome: A comparative study. *Disability and Rehabilitation, 26,* 1263–1267.

Dietz, A., McKelvey, M., & Beukelman, D.R. (2006). Visual scene displays (VSD): New AAC interfaces for persons with aphasia. *Perspectives on Augmentative and Alternative Communication, 15,* 13–17.

Dixon, L.S. (1981). A functional analysis of photo-object matching skills of severely retarded adolescents. *Journal of Applied Behavior Analysis, 14,* 465–478.

Doherty, J. (1985). The effects of sign characteristics on sign acquisition and retention: An integrative review of the literature. *Augmentative and Alternative Communication, 1,* 108–121.

Doherty, J., Daniloff, J., & Lloyd, L. (1985). The effect of categorical presentation on Amer-Ind transparency. *Augmentative and Alternative Communication, 1,* 10–16.

Dollaghan, C. (1987). Fast mapping in normal and language impaired children. *Journal of Speech and Hearing Disorders, 52,* 218–222.

Dongilli, P., Hakel, M., & Beukelman, D.R. (1992). Recovery of functional speech following traumatic brain injury. *Journal of Head Trauma Rehabilitation, 7,* 91–101.

Donnellan, A. (1984). The criterion of the least dangerous assumption. *Behavior Disorders, 9,* 141–150.

Donnellan, A., Mirenda, P., Mesaros, R., & Fassbender, L. (1984). Analyzing the communicative functions of aberrant behavior. *Journal of the Association for Persons with Severe Handicaps, 9,* 201–212.

Dowden, P. (1997). Augmentative and alternative communication decision making for children with severely unintelligible speech. *Augmentative and Alternative Communication, 13,* 48–58.

Dowden, P., Beukelman, D.R., & Lossing, C. (1986). Serving non-speaking patients in acute care settings: Intervention outcomes. *Augmentative and Alternative Communication, 2,* 38–44.

Dowden, P., & Cook, A.M. (2002). Choosing effective selection techniques for beginning communicators. In J. Reichle, D.R. Beukelman, & J.C. Light (Eds.), *Exemplary practices for beginning communicators: Implications for AAC* (pp. 395–429). Baltimore: Paul H. Brookes Publishing Co.

Downie, A.W., Low, J.M., & Lindsay, D.D. (1981). Speech disorders in parkinsonism: Usefulness of delayed auditory feedback in selected cases. *British Journal of Disorders of Communication, 16,* 135–139.

Downing, J. (2002). *Including students with severe and multiple disabilities in typical classrooms: Practical strategies for teachers* (2nd ed.). Baltimore: Paul H. Brookes Publishing Co.

Downing, J. (2005). *Teaching communication skills to students with severe disabilities* (2nd ed.). Baltimore: Paul H. Brookes Publishing Co.

Doyle, M., Kennedy, M.R.T., Jausalaitis, G., & Phillips, B. (2000). AAC and traumatic brain injury. In D.R. Beukelman, K.M. Yorkston, & J. Reichle (Eds.), *Augmentative and alternative communication for adults with acquired neurologic disorders* (pp. 271–304). Baltimore: Paul H. Brookes Publishing Co.

Drager, K., Hustad, K., & Gable, K. (2004). Telephone communication: Synthetic and dysarthric speech intelligibility and listener preferences. *Augmentative and Alternative Communication, 20,* 103–112.

Drager, K., Light, J., Carlson, R., D'Silva, K., Larsson, B., Pitkin, L., & Stopper, G. (2004). Learning of dynamic display technologies by typically developing 3-year-olds. *Journal of Speech, Language, and Hearing Research, 47,* 1133–1148.

Drager, K., Light, J., & Finke, E. (2009). Using AAC technologies to build social interaction with young children with autism spectrum disorders. In P. Mirenda & T. Iacono (Eds.), *Autism spectrum disorders and AAC* (pp. 247–278). Baltimore: Paul H. Brookes Publishing Co.

Drager, K., Light, J., Speltz, J., Fallon, K., & Jeffries, L. (2003). The performance of typically developing 2 1/2-year-olds on dynamic display AAC technologies with different system layouts and language organizations. *Journal of Speech, Language, and Hearing Research, 46,* 298–312.

Drager, K., Postal, V., Carrolus, L., Castellano, M., Gagliano, C., & Glynn, J. (2006). The effect of aided language modeling on symbol comprehension and production in 2 preschoolers with autism. *American Journal of Speech-Language Pathology, 15,* 112–125.

Drasgow, E., Halle, J.W., & Ostrosky, M.M. (1998). Effects of differential reinforcement on the generalization of a replacement mand in three children with severe language delays. *Journal of Applied Behavior Analysis, 31,* 357–374.

Drasgow, E., Halle, J.W., Ostroksy, M., & Harbers, H. (1996). Using behavioral indication and functional communication training to establish an initial sign repertoire with a young child with severe disabilities. *Topics in Early Childhood Special Education, 16,* 500–521.

Druin, A. (1999). Beginning a discussion about kids, technology, and design. In A. Druin (Ed.), *The design of children's technology* (pp. xiii–xxiii). San Francisco: Morgan Kaufmann.

Druin, A., Bederson, B., Boltman, A., Miura, A., Knotts-Callahan, D., & Platt, M. (1999). Children as our technology design partners. In A. Druin (Ed.), *The design of children's technology* (pp. 51–72). San Francisco: Morgan Kaufmann.

Duchan, J. (1987). Perspectives for understanding children with communicative disorders. In P. Knoblock (Ed.), *Understanding exceptional children and youth* (pp. 163–199). Boston: Little, Brown.

Duchan, J. (1995). *Supporting language learning in everyday life.* San Diego: Singular.

Dudek, K., Beck, A.R., & Thompson, J.R. (2006). The influence of AAC device type, dynamic vs. static screen, on peer attitudes. *Journal of Special Education Technology, 21,* 17–27.

Duffy , J. (2000). Primary progressive aphasia. *ASHA Leader, 5,* 94.

Duffy, J. (2005). Primary progressive aphasia and primary progressive apraxia of speech: An update. *ASHA Leader, 9,* 120.

Duffy, J.R., Peach, R.K., & Strand, E.A. (2007). Progressive apraxia of speech as a sign of motor neuron disease. *American Journal of Speech-Language Pathology, 16,* 198–208.

Dugan, E., Kamps, D., Leonard, B., Watkins, N., Rheinberger, A., & Stackhaus, J. (1995). Effects of cooperative learning groups during social studies for students with autism and fourth-grade peers. *Journal of Applied Behavior Analysis, 28,* 175–188.

Duker, P., & Jutten, W. (1997). Establishing gestural yes-no responding with individuals with profound mental retardation. *Education and Training in Mental Retardation and Developmental Disabilities, 32,* 59–67.

Duker, P.C., Kraaykamp, M., & Visser, E. (1994). A stimulus control procedure to increase requesting with individuals who are severely/profoundly intellectually disabled. *Journal of Intellectual Disability Research, 38,* 177–186.

Dunham, J. (1989). The transparency of manual signs in a linguistic and an environmental nonlinguistic context. *Augmentative and Alternative Communication, 5,* 214–225.

Dunlap, G., Iovannone, R., Kincaid, D., Wilson, K., Christiansen, K., Strain, P., & English, C. (2010). *Prevent-Teach-Reinforce: The school-based model of individualized positive behavior support.* Baltimore: Paul H. Brookes Publishing Co.

Dunn, L.M., & Dunn, L.M. (1981). *Peabody Picture Vocabulary Test–Revised.* Circle Pines, MN: American Guidance Service.

Dunn, L.M., & Dunn, L.M. (2007). *Peabody Picture Vocabulary Test–Fourth Edition (PPVT-4)*. San Antonio, TX: Pearson Assessments.

Durand, V.M. (1990). *Severe behavior problems.* New York: Guilford Press.

Durand, V.M. (1993). Functional communication training using assistive devices: Effects on challenging behavior. *Augmentative and Alternative Communication, 9,* 168–176.

Durand, V.M. (1999). Functional communication training using assistive devices: Recruiting natural communities of reinforcement. *Journal of Applied Behavior Analysis, 32,* 247–267.

Durand, V.M., & Carr, E.G. (1987). Social influences on self-stimulatory behavior: Analysis and treatment application. *Journal of Applied Behavior Analysis, 20,* 119–132.

Durand, V.M., & Carr, E. (1991). Functional communication training to reduce challenging behavior: Maintenance and application in new settings. *Journal of Applied Behavior Analysis, 24,* 251–264.

Durand, V.M., & Kishi, G. (1987). Reducing severe behavior problems among persons with dual sensory impairments: An evaluation of a technical assistance model. *Journal of the Association for Persons with Severe Handicaps, 12,* 2–10.

Dykens, E.M., Hodapp, R.M., & Finucane, B.M. (2000). *Genetics and mental retardation syndromes: A new look at behavior and interventions.* Baltimore: Paul H. Brookes Publishing Co.

Edmonds, R. (1979). Some schools work and more can. *Social Policy, 9*(5), 25–29.

Ehri, L., Nunes, S., Willows, D., Schuster, B., Yaghoub-Zadeh, Z., & Shanahan, T. (2001). Phonemic awareness instruction helps children learn to read: Evidence from the National Reading Panel's meta-analysis. *Reading Research Quarterly, 36,* 250–287.

Ekman, P. (1976). Movements with precise meanings. *Journal of Communication, 26,* 14–26.

Ekman, P., & Friesen, W. (1969). The repertoire of nonverbal behavior: Categories, origin, usage, and coding. *Semiotica, 1,* 49–98.

Elder, P., & Goossens', C. (1994). *Engineering training environments for interactive augmentative communication: Strategies for adolescents and adults who are moderately/severely developmentally delayed.* Birmingham, AL: Southeast Augmentative Communication Conference Publications.

Elder, P., & Goossens', C. (1996). *Communication overlays for engineering training environments: Overlays for adolescents and adults who are moderately/severely developmentally delayed.* Solana Beach, CA: Mayer-Johnson.

Ellis, E., Deshler, D., Lenz, B., Schumaker, J., & Clark, F. (1991). An instructional model for teaching learning strategies. *Focus on Exceptional Children, 23*(6), 1–24.

Emery, M.-P., Perrier, L.-L., & Acquadro, C. (2005). Patient-reported outcome and quality of life instruments database (PROQOLID): Frequently asked questions. *Health and Quality of Life Outcomes, 3,* 1–6.

Enderby, P., & Crow, E. (1990). Long-term recovery patterns of severe dysarthria following head injury. *British Journal of Disorders of Communication, 25,* 341–354.

Enderby, P., & Philipp, R. (1986). Speech and language handicap: Towards knowing the size of the problem. *British Journal of Disorders of Communication, 21,* 151–165.

Erickson, K. (2003, June 24). Reading comprehension in AAC. *ASHA Leader, 8*(12), 6–9.

Erickson, K.A., & Clendon, S.A. (2009). Addressing the literacy demands of the curriculum for beginning readers and writers. In G. Soto & C. Zangari (Eds.), *Practically speaking: Language, literacy, and academic development for students with AAC needs* (pp. 195–215). Baltimore: Paul H. Brookes Publishing Co.

Erickson, K.A., Clendon, S., Abraham, L., Roy, V., & Van de Carr, H. (2005). Toward positive literacy outcomes for students with significant developmental disabilities. *Assistive Technology Outcomes and Benefits, 2,* 45–54.

Erickson, K.A., & Koppenhaver, D.A. (1995). Developing a literacy program for children with severe disabilities. *Reading Teacher, 48,* 676–684.

Erickson, K.A., & Koppenhaver, D. (2007). *Children with disabilities: Reading and writing the four-blocks way.* Greensboro, NC: Carson-Dellosa.

Erickson, K.A., Koppenhaver, D.A., Yoder, D.E., & Nance, J. (1997). Integrated communication and literacy instruction for a child with multiple disabilities. *Focus on Autism and Other Developmental Disabilities, 12,* 142–150.

Erickson, R.J., Goldinger, S.D., & LaPointe, L.L. (1996). Auditory vigilance in aphasia individuals: Detecting nonlinguistic stimuli with full or divided attention. *Brain and Cognition, 30,* 244–253.

Eskildsen, M. (2007). Long-term acute care: A review of literature. *Journal of the American Geriatrics Society, 55,* 775–779.

Estrella, G. (2000). Confessions of a blabber finger. In M. Fried-Oken & H.A. Bersani, Jr. (Eds.), *Speaking up and spelling it out: Personal essays on augmentative and alternative communication* (pp. 31–45). Baltimore: Paul H. Brookes Publishing Co.

Fager, S. (2003, November). *AAC use across multiple settings.* Presentation at the annual convention of the American Speech-Language-Hearing Association, Philadelphia.

Fager, S., & Beukelman, D. (2009). *Supporting communication of individuals with minimal movement* [Webcast]. Retrieved from http://aac-rerc.psu.edu/index.php/webcasts/show/id/14

Fager, S., Beukelman, D., Jakobs, T., & Hossum, J.P. (2010). Evaluation of a speech recognition prototype for speakers with moderate and severe dysarthria: A preliminary report. *Augmentative and Alternative Communication, 26,* 267–277.

Fager, S., Doyle, M., & Karantounis, R. (2007). Traumatic brain injury. In D.R. Beukelman, K.L. Garrett, & K.M. Yorkston (Eds.), *Augmentative communication strategies for adults with acute or chronic medical conditions* (pp. 131–162. Baltimore: Paul H. Brookes Publishing Co.

Fager, S., Hux, K., Karantounis, R., & Beukelman, D.R. (2004). Augmentative and alternative communication use and acceptance by adults with traumatic brain injury. *Augmentative and Alternative Communication, 22,* 37–47.

Fager, S., & Karantounis, R. (2011). AAC assessment and intervention in TBI. In K. Hux (Ed.), *Assisting survivors of traumatic brain injury: The role of speech-language pathologists* (2nd ed.). Austin, TX: PRO-ED.

Fallon, K., Light, J., & Achenbach, A. (2003). The semantic organization patterns of young children: Implications for augmentative and alternative communication. *Augmentative and Alternative Communication, 19,* 74–85.

Fallon, K.A., Light, J., McNaughton, D., Drager, K., & Hammer, C. (2004). The effects of direct instruction on the single-word reading skills of children who require augmentative and alternative communication. *Journal of Speech, Language, and Hearing Research, 47,* 1424–1439.

Fallon, K., Light, J., & Paige, T. (2001). Enhancing vocabulary selection for preschoolers who require augmentative and alternative communication (AAC). *American Journal of Speech-Language Pathology, 10,* 81–94.

Falvey, M.A. (1989). *Community-based curriculum: Instructional strategies for students with severe handicaps.* Baltimore: Paul H. Brookes Publishing Co.

Farrier, L., Yorkston, K., Marriner, N., & Beukelman, D.R. (1985). Conversational control in nonimpaired speakers using an augmentative communication system. *Augmentative and Alternative Communication, 1,* 65–73.

Fay, W., & Schuler, A. (1980). *Emerging language in autistic children.* Baltimore: University Park Press.

Fenson, L., Dale, P.S., Reznick, J.S., Bates, E., Thal, D., & Pethick, S. (1994). Variability in early communicative development. *Monographs of the Society for Research in Child Development, 59,* 1–173.

Fenson, L., Marchman, V.A., Thal, D.J., Dale, P.S., Reznick, J.S., & Bates, E. (2007). *MacArthur-Bates Communicative Development Inventories* (2nd ed.). Baltimore: Paul H. Brookes Publishing Co.

Ferm, U., Sahlin, A., Sundin, L., & Hartelius, L. (2010). Using Talking Mats to support communication in persons with Huntington's disease. *International Journal of Language and Communication Disorders, 45,* 523–536.

Fey, M. (2008). Thoughts on grammar intervention in AAC. *Perspectives on Augmentative and Alternative Communication, 17,* 43–49.

Feys, P., Romberg, A., Ruutiainen, J., Davies-Smith, A., Jones, R., Avizzano, C.,…Ketelaer, P. (2001). Assistive technology to improve PC interaction for people with intention tremor. *Journal of Rehabilitation Research and Development, 38,* 235–243.

File, P., & Todman, J. (2002). Evaluation of the coherence of computer-aided conversations. *Augmentative and Alternative Communication, 18,* 228–241.

Finke, E., Light, J., & Kitko, L. (2008). A systematic review of the effectiveness of nurse communication with patients with complex communication needs with a focus on the use of augmentative and alternative communication. *Journal of Clinical Nursing, 17,* 2102–2115.

Fitzgerald, M.M., Sposato, B., Politano, P., Hetling, J., & O'Neill, W. (2009). Three head-controlled mouse emulators in three light conditions. *Augmentative and Alternative Communication, 25,* 32–41.

Flannery, B., & Horner, R. (1994). The relationship between predictability and problem behavior for students with severe disabilities. *Journal of Behavioral Education, 4,* 157–176.

Flippin, M., Reszka, S., & Watson, L. (2010). Effectiveness of the Picture Exchange Communication Systems (PECS) on communication and speech for children with autism spectrum disorders: A meta-analysis. *American Journal of Speech-Language Pathology, 19,* 178–195.

Foley, B.E. (1993). The development of literacy in individuals with severe congenital speech and motor impairments. *Topics in Language Disorders, 13*(2), 16–32.

Foley, B., & Pollatsek, A. (1999). Phonological processing and reading abilities in adolescents and adults with severe congenital speech impairments. *Augmentative and Alternative Communication, 15,* 156–173.

Foley, B.E., & Wolter, J. (2010). Literacy intervention for transition-aged youth: What is and what could be. In D.B. McNaughton & D.R. Beukelman (Eds.), *Transition strategies for adolescents and young adults who use AAC* (pp. 35–68). Baltimore: Paul H. Brookes Publishing Co.

Folstein, S.E. (1990). *Huntington disease: A disorder of families.* Baltimore: Johns Hopkins University Press.

Ford, A., & Mirenda, P. (1984). Community instruction: A natural cues and corrections decision model. *Journal of the Association for Persons with Severe Handicaps, 9,* 79–87.

Ford, H., Trigwell, P., & Johnson, M. (1998). The nature of fatigue in multiple sclerosis. *Journal of Psychosomatic Research, 45*(1), 33–38.

Fossett, B., & Mirenda, P. (2006). Sight word reading in children with developmental disabilities: A comparison of paired associate and picture-to-text matching instruction. *Research in Developmental Disabilities, 27,* 411–429.

Foulks, B., & Morrow, R. (1989). Academic survival skills for the young child at risk for school failure. *Journal of Educational Research, 82,* 158–165.

Fox, L., & Fried-Oken, M. (1996). AAC aphasiology: Partnership for future research. *Augmentative and Alternative Communication, 12,* 257–271.

Fox, L.E., Ginley, S., & Poulsen, S. (2004). A residential approach to conversational intervention. *Special Interest Division 2 Newsletter: Neurophysiology and Neurogenic Speech and Language Disorders, 14*(4), 4–10.

Fox, L., Sohlberg, M.M., & Fried-Oken, M. (2001). Effects of conversational topic choice on outcomes of an augmentative communication intervention for adults with aphasia. *Aphasiology, 15,* 171–200.

Fox, M.J. (2002). *Lucky man: A memoir.* New York: Random House.

Franklin, N.K., Mirenda, P., & Phillips, G. (1996). Comparisons of five symbol assessment protocols with nondisabled preschoolers and learners with severe intellectual disabilities. *Augmentative and Alternative Communication, 12,* 73–77.

Frattali, C.M., Holland, A.L., Thompson, C.K., Wohl, C., & Ferketic, M. (2003). *Functional Assessment of Communication Skills for Adults (ASHA FACS).* Rockville, MD: American Speech-Language-Hearing Association.

Frea, W.D., Arnold, C.L., & Vittemberga, G.L. (2001). A demonstration of the effects of augmentative communication on extreme aggressive behavior of a child with autism within an integrated preschool setting. *Journal of Positive Behavior Interventions, 3,* 194–198.

French, J.L. (2001). *Pictorial Test of Intelligence–Second Edition (PTI-2).* Austin, TX: PRO-ED.

Fried-Oken, M. (2001). Been there, done that: A very personal introduction to the special issue on augmentative and alternative communication and acquired disorders. *Augmentative and Alternative Communication, 17,* 138–140.

Fried-Oken, M., Ball, L., Golinker, L., Lasker, J., Mathy, P., & Ourand, P. (2002, November). *AAC challenges in adults with acquired neurological impairment.* Session presented at the American Speech-Language-Hearing Association Convention, Atlanta, GA.

Fried-Oken, M., & Bersani, H.A., Jr. (Eds.). (2000). *Speaking up and spelling it out: Personal essays on augmentative and alternative communication.* Baltimore: Paul H. Brookes Publishing Co.

Fried-Oken, M., & Doyle, M. (1992). Language representation for the augmentative and alternative communication of adults with traumatic brain injury. *Journal of Head Trauma Rehabilitation, 7*(3), 59–69.

Fried-Oken, M., Howard, J., & Stewart, S. (1991). Feedback on AAC intervention from adults who are temporarily unable to speak. *Augmentative and Alternative Communication, 7,* 43–50.

Fried-Oken, M., & More, L. (1992). An initial vocabulary for nonspeaking preschool children based on developmental and environmental language sources. *Augmentative and Alternative Communication, 8,* 41–56.

Fried-Oken, M., Rau, M., Fox, L., Tulman, J., & Hindal, M. (2004). ALS, AAC technology and caregivers: Attitudes, skills, and role strain. *ASHA Leader, 9,* 98.

Fried-Oken, M., Rau, M.T., & Oken, B.S. (2000). AAC and dementia. In D.R. Beukelman, K.M. Yorkston, & J. Reichle (Eds.), *Augmentative and alternative communication for adults with acquired neurologic disorders* (pp. 375–405). Baltimore: Paul H. Brookes Publishing Co.

Fried-Oken, M., Rowland, C., Baker, G., Dixon, M., Mills, C., Schultz, D., & Oken, B. (2009). The effect of voice output on the AAC-supported conversations of persons with Alzheimer's disease. *ACM Transactions on Accessible Computing, 1*(3), 15.

Fried-Oken, M., Rowland, C., & Gibbon, C. (2010). Providing augmentative and alternative communication treatment to persons with progressive nonfluent aphasia. *Perspectives on Neurophysiology and Neurogenic Speech and Language Disorders, 20,* 21–25.

Frost, L., & Bondy, A. (2002). *Picture Exchange Communication System training manual* (2nd ed.). Newark, DE: Pyramid Education Products.

Fuchs, L.S., Fuchs, D., Hosp, M., & Jenkins, J. (2001). Oral reading fluency as an indicator of reading competence: A theoretical, empirical, and historical analysis. *Scientific Studies of Reading, 5,* 239–256.

Fujisawa, K., Inoue, T., Yamana, Y., & Hayashi, H. (2011). The effect of animation on learning action symbols by individuals with intellectual disabilities. *Augmentative and Alternative Communication, 27,* 53–60.

Fuller, D., & Lloyd, L. (1991). Toward a common usage of iconicity terminology. *Augmentative and Alternative Communication, 7,* 215–220.

Fuller, D., Lloyd, L., & Schlosser, R. (1992). Further development of an augmentative and alternative communication symbol taxonomy. *Augmentative and Alternative Communication, 8,* 67–74.

Fuller, D., Lloyd, L., & Stratton, M. (1997). Aided AAC symbols. In L. Lloyd, D. Fuller, & H. Arvidson (Eds.), *Augmentative and alternative communication: Principles and practice* (pp. 48–79). Needham Heights, MA: Allyn & Bacon.

Gallagher, K.C., & Mayer, K. (2008). Enhancing development and learning through teacher-child relationships. *Young Children, 63,* 80–87.

Galvin, J., & Donnell, C. (2002). Educating the consumer and caretaker on assistive technology. In M. Scherer (Ed.), *Assistive technology: Matching device and consumer for successful rehabilitation* (pp. 153–167). Washington, DC: American Psychological Association.

Galvin, J., & Scherer, M. (1996). *Evaluating, selecting, and using appropriate assistive technology.* Gaithersburg, MD: Aspen.

Gardner, H. (2006). Training others in the art of therapy for speech sound disorders: An interactional approach. *Child Language Teaching and Therapy, 22,* 27–46.

Garrett, K. (1995). Changes in the interaction patterns of individuals with severe aphasia given three types of partner support. *Clinical Aphasiology, 23,* 237–251.

Garrett, K., & Beukelman, D.R. (1992). Augmentative communication approaches for persons with severe aphasia. In K. Yorkston (Ed.), *Augmentative communication in the medical setting* (pp. 245–338). Tucson, AZ: Communication Skill Builders.

Garrett, K., & Beukelman, D.R. (1995). Changes in the interaction patterns of an individual with severe aphasia given three types of partner support. In M. Lemme (Ed.), *Clinical aphasiology* (Vol. 23, pp. 237–251). Austin, TX: PRO-ED.

Garrett, K., & Beukelman, D. (1998). Adults with severe aphasia. In D.R. Beukelman & P. Mirenda (Eds.), *Augmentative and alternative communication: Management of severe communication disorders in children and adults* (pp. 465–499). Baltimore: Paul H. Brookes Publishing Co.

Garrett, K., Beukelman, D.R., & Low-Morrow, D. (1989). A comprehensive augmentative communication system for an adult with Broca's aphasia. *Augmentative and Alternative Communication, 5,* 55–61.

Garrett, K., Happ, B., Costello, J., & Fried-Oken, M. (2007). AAC in the intensive care unit. In D.R. Beukelman, K.L. Garrett, & K.M. Yorkston (Eds.), *Augmentative communication strategies for adults with acute or chronic medical conditions* (pp. 17–57). Baltimore: Paul H. Brookes Publishing Co.

Garrett, K.L., & Huth, C. (2002). The impact of graphic contextual information and instruction on the conversational behaviors of an individual with severe aphasia. *Aphasiology, 16,* 523–536.

Garrett, K.L., & Kimelman, M.D.Z. (2000). AAC and aphasia: Cognitive-linguistic considerations. In D.R. Beukelman, K.M. Yorkston, & J. Reichle (Eds.), *Augmentative and alternative communication for adults with acquired neurologic disorders* (pp. 339–374). Baltimore: Paul H. Brookes Publishing Co.

Garrett, K.L., & Lasker, J. (2004). Aphasia assessment materials. Retrieved from http://aac.unl.edu/screen/screen.html

Garrett, K., Schutz-Muehling, L., & Morrow, D. (1990). Low level head injury: A novel AAC approach. *Augmentative and Alternative Communication, 6,* 124.

Garrett, K., Staab, L., & Agocs, L. (1996, November). *Perceptions of scaffolded letters generated by a person with aphasia.* Paper presented at the annual convention of the American Speech-Language-Hearing Association, Seattle.

Gee, K., Graham, N., Goetz, L., Oshima, G., & Yoshioka, K. (1991). Teaching students to request the continuation of routine activities by using time delay and decreasing physical assistance in the context of chain interruption. *Journal of the Association for Persons with Severe Handicaps, 16,* 154–167.

Gerra, L., Dorfman, S., Plaue, E., Schlackman, S., & Workman, D. (1995). Functional communication as a means of decreasing self-injurious behavior: A case study. *Journal of Visual Impairment and Blindness, 89,* 343–347.

Gersten, R., Fuchs, L.S., Williams, J.P., & Baker, S. (2001). Teaching reading comprehension strategies to students with learning disabilities: A review of research. *Review of Educational Research, 71,* 279–320.

Giangreco, M.F. (1996). Choosing options and accommodations for children (COACH): Curriculum planning for students with disabilities in general education. In S. Stainback & W. Stainback (Eds.), *Inclusion: A guide for educators* (pp. 237–254). Baltimore: Paul H. Brookes Publishing Co.

Giangreco, M.F., Cloninger, C.J., & Iverson, V.S. (2011). *Choosing options and accommodations for children: A guide to educational planning for students with disabilities* (3rd ed.). Baltimore: Paul H. Brookes Publishing Co.

Gierach, J. (2009). *Assessing students' needs for assistive technology: A resource manual for school district teams* (5th ed.). Milton, WI: Wisconsin Assistive Technology Initiative.

Glennen, S. (1997). Augmentative and alternative communication assessment strategies. In S.L. Glennen & D. DeCoste (Eds.), *The handbook of augmentative and alternative communication* (pp. 149–192). San Diego: Singular.

Glennen, S.L., & DeCoste, D. (1997). *The handbook of augmentative and alternative communication.* San Diego: Singular.

Gleser, G., Gottschalk, L., & John, W. (1959). The relationship of sex and intelligence to choice words: A normative study of verbal behavior. *Journal of Clinical Psychology, 15,* 182–191.

Goetz, L., Gee, K., & Sailor, W. (1983). Crossmodal transfer of stimulus control: Preparing students with severe multiple disabilities for audiological assessment. *Journal of the Association for Persons with Severe Handicaps, 8,* 3–13.

Goldbart, J., & Marshall, J. (2004). "Pushes and pulls" on the parents of children who use AAC. *Augmentative and Alternative Communication, 20,* 194–208.

Goldman-Eisler, F. (1986). *Cycle linguistics: Experiments in spontaneous speech.* New York: Academic Press.

Goldstein, H. (2002). Communication intervention for children with autism: A review of treatment efficacy. *Journal of Autism and Developmental Disorders, 32,* 373–396.

Goodglass, H. (1980). Naming disorders and aging. In L. Obler & M. Alberts (Eds.), *Language and communication* (pp. 35–47). Lexington, MA: Lexington Books.

Goodglass, H., & Kaplan, E. (1983). *Boston Diagnostic Aphasia Examination* (2nd ed.). Philadelphia: Lea & Febiger.

Goodglass, H., Kaplan, E., & Barresi, B. (2000). *The Boston Diagnostic Aphasia Examination: Short form record booklet* (3rd ed.). Philadelphia: Lippincott, Williams & Wilkins.

Goossens', C. (1989). Aided communication intervention before assessment: A case study of a child with cerebral palsy. *Augmentative and Alternative Communication, 5,* 14–26.

Goossens', C. (2010). *Aided language stimulation update.* Paper presented at the biennial conference of the International Society for Augmentative and Alternative Communication, Barcelona, Spain.

Goossens', C., & Crain, S. (1986a). *Augmentative communication assessment resource.* Wauconda, IL: Don Johnston.

Goossens', C., & Crain, S. (1986b). *Augmentative communication intervention resource.* Wauconda, IL: Don Johnston.

Goossens', C., & Crain, S. (1987). Overview of nonelectronic eye-gaze communication devices. *Augmentative and Alternative Communication, 3,* 77–89.

Goossens', C., & Crain, S. (1992). *Utilizing switch interfaces with children who are severely physically challenged*. Austin, TX: PRO-ED.

Goossens', C., Crain, S., & Elder, P. (1992). *Engineering the preschool environment for interactive symbolic communication*. Birmingham, AL: Southeast Augmentative Communication Conference Publications.

Goossens', C., Crain, S., & Elder, P. (1994). *Communication displays for engineered preschool environments: Books 1 and 2*. Solana Beach, CA: Mayer-Johnson.

Goossens', C., Crain, S., & Elder, P. (1995). *Engineering the preschool environment for interactive symbolic communication: 18 months to 5 years developmentally* (3rd ed.). Birmingham, AL: Southeast Augmentative Communication Conference Publications.

Gorenflo, C., & Gorenflo, D. (1991). The effects of information and augmentative communication technique on attitudes toward nonspeaking individuals. *Journal of Speech and Hearing Research, 34*, 19–26.

Graham, S., & Perin, D. (2007). *Writing next: Effective strategies to improve writing of adolescents in middle and high school: A report to the Carnegie Corporation of New York*. New York: Alliance for Excellent Education.

Grandin, T. (1995). *Thinking in pictures and other reports from my life with autism*. New York: Vintage Books.

Grandin, T., & Scariano, M. (1986). *Emergence: Labeled autistic*. Novato, CA: Arena Press.

Granlund, M., & Blackstone, S. (1999). Outcomes measurement in AAC. In F.T. Loncke, J. Clibbens, H. Arvidson, & L.L. Lloyd (Eds.), *Augmentative and alternative communication: New directions in research and practice* (pp. 207–227). London: Whurr.

Granlund, M., & Olsson, C. (1987). Talspråksalternativ kommunikation och begåvningshandikapp [Alternative communication and mental retardation]. Stockholm: Stiftelsen ALA.

Green, V., O'Reilly, M., Itchon, J., & Sigafoos, J. (2005). Persistence of early emerging aberrant behavior in children with developmental disabilities. *Research in Developmental Disabilities, 26*, 47–55.

Greenspan, S., & Weider, S. (1999). A functional developmental approach to autism spectrum disorders. *Journal of the Association for Persons with Severe Handicaps, 24*, 147–161.

Gregory, M., DeLeon, I., & Richman, D. (2009). The influence of matching and motor-imitation abilities on rapid acquisition of manual signs and exchanged-based communicative responses. *Journal of Applied Behavior Analysis, 42*, 399–404.

Gregory, C., & McNaughton, S. (1993, September). Language! Welcoming a parent's perspective. *Communicating Together, 11*(3), 21–23.

Grove, N., & Walker, M. (1990). The Makaton Vocabulary: Using manual signs and graphic symbols to develop interpersonal communication. *Augmentative and Alternative Communication, 6*, 15–28.

Guralnick, M.J. (2001). Social competence with peers and early childhood inclusion: Need for alternative approaches. In M.J. Guralnick (Ed.), *Early childhood inclusion: Focus on change* (pp. 481–502). Baltimore: Paul H. Brookes Publishing Co.

Gustason, G., & Zawolkow, E. (1993). *Signing exact English*. Los Alamitos, CA: Modern Signs Press.

Gutmann, M. (1999, November). *The communication continuum in ALS: Client preferences and communication competence*. Paper presented at the annual convention of the American Speech-Language-Hearing Association, San Francisco.

Gutmann, M., & Gryfe, P. (1996, August). *The communication continuum in ALS: Critical paths and client preferences*. Proceedings of the seventh biennial conference of the International Society of Augmentative and Alternative Communication (ISAAC), Vancouver, Canada.

Hagen, C. (1984). Language disorders in head trauma. In A. Holland (Ed.), *Language disorders in adults* (pp. 245–281). Austin, TX: PRO-ED.

Hains, A.H., Fowler, S., Schwartz, I., Kottwitz, E., & Rosenkoetter, S. (1989). A comparison of preschool and kindergarten teacher expectations for school readiness. *Early Childhood Education Quarterly, 4*, 75–88.

Hall, P. (2000a). A letter to the parent(s) of a child with developmental apraxia of speech, Part 1: Speech characteristics of the disorder. *Language, Speech, and Hearing Services in Schools, 31*, 169–172.

Hall, P. (2000b). A letter to the parent(s) of a child with developmental apraxia of speech, Part 2: The nature and causes of DAS. *Language, Speech, and Hearing Services in Schools, 31*, 173–175.

Hall, P. (2000c). A letter to the parent(s) of a child with developmental apraxia of speech, Part 3: Other problems often associated with DAS. *Language, Speech, and Hearing Services in Schools, 31,* 176–178.

Hall, P. (2000d). A letter to the parent(s) of a child with developmental apraxia of speech, Part 4: Treatment of DAS. *Language, Speech, and Hearing Services in Schools, 31,* 179–181.

Halle, J., Baer, D., & Spradlin, J. (1981). Teacher's generalized use of delay as a stimulus control procedure to increase language use in handicapped children. *Journal of Applied Behavior Analysis, 14,* 389–409.

Halle, J., Brady, N., & Drasgow, E. (2004). Enhancing socially adaptive communicative repairs of beginning communicators with disabilities. *American Journal of Speech-Language Pathology, 13,* 43–54.

Halle, J., & Drasgow, E. (1995). Teaching social communication to young children with severe disabilities. *Topics in Early Childhood Special Education, 15,* 164–186.

Hamm, B., & Mirenda, P. (2006). Post-school quality of life of individuals with complex communication needs. *Augmentative and Alternative Communication, 22,* 134–147.

Hammill, D., Pearson, N., & Wiederholt, J.L. (2009). *Comprehensive Test of Nonverbal Intelligence–Second Edition (CTONI-2).* Austin, TX: PRO-ED.

Hamre, B.K., & Pianta, R.C. (2001). Early teacher–child relationships and the trajectory of children's school outcomes through eighth grade. *Child Development, 72,* 625–638.

Hanley, G., Iwata, B., & Thompson, R. (2001). Reinforcement schedule thinning following treatment with functional communication training. *Journal of Applied Behavior Analysis, 34,* 17–38.

Hanser, G.A., & Erickson, K.A. (2007). Integrated word identification and communication instruction for students with complex communication needs. *Focus on Autism and Other Developmental Disabilities, 22,* 268–278.

Hanson, E. (2007). Documentation in AAC using goal attainment scaling. *Perspectives on Augmentative and Alternative Communication, 16,* 6–9.

Hanson, E.K., & Sundheimer, C. (2009). Telephone talk: Effects of timing and use of a floorholder message on telephone conversations using synthesized speech. *Augmentative and Alternative Communication, 25,* 90–98.

Hanson, E., Yorkston, K., & Beukelman, D.R. (2004). Speech supplementation techniques for dysarthria: A systematic review. *Journal of Medical Speech Language Pathology, 12,* ix–xxix.

Hanson, E., Yorkston, K., & Britton, D. (2011). Dysarthria in amyotrophic lateral sclerosis: A systematic review of the characteristics, speech treatment, and AAC options. *Journal of Medical Speech Language Pathology, 19,* 2–30.

Hanson, W., & Metter, E. (1983). DAF speech rate modification in Parkinson's disease: A report of two cases. In W. Berry (Ed.), *Clinical dysarthria* (pp. 231–254). Austin, TX: PRO-ED.

Harradine, C., & Clifford, R. (1996). *When are children ready for kindergarten? Views of families, kindergarten teachers, and child care providers.* Paper presented at the Annual Meeting of the American Educational Research Association, New York.

Harris, L., Doyle, E.S., & Haaf, R. (1996). Language treatment approach for users of AAC: Experimental single-subject investigation. *Augmentative and Alternative Communication, 12,* 230–243.

Harris, M., & Reichle, J. (2004). The impact of aided language stimulation on symbol comprehension and production in children with moderate cognitive disabilities. *American Journal of Speech-Language Pathology, 13,* 155–167.

Harrison-Harris, O. (2002, November 5). AAC, literacy and bilingualism. *ASHA Leader Online, 20.* Retrieved from http://www.asha.org/Publications/leader/2002/021105/f021105.htm

Hart, B., & Risley, T. (1982). *How to use incidental teaching for elaborating language.* Lawrence, KS: H & H.

Hart, B., & Risley, T.R. (1995). *Meaningful differences in the everyday experience of young American children.* Baltimore: Paul H. Brookes Publishing Co.

Hart, B., & Risley, T.R. (1999). *The social world of children learning to talk.* Baltimore: Paul H. Brookes Publishing Co.

Hart, P., Scherz, J., Apel, K., & Hodson, B. (2007). Analysis of spelling error patterns of individuals with complex communication needs and physical impairments. *Augmentative and Alternative Communication, 23,* 16–29.

Hartelius, L., Runmarker, B., & Andersen, O. (2000). Prevalence and characteristics of dysarthria in a multiple sclerosis incidence cohort: In relation to neurological data. *Folia Phoniatrica et Logopaedica, 52,* 160–177.

Hartelius, L., & Svensson, P. (1994). Speech and swallowing symptoms associated with Parkinson's disease and multiple sclerosis: A survey. *Folia Phoniatrica et Logopaedica, 46,* 9–17.

Haupt, L., & Alant, E. (2002). The iconicity of picture communication symbols for rural Zulu children. *South African Journal of Communication Disorders, 49,* 40–49.

Hawking, S. (2003). Intel Worldwide Employee Communications [Interview].

Hayes, J.R. (2000). A new framework for understanding cognition and affect in writing. In R. Indrisano & J. Squire (Eds.), *Perspectives on writing: Research, theory, and practice* (pp. 6–44). Newark, DE: International Reading Association.

Heaton, E., Beliveau, C., & Blois, T. (1995). Outcomes in assistive technology. *Journal of Speech-Language Pathology and Audiology, 19,* 233–240.

Hedrick, D., Prather, E., & Tobin, A. (1984). *Sequenced Inventory of Communication Development–Revised.* Torrance, CA: Western Psychological Services.

Heine, K., Wilkerson, R., & Kennedy, T. (1996, May). *Unity now and later: Equipping a two-year-old now, while preparing in the future.* Paper presented at the 1996 Minspeak conference, Wooster, OH.

Heller, K., Allgood, M., Ware, S., Arnold, S., & Castelle, M. (1996). Initiating requests during community-based vocational training by students with mental retardation and sensory impairments. *Research in Developmental Disabilities, 17,* 173–184.

Heller, K.W., Fredrick, L.D., Tumlin, J., & Brineman, D.G. (2002). Teaching decoding for generalization using the nonverbal reading approach. *Journal of Developmental and Physical Disabilities, 14,* 19–35.

Heller, K., Ware, S., Allgood, M., & Castelle, M. (1994). Use of dual communication boards with students who are deaf-blind. *Journal of Visual Impairment and Blindness, 88,* 368–376.

Helm-Estabrooks, N. (1984). Severe aphasia. In A. Holland (Ed.), *Language disorders in adults* (pp. 159–176). San Diego: College-Hill Press.

Helm-Estabrooks, N. (2001). *Cognitive Linguistic Quick Test.* San Antonio, TX: Harcourt Assessment.

Helm-Estabrooks, N. (2002, March–April). Cognition and aphasia: A discussion and a study. *Journal of Communication Disorders, 35,* 171–186.

Helm-Estabrooks, N., Ramsberger, G., Morgan, A.R., & Nicholas, M. (1989). *Boston Assessment of Severe Aphasia (BASA).* Austin, TX: PRO-ED.

Herbert, L.E., Scherr, P.A., Bienias, J.L., Bennet, D.A., & Evans, D.A. (2003). Alzheimer disease in the US population: Prevalence estimates using the 2000 census. *Archives of Neurology, 60,* 1119–1122.

Hetzroni, O. (2002). Augmentative and alternative communication in Israel: Results from a family survey. *Augmentative and Alternative Communication, 18,* 255–266.

Hetzroni, R., & Harris, O. (1996). Cultural aspects in the development of AAC users. *Augmentative and Alternative Communication, 12,* 52–58.

Hieneman, M., Childs, K., & Sergay, J. (2006). *Parenting with positive behavior support: A practical guide to resolving your child's difficult behavior.* Baltimore: Paul H. Brookes Publishing Co.

Higginbotham, D. (1989). The interplay of communication device output mode and interaction style between nonspeaking persons and their speaking partners. *Journal of Speech and Hearing Disorders, 54,* 320–333.

Higginbotham, D.J., Bisantz, A., Sunm, M., Adams, K., & Yik, F. (2009). The effect of context priming and task type on augmentative communication performance. *Augmentative and Alternative Communication, 25,* 19–31.

Higginbotham, D.J., Moulton, B., Lesher, G., Wilkins, D., & Cornish, J. (2000). Frametalker: Development of a frame-based communication system. In *Proceedings of the 2000 CSUN Annual Conference.* Northridge: California State University at Northridge. Retrieved from http://www.csun.edu/cod/conf/2000/proceedings/0156Higginbotham.htm

Higginbotham, D.J., & Wilkins, D. (2006). The short story of Frametalker: An interactive AAC device. *Perspectives on Augmentative and Alternative Communication, 15,* 18–22.

Hill, K. (2004). Augmentative and alternative communication and language: Evidence-based practice and language activity monitoring. *Topics in Language Disorders, 245,* 18–30.

Hirdes, J., Ellis-Hale, K., & Pearson Hirdes, B. (1993). Prevalence and policy implications of communication disabilities among adults. *Augmentative and Alternative Communication, 9,* 273–280.

Ho, K., Weiss, S., Garrett, K., & Lloyd, L.L. (2005). The effect of remnant and pictographic books on the communicative interaction of individuals with global aphasia. *Augmentative and Alternative Communication, 21,* 218–232.

Hoag, L., & Bedrosian, J. (1992). The effects of speech output type, message length, and reauditorization on perceptions of communicative competence of an adult AAC user. *Journal of Speech and Hearing Research, 35,* 1363–1366.

Hoag, L., Bedrosian, J., Johnson, D., & Molineux, B. (1994). Variables affecting perceptions of social aspects of the communicative competence of an adult AAC user. *Augmentative and Alternative Communication, 10,* 129–137.

Hoag, L., Bedrosian, J., & McCoy, K. (2009). Theory-driven AAC practices with adults who use utterance-based systems: The case of conversational rule violations. *Perspectives on Augmentative and Alternative Communication, 18,* 103–109.

Hochstein, D., McDaniel, M., Nettleton, S., & Neufeld, K. (2003). The fruitfulness of a nomothetic approach to investigating AAC: Comparing two speech encoding schemes across cerebral palsied and nondisabled children. *American Journal of Speech-Language Pathology, 12,* 110–122.

Hodgdon, L. (1996). *Visual strategies for improving communication.* Troy, MI: QuirkRoberts.

Hodges, P., & Schwethelm, B. (1984). A comparison of the effectiveness of graphic symbol and manual sign training with profoundly retarded children. *Applied Psycholinguistics, 5,* 223–253.

Hoffmeister, R. (1990). ASL and its implications for education. In H. Bornstein (Ed.), *Manual communication: Implications for education* (pp. 81–107). Washington, DC: Gallaudet University Press.

Holbrook, C.M., D'Andrea, F., & Sanford, L. (2011). *Ashcroft's programmed instruction in Braille* (4th ed.). Germantown, TN: Scalars.

Honsinger, M. (1989). Midcourse intervention in multiple sclerosis: An inpatient model. *Augmentative and Alternative Communication, 5,* 71–73.

Hooper, J., Connell, T., & Flett, P. (1987). Blissymbols and manual signs: A multimodal approach to intervention in a case of multiple disability. *Augmentative and Alternative Communication, 3,* 68–76.

Hopper, T.L. (2003). "They're just going to get worse anyway": Perspectives on rehabilitation for nursing home residents with dementia. *Journal of Communication Disorders, 36,* 345–359.

Horn, C., & May, R.J. (2010). Post-high school transition supports and programs in postsecondary education for young adults who use AAC. In D.B. McNaughton & D.R. Beukelman (Eds.), *Transition strategies for adolescents and young adults who use AAC* (pp. 93–110). Baltimore: Paul H. Brookes Publishing Co.

Horn, E., & Jones, H. (1996). Comparison of two selection techniques used in augmentative and alternative communication. *Augmentative and Alternative Communication, 12,* 23–31.

Horner, R.H., McDonnell, J.J., & Bellamy, G.T. (1986). Teaching generalized skills: Instruction in simulation and community settings. In R.H. Horner, L.H. Meyer, & H.D.B. Fredericks (Eds.), *Education of learners with severe handicaps: Exemplary service strategies* (pp. 289–314). Baltimore: Paul H. Brookes Publishing Co.

Hoskins, B. (1990). Collaborative consultation: Designing the role of the speech-language pathologist in a new educational context. In W. Secord (Ed.), *Best practices in school speech-language pathology* (pp. 29–38). San Antonio, TX: Harcourt Assessment.

Hough, M., & Johnson, R.K. (2009). Use of AAC to enhance linguistic communication skills in an adult with chronic severe aphasia. *Aphasiology, 23*(7–8), 965–976.

Hsieh, M.-C., & Luo, C.-H. (1999). Morse code typing of an adolescent with cerebral palsy using microcomputer technology: Case study. *Augmentative and Alternative Communication, 15,* 216–221.

Huer, M.B. (1997). Culturally inclusive assessments for children using augmentative and alternative communication (AAC). *Journal of Children's Communication Development, 19,* 23–34.

Huer, M.B. (2000). Examining perceptions of graphic symbols across cultures: Preliminary study of the impact of culture/ethnicity. *Augmentative and Alternative Communication, 16,* 180–185.

Huer, M.B., & Miller, L. (2011). *Test of Early Communication and Emerging Language (TECEL).* Austin, TX: PRO-ED.

Huer, M.B., Parette, H.P., & Saenz, T. (2001). Conversations with Mexican Americans regarding children with disabilities and augmentative and alternative communication. *Communication Disorders Quarterly, 22,* 197–206.

Huer, M.B., Saenz, T., & Doan, J.H. D. (2001). Understanding the Vietnamese American community: Implications for training educational personnel providing services to children with disabilities. *Communication Disorders Quarterly, 23,* 27–39.

Huer, M.B., & Wyatt, T. (1999). Cultural factors in the delivery of AAC services to the African-American community. *Multicultural Electronic Journal of Communication Disorders, 2.* Retrieved from http://www.asha.ucf.edu/huer.wyatt.html

Hughes, C.A., Schumaker, J.B., McNaughton, D., Deshler, D.D., & Nolan, S.M. (2010). *The EDIT Strategy.* Lawrence: University of Kansas.

Hunt, P., Alwell, M., & Goetz, L. (1988). Acquisition of conversation skills and the reduction of inappropriate social interaction behaviors. *Journal of the Association for Persons with Severe Handicaps, 13,* 20–27.

Hunt, P., Alwell, M., & Goetz, L. (1990). *Teaching conversation skills to individuals with severe disabilities with a communication book adaptation.* Retrieved from http://www.eric.ed.gov/ERICWebPortal/search/detailmini.jsp?_nfpb=true&_&ERICExtSearch_SearchValue_0=ED335862&ERICExtSearch_SearchType_0=no&accno=ED335862

Hunt, P., Alwell, M., & Goetz, L. (1991a). Establishing conversational exchanges with family and friends: Moving from training to meaningful communication. *Journal of Special Education, 25,* 305–319.

Hunt, P., Alwell, M., & Goetz, L. (1991b). Interacting with peers through conversation turn taking with a communication book adaptation. *Augmentative and Alternative Communication, 7,* 117–126.

Hunt, P., Staub, D., Alwell, M., & Goetz, L. (1994). Achievement by all students within the context of cooperative learning groups. *Journal of the Association for Persons with Severe Handicaps, 19,* 290–301.

Hurlbut, B., Iwata, B., & Green, J. (1982). Nonvocal language acquisition in adolescents with severe physical disabilities: Blissymbol versus iconic stimulus formats. *Journal of Applied Behavior Analysis, 15,* 241–258.

Hurtig, R., & Downey, D. (2006). *The use of augmentative & alternative communication in acute care settings.* Presentation at the Iowa Speech and Hearing Association Conference.

Hurtig, R., & Downey, D. (2009). *Augmentative and alternative communication in acute and critical care settings.* San Diego: Plural.

Hustad, K.C., & Shapley, K.L. (2003). AAC and natural speech in individuals with developmental disabilities. In J.C. Light, D.R. Beukelman, & J. Reichle (Eds.), *Communicative competence for individuals who use AAC: From research to effective practice* (pp. 41–62). Baltimore: Paul H. Brookes Publishing Co.

Hux, K. (Ed.). (2011). *Assisting survivors of traumatic brain injury: The role of speech-language pathologists* (2nd ed.). Austin, TX: PRO-ED.

Hwa-Froelich, D., & Westby, C. (2003). Frameworks of education: Perspectives of Southeast Asian parents and Head Start staff. *Language, Speech, and Hearing Services in Schools, 34,* 299–319.

Hymes, D. (1972). On communicative competence. In J.B. Pride & J. Holmes (Eds.), *Sociolinguistics* (pp. 269–293). London: Penguin Books.

Iacono, T.A. (2003). Pragmatic development in individuals with developmental disabilities who use AAC. In J.C. Light, D.R. Beukelman, & J. Reichle (Eds.), *Communicative competence for individuals who use AAC: From research to effective practice* (pp. 323–360). Baltimore: Paul H. Brookes Publishing Co.

Iacono, T., & Caithness, T. (2009). Assessment issues. In P. Mirenda & T. Iacono (Eds.), *Autism spectrum disorders and AAC* (pp. 23–48). Baltimore: Paul H. Brookes Publishing Co.

Iacono, T., Carter, M., & Hook, J. (1998). Identification of intentional communication in students with severe and multiple disabilities. *Augmentative and Alternative Communication, 14,* 102–114.

Iacono, T., & Cupples, L. (2004). Assessment of phonemic awareness and word reading skills of people with complex communication needs. *Journal of Speech, Language, and Hearing Research, 47,* 437–449.

Iacono, T., & Duncum, J. (1995). Comparisons of sign alone and in combination with an electronic communication device in early language intervention: A case study. *Augmentative and Alternative Communication, 11,* 249–259.

Iacono, T., Mirenda, P., & Beukelman, D.R. (1993). Comparison of unimodal and multimodal AAC techniques for children with intellectual disabilities. *Augmentative and Alternative Communication, 9,* 83–94.

Iacono, T., & Parsons, C. (1986). A survey of the use of signing with the intellectually disabled. *Australian Communication Quarterly, 2,* 21–25.

Iacono, T., & Waring, R. (1996, August). *A case study of a parent-implemented AAC language intervention comparing signs versus sign+aid.* Paper presented at the seventh biennial conference of the International Society for Augmentative and Alternative Communication, Vancouver, British Columbia, Canada.

Individuals with Disabilities Education Improvement Act (IDEA) of 2004, PL 108-446, 20 U.S.C. §§ 1400 *et seq.*

Inglebret, E., Jones, C., & Pavel, D.M.P. (2008). Integrating American Indian/Alaska Native culture into shared storybook intervention. *Language, Speech, and Hearing Services in Schools, 39,* 521–527.

Ittelson, W.H. (1996). Visual perception of markings. *Psychonomic Bulletin & Review, 3*(2), 171–187.

Jackson-Waite, K., Robson, J., & Pring, T. (2003). Written communication using a Lightwriter in undifferentiated jargon aphasia: A single case study. *Aphasiology, 17,* 767–780.

Jacobs, B., Drew, R., Ogletree, B.T., & Pierce, K. (2004). Augmentative and alternative communication (AAC) for adults with severe aphasia: Where we stand and how we can go further. *Disability and Rehabilitation, 26*(21–22), 1231–1240.

Jagaroo, V., & Wilkinson, K. (2008). Further considerations of visual cognitive neuroscience in aided AAC: The potential role of motion perception systems in maximizing design display. *Augmentative and Alternative Communication, 24,* 29–42.

Jensema, C. (1982). Communication methods and devices for deaf-blind persons. *Directions, 3,* 60–69.

Johnson, C.P. (2004). Early clinical characteristics of children with autism. In V.B. Gupta (Ed.), *Autistic spectrum disorders in children* (pp. 85–123). New York: Marcel Dekker.

Johnson, D., & Johnson, R. (1987). *Learning together and alone: Cooperation, competition, and individualization* (2nd ed.). Upper Saddle River, NJ: Prentice Hall.

Johnson, E.M., Inglebret, E., Jones, C., & Ray, J. (2006). Perspectives of speech language pathologists regarding success versus abandonment of AAC. *Augmentative and Alternative Communication, 22,* 85–89.

Johnson, R.K., Strauss Hough, M., King, K.A., Vos, P., & Jeffs, T. (2008). Functional communication in individuals with chronic severe aphasia using augmentative communication. *Augmentative and Alternative Communication, 24,* 269–280.

Johnson, S., Meyer, L., & Taylor, B. (1996). Supported inclusion. In C. Maurice (Ed.), *Behavioral intervention for young children with autism* (pp. 331–342). Austin, TX: PRO-ED.

Johnston, J., & Wong, M.-Y. (2002). Cultural differences in beliefs and practices concerning talk to children. *Journal of Speech, Language, and Hearing Research, 42,* 916–926.

Johnston, S.S., Buchanan, S., & Davenport, L. (2009). Comparison of fixed and gradual array when teaching sound-letter correspondence to two children with autism who use AAC. *Augmentative and Alternative Communication, 25,* 136–144.

Johnston, S.S., Davenport, L., Kanarowski, B., Rhodehouse, S., & McDonnell, A.P. (2009). Teaching sound letter correspondence and consonant-vowel-consonant combinations to young children who use augmentative and alternative communication. *Augmentative and Alternative Communication, 25,* 123–135.

Johnston, S., Nelson, C., Evans, J., & Palazolo, K. (2003). The use of visual supports in teaching young children with autism spectrum disorder to initiate interactions. *Augmentative and Alternative Communication, 19,* 86–103.

Johnston, S., Reichle, J., Feeley, K., & Jones, E. (2012). *AAC strategies for individuals with moderate to severe disabilities.* Baltimore: Paul H. Brookes Publishing Co.

Joint Commission. (2010). *Advancing effective communication, cultural competence, and patient- and family-centered care: A roadmap for hospitals.* Oakbrook Terrace, IL: Joint Commission. Retrieved from http://www.jointcommission.org/assets/1/6/ARoadmapforHospitals-finalversion727.pdf

Jolleff, N., & Ryan, M. (1993). Communication development in Angelman syndrome. *Archives of Disease in Childhood, 69,* 148–150.

Jolly, A., Test, D., & Spooner, F. (1993). Using badges to increase initiations of children with severe disabilities in a play setting. *Journal of the Association for Persons with Severe Handicaps, 18,* 46–51.

Jonsson, A., Kristoffersson, L., Ferm, U., & Thunberg, G. (2011). The ComAlong communication boards: Parents' use and experiences of aided language stimulation. *Augmentative and Alternative Communication, 27,* 103–116.

Jordan, F., & Murdoch, B. (1990). Unexpected recovery of functional communication following a prolonged period of mutism post-head injury. *Brain Injury, 4,* 101–108.

Jordan, F.M., & Murdoch, B.E. (1994). Severe closed-head injury in childhood: Linguistic outcomes into adulthood. *Brain Injury, 8,* 501–508.

Jorgensen, C.M. (1998). *Restructuring high schools for all students: Taking inclusion to the next level.* Baltimore: Paul H. Brookes Publishing Co.

Jorgensen, C. (2006). Reconsidering assessment in inclusive education. In C. Jorgensen, M. Schuh, & J. Nisbet (Eds.), *The inclusion facilitator's guide* (pp. 139–165). Baltimore: Paul H. Brookes Publishing Co.

Jorgensen, C., McSheehan, M., & Sonnenmeier, R. (2010). *The Beyond Access Model: Promoting membership, participation, and learning for students with disabilities in the general education classroom.* Baltimore: Paul H. Brookes Publishing Co.

Jorgensen, C., Schuh, M., & Nisbet, J. (2006). *The inclusion facilitator's guide.* Baltimore: Paul H. Brookes Publishing Co.

Jorm, A., & Jolly, D. (1998). The incidence of dementia: A meta-analysis. *Neurology, 51,* 728–733.

Jose, R.T. (Ed.). (1983). *Understanding low vision.* New York: American Foundation for the Blind.

Judge, S., & Landeryou, M. (2007). Disambiguation (predictive texting) for AAC. *Communication Matters, 22*(2), 37–41.

Judge, S.L., & Parette, H.P. (Eds.). (1998). *Assistive technology for young children with disabilities.* Cambridge, MA: Brookline Books.

Jungblut, M., Suchanek, M., & Gerhard, H. (2009). Long-term recovery from chronic global aphasia: A case report. *Music and Medicine, 1,* 61.

Jutai, J., & Day, H. (2002). Psychological Impact of Assistive Devices Scale (PIADS). *Technology and Disability, 14,* 107–111.

Kagan, A. (1998). Supported conversation for adults with aphasia: Methods and resources for training conversation partners. *Aphasiology, 12,* 816–830.

Kagan, A. (2001). Training volunteers as conversation partners using "Supported Conversation for Adults with Aphasia" (SCA): A controlled trial. *Journal of Speech, Language, and Hearing Research, 44,* 3, 624–638.

Kagohara, D.M., van der Meer, L., Achmadi, D., Green, V., O'Reilly, M.F., Mulloy, A.,…Sigafoos, J. (2010). Behavioral intervention promotes successful use of an iPod-based communication device by an adolescent with autism. *Clinical Case Studies, 9,* 328–338.

Kame'enui, E., & Simmons, J. (1999). *Toward successful inclusion of students with disabilities: The architecture of instruction.* Reston, VA: Council for Exceptional Children.

Kangas, K., & Lloyd, L. (1988). Early cognitive skills as prerequisites to augmentative and alternative communication use: What are we waiting for? *Augmentative and Alternative Communication, 4,* 211, 221.

Karuth, D. (1985). If I were a car, I'd be a lemon. In A. Brightman (Ed.), *Ordinary moments: The disabled experience* (pp. 9–31). Syracuse, NY: Human Policy Press.

Kates, B., & McNaughton, S. (1975). *The first application of Blissymbolics as a communication medium for nonspeaking children: History and development, 1971–1974.* Don Mills, Ontario, Canada: Easter Seals Communication Institute.

Katz, J., & Mirenda, P. (2002). Including students with developmental disabilities in general education classrooms: Social benefits. *International Journal of Special Education, 17,* 25–35.

Katz, J., Mirenda, P., & Auerbach, S. (2002). Instructional strategies and educational outcomes for students with developmental disabilities in inclusive "multiple intelligences" and typical inclusive classrooms. *Research and Practice for Persons with Severe Disabilities, 27,* 227–238.

Katz, R., Haig, A., Clark, B., & DiPaola, R. (1992). Long-term survival, prognosis and life-care planning for 29 patients with chronic locked-in syndrome. *Archives of Physical Medical Rehabilitation, 73,* 403–408.

Keen, D., Sigafoos, J., & Woodyatt, G. (2001). Replacing prelinguistic behaviors with functional communication. *Journal of Autism and Developmental Disorders, 31,* 385–398.

Keenan, J., & Barnhart, K. (1993). Development of yes/no systems in individuals with severe traumatic brain injuries. *Augmentative and Alternative Communication, 9,* 184–190.

Kelford Smith, A., Thurston, S., Light, J., Parnes, P., & O'Keefe, B. (1989). The form and use of written communication produced by physically disabled individuals using microcomputers. *Augmentative and Alternative Communication, 5,* 115–124.

Kemper, S. (1988). Geriatric psycholinguistics: Syntactic limitations of oral and written language. In L. Light & D. Burke (Eds.), *Language, memory, and aging* (pp. 58–76). New York: Cambridge University Press.

Kennedy, C.H., Meyer, K.A., Knowles, T., & Shukla, S. (2000). Analyzing the multiple functions of stereotypical behavior for students with autism: Implications for assessment and treatment. *Journal of Applied Behavior Analysis, 33,* 559–571.

Kent, R., Miolo, G., & Bloedel, S. (1994). The intelligibility of children's speech: A review of evaluation procedures. *American Journal of Speech-Language Pathology, 3,* 81–95.

Kent-Walsh, J., Binger, C., & Hasham, Z. (2010). Effects of parent instruction on the symbolic communication of children using augmentative and alternative communication during storybook reading. *American Journal of Speech-Language Pathology, 19,* 97–107.

Kent-Walsh, J., & Light, J. (2003). General education teachers' experiences with inclusion of students who use augmentative and alternative communication. *Augmentative and Alternative Communication, 19,* 104–124.

Kent-Walsh, J., & McNaughton, D. (2005). Communication partner instruction in AAC: Present practices and future directions. *Augmentative and Alternative Communication, 21,* 195–204.

Kent-Walsh, J., Stark, C., & Binger, C. (2008). Tales from school trenches: AAC service-delivery and professional expertise. *Seminars in Speech Language, 29,* 146–154.

Keogh, W., & Reichle, J. (1985). Communication intervention for the "difficult-to-teach" severely handicapped. In S.F. Warren & A.K. Rogers-Warren (Eds.), *Teaching functional language* (pp. 157–194). Austin, TX: PRO-ED.

Kertesz, A. (1982). *Western Aphasia Battery.* San Antonio, TX: Harcourt Assessment.

Kertesz, A. (2006). *Western Aphasia Battery–Revised.* San Antonio, TX: Pearson.

Kiernan, C. (1983). The use of nonvocal communication techniques with autistic individuals. *Journal of Child Psychology and Psychiatry, 24,* 339–375.

Kiernan, C., Reid, B., & Jones, M. (1982). *Signs and symbols: Use of non-vocal communication systems.* Portsmouth, NH: Heinemann.

Kiernan, J.A., & Hudson, A.J. (1994). Frontal lobe atrophy in motor neuron diseases. *Brain, 117,* 747–757.

King, J., Alarcon, N., & Rogers, M. (2007). Primary progressive aphasia. In D.R. Beukelman, K.L. Garrett, & K.M. Yorkston (Eds.), *Augmentative communication strategies for adults with acute or chronic medical conditions* (pp. 207–242). Baltimore: Paul H. Brookes Publishing Co.

King, J., & Hux, K. (1995). Intervention using talking word processing software: An aphasia case study. *Augmentative and Alternative Communication, 11,* 187–192.

King, J., Spoeneman, T., Stuart, S., & Beukelman, D.R. (1995). Small talk in adult conversations. *Augmentative and Alternative Communication, 11,* 244–248.

King-DeBaun, P. (1993). *Storytime! Just for fun: stories, symbols, and emergent literacy activities for young children.* Park City, UT: Creative Communicating.

King-DeBaun, P. (1999). *Storytime. Stories, symbols, and emergent literacy activities for young, special needs children.* Park City, UT: Creative Communicating.

Kitwood, T. (1997). *Dementia reconsidered: The person comes first.* Philadelphia: Open University Press.

Klasner, E.R., & Yorkston, K.M. (2000). AAC for Huntington disease and Parkinson's disease: Planning for change. In D.R. Beukelman, K.M. Yorkston, & J. Reichle (Eds.), *Augmentative and alternative communication for adults with acquired neurologic disorders* (pp. 233–270). Baltimore: Paul H. Brookes Publishing Co.

Klasner, E.R., & Yorkston, K.M. (2001). Linguistic and cognitive supplementation strategies as augmentative and alternative communication techniques in Huntington's disease: Case report. *Augmentative and Alternative Communication, 17,* 154–160.

Kluth, P. (2010). *"You're going to love this kid!": Teaching students with autism in the inclusive classroom* (2nd ed.). Baltimore: Paul H. Brookes Publishing Co.

Kluth, P., & Chandler-Olcott, L. (2008). *"A land we can share": Teaching literacy to students with autism.* Baltimore: Paul H. Brookes Publishing Co.

Knapp, M. (1980). *Essentials of nonverbal communication.* New York: Holt, Rinehart & Winston.

Knudsen-Lindauer, S., & Harris, K. (1989). Priorities for kindergarten curricula: Views of parents and teachers. *Journal of Research in Childhood Education, 4,* 51–61.

Koehler, L., Lloyd, L., & Swanson, L. (1994). Visual similarity between manual and printed alphabet letters. *Augmentative and Alternative Communication, 10,* 87–95.

Koester, H., & Levine, S. (1996). Effect of a word prediction feature on user performance. *Augmentative and Alternative Communication, 12,* 155–168.

Koester, H., & Levine, S. (1998). Model simulations of user performance with word prediction. *Augmentative and Alternative Communication, 14,* 25–35.

Konstantareas, M. (1984). Sign language as a communication prosthesis with language-impaired children. *Journal of Autism and Developmental Disorders, 14,* 9–23.

Konstantareas, M., Oxman, J., & Webster, C. (1978). Iconicity: Effects of the acquisition of sign language by autistic and other severely dysfunctional children. In P. Siple (Ed.), *Understanding language through sign language research* (pp. 213–237). New York: Academic Press.

Koppenhaver, D.A. (1991). *A descriptive analysis of classroom literacy instruction provided to children with severe speech and physical impairments* (Unpublished doctoral dissertation). University of North Carolina at Chapel Hill.

Koppenhaver, D.A., & Erickson, K.A. (2009). Literacy in individuals with autism spectrum disorders who use AAC. In P. Mirenda & T. Iacono (Eds.), *Autism spectrum disorders and AAC* (pp. 385–412). Baltimore: Paul H. Brookes Publishing Co.

Koppenhaver, D.A., Erickson, K.A., Harris, B., McLellan, J., Skotko, B.G., & Newton, R.A. (2001). Storybook-based communication intervention for girls with Rett syndrome and their mothers. *Disability and Rehabilitation, 23*(3/4), 149–159.

Koppenhaver, D., Erickson, K., & Skotko, B. (2001). Supporting communication of girls with Rett syndrome and their mothers in storybook reading. *International Journal of Disability, Development, and Education, 48*, 395–410.

Koppenhaver, D., Evans, D., & Yoder, D. (1991). Childhood reading and writing experiences of literate adults with severe speech and motor impairments. *Augmentative and Alternative Communication, 7*, 20–33.

Koppenhaver, D., & Yoder, D. (1992). Literacy issues in persons with severe physical and speech impairments. In R. Gaylord-Ross (Ed.), *Issues and research in special education* (Vol. 2, pp. 156–201). New York: Teachers College Press.

Koppenhaver, D., & Yoder, D. (1993). Classroom literacy instruction for children with severe speech and physical impairments (SSPI): What is and what might be. *Topics in Language Disorders, 13*(2), 1–15.

Koul, R. (2003). Synthetic speech perception in individuals with and without disabilities. *Augmentative and Alternative Communication, 19*, 29–36.

Koul, R., & Corwin, M. (2003). Efficacy of AAC intervention in individuals with chronic severe aphasia. In R. Schlosser (Ed.), *The efficacy of augmentative and alternative communication: Toward evidence-based practice* (pp. 449–470). New York: Elsevier.

Koul, R., & Harding, R. (1998). Identification and production of graphic symbols by individuals with aphasia: Efficacy of a software application. *Augmentative and Alternative Communication, 14*, 11–23.

Koul, R., & Schlosser, R. (2004). Effects of synthetic speech output in the learning of graphic symbols of varied iconicity. *Disability Rehabilitation, 26*, 1278–1285.

Kovach, T. (2009). *Augmentative and alternative communication profile: A continuum of learning*. East Moline, IL: LinguiSystems.

Kovach, T.M., & Kenyon, P.B. (2003). Visual issues and access to AAC. In J.C. Light, D.R. Beukelman, & J. Reichle (Eds.), *Communicative competence for individuals who use AAC: From research to effective practice* (pp. 277–319). Baltimore: Paul H. Brookes Publishing Co.

Kozleski, E. (1991a). Expectant delay procedure for teaching requests. *Augmentative and Alternative Communication, 7*, 11–19.

Kozleski, E. (1991b). Visual symbol acquisition by students with autism. *Exceptionality, 2*, 175–194.

Kraat, A. (1985). *Communication interaction between aided and natural speakers: A state of the art report*. Toronto: Canadian Rehabilitation Council for the Disabled.

Kraat, A. (1990). Augmentative and alternative communication: Does it have a future in aphasia rehabilitation? *Aphasiology, 4*, 321–338.

Kraft, G. (1981). Multiple sclerosis. In W. Stolov & M. Clowers (Eds.), *Handbook of severe disability* (pp. 111–118). Washington, DC: U.S. Department of Education.

Kravitz, E., & Littman, S. (1990). A communication system for a nonspeaking person with hearing and cognitive impairments. *Augmentative and Alternative Communication, 6*, 100.

Kunc, N., & Van der Klift, E. (1995). *A credo for support* [poster]. Nanaimo, BC: Axis Consulting.

Kurland, J., Naeser, M.A., Baker, E.H., Doron, K., Martin, P.I., Seekins, H.E.,…Yurgelun-Todd, D. (2004). Test-retest reliability of fMRI during nonverbal semantic decision in moderate-severe nonfluent aphasia patients. *Behavioural Neurology, 15*, 87–97.

Kynette, D., & Kemper, S. (1986). Aging and loss of grammatical forms: A cross-sectional study of language performance. *Language and Communication, 6*(1/2), 65–72.

Ladd, P. (2003). *Understanding deaf culture: In search of deafhood*. Clevedon, UK: Multilingual Matters.

Ladtkow, M., & Culp, D. (1992). Augmentative communication with the traumatically brain injured population. In K. Yorkston (Ed.), *Augmentative communication in the medical setting* (pp. 139–243). Tucson, AZ: Communication Skill Builders.

Lafontaine, L., & DeRuyter, F. (1987). The nonspeaking cerebral palsied: A clinical and demographic database report. *Augmentative and Alternative Communication, 3,* 153–162.

Lahey, M., & Bloom, L. (1977). Planning a first lexicon: Which words to teach first. *Journal of Speech and Hearing Disorders, 42,* 340–349.

Lalli, J., Browder, D., Mace, C., & Brown, D. (1993). Teacher use of descriptive analysis data to implement interventions to decrease students' problem behaviors. *Journal of Applied Behavior Analysis, 25,* 227–238.

Lalli, J., Casey, S., & Kates, K. (1995). Reducing escape behavior and increasing task completion with functional communication training, extinction, and response chaining. *Journal of Applied Behavior Analysis, 28,* 261–268.

Lancioni, G., Bosco, A., Belardinelli, M., Singh, N., O'Reilly, M., & Sigafoos, J. (2010). An overview of intervention options for promoting adaptive behavior of persons with acquired brain injury and minimally conscious state. *Research in Developmental Disabilities, 31,* 1121–1134.

Lancioni, G., O'Reilly, M., & Basili, G. (2001). Use of microswitches and speech output systems with people with severe/profound intellectual or multiple disabilities: A literature review. *Research in Developmental Disabilities, 22,* 21–40.

Lancioni, G., O'Reilly, M., Cuvo, A., Singh, N., Sigafoos, J., & Didden, R. (2007). PECS and VOCAs to enable students with developmental disabilities to make requests: An overview of the literature. *Research in Developmental Disabilities, 28,* 468–488.

Lancioni, G., O'Reilly, M., Singh, N., Sigofoos, J., Oliva, D., Antonucci, M.,…Basilli, G. (2008). Microswitch-based programs for persons with multiple disabilities: An overview of some recent developments. *Perceptual and Motor Skills, 106,* 355–370.

Lancioni, G., Singh, N., O'Reilly, M., & Oliva, D. (2003). Extending microswitch-based programs for people with multiple disabilities: Use of words and choice opportunities. *Research in Developmental Disabilities, 24,* 139–148.

Lancioni, G., Singh, N., O'Reilly, M., & Oliva, D. (2005). Microswitch programs for persons with multiple disabilities: An overview of the responses adopted for microswitch activation. *Cognitive Processes, 6,* 177–188.

Lancioni, G., Singh, N., O'Reilly, M., Oliva, D., Dardanelli, E., & Pirani, P. (2003). Adapting the use of microswitches to foster response awareness and word association: Two case evaluations. *Journal of Positive Behavior Interventions, 5,* 153–157.

Lancioni, G., Singh, N., O'Reilly, M., Sigafoos, J., Didden, R., Oliva, D.,…Lamartire, A. (2007). Effects of microswitch-based programs on indices of happiness of students with multiple disabilities: A new research evaluation. *American Journal on Mental Retardation, 112,* 167–176.

Lancioni, G., Singh N., O'Reilly, M., Sigafoos, J., Oliva, D., Signorino, M., & Tommaso, M. (2010). Helping a man with acquired brain injury and multiple disabilities manage television use via assistive technology. *Clinical Case Studies, 9,* 4285–4293.

Lancioni, G., Singh N., O'Reilly, M., Sigafoos, J., Signorino, M., Oliva, D.,…Tommaso, M. (2010). A special messaging technology for two persons with acquired brain injury and multiple disabilities. *Brain Injury, 24,* 1236–1243.

Landman, C., & Schaeffler, C. (1986). Object communication boards. *Communication Outlook, 8*(1), 7–8.

Larsson, M., & Dahlgren Sandberg, A. (2008). Memory ability of children with complex communication needs. *Augmentative and Alternative Communication, 24,* 139–148.

Lasker, J.P. (2008). AAC language assessment: Considerations for adults with aphasia. *Perspectives on Augmentative and Alternative Communication, 17*(3), 105–112.

Lasker, J., Ball, L., Bringewatt, J., Stuart, S., & Marvin, M. (1996, November). *Small talk across the lifespan: AAC vocabulary selection.* Paper presented at the annual convention of the American Speech-Language-Hearing Association, Seattle.

Lasker, J.P., & Bedrosian, J.L. (2001). Promoting acceptance of augmentative and alternative communication by adults with acquired communication disorders. *Augmentative and Alternative Communication, 17,* 141–153.

Lasker, J., & Beukelman, D.R. (1999). Peers' perceptions of storytelling by an adult with aphasia. *Aphasiology, 13,* 857–869.

Lasker, J.P., & Garrett, K.L. (2006). Using the Multimodal Communication Screening Test for Persons with Aphasia (MCST-A) to guide the selection of alternative communication strategies for people with aphasia. *Aphasiology, 20*(2/3/4), 217–232.

Lasker, J.P., Garrett, K.L., & Fox, L.E. (2007). Severe aphasia. In D.R. Beukelman, K.L. Garrett, & K.M. Yorkston (Eds.), *Augmentative communication strategies for adults with acute or chronic medical conditions* (pp. 163–206). Baltimore: Paul H. Brookes Publishing Co.

Lasker, J., Hux, K., Garrett, K., Moncrief, E., & Eischeid, T. (1997). Variations on the written choice communication strategy for individuals with severe aphasia. *Augmentative and Alternative Communication, 13,* 108–116.

Lasker, J.P., LaPointe, L.L., & Kodras, J. (2005). Helping a professor with aphasia resume teaching through multimodal approaches. *Aphasiology, 19*(3/4/5), 399–410.

Lasker, J.P., Stierwalt, J.A. G., Hageman, C.F., & LaPointe, L.L. (2008). Using Motor Learning Guided theory and augmentative and alternative communication to improve speech production in profound apraxia: A case example. *Journal of Medical Speech-Language Pathology, 16,* 225–234.

Leaf, R., & McEachin, J. (1999). *A work in progress: Behavior management strategies and a curriculum for intensive behavioral treatment of autism.* New York: DRL Books.

Lee, K., & Thomas, D. (1990). *Control of computer-based technology for people with physical disabilities: An assessment manual.* Toronto: University of Toronto Press.

Lehoux, P., & Blume, S. (2000). Technology assessment and the sociopolitics of health technologies. *Journal of Health Politics, Policy and Law, 25,* 1083–1120.

Lenhart, A., Ling, R., Campbell, S., & Purcell, K. (2010, April 20). *Text messaging explodes as teens embrace it as the centerpiece of their communication strategies with friends.* Retrieved from Pew Internet & American Life Project web site: http://pewinternet.org/Reports/2010/Teens-and-Mobile-Phones/Summary-of-findings.aspx

Leonhart, W., & Maharaj, S. (1979). *A comparison of initial recognition and rate of acquisition of Pictogram Ideogram Communication (PIC) and Blissymbols with institutionalized severely retarded adults.* Unpublished manuscript, Pictogram Centre, Saskatoon, Saskatchewan, Canada.

Lesher, G., Moulton, B., & Higginbotham, D.J. (1998a). Optimal character arrangements for ambiguous keyboards. *IEEE Transactions on Rehabilitation Engineering, 6,* 415–423.

Lesher, G., Moulton, B., & Higginbotham, D.J. (1998b). Techniques for augmenting scanning communication. *Augmentative and Alternative Communication, 14,* 81–101.

Levine, S., Goodenough-Trepagnier, C., Getschow, C., & Minneman, S. (1987). Multi-character key text entry using computer disambiguation. In *Proceedings of the 10th Annual Conference on Rehabilitation Engineering* (pp. 177–179). Washington, DC: RESNA Press.

Lewis, B., Freebairn, L., Hansen, A., Iyengar, S., & Taylor, H.G. (2004). School-age follow-up of children with childhood apraxia of speech. *Language, Speech, and Hearing Services in Schools, 35,* 122–140.

Liboiron, N., & Soto, G. (2006). Shared storybook reading with a student who uses alternative and augmentative communication: A description of scaffolding practices. *Child Language Teaching and Therapy, 22,* 69–95.

Light, J. (1988). Interaction involving individuals using augmentative and alternative communication systems: State of the art and future directions. *Augmentative and Alternative Communication, 4,* 66–82.

Light, J. (1989a). *Encoding techniques for augmentative communication systems: An investigation of the recall performance of nonspeaking physically disabled adults* (Unpublished doctoral dissertation). University of Toronto.

Light, J. (1989b). Toward a definition of communicative competence for individuals using augmentative and alternative communication systems. *Augmentative and Alternative Communication, 5,* 137–144.

Light, J. (1993). Teaching automatic linear scanning for computer access: A case study of a preschooler with severe physical and communication disabilities. *Journal of Special Education Technology, 2,* 125–134.

Light, J. (1996). *Exemplary practices to develop the communicative competence of students who use augmentative and alternative communication: Final grant report.* University Park: Pennsylvania State University.

Light, J. (1997). Communication is the essence of human life: Reflections on communication competence. *Augmentative and Alternative Communication, 13,* 61–70.

Light, J.C., Arnold, K.B., & Clark, E.A. (2003). Finding a place in the "social circle of life." In J.C. Light, D.R. Beukelman, & J. Reichle (Eds.), *Communicative competence for individuals who use AAC: From research to effective practice* (pp. 361–397). Baltimore: Paul H. Brookes Publishing Co.

Light, J., Beesley, M., & Collier, B. (1988). Transition through multiple augmentative and alternative communication systems: A three-year case study of a head-injured adolescent. *Augmentative and Alternative Communication, 4*, 2–14.

Light, J.C., Beukelman, D.R., & Reichle, J. (Eds.). (2003). *Communicative competence for individuals who use AAC: From research to effective practice.* Baltimore: Paul H. Brookes Publishing Co.

Light, J.C., & Binger, C. (1998). *Building communicative competence with individuals who use augmentative and alternative communication.* Baltimore: Paul H. Brookes Publishing Co.

Light, J., Binger, C., Agate, T., & Ramsay, K. (1999). Teaching partner-focused questions to enhance the communicative competence of individuals who use AAC. *Journal of Speech, Language, and Hearing Research, 42*, 241–255.

Light, J., Binger, C., Bailey, M., & Millar, D. (1997). *Teaching the use of nonobligatory turns to enhance the communicative competence of individuals who use AAC.* Unpublished manuscript, Pennsylvania State University.

Light, J., Binger, C., Dilg, H., & Livelsberger, B. (1996, August). *Use of an introduction strategy to enhance communication competence.* Paper presented at the seventh biennial conference of the International Society for Augmentative and Alternative Communication, Vancouver, British Columbia, Canada.

Light, J., Binger, C., & Kelford Smith, A. (1994). Story reading interactions between preschoolers who use AAC and their mothers. *Augmentative and Alternative Communication, 10*, 255–268.

Light, J., Collier, B., & Parnes, P. (1985a). Communication interaction between young nonspeaking physically disabled children and their primary caregivers: Part I. Discourse patterns. *Augmentative and Alternative Communication, 1*, 74–83.

Light, J., Collier, B., & Parnes, P. (1985b). Communication interaction between young nonspeaking physically disabled children and their primary caregivers: Part II. Communicative functions. *Augmentative and Alternative Communication, 1*, 98–107.

Light, J., Collier, B., & Parnes, P. (1985c). Communication interaction between young nonspeaking physically disabled children and their primary caregivers: Part III. Modes of communication. *Augmentative and Alternative Communication, 1*, 125–133.

Light, J., Corbett, M.B., Gullapalli, G., & Lepowski, S. (1995, December). *Other orientation and the communicative competence of AAC users.* Poster presented at the annual convention of the American Speech-Language-Hearing Association, Orlando, FL.

Light, J., Dattilo, J., English, J., Gutierrez, L., & Hartz, J. (1992). Instructing facilitators to support the communication of people who use augmentative communication systems. *Journal of Speech and Hearing Research, 35*, 865–875.

Light, J., & Drager, K. (2002). Improving the design of augmentative and alternative communication technologies for young children. *Assistive Technology, 14*, 17–32.

Light, J., & Drager, K. (2011, February). *Early intervention for young children with autism, cerebral palsy, Down syndrome, and other disabilities.* Retrieved from http://aackids.psu.edu

Light, J., & Drager, K., McCarthy, J., Mellott, S., Millar, D., Parrish, C.,...Welliver, M. (2004). Performance of typically developing four- and five-year-old children with AAC systems using different language organization techniques. *Augmentative and Alternative Communication, 20*, 63–88.

Light, J., Drager, K., & Nemser, J. (2004). Enhancing the appeal of AAC technologies for young children: Lessons from the toy manufacturers. *Augmentative and Alternative Communication, 20*, 137–149.

Light, J., & Kelford Smith, A. (1993). The home literacy experiences of preschoolers who use augmentative communication systems and their nondisabled peers. *Augmentative and Alternative Communication, 9*, 10–25.

Light, J., & Kent-Walsh, J. (2003, May 27). Fostering emergent literacy for children who require AAC. *ASHA Leader, 8*, 4–5, 28–29.

Light, J., & Lindsay, P. (1991). Cognitive science and augmentative and alternative communication. *Augmentative and Alternative Communication, 7*, 186–203.

Light, J., & Lindsay, P. (1992). Message-encoding techniques for augmentative communication systems: The recall performances of adults with severe speech impairments. *Journal of Speech and Hearing Research, 35*, 853–864.

Light, J., Lindsay, P., Siegel, L., & Parnes, P. (1990). The effects of message and coding techniques on recall by literate adults using AAC systems. *Augmentative and Alternative Communication, 6*, 184–201.

Light, J., & McNaughton, D. (1993). Literacy and augmentative and alternative communication (AAC): The expectations and priorities of parents and teachers. *Topics in Language Disorders, 13*(2), 33–46.

Light, J., & McNaughton, D. (2005, November). *Augmentative and alternative communication (AAC): Maximizing the literacy skills of individuals who require AAC.* Presented at the annual convention of the American Speech-Language-Hearing Association Convention, San Diego.

Light, J., & McNaughton, D. (2009a). *Accessible Literacy Learning (ALL): Evidence-based reading instruction for learners with autism, cerebral palsy, Down syndrome, and other disabilities.* Pittsburgh: Mayer-Johnson.

Light, J., & McNaughton, D. (2009b). Addressing the literacy demands of the curriculum for conventional and more advanced readers and writers who require AAC. In G. Soto & C. Zangari (Eds.), *Practically speaking: Language, literacy, and academic development for students with AAC needs* (pp. 217–245). Baltimore: Paul H. Brookes Publishing Co.

Light, J., & McNaughton, D. (2010). *Improving literacy outcomes for individuals with autism spectrum disorders and limited speech* [Webcast]. Retrieved from http://aac.psu.edu/?p=157

Light, J., & McNaughton, D. (2011). *Literacy instruction for individuals with autism, cerebral palsy, Down syndrome, and other disabilities.* Retrieved from http://aacliteracy.psu.edu/

Light, J., McNaughton, D., & Fallon, K.A. (2009a). Single word decoding. In J. Light & D. McNaughton (Eds.), *Accessible Literacy Learning (ALL): Evidence-based reading instruction for learners with autism, cerebral palsy, Down syndrome, and other disabilities* (pp. 105–118). Pittsburgh: Mayer-Johnson.

Light, J., McNaughton, D., & Fallon, K.A. (2009b). Sound blending. In J. Light & D. McNaughton (Eds.), *Accessible Literacy Learning (ALL): Evidence-based reading instruction for learners with autism, cerebral palsy, Down syndrome, and other disabilities* (pp. 65–74). Pittsburgh: Mayer-Johnson.

Light, J., McNaughton, D., Fallon, K.A., & Millar, D. (2009). Phoneme segmentation. In J. Light & D. McNaughton (Eds.), *Accessible Literacy Learning (ALL): Evidence-based reading instruction for learners with autism, cerebral palsy, Down syndrome, and other disabilities* (pp. 75–85). Pittsburgh: Mayer-Johnson.

Light, J., McNaughton, D., Krezman, C., Williams, M., & Gulens, M. (2000). The mentor project. *Proceedings of the International Society of Augmentative and Alternative Communication, 9,* 73–75.

Light, J., McNaughton, D., & Parnes, P. (1986). *A protocol for the assessment of the communicative interaction skills of nonspeaking severely handicapped adults and their facilitators.* Toronto: Augmentative Communication Service, Hugh MacMillan Medical Centre.

Light, J., McNaughton, D., Weyer, M., & Karg, L. (2008). Evidence-based literacy instruction for individuals who require augmentative and alternative communication: A case study of a student with multiple disabilities. *Seminars in Speech and Language, 29,* 12–32.

Light, J.C., Page, R., Curran, J., & Pitkin, L. (2007). Children's ideas for the design of AAC assistive technologies for young children with complex communication needs. *Augmentative and Alternative Communication, 23,* 274–287.

Light, J.C., Parsons, A.R., & Drager, K. (2002). "There's more to life than cookies": Developing interactions for social closeness with beginning communicators who use AAC. In J. Reichle, D.R. Beukelman, & J.C. Light (Eds.), *Exemplary practices for beginning communicators: Implications for AAC* (pp. 187–218). Baltimore: Paul H. Brookes Publishing Co.

Light, J., Roberts, B., Dimarco, R., & Greiner, N. (1998). Augmentative and alternative communication to support receptive and expressive communication for people with autism. *Journal of Communication Disorders, 31,* 153–180.

Light, J., Worah, S., Bowker, A., Burki, B., Drager, K., D'Silva, K.,…et al. (2008, November). *Children's representations of early language concepts: Implications for AAC symbols.* Paper presented at the annual conference of the American Speech-Language-Hearing Association, Chicago.

Light, J., Worah, S., Drager, K., Burki, B., D'Silva, K., & Kristiansen, L. (2007). *Graphic representations of early emerging language concepts by young children from different cultural backgrounds: Implications for AAC symbols.* State College: Pennsylvania State University.

Lilienfeld, M., & Alant, E. (2002). Attitudes of children toward an unfamiliar peer using an AAC device with and without voice output. *Augmentative and Alternative Communication, 18,* 91–101.

Lindsay, P. (1989, April). *Literacy and the disabled: An unfulfilled promise or the impossible dream?* Presentation at the Pacific Conference on Technology in Education and Rehabilitation, Vancouver, British Columbia, Canada.

Linebarger, M.C., Romania, J.F., Fink, R.B., Bartlett, M.R., & Schwartz, M.F. (2008). Building on residual speech: a portable processing prosthesis for aphasia. *Journal of Rehabilitation Research and Development, 45,* 1401–1414.

Lloyd, C.M., Richardson, M.P., Brooks, D.J., Al-Chalabi, A., & Leigh, P.N. (2000). Extramotor involvement in ALS: PET studies with the GABAa ligand [11C]flumazenil. *Brain, 123*(11), 2289–2296.

Lloyd, L., & Blischak, D. (1992). AAC terminology policy and issues update. *Augmentative and Alternative Communication, 8,* 104–109.

Lloyd, L., & Fuller, D. (1986). Toward an augmentative and alternative communication symbol taxonomy: A proposed superordinate classification. *Augmentative and Alternative Communication, 2,* 165–171.

Lloyd, L., & Karlan, G. (1984). Nonspeech communication symbols and systems: Where have we been and where are we going? *Journal of Mental Deficiency Research, 38,* 3–20.

Locke, P., & Mirenda, P. (1988). A computer-supported communication approach for a non-speaking child with severe visual and cognitive impairments: A case study. *Augmentative and Alternative Communication, 4,* 15–22.

Loeding, B., Zangari, C., & Lloyd, L. (1990). A "working party" approach to planning inservice training in manual signs for an entire public school staff. *Augmentative and Alternative Communication, 6,* 38–49.

Lomen-Hoerth, C. (2004). Characterization of amyotrophic lateral sclerosis and frontotemporal dementia. *Dementia and Geriatric Cognitive Disorders, 17*(4), 337–341.

Lomen-Hoerth, C., Murphy, J., Langmore, S., Kramer, J.H., Olney, R.K., & Miller, B. (2003). Are amyotrophic lateral sclerosis patients cognitively normal? *Neurology, 60,* 1094–1097.

Lovaas, O.I. (2003). *Teaching individuals with developmental delays.* Austin, TX: PRO-ED.

Lueck, A. (2004). *Functional vision: A practitioner's guide to evaluation and intervention.* New York: AFB Press.

Luftig, R. (1984). An analysis of initial sign lexicons as a function of eight learnability variables. *Journal of the Association for Persons with Severe Handicaps, 9,* 193–200.

Lund, S.K., & Light, J. (2003). The effectiveness of grammar instruction for individuals who use augmentative and alternative communication systems: A preliminary study. *Journal of Speech, Language, and Hearing Research, 46,* 1110–1123.

Lund, S., & Light, J. (2006). Long-term outcomes for individuals who use augmentative and alternative communication: Part I. What is a "good" outcome? *Augmentative and Alternative Communication, 22,* 284–299.

Lund, S.K., & Light, J.C. (2007). Long-term outcomes for individuals who use augmentative and alternative communication: Part III. Contributing factors. *Augmentative and Alternative Communication, 23,* 323–335.

Lund, S., Millar, D., Herman, M., Hinds, A., & Light, J. (1998, November). *Children's pictorial representations of early emerging concepts: Implications for AAC.* Paper presented at the annual convention of the American Speech-Language-Hearing Association, San Antonio, TX.

Lund, S., & Troha, J. (2008). Teaching young people who are blind and have autism to make requests using a variation of the Picture Exchange Communication System with tactile symbols: A preliminary investigation. *Journal of Autism and Developmental Disorders, 38,* 719–730.

Luo, F., Higginbotham, D.J., & Lesher, G. (2007, March). *Webcrawler: Enhanced augmentative communication.* Paper presented at CSUN Conference on Disability Technology, Los Angeles.

MacDonald, J. (2004). *Communicating partners: Developmental guidelines for professionals and parents.* London: Jessica Kingsley.

MacDonald, J., & Gillette, Y. (1986). *Ecological communication system (ECO).* Columbus: Ohio State University, Nisonger Center.

MacGinitie, W., MacGinitie, R., Maria, K., Dreyer, L., & Hughes, K. (2006). *Gates-MacGinitie Reading Tests–Fourth Edition.* Rolling Meadows, IL: Riverside.

Machalicek, W., Sanford, A., Lang, R., Rispoli, M., Molfenter, N., & Mbeseha, M. (2010). Literacy interventions for students with physical and developmental disabilities who use aided AAC devices: A systematic review. *Journal of Developmental and Physical Disabilities, 22,* 219–240.

Magito-McLaughlin, D., Mullen-James, K., Anderson-Ryan, K., & Carr, E.G. (2002). Best practices: Finding a new direction for Christos. *Journal of Positive Behavior Interventions, 4,* 156–164.

Maharaj, S. (1980). *Pictogram ideogram communication.* Regina, Saskatchewan, Canada: George Reed Foundation for the Handicapped.

Mandell, A. (2002, Fall). Diagnosing primary progressive aphasia. *National Aphasia Association Newsletter, 14*(2). Retrieved from http://www.aphasia.org/Aphasia%20Facts/diagnosing_ primary_progressive_aphasia.html

Markwardt, F., Jr. (1998). *Peabody Individual Achievement Test–Revised–Normative Update (PIAT-R/ NU).* Austin, TX: Pearson Assessments.

Marriner, N., Beukelman, D.R., Wilson, W., & Ross, A. (1989). *Implementing Morse code in an augmentative communication system for ten nonspeaking individuals.* Unpublished manuscript, University of Washington, Seattle.

Martin, N., & Brownell, R. (2010). *Receptive One-Word Picture Vocabulary Test–Fourth Edition (ROWPVT-4).* San Antonio, TX: Pearson Assessments.

Martin, P.I., Naeser, M.A., Ho, M., Doron, K.W., Kurland, J., Kaplan, J.,…Pascual-Leone, A. (2009). Overt naming fMRI pre- and post-TMS: Two nonfluent aphasia patients, with and without improved naming post-TMS. *Brain & Language, 111,* 20–35.

Marvin, C.A., Beukelman, D.R., & Bilyeu, D. (1994). Vocabulary-use patterns in preschool children: Effects of context and time sampling. *Augmentative and Alternative Communication, 10,* 224–236.

Marvin, C., & Mirenda, P. (1993). Home literacy experiences of preschoolers enrolled in Head Start and special education programs. *Journal of Early Intervention, 17,* 351–367.

Marvin, C., & Privratsky, A. (1999). After-school talk: The effects of materials sent home from preschool. *American Journal of Speech-Language Pathology, 8,* 231–240.

Matas, J., Mathy-Laikko, P., Beukelman, D.R., & Legresley, K. (1985). Identifying the nonspeaking population: A demographic study. *Augmentative and Alternative Communication, 1,* 17–31.

Mathy, P., Yorkston, K.M., & Gutmann, M.L. (2000). AAC for individuals with amyotrophic lateral sclerosis. In D.R. Beukelman, K.M. Yorkston, & J. Reichle (Eds.), *Augmentative and alternative communication for adults with acquired neurologic disorders* (pp. 183–232). Baltimore: Paul H. Brookes Publishing Co.

Mathy-Laikko, P., Iacono, T., Ratcliff, A., Villarruel, F., Yoder, D., & Vanderheiden, G. (1989). Teaching a child with multiple disabilities to use a tactile augmentative communication device. *Augmentative and Alternative Communication, 5,* 249–256.

Mathy-Laikko, P., Ratcliff, A.E., Villarruel, F., & Yoder, D.E. (1987). Augmentative communication systems. In M. Bullis (Ed.), *Communication development in young children with deaf-blindness: III. Literature review* (pp. 205–241). Monmouth: Communication Skills Center for Young Children with Deaf-Blindness, Teaching Research Division, Oregon State System of Higher Education.

Mayer-Johnson LLC. (1981–2011). *The Picture Communication Symbols.* Pittsburgh: Author.

McBride, D. (2008a). *ACES High-Tech Evaluation Toolkit.* Evergreen, CO: AAC TechConnect.

McBride, D. (2008b). *ACES Low-to-Lite Tech Evaluation Toolkit.* Evergreen, CO: AAC TechConnect.

McCarthy, J., & Light, J.C. (2005). Attitudes toward individuals who use augmentative and alternative communication: Research review. *Augmentative and Alternative Communication, 21,* 41–55.

McCarthy, J., Light, J., Drager, K., McNaughton, D., Grodzicki, L., Jones, J.,…Parkin, E. (2006). Re-designing scanning to reduce learning demands: The performance of typically developing 2-year-olds. *Augmentative and Alternative Communication, 22,* 269–283.

McCarthy, C.F., McLean, L.K., Miller, J., Paul-Brown, D., Romski, M.A., Rourk, J.D., & Yoder, D.E. (1998). *Communication supports checklist for programs serving individuals with severe disabilities.* Baltimore: Paul H. Brookes Publishing Co.

McClannahan, L.E., & Krantz, P.J. (1999). *Activity schedules for children with autism: Teaching independent behavior.* Bethesda, MD: Woodbine House.

McCord, M.S., & Soto, G. (2004). Perceptions of AAC: An ethnographic investigation of Mexican-American families. *Augmentative and Alternative Communication, 20,* 209–227.

McDonald, E., & Schultz, A. (1973). Communication boards for cerebral palsied children. *Journal of Speech and Hearing Disorders, 38,* 73–88.

McEwen, I., & Lloyd, L.L. (1990). Positioning students with cerebral palsy to use augmentative and alternative communication. *Language, Speech, and Hearing Services in Schools, 21,* 15–21.

McGee, G., Morrier, M., & Daly, T. (1999). An incidental teaching approach to early intervention for toddlers with autism. *Journal of the Association for Persons with Severe Handicaps, 24,* 133–146.

McGinnis, J. (1991). *Development of two source lists for vocabulary selection in augmentative communication: Documentation of the spoken and written vocabulary of third grade students* (Unpublished doctoral dissertation). University of Nebraska–Lincoln.

McKelvey, M., Dietz, A., Hux, K., Weissling, K., & Beukelman, D.R. (2007). Performance of a person with chronic aphasia using personal and contextual pictures in a visual scene display prototype. *Journal of Medical Speech-Language Pathology, 15,* 305–317.

McKelvey, M., Evans, D., Kawai, N., & Beukelman, D. (2012). *Communication styles of persons with amyotrophic lateral sclerosis as recounted by surviving partners: A phenomenological study.* Manuscript submitted for publication.

McKelvey, M., Hux, K., Dietz, A., & Beukelman, D.R. (2010). Impact of personal relevance and contextualization on comprehension by people with chronic aphasia. *American Journal of Speech-Language Pathology, 19,* 22–33.

McLean, J., McLean, L., Brady, N., & Etter, R. (1991). Communication profiles of two types of gestures using nonverbal persons with severe to profound mental retardation. *Journal of Speech and Hearing Research, 34,* 294–308.

McLean, J., & Snyder McLean, L. (1988). Applications of pragmatics to severely mentally retarded children and youth. In R.L. Schiefelbusch & L.L. Lloyd (Eds.), *Language perspectives: Acquisition, retardation, and intervention* (2nd ed., pp. 255–288). Austin, TX: PRO-ED.

McNaughton, D., Arnold, A., Sennott, S., & Serpentine, E. (2010). Employment and individuals who use AAC. In D.B. McNaughton & D.R. Beukelman (Eds.), *Transition strategies for adolescents and young adults who use AAC* (pp. 111–127). Baltimore: Paul H. Brookes Publishing Co.

McNaughton, D.B., & Beukelman, D.R. (Eds.). (2010). *Transition strategies for adolescents and young adults who use AAC.* Baltimore: Paul H. Brookes Publishing Co.

McNaughton, D., & Bryen, D. (2007). AAC technologies to enhance participation and access to meaningful societal roles for adolescents and adults with developmental disabilities who require AAC. *Augmentative and Alternative Communication, 23,* 217–229.

McNaughton, D., & Kennedy, P. (2010). Introduction: Key components of successful transitions. In D.B. McNaughton & D.R. Beukelman (Eds.), *Transition strategies for adolescents and young adults who use AAC* (pp. 3–15). Baltimore: Paul H. Brookes Publishing Co.

McNaughton, D., & Light, J. (1989). Teaching facilitators to support the communication skills of an adult with severe cognitive disabilities: A case study. *Augmentative and Alternative Communication, 5,* 35–41.

McNaugthon, D., Light, J., & Arnold, K. (2002). "Getting your wheel in the door": Successful full-time employment experiences of individuals with cerebral palsy who use augmentative and alternative communication. *Augmentative and Alternative Communication, 18,* 59–76.

McNaughton, D., Light, J., & Groszyk, L. (2001). "Don't give up": Employment experiences of individuals with amyotrophic lateral sclerosis who use augmentative and alternative communication. *Augmentative and Alternative Communication, 17,* 179–195.

McNaughton, D., Rackensperger, T., Benedek-Wood, E., Williams, M.B., & Light, J.C. (2008). "A child needs to be given a chance to succeed": Parents of individuals who use AAC describe the benefits and challenges of learning AAC technologies. *Augmentative and Alternative Communication, 24,* 43–55.

McNaughton, D., & Tawney, J. (1993). Comparison of two spelling instruction techniques for adults who use augmentative and alternative communication. *Augmentative and Alternative Communication, 9,* 72–82.

McNaughton, S. (1990a). Introducing AccessBliss. *Communicating Together, 8*(2), 12–13.

McNaughton, S. (1990b). StoryBliss. *Communicating Together, 8*(1), 12–13.

Medicare funding of AAC technology, assessment/application protocol. (2004). Retrieved from the AAC-RERC web site, supported in part by the National Institute on Disability and Rehabilitation Research (NIDRR): http://aac-rerc.psu.edu/index.php/pages/show/id/27

Mergler, N., & Goldstein, M. (1983). Why are there old people? *Human Development, 26,* 130–143.

Mesibov, G., Browder, D., & Kirkland, C. (2002). Using individualized schedules as a component of positive behavioral support for students with developmental disabilities. *Journal of Positive Behavior Interventions, 4,* 73–79.

Mesulam, M. (2001). Primary progressive aphasia. *Annals of Neurology, 49,* 425–432.

Mesulam, M. (2007). Primary progressive aphasia: A 25-year retrospective. *Alzheimer Disease & Associated Disorders, 21,* 7–11.

Meyer, L.H., Peck, C.A., & Brown, L. (Eds.). (1991). *Critical issues in the lives of people with severe disabilities.* Baltimore: Paul H. Brookes Publishing Co.

Michelsen, S.I., Uldall, P., Mette, A., & Madsen, M. (2005). Employment prospects in cerebral palsy. *Developmental Medicine & Child Neurology, 47,* 511–517.

Mike, D.G. (1995). Literacy and cerebral palsy: Factors influencing literacy learning in a self-contained setting. *Journal of Literacy Research, 27,* 627–642.

Miles, B. (2008, October). Overview on deaf-blindness. *DB-Link*, 1–6.

Millar, D.C. (2009). Effects of AAC on natural speech development of individuals with autism. In P. Mirenda & T. Iacono (Eds.), *Autism spectrum disorders and AAC* (pp. 171–192). Baltimore: Paul H. Brookes Publishing Co.

Millar, D., Light, J., & McNaughton, D. (2004). The effect of direct instruction and writers workshop on the early writing skills of children who use augmentative and alternative communication. *Augmentative and Alternative Communication, 20,* 164–178.

Millar, D.C., Light, J.C., & Schlosser, R.W. (2006). The impact of augmentative and alternative communication intervention on the speech production of individuals with developmental disabilities: A research review. *Journal of Speech, Language, and Hearing Research, 49,* 248–264.

Millin, N. (1995). Developing our own voices. *Communicating Together, 12*(1), 2–4.

Mims, P.J., Browder, D.M., Baker, J.N., Lee, A., & Spooner, F. (2009). Increasing comprehension of students with significant intellectual disabilities and visual impairments during shared stories. *Education and Training in Developmental Disabilities, 44,* 409–420.

Mineo, B., Peischl, D., & Pennington, C. (2008). Moving targets: The effect of animation on identification of action word representations. *Augmentative and Alternative Communication, 24,* 162–173.

Mineo Mollica, B. (2003). Representational competence. In J.C. Light, D.R. Beukelman, & J. Reichle (Eds.), *Communicative competence for individuals who use AAC: From research to effective practice* (pp. 107–145). Baltimore: Paul H. Brookes Publishing Co.

Mirenda, P. (1985). Designing pictorial communication systems for physically able-bodied students with severe handicaps. *Augmentative and Alternative Communication, 1,* 58–64.

Mirenda, P. (1993). AAC: Bonding the uncertain mosaic. *Augmentative and Alternative Communication, 9,* 3–9.

Mirenda, P. (1997). Supporting individuals with challenging behaviour through functional communication training and AAC: A research review. *Augmentative and Alternative Communication, 13,* 207–225.

Mirenda, P. (2003a). "He's not really a reader….": Perspectives on supporting literacy development in individuals with autism. *Topics in Language Disorders, 23,* 270–281.

Mirenda, P. (2003b). Toward functional augmentative and alternative communication for students with autism: Manual signs, graphic symbols, and voice output communication aids. *Language, Speech, and Hearing Services in Schools, 34,* 202–215.

Mirenda, P. (2003c). Using AAC to replace problem behavior. *Augmentative Communication News, 15*(4), 10–11.

Mirenda, P., & Bopp, K.D. (2003). "Playing the game": Strategic competence in AAC. In J.C. Light, D.R. Beukelman, & J. Reichle (Eds.), *Communicative competence for individuals who use AAC: From research to effective practice* (pp. 401–437). Baltimore: Paul H. Brookes Publishing Co.

Mirenda, P., & Brown, K. (2007, June). Supporting individuals with autism and problem behavior using AAC. *Perspectives on Augmentative and Alternative Communication, 16* (2), 26–31.

Mirenda, P., & Brown, K. (2009). A picture is worth a thousand words: Using visual supports for augmented input with individuals with autism spectrum disorders. In P. Mirenda & T. Iacono (Eds.), *Autism spectrum disorders and AAC* (pp. 303–332). Baltimore: Paul H. Brookes Publishing Co.

Mirenda, P., & Dattilo, J. (1987). Instructional techniques in alternative communication for learners with severe intellectual disabilities. *Augmentative and Alternative Communication, 3,* 143–152.

Mirenda, P., & Erickson, K. (2000). Augmentative communication and literacy. In A.M. Wetherby & B.M. Prizant (Eds.), *Autism spectrum disorders: A transactional developmental perspective* (pp. 333–367). Baltimore: Paul H. Brookes Publishing Co.

Mirenda, P., & Iacono, T. (Eds.) (2009). *Autism spectrum disorders and AAC.* Baltimore: Paul H. Brookes Publishing Co.

Mirenda, P., & Locke, P. (1989). A comparison of symbol transparency in nonspeaking persons with intellectual disabilities. *Journal of Speech and Hearing Disorders, 54,* 131–140.

Mirenda, P., & Santogrossi, J. (1985). A prompt-free strategy to teach pictorial communication system use. *Augmentative and Alternative Communication, 1,* 143–150.

Mirenda, P., & Schuler, A. (1988). Teaching individuals with autism and related disorders to use visual-spatial symbols to communicate. In S.W. Blackstone, E.L. Cassatt-James, & D. Bruskin (Eds.), *Augmentative communication: Implementation strategies* (pp. 5.1:17–5.1:25). Rockville, MD: American Speech-Language-Hearing Association.

Mirenda, P., & Schuler, A. (1989). Augmenting communication for persons with autism: Issues and strategies. *Topics in Language Disorders, 9,* 24–43.

Mitchell, J.D., & Borasio, G.D. (2007). Amyotrophic lateral sclerosis. *The Lancet, 369,* 2031–2041.

Mitsuyama, Y., Kogoh, H., & Ata, K. (1985). Progressive dementia with motor neuron disease: An additional case report and neuropathological review of 20 cases in Japan. *European Archives of Psychiatry and Neurological Sciences, 235*(1), 1–8.

Mizuko, M. (1987). Transparency and ease of learning of symbols represented by Blissymbols, PCS, and Picsyms. *Augmentative and Alternative Communication, 3,* 129–136.

Mizuko, M., & Reichle, J. (1989). Transparency and recall of symbols among intellectually handicapped adults. *Journal of Speech and Hearing Disorders, 54,* 627–633.

Mizuko, M., Reichle, J., Ratcliff, A., & Esser, J. (1994). Effects of selection techniques and array sizes on short-term visual memory. *Augmentative and Alternative Communication, 10,* 237–244.

Moes, D.R. (1998). Integrating choice-making opportunities within teacher-assigned academic tasks to facilitate the performance of children with autism. *Journal of the Association for Persons with Severe Handicaps, 23,* 319–328.

Moje, E.B. (1996). "I teach students, not subjects": Teacher-student relationships as contexts for secondary literacy. *Reading Research Quarterly, 31,* 172–195.

Montgomery, G.K., & Erickson, L.M. (1987). Neuropsychological perspectives in amyotrophic lateral sclerosis. *Neurologic Clinics, 5*(1), 61–81.

Moore, D.W., Bean, T.W., Birdyshaw, D., & Rycik, J.A. (1999). Adolescent literacy: A position statement. *Journal of Adolescent & Adult Literacy, 43,* 97–112.

Morrow, D., Beukelman, D.R., Mirenda, P., & Yorkston, K. (1993). Vocabulary selection for augmentative communication systems: A comparison of three techniques. *American Journal of Speech-Language Pathology, 2,* 19–30.

Moster, D., Lie, R., Irgens, L., Bjerkedal, T., & Markestad, T. (2001). The association of Apgar score with subsequent death and cerebral palsy: A population-based study in infants. *Journal of Pediatrics, 138,* 791–792.

Mount, B., & Zwernik, K. (1988). *It's never too early, it's never too late* (Pub. No. 421). St. Paul, MN: Metropolitan Council.

Müller, E., & Soto, G. (2002). Conversation patterns of three adults using aided speech: Variations across partners. *Augmentative and Alternative Communication, 18,* 77–90.

Munroe, S. (2001). *Developing a national volunteer registry for persons with deafblindness in Canada: Results from the study, 1999–2001.* Brantford, ON: Canadian Deafblind and Rubella Association.

Murdoch, B.E., & Lethlean, J.B. (2000). High-level language, naming and discourse abilities in multiple sclerosis. In B. Murdoch & D.G. Theodoros (Eds.), *Speech and language disorders in multiple sclerosis* (pp. 131–155). London: Whurr.

Murphy, J., & Cameron, L. (2008). The effectiveness of Talking Mats® with people with intellectual disability. *British Journal of Learning Disabilities, 36,* 232–241.

Murphy, J., Markova, I., Moodie, E., Scott, J., & Boa, S. (1995). Augmentative and alternative communication systems used by people with cerebral palsy in Scotland: Demographic survey. *Augmentative and Alternative Communication, 11,* 26–36.

Murphy, J., Tester, S., Hubbard, G., Downs, M., & McDonald, C. (2005). Enabling frail older people with a communication difficulty to express their views: The use of Talking Mats as an interview tool. *Health and Social Care in the Community, 13,* 95–107.

Murray, L.L. (2000). Spoken language production in Huntington's and Parkinson's diseases. *Journal of Speech, Language, and Hearing Research, 43,* 1350–1366.

Murray, L.L., Holland, A.L., & Beeson, P.M. (1997). Auditory processing in individuals with mild aphasia: A study of resource allocation. *Journal of Speech Language and Hearing Research, 40,* 792–808.

Murray-Branch, J., Udvari-Solner, A., & Bailey, B. (1991). Textured communication systems for individuals with severe intellectual and dual sensory impairments. *Language, Speech, and Hearing Services in Schools, 22,* 260–268.

Musselwhite, C. (1985). *Songbook: Signs and symbols for children.* Wauconda, IL: Don Johnston.

Musselwhite, C. (1986). *Adaptive play for special needs children: Strategies to enhance communication and learning.* San Diego: Singular.

Musselwhite, C., & King-DeBaun, P. (1997). *Emerging success.* Volo, IL: Don Johnston.

Musselwhite, C., & St. Louis, K. (1988). *Communication programming for persons with severe handicaps* (2nd ed.). Austin, TX: PRO-ED.

Nagi, S. (1991). Disability concepts revisited: Implications for prevention. In A. Pope & A. Tarlov (Eds.), *Disability in America: Toward a national agenda for prevention* (pp. 309–327). Washington, DC: National Academy Press.

Naglieri, J. (2003). *Naglieri Nonverbal Ability Test–Individual Administration*. San Antonio, TX: Pearson Assessments..

Nakamura, K., Newell, A., Alm, N., & Waller, A. (1998). How do members of different language communities compose sentences with a picture-based communication system? A cross-cultural study of picture-based sentences constructed by English and Japanese speakers. *Augmentative and Alternative Communication, 14,* 71–80.

Namy, L. (2001). What's in a name when it isn't a word? 17-month-olds' mapping of nonverbal symbols to object categories. *Infancy, 2,* 1–122.

Namy, L., Campbell, A.L., & Tomasello, M. (2004). The changing role of iconicity in non-verbal symbol learning: A U-shaped trajectory in the acquisition of arbitrary gestures. *Journal of Cognition and Development, 5,* 37–57.

National Consortium on Deaf-Blindness (2011). *The importance of communication.* Retrieved from http://www.nationaldb.org/FFCommunication.php

National Institute of Neurological Disorders and Stroke. (2009, September 15). *Guillain-Barré Syndrome Fact Sheet.* Retrieved from http://www.ninds.nih.gov/disorders/gbs/detail_gbs.htm

National Institute on Deafness and Other Communication Disorders. (2008, October). *Aphasia* (NIH Pub. No. 97–4257). Retrieved from http://www.nidcd.nih.gov/health/voice/pages/aphasia.aspx

National Joint Committee for the Communication Needs of Persons with Severe Disabilities. (1992). Guidelines for meeting the communication needs of persons with severe disabilities. *ASHA, 34*(Suppl. 7), 2–3.

National Joint Committee for the Communication Needs of Persons with Severe Disabilities. (2003a). Position statement on access to communication services and supports: Concerns regarding the application of restrictive eligibility policies. *ASHA Supplement, 23,* 19–20.

National Joint Committee for the Communication Needs of Persons with Severe Disabilities. (2003b). Supporting documentation for the position statement on access to communication services and supports: Concerns regarding the application of restrictive eligibility policies. *ASHA Supplement, 23,* 73–81.

National Reading Panel. (2000). *Report of the National Reading Panel. Teaching children to read: An evidence-based assessment of the scientific research literature on reading and its implications for reading instruction: Reports of the subgroups* (NIH Publication No. 00–4754). Washington, DC: U.S. Government Printing Office.

National Research Council Committee on Educational Interventions for Children with Autism, Division of Behavioral and Social Sciences and Education. (2001). *Educating children with autism.* Washington, DC: National Academy Press.

Nelson, C., van Dijk, J., Oster, T., & McDonnell, A. (2009). *Child-guided strategies: The van Dijk approach to assessment.* Louisville, KY: American Printing House for the Blind.

Nelson, K. (1988). Acquisition of words by first language learners. In M.B. Franklin & S.S. Barten (Eds.), *Child language: A reader* (pp. 50–59). New York: Oxford University Press.

Nelson, N. (1992). Performance is the prize: Language competence and performance among AAC users. *Augmentative and Alternative Communication, 8,* 3–18.

Newman, T.M., Macomber, D., Naples, A.J., Babitz, T., Volkmar, F., Grigorenko, E.L. (2007). Hyperlexia in children with autism spectrum disorders. *Journal of Autism and Developmental Disorders, 37,* 760–774.

Nicholas, M., Sinotte, M., & Helm-Estabrooks, N. (2005). Using a computer to communicate: Effect of executive function impairments in people with severe aphasia. *Aphasiology, 19*(10/11), 1052–1065.

Nicholas, M., Sinotte, M.P., & Helm-Estabrooks, N. (2011). C-Speak Aphasia alternative communication program for people with severe aphasia: Importance of executive functioning and semantic knowledge. *Neuropsychological Rehabilitation, 21,* 322–366.

Nigam, R. (2003). Do individuals from diverse cultural and ethnic backgrounds perceive graphic symbols differently? *Augmentative and Alternative Communication, 19,* 135–136.

Nigam, R., Schlosser, R., & Lloyd, L.L. (2006). Concomitant use of the matrix strategy and the mand-model procedure in teaching graphic symbol combinations. *Augmentative and Alternative Communication, 22,* 160–177.

No Child Left Behind Act of 2001, PL 107-110, 115 Stat. 1425, 20 U.S.C. §§ 6301 *et seq.*

Nolan, C. (1987). *Under the eye of the clock.* New York: St. Martin's Press.

Nordness, A., & Beukelman, D.R. (2010). Speech practice patterns of children with speech sound disorders: The impact of parental record keeping and computer-led practice. *Journal of Medical Speech-Language Pathology, 18,* 104–108.

Northup, J., Wacker, D., Berg, W., Kelly, L., Sasso, G., & DeRaad, A. (1994). The treatment of severe behavior problems in school settings using a technical assistance model. *Journal of Applied Behavior Analysis, 27,* 33–48.

O'Brien, J., & Lyle O'Brien, C. (2002). *Implementing person-centered planning: Voices of experience.* Toronto: Inclusion Press.

O' Brien, J., & Pearpoint, J. (2007). *Person-centered planning using MAPS & PATH: A workbook for facilitators.* Toronto: Inclusion Press.

Ogletree, B. (2010). A causal relationship between pre-treatment matching or motor imitation skills and later acquisition of manual signing or picture exchange communication in children with ASD remains to be established. *Evidence-based Communication Assessment and Intervention, 4,* 105–108.

Ogletree, B., Bruce, S., Finch, A., Fahey, R., & McLean, L. (2011). Recommended communication-based interventions for individuals with severe intellectual disabilities. *Communication Disorders Quarterly, 32,* 164–175.

Okalidou, A., & Malandraki, G. (2007). The application of PECS in children with autism and deafness: A case study. *Focus on Autism and Other Developmental Disabilities, 22,* 23–32.

O'Keefe, B., Brown, L., & Schuller, R. (1998). Identification and rankings of communication aid features by five groups. *Augmentative and Alternative Communication, 14,* 37–50.

O'Keefe, B., & Dattilo, J. (1992). Teaching the response-recode form to adults with mental retardation using AAC systems. *Augmentative and Alternative Communication, 8,* 224–233.

Oliver, J., Ponford, J., & Curren, C. (1996). Outcomes following traumatic brain injury. A comparison between 2 and 5 years after injury. *Brain Injury, 10,* 841–848.

Olmos-Lau, N., Ginsberg, M., & Geller, J. (1977). Aphasia in multiple sclerosis. *Neurology, 27,* 623–626.

Olsson, C., & Granlund, M. (2003). Pre-symbolic communication intervention. In R. Schlosser (Ed.), *Efficacy research in augmentative and alternative communication* (pp. 299–322). New York: Elsevier.

Orel-Bixler, D. (1999). Clinical vision assessment for infants. In D. Chen (Ed.), *Essential elements in early intervention* (pp. 107–156). New York: AFB Press.

Orelove, F.P., & Sobsey, D. (1996). *Educating children with multiple disabilities: A transdisciplinary approach* (3rd ed.). Baltimore: Paul H. Brookes Publishing Co.

Oxley, J., & Norris, J. (2000). Children's use of memory strategies: Relevance to voice output communication aid use. *Augmentative and Alternative Communication, 16,* 79–94.

Pakula, A.T., Van Naarden Braun, K., & Yeargin-Allsopp, M. (2009). Cerebral palsy: classification and epidemiology. *Physical Medicine and Rehabilitation Clinics of North America, 20,* 425–452.

Pappas, N.W., McLeod, S., McAllister, L., & McKinnon, D.H. (2008). Parental involvement in speech intervention: A national survey. *Clinical Linguistics & Phonetics, 22,* 335–344.

Parette, P., Chuang, S.J., & Huer, M.B. (2004). First generation Chinese family attitudes regarding disabilities and educational interventions. *Focus on Autism and Other Developmental Disabilities, 19,* 114–123.

Parette, P., & Huer, M.B. (2002). Working with Asian American families whose children have augmentative and alternative communication needs. *Journal of Special Education Technology, 17*(4), 5–13.

Parette, H., Huer, M.B., & Scherer, M. (2004). Effects of acculturation on assistive technology service delivery. *Journal of Special Education Technology, 19,* 31–42.

Parette, P., Huer, M.B., & Wyatt, T. (2002). Young African American children with disabilities and augmentative and alternative communication issues. *Early Childhood Journal, 29,* 210–227.

Park, C.C. (1982). *The siege.* Boston: Little, Brown.

Parnes, P. (1995). "Oh, Wow Days are gone forever," Canadian administrator reports. In S. Blackstone & H. Pressman (Eds.), *Outcomes in AAC conference report: Alliance '95* (pp. 21–22). Monterey, CA: Augmentative Communication.

Paul, D., Frattali, C., Holland, A., Thompson, C., Caperton, C., & Slater, S. (2004). *Quality of Communication Life Scale (ASHA QCL).* Rockville, MD: American Speech-Language-Hearing Association.

Paul, R. (1997). Facilitating transitions in language development for children using AAC. *Augmentative and Alternative Communication, 13,* 141–148.

Pearpoint, J., O'Brien, J., & Forest, M. (2008). PATH: *A workbook for planning positive possible futures for schools, organizations, businesses, and families.* Toronto: Inclusion Press.

Peck, S., Wacker, D., Berg, W., Cooper, L., Brown, K., Richman, D.,…Millard, T. (1996). Choice-making treatment of young children's severe behavior problems. *Journal of Applied Behavior Analysis, 29,* 263–290.

Peck Peterson, S.M., Derby, K.M., Harding, J.W., Weddle, T., & Barretto, A. (2002). Behavioral support for school-age children with developmental disabilities and problem behavior. In J.M. Lucyshyn, G. Dunlap, & R.W. Albin (Eds.), *Families and positive behavior support: Addressing problem behavior in family contexts* (pp. 287–304). Baltimore: Paul H. Brookes Publishing Co.

Pellegrino, L. (2002). Cerebral palsy. In M.L. Batshaw (Ed.), *Children with disabilities* (5th ed., pp. 443–466). Baltimore: Paul H. Brookes Publishing Co.

Pepper, J., & Weitzman, E. (2004). *It takes two to talk: A practical guide for parents of children with language delays.* Toronto: Hanen Centre.

Pierce, P., Steelman, J., Koppenhaver, D., & Yoder, D. (1993, March). Linking symbols with language. *Communicating Together, 11*(1), 18–19.

Piotrkowski, C., Botsko, M., & Matthews, E. (2001). Parents' and teachers' beliefs about children's school readiness in a high-need community. *Early Childhood Research Quarterly, 15,* 537–558.

Poole, M. (1979). Social class, sex, and linguistic coding. *Language and Speech, 22,* 49–67.

Porter, G. (2007). *Pragmatic Organization Dynamic Display communication books: Direct access templates.* Melbourne, Australia: Cerebral Palsy Education Centre.

Porter, G., & Cafiero, J.M. (2009, December). Pragmatic Organization Dynamic Display (PODD) communication books: A promising practice for individuals with autism spectrum disorders. *Perspectives on Augmentative and Alternative Communication, 18,* 121–129.

Porter, P. (1989). Intervention in end stage of multiple sclerosis. *Augmentative and Alternative Communication, 5,* 125–127.

Prentice, J. (2000). With communication anything is possible. In M. Fried-Oken & H. Bersani, Jr. (Eds.), *Speaking up and spelling it out: Personal essays on augmentative and alternative communication* (pp. 208–214). Baltimore: Paul H. Brookes Publishing Co.

Preston, D., & Carter, M. (2009). A review of the efficacy of the Picture Exchange Communication System intervention. *Journal of Autism and Developmental Disorders, 39,* 1471–1486.

Price, S.P. (2000). My early life and education. In M. Fried-Oken & H.A. Bersani, Jr. (Eds.), *Speaking up and spelling it out: Personal essays on augmentative and alternative communication* (pp. 105–114). Baltimore: Paul H. Brookes Publishing Co.

Prizant, B. (1983). Language and communicative behavior in autism: Toward an understanding of the "whole" of it. *Journal of Speech and Hearing Disorders, 46,* 241–249.

Prizant, B.M., Wetherby, A., Rubin, E., & Laurent, A. (2003). The SCERTS Model: A transactional, family-centered approach to enhancing communication and socioemotional abilities of children with autism spectrum disorder. *Infants and Young Children, 16,* 296–316.

Prizant, B.M., Wetherby, A.M., Rubin, E., Laurent, A.C., & Rydell, P.J. (2006a). *The SCERTS® Model: A comprehensive educational approach for children with autism spectrum disorders: Vol. I. Assessment.* Baltimore: Paul H. Brookes Publishing Co.

Prizant, B.M., Wetherby, A.M., Rubin, E., Laurent, A.C., & Rydell, P.J. (2006b). *The SCERTS® Model: A comprehensive educational approach for children with autism spectrum disorders: Vol. II. Program planning and intervention.* Baltimore: Paul H. Brookes Publishing Co.

Prouty, S., & Prouty, M. (2009, Fall). Intervenors: One key to success. *Deaf-Blind Perspectives, 17,* 1–4.

Purdy, M., & Dietz, A. (2010). Factors influencing AAC usage by individuals with aphasia. *Perspectives on Augmentative and Alternative Communication, 19,* 70–78.

Purdy, M., & Koch, A. (2006). Prediction of strategy usage by adults with aphasia. *Aphasiology, 20*(2/3/4), 337–348.

Putnam, J.W. (Ed.). (1998). *Cooperative learning and strategies for inclusion: Celebrating diversity in the classroom* (2nd ed.). Baltimore: Paul H. Brookes Publishing Co.

QIAT Consortium. (2009). *Quality indicators for assistive technology services.* Retrieved from http://natri.uky.edu/assoc_projects/qiat/index.html

Rackensperger, T., Krezman, C., McNaughton, D., Williams, M.B., & D'Silva, K. (2005). "When I first got it, I wanted to throw it off a cliff": The challenges and benefits of learning AAC technologies as described by adults who use AAC. *Augmentative and Alternative Communication, 21,* 165–186.

Rackowska, M. (2000). The different one in society. In M. Williams & C. Krezman (Eds.), *Beneath the surface: Creative expressions of augmented communicators* (p. 88). Toronto: ISAAC Press.

Radell, U. (1997). Augmentative and alternative communication assessment strategies: Seating and positioning. In S.L. Glennen & D. DeCoste (Eds.), *The handbook of augmentative and alternative communication* (pp. 193–242). San Diego: Singular.

Raney, C., & Silverman, F. (1992). Attitudes toward nonspeaking individuals who use communication boards. *Journal of Speech and Hearing Research, 35,* 1269–1271.

Rao, S.M. (1995). Neuropsychology of multiple sclerosis. *Current Opinion in Neurology, 8,* 216–220.

Raskind, M., & Bryant, B. (2002). *Functional Evaluation for Assistive Technology (FEAT).* Port Chester, NY: National Professional Resources.

Rasmussen, P., Bšrjesson, O., Wentz, E., & Gillberg, C. (2001). Autistic disorders in Down syndrome: Background factors and clinical correlates. *Developmental Medicine and Child Neurology, 43,* 750–754.

Ratcliff, A. (1994). Comparison of relative demands implicated in direct selection and scanning: Considerations from normal children. *Augmentative and Alternative Communication, 10,* 67–74.

Redmond, S., & Johnston, S. (2001). Evaluating the morphological competence of children with severe speech and physical impairments. *Journal of Speech, Language, and Hearing Research, 44,* 1362–1375.

Reed, C., Delhorne, L., Durlach, N., & Fischer, S. (1990). A study of the tactual and visual reception of fingerspelling. *Journal of Speech and Hearing Research, 33,* 786–797.

Reed, C., Delhorne, L., Durlach, N., & Fischer, S. (1995). A study of the tactual reception of sign language. *Journal of Speech and Hearing Research, 38,* 477–489.

Rees, N. (1982). Language intervention with children. In J. Miller, D. Yoder, & R. Schiefelbusch (Eds.), *Contemporary issues in language intervention* (American Speech-Language-Hearing Association Report No. 12, pp. 309–316). Rockville, MD: American Speech-Language-Hearing Association.

Rehabilitation Act of 1973, PL 93-112, 29 U.S.C. §§ 701 *et seq.*

Rehfeldt, R., Kinney, E., Root, S., & Stromer, R. (2004). Creating activity schedules using Microsoft PowerPoint. *Journal of Applied Behavior Analysis, 37,* 115–128.

Rehfeldt, R., & Root, S. (2005). Establishing derived requesting skills in adults with severe developmental disabilities. *Journal of Applied Behavior Analysis, 38,* 101–105.

Reichert Hoge, D., & Newsome, C. (2002). *The Source for augmentative alternative communication.* East Moline, IL: LinguiSystems.

Reichle, J., & Brown, L. (1986). Teaching the use of a multipage direct selection communication board to an adult with autism. *Journal of the Association for Persons with Severe Handicaps, 11,* 68–73.

Reichle, J., & Drager, K. (2010). Examining issues of aided communication display and navigational strategies for young children with developmental disabilities. *Journal of Developmental and Physical Disabilities, 22,* 289–311.

Reichle, J., & Johnston, S. (1999). Teaching the conditional use of communicative requests to two school-age children with severe developmental disabilities. *Language, Speech, and Hearing Services in Schools, 30,* 324–334.

Reichle, J., & Karlan, G. (1985). The selection of an augmentative system of communication intervention: A critique of decision rules. *Journal of the Association for Persons with Severe Handicaps, 10,* 146–156.

Reichle, J., Rogers, N., & Barrett, C. (1984). Establishing pragmatic discrimination among the communicative functions of requesting, rejecting, and commenting in an adolescent. *Journal of the Association for Persons with Severe Handicaps, 9,* 31–36.

Reichle, J., Sigafoos, J., & Piché, L. (1989). Teaching an adolescent with blindness and severe disabilities: A correspondence between requesting and selecting preferred objects. *Journal of the Association for Persons with Severe Handicaps, 14,* 75–80.

Reichle, J., & Wacker, D.P. (Eds.). (1993). *Communication and language intervention series: Vol. 3. Communicative alternatives to challenging behavior: Integrating functional assessment and intervention strategies.* Baltimore: Paul H. Brookes Publishing Co.

Reichle, J., York, J., & Sigafoos, J. (1991). *Implementing augmentative and alternative communication: Strategies for learners with severe disabilities.* Baltimore: Paul H. Brookes Publishing Co.

Remington, B. (1994). Augmentative and alternative communication and behavior analysis: A productive partnership? *Augmentative and Alternative Communication, 10,* 3–13.

Remington, B., & Clarke, S. (1993a). Simultaneous communication and speech comprehension: Part I. Comparison of two methods of teaching expressive signing and speech comprehension skills. *Augmentative and Alternative Communication, 9,* 36–48.

Remington, B., & Clarke, S. (1993b). Simultaneous communication and speech comprehension: Part II. Comparison of two methods overcoming selective attention during expressive sign training. *Augmentative and Alternative Communication, 9,* 49–60.

Remington, B., Watson, J., & Light, J. (1990). Beyond the single sign: A matrix-based approach to teaching productive sign combinations. *Mental Handicap Research, 3,* 33–50.

Renwick, R., Brown, I., & Raphael, D. (1998). *The quality of life profile: People with physical and sensory disabilities.* Toronto: University of Toronto, Centre for Health Promotion.

Rescorla, L., Alley, A., & Christine, J. (2001). Word frequencies of toddlers' lexicons. *Journal of Speech, Language, and Hearing Research, 44,* 598–609.

Richter, M., Ball, L., Beukelman, D.R., Lasker, J., & Ullman, C. (2003). Attitudes toward communication modes and message formulation techniques used for storytelling by people with amyotrophic lateral sclerosis. *Augmentative and Alternative Communication, 19,* 170–186.

Rijntjes, M. (2006). Mechanisms of recovery in stroke patients with hemiparesis or aphasia: New insights, old questions and the meaning of therapies. *Current Opinion in Neurology, 19,* 76–83.

Robbins, A.M., & Osberger, M.J. (1992). *Meaningful use of speech scale.* Indianapolis: Indiana University School of Medicine.

Robinson, N., & Solomon-Rice, P. (2009). Supporting collaborative teams and families in AAC. In G. Soto & K. Zangari (Eds.), *Practically speaking: Language, literacy, and academic development of students with AAC needs* (pp. 289–312). Baltimore: Paul H. Brookes Publishing Co.

Rochat, P., & Callaghan, T. (2005). What drives symbolic development? The case of pictorial comprehension and production. In L. Namy (Ed.), *Symbol use and symbolic representation: Developmental and comparative perspectives* (pp. 25–46). Mahwah, NJ: Lawrence Erlbaum.

Rogers, M.A., & Alarcon, N.B. (1999). Characteristics and management of primary progressive aphasia. *Neurophysiology and Neurogenic Speech and Language Disorders Newsletter, 9,* 12–26.

Rogers, S., & Dawson, G. (2010). *Early Start Denver model for young children with autism: Promoting language, learning, and engagement.* New York: Guilford Press.

Rogers-Warren, A., & Warren, S. (1980). Mands for verbalization: Facilitating the display of newly trained language in children. *Behavior Modification, 4,* 361–382.

Roid, G.H., & Miller, L.J. (1997). *Leiter International Performance Scale–Revised.* Wood Dale, IL: Stoelting.

Roid, G.H., & Miller, L.J. (1999). *Stoelting Brief Intelligence Test (S-BIT).* Wood Dale, IL: Stoelting.

Roman, A., Quach, W., Coggiola, J., & Moore, D. (2010, December). *A study comparing three low-tech communication methods for people with only eye movement.* Presentation at the International Symposium on ALS/MND, Orlando, FL.

Roman-Lantzy, C. (2007). *Cortical visual impairment: An approach to assessment and intervention.* New York: American Foundation for the Blind.

Romich, B., Hill, K., Miller, D., Adamson, J., Anthony, A., & Sunday, J. (2004). U-LAM: Universal Language Activity Monitor. *Proceedings of the 2004 RESNA Conference.* Arlington, VA: RESNA Press. Retrieved from http://www.aacinstitute.org/Resources/ProductsandServices/U-LAM/papers/Romich,et.al.(2004).html

Romski, M.A., & Ruder, K. (1984). Effects of speech and speech and sign instruction on oral language learning and generalization of object 1 action combinations by Down's syndrome children. *Journal of Speech and Hearing Disorders, 49,* 293–302.

Romski, M., & Sevcik, R. (1988a). Augmentative and alternative communication systems: Considerations for individuals with severe intellectual disabilities. *Augmentative and Alternative Communication, 4,* 83–93.

Romski, M., & Sevcik, R. (1988b, November). *Speech output communication systems: Acquisition/use by youngsters with retardation.* Miniseminar presented at the annual convention of the American Speech-Language-Hearing Association, Boston.

Romski, M.A., & Sevcik, R.A. (1992). Developing augmented language in children with severe mental retardation. In S.F. Warren & J. Reichle (Eds.), *Communication and language intervention series: Vol. 1. Causes and effects in communication and language intervention* (pp. 113–130). Baltimore: Paul H. Brookes Publishing Co.

Romski, M.A., & Sevcik, R.A. (1993). Language learning through augmented means: The process and its products. In A.P. Kaiser & D.B. Gray (Eds.), *Communication and language intervention series: Vol. 2. Enhancing children's communication: Research foundations for intervention* (pp. 85–104). Baltimore: Paul H. Brookes Publishing Co.

Romski, M.A., & Sevcik, R.A. (1996). *Breaking the speech barrier: Language development through augmented means.* Baltimore: Paul H. Brookes Publishing Co.

Romski, M.A., & Sevcik, R. (1999, May). Speech comprehension and early augmented language intervention: Concepts, measurement, and clinical considerations. *ASHA Special Interest Division 12 Newsletter, 8*(2), 7–10.

Romski, M.A., & Sevcik, R.A. (2003). Augmented input: Enhancing communication development. In J.C. Light, D.R. Beukelman, & J. Reichle (Eds.), *Communicative competence for individuals who use AAC: From research to effective practice* (pp. 147–162). Baltimore: Paul H. Brookes Publishing Co.

Romski, M.A., & Sevcik, R. (2005). Augmentative communication and early intervention: Myths and realities. *Infants & Young Children, 18,* 174–185.

Romski, M.A., Sevcik, R.A., & Adamson, L.B. (1999). Communication patterns of youth with mental retardation with and without their speech-output communication devices. *American Journal on Mental Retardation, 104,* 249–259.

Romski, M.A., Sevcik, R.A., Adamson, L.B., & Bakeman, R. (2005). Communication patterns of augmented communicators, nonspeakers and speakers: Interactions with unfamiliar partners. *American Journal on Mental Retardation, 110,* 226–239.

Romski, M.A., Sevcik, R., Adamson, L., Cheslock, M., Smith, A., Barker, R.M., & Bakeman, R. (2010). Randomized comparison of augmented and nonaugmented language interventions for toddlers with developmental delays and their parents. *Journal of Speech, Language, and Hearing Research, 53,* 350–364.

Romski, M.A., Sevcik, R.A., & Forrest, S.C. (2001). Assistive technology and augmentative and alternative communication in inclusive early childhood programs. In M.J. Guralnick (Ed.), *Early childhood inclusion: Focus on change* (pp. 465–479). Baltimore: Paul H. Brookes Publishing Co.

Romski, M., Sevcik, R., & Pate, J. (1988). Establishment of symbolic communication in persons with severe retardation. *Journal of Speech and Hearing Disorders, 53,* 94–107.

Romski, M.A., Sevcik, R., Robinson, B., Mervis, C., & Bertrand, J. (1996). Mapping the meanings of novel visual symbols by youth with moderate or severe mental retardation. *American Journal on Mental Retardation, 100,* 391–402.

Rönnberg, J., & Borg, E., (2001). A review and evaluation of research on the deaf-blind from perceptual, communicative, social and rehabilitative perspectives. *Scandinavian Audiology, 30,* 67–77.

Rosa-Lugo, L.I., & Kent-Walsh, J. (2008). Effects of parent instruction on communicative turns of Latino children using augmentative and alternative communication during storybook reading. *Communication Disorders Quarterly, 30,* 49–61.

Rose, D., & Meyer, A. (2002). *Teaching every student in the digital age: Universal design for learning.* Washington, DC: Association for Supervision and Curriculum Development (ASCD).

Roseberry-McKibbin, C. (2000). "Mirror, mirror on the wall": Reflections of a "third culture" American. *Communication Disorders Quarterly, 22,* 56–60.

Rosen, M., & Goodenough-Trepagnier, C. (1981). Factors affecting communication rate in nonvocal communication systems. *Proceedings of the Fourth Annual Conference on Rehabilitation Engineering* (pp. 194–195). Washington, DC: RESNA Press.

Rosenbaum, P.L., Paneth, N., Leviton, A., Goldstein, M., & Bax, M. (2007). A report: The definition and classification of cerebral palsy April 2006. *Developmental Medicine & Child Neurology, 49,* 8–14.

Rosenberg, S., & Beukelman, D.R. (1987). The participation model. In C.A. Coston (Ed.), *Proceedings of the national planners conference on assistive device service delivery* (pp. 159–161). Washington, DC: Association for the Advancement of Rehabilitation Technology.

Roth, F., & Cassatt-James, E. (1989). The language assessment process: Clinical implications for individuals with severe speech impairments. *Augmentative and Alternative Communication, 5,* 165–172.

Rotholz, D., Berkowitz, S., & Burberry, J. (1989). Functionality of two modes of communication in the community by students with developmental disabilities: A comparison of signing and communication books. *Journal of the Association for Persons with Severe Handicaps, 14,* 227–233.

Rowland, C. (1990). Communication in the classroom for children with dual sensory impairments: Studies of teacher and child behavior. *Augmentative and Alternative Communication, 6,* 262–274.

Rowland, C. (1996, 2004). *Communication Matrix.* Portland, OR: Design to Learn.

Rowland, C., & Schweigert, P. (1989). Tangible symbols: Symbolic communication for individuals with multisensory impairments. *Augmentative and Alternative Communication, 5,* 226–234.

Rowland, C., & Schweigert, P. (1990). *Tangible symbol systems: Symbolic communication for individuals with multisensory impairments.* Tucson, AZ: Communication Skill Builders.

Rowland, C., & Schweigert, P. (1991). *The early communication process using microswitch technology.* Tucson, AZ: Communication Skill Builders.

Rowland, C., & Schweigert, P. (1996). *Tangible symbol systems* (Rev. ed.) [Videotape]. San Antonio, TX: Harcourt Assessment.

Rowland, C., & Schweigert, P. (2000a). Tangible symbols, tangible outcomes. *Augmentative and Alternative Communication, 16,* 61–78, 205.

Rowland, C., & Schweigert, P. (2000b). *Tangible symbol systems* (2nd ed.). Portland: Oregon Health and Science University.

Rowland, C., & Schweigert, P. (2002). *Problem solving skills.* Portland, OR: Design to Learn.

Rowland, C., & Schweigert, P.D. (2003). Cognitive skills and AAC. In J.C. Light, D.R. Beukelman, & J. Reichle (Eds.), *Communicative competence for individuals who use AAC: From research to effective practice* (pp. 241–275). Baltimore: Paul H. Brookes Publishing Co.

Rowland, C., & Schweigert, P. (2004). *First things first: Early communication for the pre-symbolic child with severe disabilities.* Portland, OR: Design to Learn.

Rubin, E., Laurent, A.C., Prizant, B.M., & Wetherby, A. (2009). AAC and the SCERTS model: Incorporating AAC within a comprehensive, multidisciplinary educational program. In P. Mirenda & T. Iacono (Eds.), *Autism spectrum disorders and AAC* (pp. 195–217). Baltimore: Paul H. Brookes Publishing Co.

Rutz, L. (2005). Living with ALS. *Augmentative Communication News, 17,* 1–4.

Ryndak, D., & Alper, S. (Eds.). (2003). *Curriculum and instruction for students with significant disabilities in inclusive settings* (2nd ed.). Boston: Allyn & Bacon.

Sainato, D.M., & Morrison, R.S. (2001). Transition to inclusive environments for young children with disabilities: Toward a seamless system of service delivery. In M.J. Guralnick (Ed.), *Early childhood inclusion: Focus on change* (pp. 293–306). Baltimore: Paul H. Brookes Publishing Co.

Saito, Y., & Turnbull, A. (2007). Augmentative and alternative communication practice in the pursuit of family quality of life: A review of the literature. *Research & Practice for Persons with Severe Disabilities, 32,* 50–65.

Sarno, M., Buonaguro, A., & Levita, E. (1986). Characteristics of verbal impairment in closed head injured patients. *Archives of Physical Medicine and Rehabilitation, 67,* 400–405.

Saunders, C., Walsh, T., & Smith, M. (1981). Hospice care in the motor neuron diseases. In C. Saunders & J. Teller (Eds.), *Hospice: The living idea.* London: Edward Arnold.

Schaeffer, B. (1980). Spontaneous language through signed speech. In R. Schiefelbusch (Ed.), *Nonspeech language and communication* (pp. 421–446). Baltimore: University Park Press.

Schalock, R., Borthwick-Duffy, S., Bradley, V., Buntinx, W., Coulter, D., Craig, E.,...Yeager, M. (2010). *Intellectual disability: Definition, classification, and systems of support* (11th ed.). Washington, DC: American Association on Intellectual and Developmental Disabilities.

Schank, R. (1990). *Tell me a story: A new look at real and artificial memory.* New York: Charles Scribner's Sons.

Schepis, M., & Reid, D. (2003). Issues affecting staff enhancement of speech-generating device use among people with severe cognitive disabilities. *Augmentative and Alternative Communication, 19,* 59–65.

Scherer, M.J., Sax, C., Vanbiervliet, A., Cushman, L.A., & Scherer, J.V. (2005). Predictors of assistive technology use: The importance of personal and psychosocial factors. *Disability and Rehabilitation, 27,* 1321–1331.

Schlosser, R. (1999a). Nomenclature of category levels in graphic symbols, Part I: Is a flower a flower a flower? *Augmentative and Alternative Communication, 13,* 4–13.

Schlosser, R. (1999b). Nomenclature of category levels in graphic symbols, Part II: The role of similarity in categorization. *Augmentative and Alternative Communication, 13,* 14–29.

Schlosser, R. (2003a). Efficacy and outcomes measurement in augmentative and alternative communication. In R. Schlosser (Ed.), *The efficacy of augmentative and alternative communication: Toward evidence-based practice* (pp. 13–25). New York: Elsevier.

Schlosser, R. (Ed.). (2003b). *The efficacy of augmentative and alternative communication: Toward evidence-based practice.* New York: Elsevier.

Schlosser, R.W. (2003c). Outcomes measurement in AAC. In J.C. Light, D.R. Beukelman, & J. Reichle (Eds.), *Communicative competence for individuals who use AAC: From research to effective practice* (pp. 479–513). Baltimore: Paul H. Brookes Publishing Co.

Schlosser, R. (2003d). Roles of speech output in augmentative and alternative communication: Narrative review. *Augmentative and Alternative Communication, 19,* 5–27.

Schlosser, R. (2003e). Selecting graphic symbols for an initial request lexicon. In R. Schlosser (Ed.), *The efficacy of augmentative and alternative communication: Toward evidence-based practice* (pp. 347–402). New York: Elsevier.

Schlosser, R. (2004). Goal attainment scaling as a clinical measurement technique in communication disorders: A critical review. *Journal of Communication Disorders, 37,* 217–239.

Schlosser, R., Belfiore, P., Nigam, R., Blischak, D., & Hetzroni, O. (1995). The effects of speech output technology on the learning of graphic symbols. *Journal of Applied Behavior Analysis, 28,* 537–549.

Schlosser, R., Blischak, D., Belfiore, P., Bartley, C., & Barnett, N. (1998). The effectiveness of synthetic speech output and orthographic feedback in a student with autism: A preliminary study. *Journal of Autism and Developmental Disorders, 28,* 309–319.

Schlosser, R., Koul, R., & Costello, J. (2007). Asking well-built questions for evidence-based practice in augmentative and alternative communication. *Communication Disorders Quarterly, 40,* 235–238.

Schlosser, R., & Lee, D. (2000). Promoting generalization and maintenance in augmentative and alternative communication: A meta-analysis of 20 years of effectiveness research. *Augmentative and Alternative Communication, 16,* 208–226.

Schlosser, R., McGhie-Richmond, D., Blackstein-Adler, S., Mirenda, P., Antonius, K., & Janzen, P. (2000). Training a school team to integrate technology meaningfully into the curriculum: Effects on student participation. *Journal of Special Education Technology, 15,* 31–44.

Schlosser, R., & Raghavendra, P. (2003). Toward evidence-based practice in AAC. In R. Schlosser (Ed.), *The efficacy of augmentative and alternative communication: Toward evidence-based practice* (pp. 260–297). New York: Elsevier.

Schlosser, R., & Sigafoos, J. (2002). Selecting graphic symbols for an initial request lexicon: Integrative review. *Augmentative and Alternative Communication, 18,* 102–123.

Schlosser, R., & Sigafoos, J. (2006). Augmentative and alternative communication interventions for persons with developmental disabilities: Narrative review of comparative single-subject experimental studies. *Research in Developmental Disabilities, 27,* 1–29.

Schlosser, R., & Sigafoos, J. (2009). Navigating evidence-based information sources in augmentative and alternative communication. *Augmentative and Alternative Communication, 25,* 225–235.

Schlosser, R., Sigafoos, J., & Koul. R. (2009). Speech output and speech-generating devices in autism spectrum disorders. In P. Mirenda & T. Iacono (Eds.), *Autism spectrum disorders and AAC* (pp. 141–169). Baltimore: Paul H. Brookes Publishing Co.

Schlosser, R., & Wendt, O. (2008). Effects of augmentative and alternative communication intervention on speech production in children with autism: A systematic review. *American Journal of Speech-Language Pathology, 17,* 212–230.

Schlosser, R., Wendt, O., Angermeier, K., & Shetty, M. (2005). Searching for evidence in augmentative and alternative communication: Navigating a scattered literature. *Augmentative and Alternative Communication, 21,* 233–255.

Schlosser, R., Wendt, O., & Sigafoos, J. (2007). Not all systematic reviews are created equal: Considerations for appraisal. *Evidence-based Communication Assessment and Intervention, 1,* 138–150.

Schneider, E.D. (2004). Communication disorders in children with autism: Characteristics, assessment, treatment. In V.B. Gupta (Ed.), *Autistic spectrum disorders in children* (pp. 193–208). New York: Marcel Dekker.

Seal, B., & Bonvillian, J. (1997). Sign language and motor functioning in students with autistic disorder. *Journal of Autism and Developmental Disorders, 27,* 437–466.

Seale, J.M., Garrett, K.L., & Figley, L. (2007, September). *Quantitative differences in aphasia interactions with visual scene AAC displays.* Poster presented at the 2007 Clinical AAC Research Conference, Lexington, KY.

Seligman, M. (1975). *Helplessness: On depression, development, and death.* San Francisco: W.H. Freeman.

Semel, E., Wiig, E., & Secord, W. (2003). *Clinical Evaluation of Language Fundamentals–Fourth Edition (CELF-4)*. San Antonio, TX: Harcourt Assessment.

Semel, E., Wiig, E., & Secord, W. (2004). *Clinical Evaluation of Language Fundamentals–Fourth Edition (CELF-4) Screening test*. San Antonio, TX: Psychological Corporation.

Sennott, S., & Bowker, A. (2009). Autism, AAC, and Proloquo2Go. *Perspectives on Augmentative and Alternative Communication, 18*, 137–145.

Sevcik, R., & Romski, M. (1986). Representational matching skills of persons with severe retardation. *Augmentative and Alternative Communication, 2*, 160–164.

Sevcik, R., Romski, M.A., & Wilkinson, K. (1991). Roles of graphic symbols in the language acquisition process for persons with severe cognitive disabilities. *Augmentative and Alternative Communication, 7*, 161–170.

Shakespeare, W.T., & Muir, C.K. (Ed.). (1982). *Troilus and Cressida*. New York: Oxford University Press.

Shaman, D. (2009, June). *A team approach to cortical visual impairment in schools*. Retrieved from http://www.nationaldb.org/documents/products/TeamApproachtoCVI.pdf

Shane, H., & Cohen, C. (1981). A discussion of communicative strategies and patterns by nonspeaking persons. *Language, Speech, and Hearing Services in Schools, 12*, 205–210.

Shane, H.C., O'Brien, M., & Sorce, J. (2009). Use of a visual graphic language system to support communication for persons on the autism spectrum. *Perspectives on Augmentative and Alternative Communication, 18*, 130–136.

Shane, H.C., & Weiss-Kapp, S. (2008). *Visual language in autism*. San Diego: Plural.

Shriberg, L.D. (2006, June). *Research in idiopathic and symptomatic childhood apraxia of speech*. Paper presented at the 5th International Conference on Speech Motor Control, Nijmegen, The Netherlands.

Shriberg, L., Aram, D., & Kwiatowksi, J. (1997). Developmental apraxia of speech: I. Descriptive and theoretical perspectives. *Journal of Speech, Language, and Hearing Research, 40*, 273–285.

Shroyer, E.H. (2011). *Signs of the times* (2nd ed.). Washington, DC: Gallaudet University Press.

Siegel, E.B., & Cress, C.J. (2002). Overview of the emergence of early AAC behaviors: Progression from communicative to symbolic skills. In J. Reichle, D.R. Beukelman, & J.C. Light (Eds.), *Exemplary practices for beginning communicators: Implications for AAC* (pp. 25–57). Baltimore: Paul H. Brookes Publishing Co.

Siegel, E., & Wetherby, A. (2000). Nonsymbolic communication. In M. Snell (Ed.), *Instruction of students with severe disabilities* (5th ed., pp. 409–451). Columbus, OH: Merrill.

Siegel-Causey, E., & Guess, D. (1989). *Enhancing nonsymbolic communication interactions among learners with severe disabilities*. Baltimore: Paul H. Brookes Publishing Co.

Sienkiewicz-Mercer, R., & Kaplan, S. (1989). *I raise my eyes to say yes*. Boston: Houghton Mifflin.

Sigafoos, J. (1998). Assessing conditional use of graphic mode requesting in a young boy with autism. *Journal of Developmental and Physical Disabilities, 10*, 133–151.

Sigafoos, J. (1999). Creating opportunities for augmentative and alternative communication: Strategies for involving people with developmental disabilities. *Augmentative and Alternative Communication, 15*, 183–190.

Sigafoos, J., Arthur, M., & O'Reilly, M. (2003). *Challenging behavior and developmental disability*. Baltimore: Paul H. Brookes Publishing Co.

Sigafoos, J., Arthur-Kelly, M., & Butterfield, N. (2006). *Enhancing everyday communication for children with disabilities*. Baltimore: Paul H. Brookes Publishing Co.

Sigafoos, J., & Couzens, D. (1995). Teaching functional use of an eye gaze communication board to a child with multiple disabilities. *British Journal of Developmental Disabilities, 16*, 114–125.

Sigafoos, J., Couzens, D., Roberts, D., Phillips, C., & Goodison, K. (1996). Teaching requests for food and drink to children with multiple disabilities in a graphic communication mode. *Journal of Developmental and Physical Disabilities, 8*, 247–262.

Sigafoos, J., Didden, R., Schlosser, R., Green, V., O'Reilly, M., & Lancioni, G. (2008). A review of intervention studies on teaching AAC to individuals who are deaf and blind. *Journal of Developmental and Physical Disabilities, 20*, 71–99.

Sigafoos, J., Drasgow, E., Reichle, J., O'Reilly, M., & Tait, K. (2004). Tutorial: Teaching communicative rejecting to children with severe disabilities. *American Journal of Speech-Language Pathology, 13*, 31–42.

Sigafoos, J., Drasgow, E., & Schlosser, R. (2003). Strategies for beginning communicators. In R. Schlosser (Ed.), *The efficacy of augmentative and alternative communication: Toward evidence-based practice* (pp. 323–346). New York: Elsevier.

Sigafoos, J., Green, V., Schlosser, R., O'Reilly, M., Lancioni, G., Rispoli, M., & Lang, R. (2009). Communication intervention in Rett syndrome: A systematic review. *Research in Autism Spectrum Disorders, 3,* 304–318.

Sigafoos, J., Laurie, S., & Pennell, D. (1995). Preliminary assessment of choice making among children with Rett syndrome. *Journal of the Association for Persons with Severe Handicaps, 20,* 175–184.

Sigafoos, J., Laurie, S., & Pennell, D. (1996). Teaching children with Rett syndrome to request preferred objects using aided communication: Two preliminary studies. *Augmentative and Alternative Communication, 12,* 88–96.

Sigafoos, J., & Meikle, B. (1996). Functional communication training for the treatment of multiply determined challenging behavior in two boys with autism. *Behavior Modification, 20,* 60–84.

Sigafoos, J., & Mirenda, P. (2002). Strengthening communicative behaviors for gaining access to desired items and activities. In J. Reichle, D.R. Beukelman, & J.C. Light (Eds.), *Exemplary practices for beginning communicators: Implications for AAC* (pp. 123–156). Baltimore: Paul H. Brookes Publishing Co.

Sigafoos, J., O'Reilly, M.F., Drasgow, E., & Reichle, J. (2002). Strategies to achieve socially acceptable escape and avoidance. In J. Reichle, D.R. Beukelman, & J.C. Light (Eds.), *Exemplary practices for beginning communicators: Implications for AAC* (pp. 157–186). Baltimore: Paul H. Brookes Publishing Co.

Sigafoos, J., O'Reilly, M., Ganz, J., Lancioni, G., & Schlosser, R. (2005). Supporting self-determination in AAC interventions by assessing preference for communication devices. *Technology and Disability, 17,* 143–153.

Sigafoos, J., & Reichle, J. (1992). Comparing explicit to generalized requesting in an augmentative communication mode. *Journal of Developmental and Physical Disabilities, 4,* 167–188.

Sigafoos, J., Roberts, D., Kerr, M., Couzens, D., & Baglioni, A. (1994). Opportunities for communication in classrooms serving children with developmental disabilities. *Journal of Autism and Developmental Disabilities, 24,* 259–279.

Sigafoos, J., & Roberts-Pennell, D. (1999). Wrong-item format: A promising intervention for teaching socially appropriate forms of rejecting to children with developmental disabilities. *Augmentative and Alternative Communication, 15,* 135–140.

Silverman, F. (1995). *Communication for the speechless* (3rd ed.). Needham Heights, MA: Allyn & Bacon.

Simmons, N., & Johnston, J. (2004, February). *Cultural differences in beliefs and practices concerning talk to children: East-Indian and Western mothers.* Poster presented at the 4th Early Years Conference, Vancouver, British Columbia.

Simpson, K. (1996). *Interaction patterns of four students with severe expressive communication impairments in regular classroom settings* (Unpublished doctoral dissertation). University of Nebraska–Lincoln.

Simpson, K., Beukelman, D.R., & Sharpe, T. (2000). An elementary student with severe expressive communication impairment in a general education classroom: Sequential analysis of interactions. *Augmentative and Alternative Communication, 16,* 107–121.

Singh, N., Lancioni, G., O'Reilly, M., Molina, E., Adkins, A., & Oliva, D. (2003). Self-determination during mealtimes through microswitch choice-making by an individual with complex multiple disabilities and profound mental retardation. *Journal of Positive Behavior Interventions, 5,* 209–215.

Skotko, B., Koppenhaver, D., & Erickson, K. (2004). Parent reading behaviors and communication outcomes in girls with Rett syndrome. *Exceptional Children, 70,* 145–166.

Slesaransky-Poe, G.L. (1997). Does the use of voice output communication make a difference in the communicative effectiveness and the quality of life of people with significant speech disabilities? *Dissertation Abstracts International* (UMI No. 9724281).

Small, J.A., Gutman, G., Makela, S., & Hillhouse, B. (2003). Effectiveness of communication strategies used by caregivers of persons with Alzheimer's disease during activities of daily living. *Journal of Speech, Language, and Hearing Research, 46,* 353–367.

Small, J.A., Kemper, S., & Lyons, K. (1997). Sentence comprehension in Alzheimer's disease: Effects of grammatical complexity, speech rate and repetition. *Psychology and Aging, 12*(1), 3–11.

Smebye, H. (1990, August). *A theoretical basis for early communication intervention.* Paper presented at the fifth biennial conference of the International Society for Augmentative and Alternative Communication, Stockholm.

Smith, C., & Uttley, W. (2008). *Let's sign and Down syndrome: Signs for children with special needs.* Stockton-on-Tees, UK: Co-Sign Communications.

Smith, K.L., Crete-Nishihata, M., Damioanakis, T., Baecker, R.M., & Marziali, E. (2009). Multimedia biographies: A reminiscence and social stimulus tool for persons with cognitive impairment. *Journal of Technology in Human Services, 27,* 287–306.

Smith, J., McCarthy, J., & Benigno, J. (2009). The effect of high-tech AAC system position on the joint attention of infants without disabilities. *Augmentative and Alternative Communication, 25,* 165–175.

Smith, M. (1996). The medium or the message: A study of speaking children using communication boards. In S. von Tetzchner & M.H. Jensen (Eds.), *Augmentative and alternative communication: European perspectives* (pp. 119–136). London: Whurr.

Smith, M., Garrett, K.L., & Lasker, J.P. (2007, September). *Comparing decontextualized reading to Written Choice Conversation Strategy in people with severe aphasia.* Platform session at the Clinical AAC Conference, Lexington, KY.

Smith, M., & Grove, N. (1999). The bimodal situation of children learning language using manual and graphic signs. In F.T. Loncke, J. Clibbens, H. Arvidson, & L.L. Lloyd (Eds.), *Augmentative and alternative communication: New directions in research and practice* (pp. 8–30). London: Whurr.

Smith, M.M., & Grove, N.C. (2003). Asymmetry in input and output for individuals who use AAC. In J.C. Light, D.R. Beukelman, & J. Reichle (Eds.), *Communicative competence for individuals who use AAC: From research to effective practice* (pp. 163–195). Baltimore: Paul H. Brookes Publishing Co.

Smith, T. (2001). Discrete trial training in the treatment of autism. *Focus on Autism and Other Developmental Disabilities, 16,* 86–92.

Snell, M. (2002). Using dynamic assessment with learners who communicate nonsymbolically. *Augmentative and Alternative Communication, 18,* 163–176.

Snell, M., Brady, N., McLean, L., Ogletree, B., Siegel, E., Sylvester, L.,...Romski, M.A. (2010). Twenty years of communication intervention research with individuals who have severe intellectual and developmental disabilities. *American Journal of Intellectual and Developmental Disabilities, 115,* 364–380.

Snell, M., Caves, K., McLean, L., Mineo Mollica, B., Mirenda, P., Paul-Brown, D.,...Yoder, D. (2003). Concerns regarding the application of restrictive "eligibility" policies to individuals who need communication services and supports: A response by the National Joint Committee for the Communication Needs of Persons with Severe Disabilities. *Research and Practice for Persons with Severe Disabilities, 28,* 70–78.

Snell, M., Chen, L.-Y., & Hoover, K. (2006). Teaching augmentative and alternative communication to students with severe disabilities: A review of intervention research 1997–2003. *Research and Practice for Persons with Severe Disabilities, 31,* 203–214.

Snyder-McLean, L., Solomonson, B., McLean, J., & Sack, S. (1984). Structuring joint action routines: A strategy for facilitating language and communication development in the classroom. *Seminars in Speech and Language, 5,* 213–228.

Sobsey, D., & Wolf-Schein, E. (1996). Children with sensory impairments. In F.P. Orelove & D. Sobsey (Eds.), *Educating children with multiple disabilities: A transdisciplinary approach* (3rd ed., pp. 411–450). Baltimore: Paul H. Brookes Publishing Co.

Soderholm, S., Meinander, M., & Alaranta, H. (2001). Augmentative and alternative communication methods in locked-in syndrome. *Journal of Rehabilitation Medicine, 33,* 235–239.

Sohlberg, M.M., Fickas, S., Ehlhardt, L., & Todis, B. (2005). The longitudinal effects of accessible email for individuals with severe cognitive impairments. *Aphasiology, 19,* 651–681.

Son, H.-S., Sigafoos, J., O'Reilly, M., & Lancioni, G.E. (2006). Comparing two types of augmentative and alternative communication systems for children with autism. *Pediatric Rehabilitation, 9,* 389–395.

Soto, G. (1999). Understanding the impact of graphic sign use on the message structure. In F.T. Loncke, J. Clibbens, H. Arvidson, & L.L. Lloyd (Eds.), *Augmentative and alternative communication: New directions in research and practice* (pp. 40–48). London: Whurr.

Soto, G., & Dukhovny, E. (2008). The effect of shared book reading on the acquisition of expressive vocabulary of a 7 year old who uses AAC. *Seminars in Speech and Language, 29,* 133–145.

Soto, G., Solomon-Rice, P., & Caputo, M. (2009). Enhancing the personal narrative skills of elementary school-aged students who use AAC: The effectiveness of personal narrative intervention. *Journal of Communication Disorders, 42,* 43–57.

Soto, G., & Toro-Zambrana, W. (1995). Investigation of Blissymbol use from a language research paradigm. *Augmentative and Alternative Communication, 11,* 118–130.

Soto, G., Yu, B., & Henneberry, S. (2007). Supporting the development of narrative skills of an eight-year-old child who uses an augmentative and alternative communication device. *Child Language Teaching and Therapy, 23,* 27–45.

Soto, G., Yu, B., & Kelso, J. (2008). Effectiveness of multifaceted narrative intervention on the stories told by a 12-year-old girl who uses AAC. *Augmentative and Alternative Communication, 24,* 76–87.

Soto, G., & Zangari, C. (Eds.). (2009). *Practically speaking: Language, literacy, and academic development of students with AAC needs.* Baltimore: Paul H. Brookes Publishing Co.

Spencer, K.A., Yorkston, K.M., & Duffy, J.R. (2003). Behavioral management of respiratory/phonatory dysfunction from dysarthria: A flowchart for guidance in clinical decision-making. *Journal of Medical Speech-Language Pathology, 11*(2), xxxix–lxi.

Spiegel, B., Benjamin, B., & Spiegel, S. (1993). One method to increase spontaneous use of an assistive communication device: A case study. *Augmentative and Alternative Communication, 9,* 111–118.

Spragale, D., & Micucci, S. (1990). Signs of the week: A functional approach to manual sign training. *Augmentative and Alternative Communication, 6,* 29–37.

Srinivasan, S., Mathew, S., & Lloyd, L.L. (2011). Insights into communication intervention and AAC in South India: A mixed-methods study. *Communication Disorders Quarterly, 32,* 232–246.

Staehely, J. (2000). Prologue: The communication dance. In M. Fried-Oken & H.A. Bersani, Jr. (Eds.), *Speaking up and spelling it out: Personal essays on augmentative and alternative communication* (pp. 1–12). Baltimore: Paul H. Brookes Publishing Co.

Stanford, A. (2002). *Asperger syndrome and long-term relationships.* London: Jessica Kingsley.

Stedt, J., & Moores, D. (1990). Manual codes on English and American Sign Language: Historical perspectives and current realities. In H. Bornstein (Ed.), *Manual communication: Implications for education* (pp. 1–20). Washington, DC: Gallaudet University Press.

Steege, M., Wacker, D., Cigrand, K., Berg, W., Novak, C., Reimers, T.,…DeRaad, A. (1990). Use of negative reinforcement in the treatment of self-injurious behavior. *Journal of Applied Behavior Analysis, 23,* 459–468.

Stephenson, J. (2007). The effect of color on the recognition and use of line drawings by children with severe intellectual disabilities. *Augmentative and Alternative Communication, 23,* 44–55.

Stephenson, J. (2009a). Iconicity in the development of picture skills: Typical development and implications for individuals with severe intellectual disabilities. *Augmentative and Alternative Communication, 25,* 187–201.

Stephenson, J. (2009b). Picture-book reading as an intervention to teach the use of line drawings for communication with students with severe intellectual disabilities. *Augmentative and Alternative Communication, 25,* 202–214.

Stewart, F., Worrall, L., Egan, J., & Oxenham, D. (2004). Addressing Internet training issues for people with Parkinson's disease. *Advances in Speech Language Pathology, 6*(4), 209–220.

Stiliman, R., & Battle, C. (1984). Developing prelanguage communication in the severely handicapped: An interpretation of the Van Dijk method. *Seminars in Speech and Language, 5,* 159–170.

Stoner, J., Beck, A., Bock, S., Hickey, K., Kosuwan, K., & Thompson, J. (2006). The effectiveness of the Picture Exchange Communication System with nonspeaking adults. *Remedial and Special Education, 27,* 154–165.

Storey, K., & Provost, O. (1996). The effect of communication skills instruction on the integration of workers with severe disabilities in supported employment settings. *Education and Training in Mental Retardation and Developmental Disabilities, 31,* 123–141.

Strand, E.A., & Skinder, A. (1999). Treatment of developmental apraxia of speech: Integral stimulation methods. In A.J. Caruso & E.A. Strand (Eds.), *Clinical management of motor speech disorders in children.* New York: Thieme.

Strauss, D., & Shavelle, R. (1998). Life expectancy of adults with cerebral palsy. *Developmental Medicine and Child Neurology, 40,* 369–375.

Stromswold, K. (1994, January). *Language comprehension without production: Implications for theories of language acquisition.* Paper presented at the Boston University Conference on Language Development, Boston.

Stuart, S. (1988). Expanding sequencing, turn-taking and timing skills through play acting. In S.W. Blackstone, E.L. Cassatt-James, & D. Bruskin (Eds.), *Augmentative communication: Implementation strategies* (pp. 5.8:21–5.8:26). Rockville, MD: American Speech-Language-Hearing Association.

Stuart, S. (1991). *Topic and vocabulary use patterns of elderly men and women in two age cohorts* (Unpublished doctoral dissertation). University of Nebraska–Lincoln.

Stuart, S., Lasker, J.P., & Beukelman, D.R. (2000). AAC message management. In D.R. Beukelman, K.M. Yorkston, & J. Reichle (Eds.), *Augmentative and alternative communication for adults with acquired neurologic disorders* (pp. 25–54). Baltimore: Paul H. Brookes Publishing Co.

Stuart, S., Vanderhoof, D., & Beukelman, D.R. (1993). Topic and vocabulary use patterns of elderly women. *Augmentative and Alternative Communication, 9,* 95–110.

Sturm, J.M., & Clendon, S.A. (2004). AAC, language, and literacy: Fostering the relationship. *Topics in Language Disorders, 24*(1), 76–91.

Sturm, J., & Nelson, N. (1997). Formal classroom lessons: New perspectives on a familiar discourse event. *Language, Speech, and Hearing Services in Schools, 28,* 255–273.

Sturtevant, E.G., & Linek, W.M. (2003). The instructional beliefs and decisions of middle and secondary teachers who successfully blend literacy and content. *Literacy Research and Instruction, 43,* 74–89.

Sundberg, M. (1993). Selecting a response form for nonverbal persons: Facilitated communication, pointing systems, or sign language. *Analysis of Verbal Behavior, 11,* 99–116.

Sundberg, M.L., & Partington, J.W. (1998). *Teaching language to children with autism or other developmental disabilities (version 7.1).* Pleasant Hill, CA: Behavior Analysts.

Sussman, F. (1999). *More than words: Helping parents to promote communication and social skills in children with autism spectrum disorder.* Toronto: Hanen Centre.

Sutherland, D.E., Gillon, G., & Yoder, D. (2005). AAC use and service provision: A survey of New Zealand speech-language therapists. *Augmentative and Alternative Communication, 21,* 295–307.

Sutton, A. (1999). Linking language learning experiences and grammatical acquisition. In F.T. Loncke, J. Clibbens, H. Arvidson, & L.L. Lloyd (Eds.), *Augmentative and alternative communication: New directions in research and practice* (pp. 49–61). London: Whurr.

Sutton, A., & Gallagher, T. (1993). Verb class distinctions and AAC language-encoding limitations. *Journal of Speech and Hearing Research, 36,* 1216–1226.

Sutton, A., & Gallagher, T. (1995). Comprehension assessment of a child using an AAC system. *American Journal of Speech-Language Pathology, 4,* 60–69.

Sutton, A., Gallagher, T., Morford, J., & Shahnaz, N. (2000). Constituent order patterns and syntactic distinctions in relative clause sentences produced using AAC systems. *Applied Psycholinguistics, 21,* 473–486.

Sutton, A., & Morford, J. (1998). Constituent order in picture pointing sequences produced by speaking children using AAC. *Applied Psycholinguistics, 19,* 526–536.

Sutton, A., Soto, G., & Blockberger, S. (2002). Grammatical issues in graphic symbol communication. *Augmentative and Alternative Communication, 18,* 192–204.

Swengel, K., & Marquette, J. (1997). Service delivery in AAC. In S.L. Glennen & D. DeCoste (Eds.), *The handbook of augmentative and alternative communication* (pp. 21–58). San Diego: Singular.

Swinehart-Jones, D., & Heller, K.W. (2009). Teaching students with severe speech and physical impairments a decoding strategy using internal speech and motoric indicators. *Journal of Special Education, 43,* 131–144.

Tennant, R.A., & Gluszak Brown, M. (2010). *American Sign Language hand-shape dictionary* (3rd ed.). Washington, DC: Gallaudet University Press.

Thistle, J., & Wilkinson, K. (2009). The effects of color cues on typically developing preschoolers' speed of locating a target line drawing: Implications for augmentative and alternative communication display design. *American Journal of Speech-Language Pathology, 18,* 231–240.

Thompson, J.R., Bradley, V.J., Bruntix, W.H., Schalock, R.L., Shogren, K. A, Snell, M.E....Yeager, M. (2009). Conceptualizing supports and the support needs of people with intellectual disability. *Intellectual and Developmental Disabilities, 47,* 135–146.

Thompson, J.R., Bryant, B., Campbell, E.M., Craig, E.M., Hughes, C., Rotholz, D. A.,...Wehmeyer, M. (2004). *Supports Intensity Scale.* Washington, DC: American Association on Intellectual and Developmental Disabilities.

Thousand, J.S., & Villa, R.A. (2000). Collaborative teams: A powerful tool in school restructuring. In R.A. Villa & J.S. Thousand (Eds.), *Restructuring for caring and effective education: Piecing the puzzle together* (pp. 254–292). Baltimore: Paul H. Brookes Publishing Co.

Thurman, D., Alverson, C., Dunn, K., Guerrero, J., & Sniezek, J. (1999). Traumatic brain injury in the United States: A public health perspective. *Journal of Head Trauma and Rehabilitation, 14,* 602–615.

Tien, K-C. (2008). Effectiveness of the Picture Exchange Communication System as a functional communication intervention for individuals with autism spectrum disorders: A practice-based research synthesis. *Education and Training in Developmental Disabilities, 43,* 61–76.

Tiger, J., Hanley, G., & Bruzek, J. (2008). Functional communication training: A review and practical guide. *Behavior Analysis in Practice, 1*(1), 16–23.

Tincani, M. (2004). Comparing the picture exchange communication system and sign language training for children with autism. *Focus on Autism and Other Developmental Disabilities, 19,* 152–163.

Todman, J. (2000). Rate and quality of conversations using a text-storage AAC system: Single-case training study. *Augmentative and Alternative Communication, 16,* 164–179.

Todman, J., & Alm, N. (1997). TALKboards for social conversation. *Communication Matters, 11,* 13–15.

Todman, J., & Alm, N. (2003). Modelling conversational pragmatics in communication aids. *Journal of Pragmatics, 35,* 523–538.

Todman, J., Alm, N., Higginbotham, J., & File, P. (2008). Whole utterance approaches in AAC. *Augmentative and Alternative Communication, 24,* 235–254.

Todman, J., & Lewins, E. (1996). Conversational rate of a non-vocal person with motor neurone disease using the "TALK" system. *International Journal of Rehabilitation Research, 19,* 285–287.

Todman, J., Rankin, D., & File, P. (1999). The use of stored text in computer-aided conversation: A single-case experiment. *Journal of Language and Social Psychology, 18,* 287–309.

Tomoeda, C.K., Bayles, K.A., Boone, D.R., Kaszniak, A.W., & Slauson, T.J. (1990). Speech rate and syntactic complexity effects on the auditory comprehension of Alzheimer patients. *Journal of Communication Disorders, 23,* 151–161.

Tonsing, K., & Alant, E. (2004). Topics of social conversation in the work place: A South African perspective. *Augmentative and Alternative Communication, 20,* 89–102.

Torgesen, J.K., & Bryant, B.R. (2004). *Test of Phonological Awareness–Second Edition.* Austin, TX: PRO-ED.

Torgesen, J.K., Wagner, R.K., & Rashotte, C.A. (1994). Longitudinal studies of phonological processing and reading. *Journal of Learning Disabilities, 27,* 276–286.

"Traci." (2003, January). Success comes in all sizes. *Apraxia-Kids Monthly, 4*(1), 7.

Trembath, D., Balandin, S., Togher, L., & Stancliffe, R.J. (2009). Peer-mediated teaching and augmentative and alternative communication for preschool-aged children with autism. *Journal of Intellectual & Developmental Disability, 34,* 173–186.

Trenholm, B., & Mirenda, P. (2006). Home and community literacy experiences of individuals with Down syndrome. *Down Syndrome Research and Practice, 10,* 30–40.

Treviranus, J., & Roberts, V. (2003). Supporting competent motor control of AAC systems. In J.C. Light, D.R. Beukelman, & J. Reichle (Eds.), *Communicative competence for individuals who use AAC: From research to effective practice* (pp. 199–240). Baltimore: Paul H. Brookes Publishing Co.

"Trina." (2004, March). Success comes in all sizes. *Apraxia-Kids Monthly, 5*(3), 5–6.

Trottier, N., Kamp, L., & Mirenda, P. (2011). Effects of peer-mediated instruction to teach use of speech-generating devices to students with autism in social game routines. *Augmentative and Alternative Communication, 27,* 26–39.

Trudeau, N., Cleave, P., & Woelk, E. (2003). Using augmentative and alternative communication approaches to promote participation of preschoolers during book reading: A pilot study. *Child Language Teaching and Therapy, 19,* 181–210.

Trudeau, N., Morford, J., & Sutton, A. (2010). The role of word order in the interpretation of canonical and non-canonical graphic symbol utterances: A developmental study. *Augmentative and Alternative Communication, 26,* 108–121.

Truxler, J.E., & O'Keefe, B.M. (2007). The effects of phonological awareness instruction on beginning word recognition and spelling. *Augmentative and Alternative Communication, 23,* 164–176.

Tscuchiya, K., Ozawa, E., Fukushima, J., Yasui, H., Kondo, H., Nakano, I., & Ikeda, K. (2000). Rapidly progressive aphasia and motor neuron disease: A clinical, radiological, and pathological study of an autopsy case with circumscribed lobar atrophy. *Acta Neuropathologica (Berlin), 99,* 81–87.

Turnell, R., & Carter, M. (1994). Establishing a repertoire of requesting for a student with severe and multiple disabilities using tangible symbols and naturalistic time delay. *Australia and New Zealand Journal of Developmental Disabilities, 19,* 193–207.

Udwin, O., & Yule, W. (1990). Augmentative communication systems taught to cerebral palsied children: A longitudinal study: I. The acquisition of signs and symbols, and syntactic aspects of their use over time. *British Journal of Disorders of Communication, 25,* 295–309.

Udwin, O., & Yule, W. (1991). Augmentative communication systems taught to cerebral palsied children: A longitudinal study: II. Pragmatic features of sign and symbol use. *British Journal of Disorders of Communication, 26,* 137–148.

Ulatowska, H., Cannito, M., Hayashi, M., & Fleming, S. (1985). *The aging brain: Communication in the elderly.* San Diego: College-Hill Press.

University of Kentucky Assistive Technology Project. (2002). University of Kentucky Assistive Technology (UKAT) Toolkit. Retrieved from http://serc.gws.uky.edu/www/ukatii/toolkit/index.html

U.S. Census Bureau. (2010). *American Community Survey 1-year estimates: Language spoken at home.* Washington, DC: Author.

Utley, B.L. (2002). Visual assessment considerations for the design of AAC systems. In J. Reichle, D.R. Beukelman, & J.C. Light (Eds.), *Exemplary practices for beginning communicators: Implications for AAC* (pp. 353–394). Baltimore: Paul H. Brookes Publishing Co.

Utley, B., & Rapport, M.J.K. (2002). Essential elements of effective teamwork: Shared understanding and differences between special educators and related service providers. *Physical Disabilities: Education and Related Services, 20,* 9–47.

Valentic, V. (1991). Successful integration from a student's perspective. *Communicating Together, 9*(2), 9.

van Balkom, H., & Welle Donker-Gimbrère, M. (1996). A psycholinguistic approach to graphic language use. In S. von Tetzchner & M.H. Jensen (Eds.), *Augmentative and alternative communication: European perspectives* (pp. 153–170). London: Whurr.

Vanderheiden, G., & Kelso, D. (1987). Comparative analysis of fixed-vocabulary communication acceleration techniques. *Augmentative and Alternative Communication, 3,* 196–206.

Vanderheiden, G.C., & Lloyd, L. (1986). Communication systems and their components. In S. Blackstone (Ed.), *Augmentative communication: An introduction* (pp. 49–162). Rockville, MD: American Speech-Language-Hearing Association.

Vanderheiden, G., & Yoder, D. (1986). Overview. In S. Blackstone (Ed.), *Augmentative communication: An introduction* (pp. 1–28). Rockville, MD: American Speech-Language-Hearing Association.

van der Merwe, E., & Alant, E. (2004). Associations with MinSpeak icons. *Journal of Communication Disorders, 37,* 255–274.

Vandervelden, M.C., & Siegel, L.S. (1995). Phonological recoding and phoneme awareness in early literacy: A developmental approach. *Reading Research Quarterly, 30,* 854–875.

Vandervelden, M., & Siegel, L. (1999). Phonological processing and literacy in AAC users and students with motor speech impairments. *Augmentative and Alternative Communication, 15,* 191–211.

Vandervelden, M., & Siegel, L. (2001). Phonological processing in written word learning: Assessment for children who use augmentative and alternative communication. *Augmentative and Alternative Communication, 17,* 37–51.

van de Sandt-Koenderman, W.M. (2004). High tech AAC and aphasia: Widening horizons? *Aphasiology, 18*(3), 245–263.

van de Sandt-Koenderman, W.M., Wiegers, J., Wielaert, S.M., Duivenvoorden, H.J., & Ribbers, G.M. (2007). A computerised communication aid in severe aphasia: An exploratory study. *Disability and Rehabilitation, 29,* 1701–1709.

Van Tatenhove, G. (1996). *Field of dreams: Sowing language and reaping communication.* Paper presented at the 1996 Minspeak conference, Wooster, OH.

Van Tatenhove, G. (2005). *A protocol for assessing metaphoric use of pictures.* Retrieved from http://www.vantatenhove.com/files/MetaphorProtocol.pdf

Vaughn, S., Wanzek, J., Woodruff, A.L., & Linan-Thompson, S. (2007). Prevention and early identification of students with reading disabilities. In D. Haager, J. Klingner, & S. Vaughn (Eds.), *Evidence-based reading practices for response to intervention* (pp. 11–27). Baltimore: Paul H. Brookes Publishing Co.

Venkatagiri, H. (1993). Efficiency of lexical prediction as a communication acceleration technique. *Augmentative and Alternative Communication, 12,* 161–167.

Venkatagiri, H. (1999). Efficient keyboard layouts for sequential access in augmentative and alternative communication. *Augmentative and Alternative Communication, 15,* 126–134.

Venkatagiri, H., & Ramabadran, T. (1995). Digital speech synthesis: A tutorial. *Augmentative and Alternative Communication, 11*, 14–25.

Vicker, B. (1996). *Using tangible symbols for communication purposes: An optional step in building the two-way communication process.* Bloomington: Indiana University, Indiana Resource Center for Autism.

Visser, N., Alant, E., & Harty, M. (2008). Which graphic symbols do 4-year-old children choose to represent each of the four basic emotions? *Augmentative and Alternative Communication, 24*, 302–312.

von Tetzchner, S., & Jensen, M.H. (Eds.). (1996). *Augmentative and alternative communication: European perspectives.* London: Whurr.

von Tetzchner, S., & Martinsen, H. (1992). *Introduction to symbolic and augmentative communication.* London: Whurr.

Wacker, D.P., Berg, W.K., & Harding, J.W. (2002). Replacing socially unacceptable behavior with acceptable communication responses. In J. Reichle, D.R. Beukelman, & J.C. Light (Eds.), *Exemplary practices for beginning communicators: Implications for AAC* (pp. 97–122). Baltimore: Paul H. Brookes Publishing Co.

Wacker, D., Steege, M., Northup, J., Sasso, G., Berg, W., Reimers, T.,...Donn, L.A. (1990). A component analysis of functional communication training across three topographies of severe behavior problems. *Journal of Applied Behavior Analysis, 23*, 417–429.

Wagner, R., & Torgeson, J. (1987). The nature of phonological processing skills in early literacy: A developmental approach. *Psychological Bulletin, 101*, 192–212.

Waller, A., O'Mara, D.A., Tait, L., Booth, L., Brophy-Arnott, B., & Hood, H.E. (2001). Using written stories to support the use of narrative in conversational interactions: Case study. *Augmentative and Alternative Communication, 17*, 221–232.

Watters, C., Owen, M., & Munroe, S. (2005). *A study of deafblind demographics and services in Canada: Report prepared for the Canadian National Society of the Deaf-Blind.* Ottawa: Government of Canada, Social Developments Partnership Program.

Weiss, L., Thatch, D., & Thatch, J. (1987). *I wasn't finished with life.* Dallas, TX: E-Heart Press.

Weiss, P.L., Seligman-Wine, J., Lebel, T., Arzi, N., & Yalon-Chamovitz, S. (2005). A demographic survey of children and adolescents with complex communication needs in Israel. *Augmentative and Alternative Communication, 21*, 56–66.

Weiss-Lambrou, R. (2002). Satisfaction and comfort. In M. Scherer (Ed.), *Assistive technology: Matching device and consumer for successful rehabilitation* (pp. 77–94). Washington, DC: American Psychological Association.

Wendt, O. (2009). Research on the use of graphic symbols and manual signs. In P. Mirenda & T. Iacono (Eds.), *Autism spectrum disorders and AAC* (pp. 83–137). Baltimore: Paul H. Brookes Publishing Co.

Westby, C. (1985). Learning to talk—talking to learn: Oral-literate language differences. In C. Simon (Ed.), *Communication skills and classroom success: Therapy methodologies for language-learning disabled students* (pp. 181–213). San Diego: College-Hill Press.

Wetherby, A.M., & Prizant, B.M. (1993). *Communication and Symbolic Behavior Scales™ (CSBS™).* Baltimore: Paul H. Brookes Publishing Co.

Wetherby, A.M., & Prizant, B.M. (2002). *Communication and Symbolic Behavior Scales Developmental Profile™ (CSBS DP™).* Baltimore: Paul H. Brookes Publishing Co.

Wetherby, A., & Prutting, C. (1984). Profiles of communicative and cognitive-social abilities in autistic children. *Journal of Speech and Hearing Research, 27*, 364–377.

Wijesekera, L.C., & Leigh, P.N. (2009). Amyotrophic lateral sclerosis. *Orphanet Journal of Rare Disorders, 4*(3), 1–22.

Wikstrom, J., Poser, S., & Ritter, G. (1980). Optic neuritis as an initial symptom in multiple sclerosis. *Acta Neurologica Scandinavica, 61*, 178–185.

Wilbur, R., & Peterson, L. (1998). Modality interactions of speech and signing in simultaneous communication. *Journal of Speech, Language, and Hearing Research, 41*, 200–212.

Wilcox, M.J., Bacon, C., & Shannon, M.S. (1995, December). *Prelinguistic intervention: Procedures for young children with disabilities.* Paper presented at the ASHA Annual Convention, Orlando, FL.

Wilkinson, G., & Robertson, G. (2006). *Wide Range Achievement Test–Fourth Edition.* Torrance, CA: Western Psychological Services.

Wilkinson, K. (2005). Disambiguation and mapping of new word meanings by individuals with intellectual/developmental disabilities. *American Journal on Mental Retardation, 110*, 71–86.

Wilkinson, K., & Albert, A. (2001). Adaptations of fast mapping for vocabulary intervention with augmented language users. *Augmentative and Alternative Communication, 17,* 120–132.

Wilkinson, K., Carlin, M., & Jagaroo, V. (2006). Preschoolers' speed of locating a target symbol under different color conditions. *Augmentative and Alternative Communication, 22,* 123–133.

Wilkinson, K., Carlin, M., & Thistle, J. (2008). The role of color cues in facilitating accurate and rapid location of aided symbols by children with and without Down Syndrome. *American Journal of Speech-Language Pathology, 17,* 179–193.

Wilkinson, K., Foderaro, L., Maurer, J., Weinreb, C., & O'Neill, T. (2011, November). *Constructing fun and educational children's books using desktop computer applications.* Presented at the annual convention of the American Speech-Language-Hearing Association, San Diego.

Wilkinson, K., & Green, G. (1998). Implications of fast mapping for vocabulary expansion in individuals with mental retardation. *Augmentative and Alternative Communication, 14,* 162–170.

Wilkinson, K.M., & Hennig, S. (2007). The state of research and practice in augmentative and alternative communication for children with developmental/intellectual disabilities. *Mental Retardation and Developmental Disabilities Research Reviews, 13,* 58–69.

Wilkinson, K., & Jagaroo, V. (2004). Contributions of cognitive science to AAC display design. *Augmentative and Alternative Communication, 20,* 123–136.

Wilkinson, K., & McIlvane, W. (2002). Considerations in teaching graphic symbols to beginning communicators. In J. Reichle, D.R. Beukelman, & J. Light (Eds.), *Exemplary practices for beginning communicators: Implications for AAC* (pp. 273–321). Baltimore: Paul H. Brookes Publishing Co.

Wilkinson, K., Romski, M.A., & Sevcik, R. (1994). Emergence of visual-graphic symbol combinations by youth with moderate or severe mental retardation. *Journal of Speech and Hearing Research, 37,* 883–985.

Williams, B. (2000). More than an exception to the rule. In M. Fried-Oken & H.A. Bersani, Jr. (Eds.), *Speaking up and spelling it out: Personal essays on augmentative and alternative communication* (pp. 245–254). Baltimore: Paul H. Brookes Publishing Co.

Williams, K.T. (2001). *Group Reading Assessment and Diagnostic Evaluation (GRADE).* Austin, TX: Pearson Assessments.

Williams, M. (1995, March). Whose outcome is it anyway? *Alternatively Speaking, 2*(1), 1, 2, 6.

Williams, M.B. (2006). *How far we've come, how far we've got to go: Tales from the trenches* [Webcast]. Retrieved from http://aac-rerc.psu.edu/index.php/webcasts/show/id/2

Williams, M., & Krezman, C. (Eds.). (2000). *Beneath the surface: Creative expressions of augmented communicators.* Toronto: International Society for Augmentative and Alternative Communication.

Williams, M., Krezman, C., & McNaughton, D. (2008). "Reach for the stars": Five principles for the next 25 years of AAC. *Augmentative and Alternative Communication, 24,* 194–206.

Wimo, A., Jonsson, L., & Winblad, B. (2006). An estimate of the worldwide prevalence and direct costs of dementia in 2003. *Dementia and Geriatric Cognitive Disorders, 21,* 175–181.

Windsor, J., & Fristoe, M. (1989). Key word signing: Listeners' classification of signed and spoken narratives. *Journal of Speech and Hearing Disorders, 54,* 374–382.

Windsor, J., & Fristoe, M. (1991). Key word signing: Perceived and acoustic differences between signed and spoken narratives. *Journal of Speech and Hearing Research, 34,* 260–268.

Wing, L. (1996). *The autistic spectrum: A guide for parents and professionals.* London: Constable.

Winter, S., Autry, A., Boyle, C., & Yeargin-Allsopp, M. (2002). Trends in the prevalence of cerebral palsy in a population-based study. *Pediatrics, 110,* 1220–1225.

Wiseman, N.D. (2006). *Could it be autism? A parent's guide to the first signs and next steps.* New York: Broadway Books.

Wood, L.A., Lasker, J., Siegel-Causey, E., Beukelman, D.R., & Ball, L. (1998). Input framework for augmentative and alternative communication. *Augmentative and Alternative Communication, 14,* 261–267.

Woodcock, R.W., McGrew, K.S., & Mather, N. (2006). *Woodcock-Johnson III Complete Battery.* Scarborough, Ontario, Canada: Nelson.

Wood Jackson, C., Wahlquist, J., & Marquis, C. (2011). Visual supports for shared reading with young children: The effect of static overlay design. *Augmentative and Alternative Communication, 27,* 91–102.

Woodward, J. (1990). Sign English in the education of deaf students. In H. Bornstein (Ed.), *Manual communication: Implications for education* (pp. 67–80). Washington, DC: Gallaudet University Press.

Worah, S. (2008). *The effects of redesigning the representations of early emerging concepts of identification and preference: A comparison of two approaches for representing vocabulary in augmentative and alternative communication (AAC) systems for young children* (Unpublished doctoral dissertation). Pennsylvania State University.

Workinger, M., & Netsell, R. (1988). *Restoration of intelligible speech 13 years post-head injury.* Unpublished manuscript, Boys Town National Communication Institute, Omaha, NE.

World Health Organization. (2001). *The world health report 2001—mental illness: New understanding, new hope.* Geneva: Author. Retrieved from http://www.who.int/whr/en/

Wright, H.H., & Shisler, R.J. (2005). Working memory in aphasia: Theory, measures, and clinical implications. *American Journal of Speech-Language Pathology, 14,* 107–118.

Yamamoto, J., & Mochizuki, A. (1988). Acquisition and functional analysis of manding with autistic children. *Journal of Applied Behavior Analysis, 21,* 57–64.

Yang, C.-S., Cheng, H.-Y., Chuang, L.-Y., & Yang, C.-H. (2009). A wireless Internet interface for persons with physical disabilities. *Mathematical and Computer Modelling, 50,* 72–80.

Yang, C.-H., Huang, H.-C., Chuang, L.-Y., & Yang, C.-H. (2008). A mobile communication aid system for persons with physical disabilities. *Mathematical and Computer Modelling, 47,* 318–327.

Yasuda, K., Kuwabara, K., Kuwahara, N., Abe, S., & Tetsutani, N. (2009). Effectiveness of personalized reminiscence photo videos for individuals with dementia. *Neuropsychological Rehabilitation, 19,* 603–619.

Ylvisaker, M. (1986). Language and communication disorders following pediatric head injury. *Journal of Head Trauma Rehabilitation, 1,* 48–56.

York, J., & Weimann, G. (1991). Accommodating severe physical disabilities. In J. Reichle, J. York, & J. Sigafoos (Eds.), *Implementing augmentative and alternative communication: Strategies for learners with severe disabilities* (pp. 239–256). Baltimore: Paul H. Brookes Publishing Co.

Yorkston, K., & Beukelman, D. (2007). AAC intervention for progressive conditions: Multiple sclerosis, Parkinson's disease and Huntington's disease. In D.R. Beukelman, K.L. Garrett, & K.M. Yorkston (Eds.), *Augmentative communication strategies for adults with acute or chronic medical conditions* (pp. 317–345. Baltimore: Paul H. Brookes Publishing Co.

Yorkston, K., Beukelman, D., Hakel, M., & Dorsey, M. (2007). *Speech Intelligibility Test.* Lincoln, NE: Madonna Rehabilitation Hospital.

Yorkston, K., Beukelman, D.R., Strand, E., & Bell, K. (1999). *Management of motor speech disorders in children and adults.* Austin, TX: PRO-ED.

Yorkston, K., Beukelman, D., Strand, E., & Hakel, M. (2010). *Clinical management of speakers with motor speech disorders* (3rd ed.). Austin, TX: PRO-ED.

Yorkston, K., Fried-Oken, M., & Beukelman, D.R. (1988). Single word vocabulary needs: Studies from various nonspeaking populations. *Augmentative and Alternative Communication, 4,* 149.

Yorkston, K., Honsinger, M., Mitsuda, P., & Hammen, V. (1989). The relationship between speech and swallowing disorders in head-injured patients. *Journal of Head Trauma Rehabilitation, 4,* 1–16.

Yorkston, K., & Karlan, G. (1986). Assessment procedures. In S. Blackstone (Ed.), *Augmentative communication: An introduction* (pp. 163–196). Rockville, MD: American Speech-Language-Hearing Association.

Yorkston, K.M., Klasner, E.R., Bowen, J., Ehde, D.M., Gibbons, L., Johnson, K., & Kraft, G. (2003). Characteristics of multiple sclerosis as a function of the severity of speech disorders. *Journal of Medical Speech-Language Pathology, 11*(2), 73–85.

Yorkston, K.M., Klasner, E.R., & Swanson, K.M. (2001). Communication in context: A qualitative study of the experiences of individuals with multiple sclerosis. *American Journal of Speech-Language Pathology, 10,* 126–137.

Yorkston, K., Miller, R., Strand, E., & Britton, D. (2012). *Management of speech and swallowing in degenerative diseases* (3rd ed.). Austin, TX: PRO-ED.

Yorkston, K., Smith, K., & Beukelman, D.R. (1990). Extended communication samples of augmented communicators: I. A comparison of individualized versus standard vocabularies. *Journal of Speech and Hearing Disorders, 55,* 217–224.

Yorkston, K., Spencer, K., & Duffy, J. (2003). Behavioral management of respiratory/phonatory dysfunction from dysarthria: A systematic review of the evidence. *Journal of Medical Speech-Language Pathology, 11*(2), xiii–xxxviii.

Yorkston, K., Strand, E., & Kennedy, M. (1996). Comprehensibility of dysarthric speech: Implications for assessment and treatment planning. *American Journal of Speech-Language Pathology, 5,* 55–66.

Zangari, C., Lloyd, L., & Vicker, B. (1994). Augmentative and alternative communication: An historic perspective. *Augmentative and Alternative Communication, 10,* 27–59.

Resources and Web Links

AAC Funding Help: http://aacfundinghelp.com; see also AAC-RERC: Search Results for "funding": http://aac-rerc.psu.edu/index.php/search/search/?terms= funding&submit=go

AAC Institute: http://www.aacinstitute.org/

AAC Intervention: http://aacintervention.com/

AAC-RERC (Rehabilitation Engineering Research Center on Communication Enhancement): http://aac-rerc.psu.edu/

AAC-RERC: *AAC and College Life: Just Do It!:* http://aac-rerc.psu.edu/index .php/webcasts/show/id/5

AAC-RERC: *AAC for Persons with Primary Progressive Aphasia:* http://aac-rerc.psu.edu/index.php/webcasts/show/id/18

AAC-RERC: *How Far We've Come, How Far We've Got to Go: Tales from the Trenches:* http://aac-rerc.psu.edu/index.php/webcasts/show/id/2

AAC-RERC: *Medicare Funding of AAC Technology:* http://aac-rerc.psu.edu/ index.php/pages/show/id/5

AAC-RERC: *Mobile Devices and Communication Apps:* http://aac-rerc.psu .edu/index.php/pages/show/id/46

AAC-RERC: *Seating and Positioning for Individuals Who Use AT* (Assistive Technology): http://aac-rerc.psu.edu/index.php/webcasts/show/id/9

AAC-RERC: *Supporting Communication of Individuals with Minimal Movement:* http://aac-rerc.psu.edu/index.php/webcasts/show/id/14

AAC-RERC: *AAC: A User's Perspective:* http://aac-rerc.psu.edu/index.php/ webcasts/show/id/3

AAC-RERC: *Visual Immersion Program (VIP) for Individuals with Autism:* http://aac-rerc.psu.edu/index.php/webcasts/show/id/6

AAC-RERC: Webcasts: http://aac-rerc.psu.edu/index.php/pages/show/id/44

AAC-RERC: Writers Brigade: http://aac-rerc.psu.edu/index.php/projects/ show/id/16

AAC TechConnect: http://www.aactechconnect.com; see also the AAC-RERC page about AAC TechConnect: http://aac-rerc.psu.edu/index.php/projects/ show/id/12

AapNootMuis: http://www.aapnootmuis.com/

Ability Research: http://www.skypoint.com/members/ability/

AbleData: http://www.abledata.com

AbleNet, Inc.: http://www.ablenetinc.com/

Adaptivation, Inc.: http://www.adaptivation.com/

Adaptive Design Association, Inc.: http://www.adaptivedesign.org/

Adaptive Switch Laboratories, Inc.: http://www.asl-inc.com/

Advanced Multimedia Devices, Inc.: http://www.amdi.net/

AliMed: http://www.alimed.com

ALS Association: http://www.alsa.org/

American Association of the Deaf-Blind: http://www.aadb.org

American Association on Intellectual and Developmental Disabilities (AAIDD) Supports Intensity Scale: http://www.siswebsite.org/cs/product_info

American Printing House for the Blind, Inc.: http://www.aph.org/

American Speech-Language-Hearing Association: http://www.asha.org

American Speech-Language-Hearing Association: Evidence-Based Practice (EBP): http://www.asha.org/members/ebp/

American Speech-Language-Hearing Association: Functional Assessment of Communication Skills for Adults (ASHA FACS): http://www.asha.org/eweb/OLSDynamicPage.aspx?Webcode=olsdetails&title=Functional+Assessment+of+Communication+Skills+for+Adults+%28ASHA+FACS%29

American Speech-Language-Hearing Association: *Guidelines for the Audiologic Assessment of Children from Birth to Five Years of Age:* http://www.asha.org/docs/html/GL2004-00002.html

American Speech-Language-Hearing Association: National Outcomes Measurement System (NOMS): http://www.asha.org/members/research/noms/

American Speech-Language-Hearing Association: Quality of Communication Life Scale (ASHA QCL): http://www.asha.org/eweb/OLSDynamicPage.aspx?Webcode=olsdetails&title=Quality+of+Communication+Life+Scale+%28ASHA+QCL%29

Aphasia Institute: http://aphasia.ca/

Apple, Inc.: http://www.apple.com/

APPSForAAC: http://www.appsforaac.net/

Apps for AAC by Jane Farrall: http://www.spectronicsinoz.com/article/iphoneipad-apps-for-aac

Apraxia-Kids: http://www.apraxia-kids.org

ASCD (formerly the Association for Supervision and Curriculum Development): http://www.ascd.org/

Assessment of Phonological Awareness and Reading (APAR): http://elr.com.au/apar

Assistive Technology of Alaska (ATLA):   http://atlaak.org

Assistive Technology Research Lab, University of Ottawa: http://www
.piads.net

**Assistive Technology Research Lab at the University of Ottawa:
Psychological Impact of Assistive Devices Scale:**   http://www.piads.net/9/
index1.2.html

Assistyx LLC: http://www.assistyx.com

Attainment Company: http://www.attainmentcompany.com

**Augmentative Communication Community Partnerships Canada
(ACCPC):**   http://www.accpc.ca/

Augmentative Communication, Inc.:   http://www.augcominc.com/

Augmentative Communication Online Users Group (ACOLUG):   http://listserv
.temple.edu/archives/acolug.html

Aurora Systems, Inc.:   http://www.aurora-systems.com/

Autism Speaks, Inc.:   http://www.autismspeaks.org

**Autism Spectrum Disorders Canadian-American Research Consortium
(ASD-CARC):**   http://www.autismresearch.ca/

A-Z to Deafblindness: http://www.deafblind.com

Barkley Augmentative and Alternative Communication (AAC) Center:
http://aac.unl.edu/

**Barkley Augmentative and Alternative Communication (AAC) Center:
Vocabulary Resources:**   http://aac.unl.edu/vocabulary.html

**Barkley Augmentative and Alternative Communication (AAC) Center: AAC-
Aphasia Categories of Communicators Checklist:**   http://aac.unl.edu/
screen/aphasiachecklist.pdf

**Barkley Augmentative and Alternative Communication (AAC) Center:
Aphasia Assessment Materials:**   http://aac.unl.edu/screen/screen.html

**Barkley Augmentative and Alternative Communication (AAC) Center:
Aphasia Needs Assessment:**   http://aac.unl.edu/screen/aphasianeeds.pdf

BlissOnline: http://www.blissonline.se/

Blissymbolics Communication International: http://www.blissymbolics
.org/pfw/

Braille Authority of North America (BANA):   http://www.brailleauthority.org/

Bridges: http://www.bridges-canada.com/

Canadian Deafblind Association: http://www.cdbraontario.ca

CAST, Inc. (formerly Center for Applied Special Technology):   http://www
.cast.org/

CAST Universal Design for Learning (UDL) Book Builder: http://bookbuilder
.cast.org/

Center for Effective Collaboration and Practice (CECP):   http://cecp.air.org/

**Center for Literacy and Disability Studies at the University of North
Carolina-Chapel Hill:**   http://www.med.unc.edu/ahs/clds/

Center on Positive Behavioral Interventions and Supports: http://www.pbis.org/

CIRCA (Computer Interactive Reminiscence and Conversation Aid): http://www.computing.dundee.ac.uk/projects/circa/

Closing the Gap: http://www.closingthegap.com/

Communication and Assistive Device Laboratory, State University of New York at Buffalo: http://cdswebserver.med.buffalo.edu/drupal/?q=node/69

Communication Rights Australia: http://www.caus.com.au

Computer Vision and Image Processing, School of Computing, University of Dundee: http://www.computing.dundee.ac.uk/projects/vision/index.php

Consumer Survey on Communicative Effectiveness: http://affnet.ucp.org/ucp_channeldoc.cfm/1/14/86/86-86/757

Creative Communicating: http://www.creativecommunicating.com/index.cfm

Crestwood Communication Aids, Inc.: http://www.communicationaids.com/products.htm

Crick Software, Inc.: http://www.cricksoft.com/us/home.aspx

DeafblindResources.org: http://www.deafblindresources.org

DeafBooks: http://www.deafbooks.co.uk/

Design to Learn: http://www.designtolearn.com/; see also http://www.ohsu.edu/xd/research/centers-institutes/institute-on-development-and-disability/design-to-learn/index.cfm

Disability Solutions: http://www.disabilitycompass.org/publications/back-issues-of-disability-solutions

Don Johnston, Inc.: http://www.donjohnston.com/

Do2Learn: http://www.do2learn.com/

Doug Dodgen and Associates: http://www.dougdodgen.com/index.html

Down Syndrome Education International: http://www.dseinternational.org/en/gb/

DynaVox: http://www.dynavoxtech.com/

DynaVox Mayer-Johnson: http://www.mayer-johnson.com/

e-Learning Design Lab: http://www.elearndesign.org/resources.html

elliecards: http://www.elliecards.com/index.html

EnableMart: http://www.enablemart.com/Catalog/Speech-Generating-Devices

Enabling Devices: http://enablingdevices.com/catalog

EyeTech Digital Systems: http://www.eyetechaac.com/

Family Center on Technology and Disability: http://www.fctd.info

Family Center on Technology and Disability: *Family Information Guide to Assistive Technology:* http://fctd.info/resources/fig/; for Spanish version, see http://fctd.info/resources/fig/spanish/

First Signs, Inc.: http://www.firstsigns.org

Gail Van Tatenhove: http://vantatenhove.com

Gail Van Tatenhove: *A Protocol for Assessing Metaphoric Use of Pictures:*
http://www.vantatenhove.com/files/MetaphorProtocol.pdf

Gallaudet University Press: http://gupress.gallaudet.edu/

GameBase: http://www.gamebase.info/magazine/read/top-10-head-mouse-games_295.html

Giving Greetings: http://www.givinggreetings.com/

Good Karma Applications, Inc.: http://goodkarmaapplications.com

The Great Talking Box Company: http://www.greattalkingbox.com/

Gus Communication Devices, Inc.: http://www.gusinc.com/

Handicom: http://www.handicom.nl/en/

The Hanen Centre: http://www.hanen.org/Home.aspx

Harcourt Assessment (Psychological Corporation, Canada): http://www.psych.utoronto.ca/users/dgoldst/The%20Psychological%20Corporation,%20Canada.htm

Huntington's Disease Society of America: http://www.hdsa.org/

Inclusion Press: http://www.inclusion.com/

Inclusive Technology Ltd.: http://www.inclusive.co.uk/

Inclusive Technology Ltd.: *Switch Progression Road Map:* http://www.inclusive.co.uk/articles/switch-progression-road-map

Indiana Institute on Disability and Community: http://www.iidc.indiana.edu/

Informa Healthcare: *Augmentative and Alternative Communication* journal:
http://informahealthcare.com/loi/aac

Inspiration Software, Inc.: http://www.inspiration.com/

Institute on Communication and Inclusion: http://soe.syr.edu/centers_institutes/institute_communication_inclusion/default.aspx

Institute on Disabilities, Temple University: http://www.temple.edu/instituteondisabilities/

Institute on Disabilities, Temple University: AAC Vocabulary:
http://disabilities.temple.edu/aacvocabulary/

Institute on Disability, University of New Hampshire: http://www.iod.unh.edu/Home.aspx

Institute for Matching Person and Technology, Inc.: http://matchingpersonandtechnology.com/

IntelliTools: http://www.intellitools.com/default.html

International Council on English Braille (ICEB): http://iceb.org/

International Society for Augmentative and Alternative Communication (ISAAC): http://www.isaac-online.org/

International Society for Autism Research (INSAR): http://www.autism-insar.org

InvoTek, Inc.: http://www.invotek.org/

The Joint Commission: Advancing Effective Communication, Cultural Competence, and Patient- and Family-Centered Care: A Roadmap for Hospitalss: http://www.jointcommission.org/assets/1/6/ARoadmapforHospitalsfinalversion727.pdf

Krown Manufacturing, Inc.: http://www.krownmfg.com/us/

LAB Resources: http://www.labresources-assistivetechnology.com/

LC Technologies, Inc.: http://www.eyegaze.com/

Lee Silverman Voice Treatment: http://www.lsvtglobal.com/

Let's Play! Projects: http://letsplay.buffalo.edu/

Lingraphica America, Inc.: http://www.aphasia.com/

LinguiSystems: http://www.linguisystems.com

Luminaud Inc.: http://www.luminaud.com/

Madentec, Inc.: http://www.madentec.com/

Madonna Rehabilitation Hospital: http://www.madonna.org/

Makaton Charity: http://www.makaton.org/

Marsha Forest Centre: http://www.inclusion.com/forestcentre.html

Matching Person and Technology: http://matchingpersonandtechnology.com/

Mayo Clinic: http://www.mayoclinic.com/index.cfm

Medicare Funding of AAC Technology Assessment/Application Protocol: http://aac-rerc.psu.edu/index.php/pages/show/id/27

Microsystems: http://www.microsystems.com/

Minspeak: http://www.minspeak.com/

Modern Signs Press: http://www.modernsignspress.com/

Monash University Centre for Developmental Disability Health Victoria: Accessible Word Reading Intervention: http://cddh.monash.org/access/accessability2/awri/

Nanogames: http://www.arcess.com

National Aphasia Association Newsletter: http://www.aphasia.org/

National Consortium on Deaf-Blindness: http://www.nationaldb.org

National Cued Speech Association: http://www.cuedspeech.org/

National Institute of Neurological Disorders and Stroke: http://www.ninds.nih.gov/research/parkinsonsweb/index.htm

National Joint Committee for the Communication Needs of Persons with Severe Disabilities (NJC): http://www.asha.org/NJC/

National Parkinson Foundation: http://www.parkinson.org/

National Professional Resources, Inc.: http://nprinc.com

National Technical Institute for the Deaf: http://www.ntid.rit.edu/

NaturalPoint: http://www.naturalpoint.com/

N2Y, Inc.: http://www.n2y.com/

Nuance Communications, Inc.: http://www.nuance.com/

Office of Special Education Programs (OSEP) Ideas that Work: Tangible Symbol Systems: http://www.osepideasthatwork.org/toolkit/pdf/TangibleSymbol%20Systems.pdf

Office of Special Education Programs (OSEP) Technical Assistance Center on Positive Behavioral Interventions and Supports: http://www.pbis.org/

One Switch: http://www.oneswitch.org.uk/

Origin Instruments: http://www.orin.com/

Patient-Reported Outcome and Quality of Life Instruments Database (PROQOLID): http://proqolid.org/proqolid

Paul H. Brookes Publishing Co.: http://www.brookespublishing.com/

Pearson Assessments: http://www.pearsonassessments.com/pai/

Pearson PreK–12 Education: http://www.pearsonschool.com/

Pennsylvania State University: AAC at Penn State: http://aac.psu.edu

Pennsylvania State University: AAC at Penn State: *Improving Literacy Outcomes for Individuals with Autism Spectrum Disorders and Limited Speech* **(webcast):** http://aacliteracy.psu.edu/index.php/page/show/id/17

Pennsylvania State University Early Intervention for Young Children with Autism, Cerebral Palsy, Down Syndrome, and Other Disabilities: http://aackids.psu.edu

Pennsylvania State University Early Intervention for Young Children with Autism, Cerebral Palsy, Down Syndrome, and Other Disabilities: Success Stories: http://aackids.psu.edu/index.php/page/show/id/2

Pennsylvania State University Literacy Instruction for Individuals with Autism, Cerebral Palsy, Down Syndrome and Other Disabilities: http://aacliteracy.psu.edu/index.php/page/show/id/1

Pennsylvania State University Literacy Instruction for Individuals with Autism, Cerebral Palsy, Down Syndrome and Other Disabilities: Reading Comprehension: http://aacliteracy.psu.edu/index.php/page/show/id/11

Pennsylvania State University Literacy Instruction for Individuals with Autism, Cerebral Palsy, Down Syndrome and Other Disabilities: Shared Reading: http://aacliteracy.psu.edu/index.php/page/show/id/8

Pennsylvania State University Literacy Instruction for Individuals with Autism, Cerebral Palsy, Down Syndrome and Other Disabilities: Student Success Stories: http://aacliteracy.psu.edu/index.php/page/show/id/2

Pictogram: http://pictogram.se/english/

Plural Publishing, Inc.: http://www.pluralpublishing.com

Prentke Romich Company (PRC): http://www.prentrom.com/

PRO-ED, Inc.: http://www.proedinc.com/customer/default.aspx

Program Development Associates: http://www.disabilitytraining.com/

The Prompt Institute: http://www.promptinstitute.com/

Pyramid Educational Consultants: http://www.pecs.com/

Quality Indicators for Assistive Technology (QIAT) Consortium: http://natri
.uky.edu/assoc_projects/qiat/

Quality of Life Research Projects: http://www.utoronto.ca/qol/projects.htm

**Quality of Life Projects: Instruments for People with Physical and Sensory
Disabilities:** http://www.utoronto.ca/qol/physSensDis.htm

Quality of Life Research Unit, University of Toronto: http://www.utoronto
.ca/qol/

**Rehabilitation Research and Training Center on Positive Behavior Support
(RRTC-PBS):** http://cfs.cbcs.usf.edu/projects-research/detail.cfm?id=106

Riverside Publishing: http://www.riverpub.com/

RJ Cooper and Associates, Inc.: http://www.rjcooper.com/

Saltillo Corporation: http://saltillo.com/

Scope Communication Resource Centre: http://www.scopevic.org.au/index
.php/site/whatweoffer/communicationresourcecentre

Scope (COMPIC Publishing Software): http://www.scopevic.org.au/index
.php/yiiCart/frontend/product/product/path/1_17/id/

SEDL Reading Resources: http://www.sedl.org/reading/rad

Shiny Learning Free Games and Demos: http://www.shinylearning.co.uk/
freegames/

**Signing Exact English (S.E.E.) Center for the Advancement of Deaf
Children:** http://www.seecenter.org/

Silver Lining Multimedia, Inc.: http://www.silverliningmm.com/

Simplified Technology: http://www.lburkhart.com/main.htm

Simplified Technology: Handouts: http://www.lburkhart.com/
handouts.htm

Slater Software, Inc.: http://www.slatersoftware.com/

**SPARKLE (Supporting Parent Access to Resources, Knowledge, Linkages
and Education):** http://www.sparkle.usu.edu

Speaking Differently: http://www.speakingdifferently.org/

SpeakUp!: http://www.speakup.org/

Special Needs Computers: http://www.specialneedscomputers.ca/

Speechmark Publishing: http://www.speechmark.net/

Stoelting Co.: https://www.stoeltingco.com/

**Studies to Advance Autism Research and Treatment (STAART)
Network:** http://www.nimh.nih.gov/health/topics/autism-spectrum-disorders-
pervasive-developmental-disorders/nih-initiatives/staart/index.shtml

Support Helps Others Use Technology (SHOUT): http://www.shoutaac.org/

Symbolstix Online: http://symbolstix.n2y.com/

Talk to Me Technologies LLC: http://www.talktometechnologies.com/

Talking Mats: http://www.talkingmats.com/

Tar Heel Reader: http://tarheelreader.org/

TBox Apps: http://www.tboxapps.com/

Tech Connections: http://www.techconnections.org/

Technical Assistance Center on Social Emotional Intervention for Young Children (TACSEI):   http://www.challengingbehavior.org/

Texas School for the Blind and Visually Impaired: Tactile Symbols Directory to Standard Tactile Symbol List: http://www.tsbvi.edu/tactile-symbols

Texas School for the Blind and Visually Impaired: Technology Assessment Checklist for Students with Visual Impairments: http://www.tsbvi.edu/assessment/140-technology-assessment-checklist-for-students-with-visual-impairments

Tobii Technology: http://www.tobii.com/en/

Toby Churchill Ltd.:   http://www.toby-churchill.com/

University of Kentucky Assistive Technology (UKAT) Project, UKAT Toolkit: http://serc.gws.uky.edu/www/ukatii/index.html

WesTest Engineering Corp.: Darci USB: http://www.westest.com/darci/usbindex.html

Wherify Wireless, Inc.:   http://www.wherifywireless.com/

Widgit Software: http://www.widgit.com/

Wiley: http://www.wiley.com/

Wisconsin Assistive Technology Initiative (WATI):   http://www.wati.org/

Words+, Inc.:   http://www.words-plus.com/

Yooralla: http://www.yooralla.com.au/

ZYGO-USA: http://www.zygo-usa.com/usa/

Index

Tables and figures are indicated by *t* and *f*, respectively.